Warwickshire College
* 0 0 5 0 9 8 8 2 *

Equine Stud Farm Medicine

P.D. ROSSDALE MA, FRCVS
S.W. RICKETTS BSc, BVSc, FRCVS

SECOND EDITION

BAILLIÈRE TINDALL · LONDON

A BAILLIÈRE TINDALL book published by
Cassell Ltd.
35 Red Lion Square, London WC1R 4SG

and at Sydney, Auckland, Toronto, Johannesburg

an affiliate of
Macmillan Publishing Co. Inc.
New York

First published 1974 as *The Practice of Equine Stud Medicine*
Second edition 1980

ISBN 0 7020 0754 4

French edition (Librarie Maloine, Paris) 1978
Spanish edition (Editorial Hemisferio Sur, Buenos Aires) 1979

Published in the United States of America by
Lea & Febiger, Philadelphia

Set by Scribe Design. Printed and bound in Great Britain by
William Clowes (Beccles) Limited, Beccles and London.

British Library Cataloguing in Publication Data

Rossdale, Peter Daniel
Equine stud farm medicine – 2nd ed.
1. Horse breeding 2. Horses – Diseases
I. Title II. Ricketts, Sidney W
III. Practice of equine stud medicine
636. 1'D8'54 SF291

ISBN 0-7020-0754-4

Contents

Preface vii

Acknowledgements ix

1. **Events Leading to Conception** 1

Reproductive Anatomy of the Mare 1
The Oestrous Cycle 11
Management of the Mare's Sexual Functions 42
Infertility/Subfertility in the Mare 53

2. **The Stallion** 120

Selection of Stallions 120
Reproductive Anatomy 120
Endocrinology 123
Reproductive Behaviour 128
Semen 137
Infertility 146
Artificial Insemination 158

3. **Gestation** 165

Embryology 165
Uterine Changes 181
Endocrinology 184
Fetal Environment and Metabolism 191
Abortion 195
Management of the In-foal Mare 206
Pregnancy Diagnosis 206
Gestational Length 213
Prenatal Mammary Development 213

4. **Birth** 220

Initiation and Endocrinology of Birth 220
Induction 225
The Forces of Delivery 231
Anatomy of Birth 233
Maternal Behaviour 239
Effect of Parturition on the Fetus 251
Management of the Foaling Mare 251

Dystocia and Abnormal Conditions of Birth 260
Caesarean Section Versus Embryotomy 271

5. **The Adaptive Period** 277

The Normal Newborn Foal 277
Diseases of the First Four Days after Birth 305
Differential Diagnosis of Neonatal Disease 349
Perinatal Mortality 356
Twins 357

6. **The Older Foal and Yearling** 361

Health 361
Weaning 366
Lactation 368
Orphan Foals 372
Haematological Standards 378
Biochemical Standards 381
Growth 382
Musculoskeletal Disorders 386
Other Disorders 399

7. **General Medicine** 421

Infectious Conditions 421
Parasites 438
Skin Diseases 451
Digestive System 458
Cardiovascular System 475
Respiratory System 476
Blood and Blood-forming Organs 479
Urinary System 486
Nervous System 488
Musculoskeletal System 489

8. **Clinical and Further Examinations** 501

Hygiene at Gynaecological Examinations 502
Hypodermic Injection 504
Passing a Stomach Tube 507
Rectal Examination 509
Endoscopic Examinations 512
Nerve Blocks 514
Radiography 516
Diagnostic Physiotherapy 516
Clinical Pathology 516
Parasitology 528
Urine Analysis 529
Bacteriology 530
Virology 584
Mycology 535
Cytology 536
Histology 540
Endocrinology 545
Blood and Urine Pregnancy Tests 546
Cross-matching Blood 546
Blood Transfusion 547

Index 551

Preface

This book sets out to give readers a balanced view of the problems they are likely to encounter on an equine breeding establishment and, by including references, to provide opportunities for further reading. It is written for clinicians, students and research workers interested in the problems that affect breeding horses; but many of the problems discussed are encountered by all equine practitioners, in whatever sphere they work.

The book is divided into eight chapters. Chapter 1 describes the reproductive anatomy, physiology, management and pathology of the non-pregnant mare in the period leading up to conception. Chapter 2 deals with the reproductive anatomy, physiology and pathology of the stallion, the collection and evaluation of semen samples and the management of the mating process. The technique and application of artificial insemination are discussed. Chapter 3 records normal and abnormal gestation and the problems of abortion. Chapter 4 outlines the birth processes and obstetric problems. Chapter 5 is concerned with the normal adaptation of the newborn foal to extrauterine life and the problems of the immediate post-natal period. Chapter 6 provides an account of problems encountered in growing foals and yearlings. Chapter 7 includes general medical conditions which may be encountered in, but are not confined to, horses at stud farms. Chapter 8 details the clinical and other examinations and diagnostic techniques, with emphasis on those which are particularly relevant to reproductive problems or which practitioners might find useful.

Many advances in knowledge of equine stud farm medicine have occurred since this book was first published in 1974 and we have assimilated the more important of these in this considerably enlarged second edition. The subject has attracted a wealth of new scientific literature, including two international symposia on equine reproduction, held at Cambridge, U.K., and Davis, California, USA, but in addition practical experiences, especially in the field of clinical endocrinology and venereology, have added new dimensions to routine stud farm practice. In 1977, the horse breeding industry, clinicians and scientists withstood the major challenge of a 'new' venereal disease (contagious equine metritis). This provided the need for a collaborative approach to seek answers to the questions of aetiology, diagnosis, prognosis, epidemiology, treatment and control measures. A re-evaluation of routine stud farm management, hygiene and preventive medicine followed.

Endocrinological advances have enabled the clinician to monitor and evaluate the hormonal status of individuals with greater understanding. Significant practical advances have been made, with the use of artificial light programmes, gonadotrophin-releasing hormones, oral progestagens and prostaglandins, in hastening the onset of cyclic oestrous behaviour and ovarian activity at the start of the imposed breeding season. Our knowledge and understanding of the reproductive physiology of the stallion have been improved by the publication of basic research, particularly in the fields of endocrinology and the seasonal variation and evaluation of semen quality. The techniques of endometrial biopsy and cytology have improved knowledge and understanding of the response of the mare's endometrium to the normal and abnormal challenges and changes that occur during the course of stud farm life. Basic and applied research into the adaptations of the newborn foal to extrauterine life have continued. These have enabled improvements to be made in the evaluation and treatment of abnormality during this vitally important period.

In revising the book, we have endeavoured to take account of these many important developments and hope that our readers will continue to find it of practical assistance in their work.

P.D. ROSSDALE
S.W. RICKETTS

July 1980

Acknowledgements

In writing this book we are indebted to a number of people. In particular we wish to record out thanks to our partners in practice, Michael Hunt MA, VetMB, MRCVS, Colin Peace MA, VetMB, MRCVS, Raymond Hopes BVMS, MRCVS and Nicholas Wingfield Digby BVSc, MRCVS who have, at all times, been ready to offer advice and encouragement. We gratefully acknowledge contact with many members of various veterinary schools and university departments who have provided us with direct help and with the necessary insight and determination for our labours.

Some of the data that we have presented was obtained during the course of work partly financed by the Wellcome Trust and the Horserace Betting Levy Board, to whom we are very grateful.

We thank the staff of Beaufort Cottage Laboratories, especially Robert Cash, Kath Gifkins, Hazel Heathershaw and Amanda Cheese, for technical help and in the preparation of statistical data. We thank Robert Patman for help with photographic processing and Derek Thurlbourn and John Fuller for the preparation of some graphs and figures. The staff of the Royal College of Veterinary Surgeons Library gave valuable assistance in the investigation of literature and checking of references.

All photographs, other than those specified, were taken by the authors and we would like to thank those who have helped us in this task, notably the staff of Ashley Heath, Banstead Manor, Cheveley Park, Derisley Wood, Glebe House, Northmore and Woodlands studs at Newmarket. Permission to reproduce many other illustrations has been given by various authors and editors, as recognized in the text, and we thank them all.

We thank Jenny Ricketts, Sonia Steer and Janette Wade for typing the manuscript.

P.D.R.
S.W.R.

Events Leading to Conception 1

Conception is based on a sequence of events culminating in the entry of a spermatozoon into the ovum. This union depends on the participation of stallion and mare in behavioural patterns which are closely linked with endocrinological changes of a complex but integrated nature. In this chapter we discuss the significance of these changes in the context of modern stud farm management and the need to achieve high conception rates under economic conditions. Our description is concerned with the anatomy and physiology of the sexual organs and glands of the mare, with particular reference to the practical application of available information to the diagnosis and therapy of infertility. Emphasis is also given to sexual behaviour which is the outward expression of the fundamental physiological changes in the body and which is a common denominator of veterinary and managerial interests. In free-range breeding, behavioural patterns are the basis of conception; but where mares and stallions are bred in hand, behaviour becomes more a matter of human opinion and decision. It is this last consideration which lends particular importance to the understanding of day-to-day problems in stud farms during the breeding season.

REPRODUCTIVE ANATOMY OF THE MARE

The ovaries

The ovaries contain the female gametes (ova). Many thousands of these are present in the two ovaries at birth and no more develop during the animal's lifetime. After puberty, ova are extruded from the ovaries at intervals determined by secretions of anterior pituitary hormones.

The ovaries are typically bean-shaped and vary in size, depending on age and season of the year. Individual variations also occur. The ovaries of maiden mares in winter are usually about 2–4 cm long and 2–3 cm wide. The ovaries increase in spring to 5–8 cm × 3–4 cm. In winter they may feel hard and in spring, i.e. during sexual activity, they usually feel softer.

The size of older mares' ovaries varies considerably, irrespective of the season of the year. During sexual quiescence (anoestrus) their size is minimal, i.e. 3–6 cm long. During seasons of sexual activity they grow, but do not normally become larger than about 10 × 5 cm. In many cases, the ovaries lose their typical bean shape and become rounded or irregular in contour and one ovary may be much larger than the other.

Typically the ovary has a medial and lateral surface and a convex border to which the broad ligament containing blood vessels and nerves is attached. The opposite or free border has a narrow depression (the ovulation fossa) through which the ova are shed.

The clinician can easily pick up the ovaries on rectal examination (see p. 48) and recognize by feel and identify by palpation the rounded extremities which, depending on the plane in which the ovary is held, may be left or right, anterior or posterior.

The ovaries are situated in the sublumbar region ventral to the fourth or fifth lumbar vertebra. The average distance from the ovaries to the vulva is 50–55 cm in a mare of medium size (Sisson 1953).

The ovary is covered by peritoneum except at the attached border (hilus) where nerves and vessels enter. The ovarian stroma is composed of spindle-shaped connective tissue cells and intercellular substance. Bundles of cells and fibres run in various directions giving a 'swirly' appearance. The stroma is organized into a tough fibrous capsule which encloses the ovary except at a point opposite the hilus, the ovulation fossa. The stroma contains small bodies consisting of a central cell (primordial germ cell) enclosed by a single layer of epithelial cells known as the primordial follicle. There are several hundred thousand of these structures in the two ovaries at birth. In the immature ovary the germ cell (oogonium) is surrounded by a layer of follicular epithelial cells (granulosa). Soon some of the oogonia develop into larger cells (primary oocytes) which undergo the first stage of meiosis. They do not complete meiosis until after puberty and when the follicle is mature.

Of the many primary follicles present in the two ovaries at birth only a fraction reach maturity and liberate ova. Most of the follicles degenerate or undergo partial development followed by regression (atresia).

The primary follicle is about 45 μm in diameter. As it develops the epithelial cells surrounding the oocyte change from a flat to a stratified columnar shape. The oocyte increases in size and develops a thick outer membrane, the zone pellucida.

Fluid accumulates among the follicular epithelial cells and eventually fills a central cavity lined by follicular cells. The oocyte is attached to one side of the cavity on a mound of follicular cells known as the cumulus oophorus (*cumulus* = heap; *oon* = egg; *phoros* = bearer).

The stroma immediately adjacent to the follicle becomes organized into a membrane (theca), the inner lining of which is vascular and the outer lining non-vascular.

Follicular development continues until the follicle reaches about 3–5 cm in diameter. The 3 cm diameter size appears to represent an important stage in maturation of the follicle related to a three-fold increase in concentration of oestrogens and androgens (Kenney et al. 1979). It seems that oestrogens tend to prevent regression, although Kenney et al. did not find evidence that a drop in oestrogen levels was the cause of atresia and degeneration started when levels were high. Nor, in their opinion, did a rise in androgen levels precipitate spontaneous atresia. In our present state of knowledge the cause of follicular atresia in the mare is unknown. Kenney et al. (1979) described three stages in the atretic process in which the granulosa cell nuclei underwent karyorrhexis and pyknosis, lysis and, in the final stage, the separate identity of the granulosa and thecal cells were lost. During the process of atresia the steroid levels in follicular fluid diminish. It seems that follicular atresia in the mare is a process involving a gradual loss of 'viability'. Kenney's findings indicate that, once atresia starts, it proceeds in a gradual and methodical manner. Clinical experience, however, suggests that some follicles may ovulate at a less than 3 cm size, but this is the exception, not the rule.

The mature ('ripe') follicle bursts at the ovulation fossa (Witherspoon 1975) and discharges its contents towards the open end of the fallopian tube. After the ovum and part of the follicular wall have been extruded the follicle collapses and the thecal lining and remaining epithelial cells are thrown into folds. Bleeding occurs into the centre of the follicle and a clot forms. The follicular or granulosa cells grow into the clot and together with thecal cells constitute the corpus luteum (CL). Blood vessels and fibroblasts enter the CL which changes from a soft consistency and reddish-purple colour to a firm consistency and reddish-brown. As the CL becomes non-functional it turns yellow and eventually brown or white as the active luteal cells are replaced by scar tissue. Histological changes in the corpus luteum and their relationship with the production of progesterone have been described by Van Niekerk et al. (1975). Fibroblast cells in the theca proliferate and enlarge during pro-oestrus to form large thecal cells which, at ovulation, are in various stages of degeneration. These cells are replaced by hypertrophied fibroblasts. The granulosa cells cease dividing three days before ovulation and just before rupture the membrana granulosa changes from a compact to an open lace-like layer. About two hours after ovulation, the granulosa cells are 10 μm in diameter and have a dark-staining nucleus 5–6 μm in diameter. They then enlarge very quickly and ten hours later the nuclei of some become vesicular and increase to 7.5 μm in diameter. Within 24 hours of ovulation these cells measure 15 μm in diameter and start to secrete progesterone. By Day 3, all these cells are luteinized, although maximum hypertrophy is not attained until Day 9 when the cells measure 37.5 μm and the nuclei 10 μm in diameter. These dimensions decrease after Day 12 and by Day 20, when the follicle of the next cycle is on the point of rupture, they are in an advanced stage of regression. There is also a large number of homogeneously eosinophilic small cells with a condensed, darkly stained nucleus, 5–6 μm in diameter. These cells increase in number and on Day 7 account for about 15% of the total lutein cell population, the proportion increasing up to 60% on Day 14. Van Niekerk considers that these small dark cells are in a resting stage and that they cease to be converted into the large, light variety when the latter begin to degenerate from Day 12 onwards. This author also studied the lutein cells of the pregnant

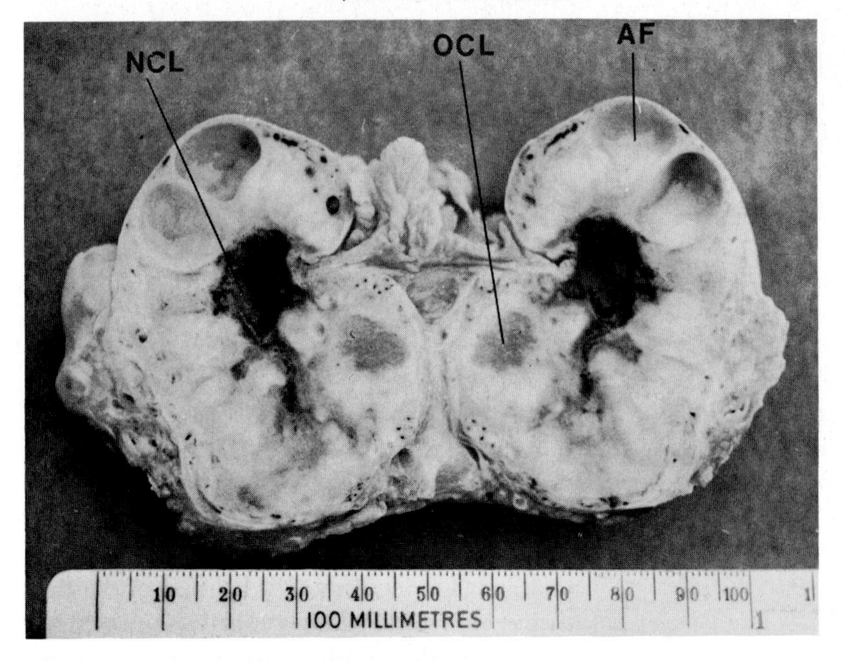

(a)

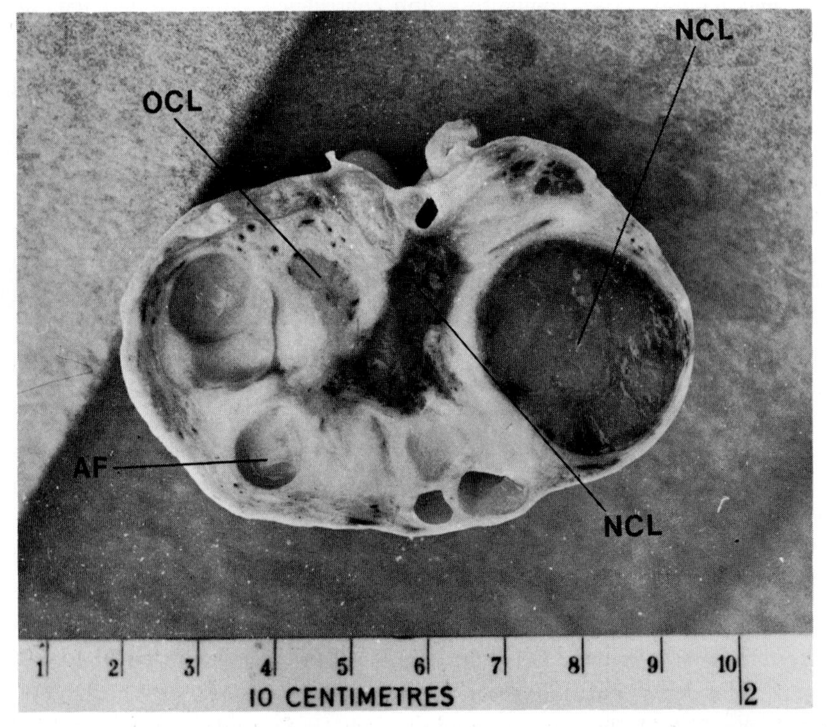

(b)

Fig. 1.1. Ovaries cut in cross-section to show old and new corpora lutea (OCL and NCL), atretic follicle (AF) and ripe follicle (RF).

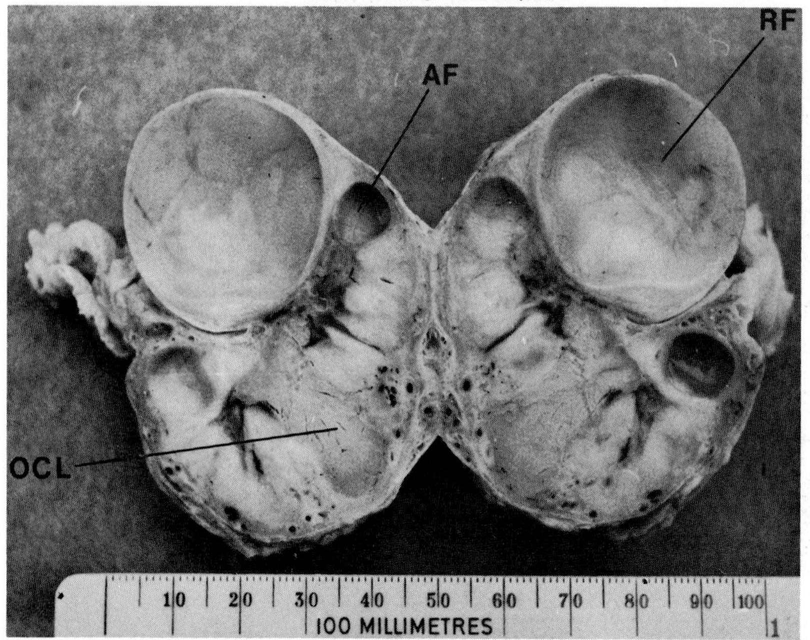

(c)

mare and found that the large lutein cells reach a maximum of 40 μm on Day 30, before regression sets in between Days 38 and 40, and that the small dark cells increase very rapidly, in proportion, between Day 36 and 44, shortly before the formation of a secondary CL.

On section of an ovary, some or all of the gross structures described may be present (Fig. 1.1).

The follicles are distributed throughout the stroma; they may have thick non-vascular or thin vascular walls. CLs of varying ages and colour may be found. Recent CLs are usually wedge-shaped with the base distal to the ovulation fossa.

The CL does not project from the surface of the ovary, as in the cow and pig, but is embedded in the ovarian stroma. The ovary acts as an endocrine gland forming the hormones oestrogen and progesterone in addition to its role of ovum producer.

The pituitary gland

The pituitary gland lies immediately below the base of the brain, to which it is attached, and rests in a depression in the upper surface of the sphenoid bone. From a functional viewpoint the pituitary is divided into the posterior lobe, which is innervated by nerve tracts originating in the hypothalamus, and the anterior lobe, which has no direct nerve supply. The posterior lobe secretes the hormones oxytocin and vasopressin, and the anterior lobe secretes the gonad-stimulating (gonadotrophic) hormones, follicle-stimulating hormone (FSH), luteinizing hormone (LH) and prolactin. The character and actions of these hormones are discussed below. The anterior pituitary also secretes adrenocorticotrophic hormones (ACTH) and thyroid-stimulating hormone (TSH) which influence the reproductive system indirectly but are not usually considered true reproductive hormones.

The posterior pituitary develops from a ventral outgrowth of the forebrain and is composed of nervous tissue. The nerve cells are situated in the supraoptic and paraventricular nuclei of the hypothalamus (Fig. 1.2). Besides conducting nervous

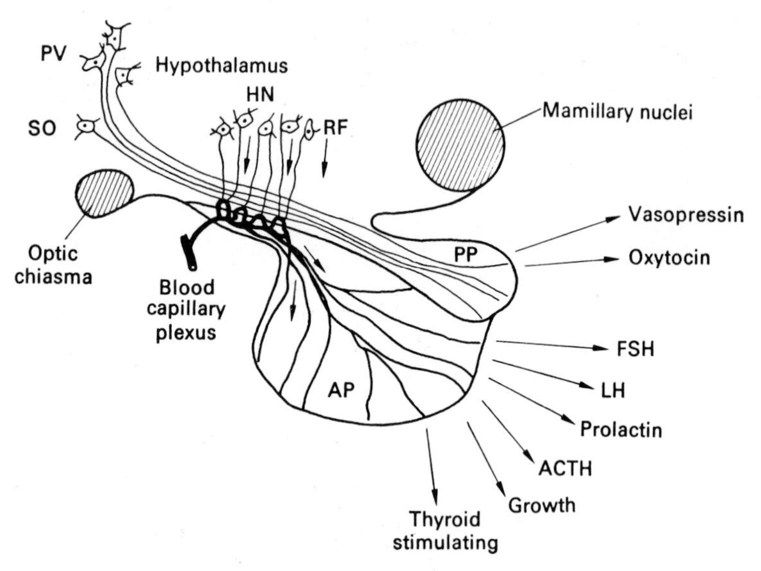

Fig. 1.2. The relationship of nervous control of posterior pituitary (PP) and neurohumoral control of anterior pituitary (AP). Hypothalamic (HN), paraventricular (PV) + supraoptic (SO) cells; RF, releasing factor; ↓, pathway of releasing factor. For full details see text. (*Adapted from Cross 1972*)

impulses, these cells manufacture the polypeptide hormones vasopressin and oxytocin (Cross 1972). The hormones travel down the axons of the nerve cells to the posterior lobe where they are stored until released by appropriate nervous stimuli. For example, oxytocin is released by reflexes initiated during parturition by stretching of the vaginal wall and, later, when the foal approaches the mammary region (milk ejection reflex).

The anterior pituitary develops from the ectoderm of the roof of the buccal cavity and has no direct nervous control. It is, however, connected indirectly to the hypothalamus by a portal system of blood vessels (Fig. 1.2) which conveys releasing and inhibiting factors secreted by hypothalamic cells. There are about ten of these factors (Cross 1972). The FSH- and LH-releasing factors and the prolactin-inhibiting factors are of particular interest because of their effects on the oestrous cycle and mammary development. Although work on the practical application of these substances is in its infancy, future development could have far-reaching significance in equine medicine and the management of the reproductive process (see p. 33).

The genital tract

The genital tract consists of fallopian tubes, uterus, cervix and vagina (Fig. 1.3). It extends from the vulval orifice to the ovaries, receives the male organ, forms a pathway up which the spermatozoa travel to meet the ovum, 'houses' the developing embryo and provides a passage for expulsion of the fetus to the exterior.

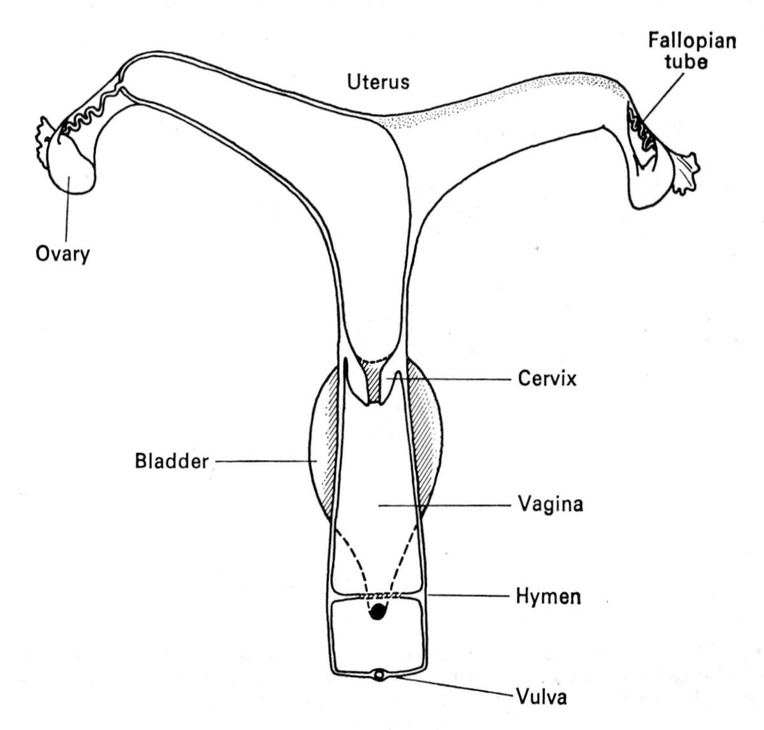

Fig. 1.3. The composition of the genital tract: the fallopian tubes, uterus, cervix and vagina.

The oviducts or fallopian tubes are two tortuous tubes 20–30 cm long extending from the uterine horns to the ovaries. They are 2–3 mm in diameter at their uterine end and 4–8 mm in diameter at their ovarian end. Each tube is enclosed in a peritoneal fold (mesosalpinx); the ovarian extremity is funnel-shaped and its edge irregular with projections (fimbriae) attached to the ovulation fossa. The tube communicates with the peritoneal cavity via a small opening through which the ovum can pass at ovulation. Cysts and embryological remnants are sometimes present in the fimbriae and mesosalpinx, e.g. parovarian cysts may be present and palpated rectally as small fluctuant cysts, often at one pole of the ovary (Osborne 1966). The tube consists of three layers: an outer fibrous and serous coat, a middle muscular coat of circular and longitudinal fibres and an inner mucous membrane composed of single-layer columnar ciliated and secretory cells.

The uterus is a hollow muscular organ continuous with the fallopian tubes anteriorly and opening posteriorly through the cervix into the vagina. It is attached to the sublumbar region by two folds of peritoneum (the broad ligaments) and consists of two horns, a body and a neck (cervix). The horns are about 25 cm long and the body 18–20 cm in length and 10 cm in diameter.

The wall of the uterus consists of three coats: an outer serous layer continuous with the broad ligaments; a muscular layer (myometrium) containing an external layer of longitudinal fibres and an internal layer of circular fibres; and a mucous membrane (endometrium) comprising luminal epithelium, a stroma of connective tissue, glands and their ducts.

The uterus is supplied by the uterine artery and the uterine branch of the utero-ovarian artery and its nerves are derived from the uterine and pelvic sympathetic plexuses.

The cervix is the constricted posterior part of the uterus. It is about 7 cm long and 4 cm in diameter in the sexually inactive phase and projects into the anterior vagina.

The vagina extends horizontally through the pelvic cavity from the cervix to the vulva. It is about 20 cm long and up to 12 cm in diameter but its walls are normally in apposition. Most of the vagina is uncovered by peritoneum and it is surrounded by loose connective tissue, veins and fat. Its wall is composed of muscular and mucous coats. The mucous coat is very elastic and covered with stratified epithelium. The vagina is divided into anterior and posterior parts by a transverse fold (hymen) which is usually patent. The arterial supply comes from the pudic arteries and the nerves are derived from the sympathetic pelvic plexus.

The vulva is covered by mucous membrane and is continuous in front with the vagina and opens externally about 7 cm below the anus. It consists of two lips connected by a dorsal and ventral commissure. Immediately inside the ventral commissure is the glans clitoridis (Fig. 1.4). The clitoris lies within a pouch or fossa which may contain a variable quantity of smegma-like inspissated material. The clitoris itself contains three sinuses, which may also contain inspissated material and may be a reservoir of 'infection' for some venereal-disease-producing organisms (Powell et al. 1978; Simpson & Eaton-Evans 1978*a*, *b*). The sinuses are situated towards the dorsal aspect of the clitoris. The central sinus is the largest and the lateral ones may not be present in all cases. The vulval lips are covered by thin pigmented skin which is supplied with sebaceous and sweat glands. Beneath the skin are muscles that fuse above with the anal sphincter.

The perineum (Greek: *perineas* = space between anus and scrotum) is a loosely defined region in the mare, including the anus, vulva and adjacent skin. Its conformation is of clinical importance because of the part it plays in protecting the genital tract from the entrance of air (pneumovagina) and bacteria through the vulva. It is also subject to lacerations, wounds and bruising during birth or from kicking by other mares.

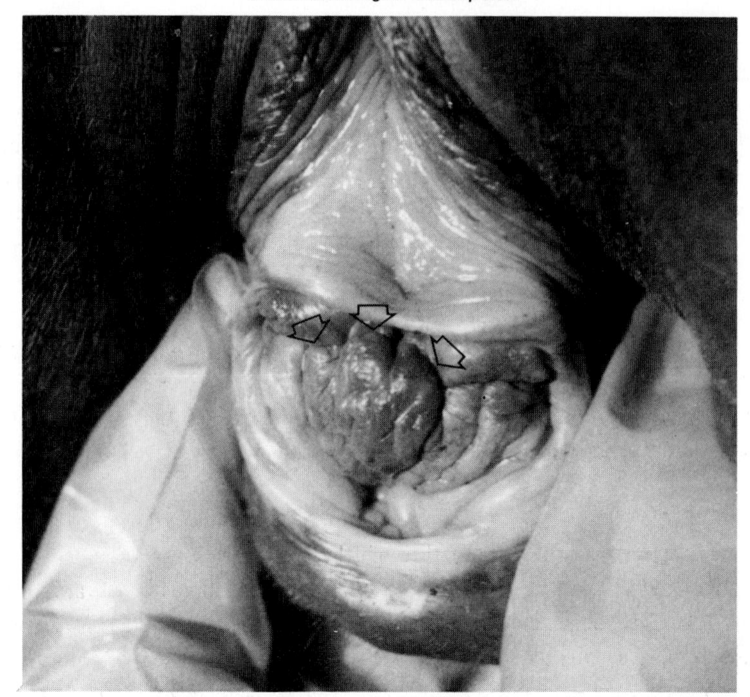

Fig. 1.4. The clitoris everted by digital manipulation to show the folds of the clitoral fossa and the position of the entrances to the clitoral sinuses (arrowed).

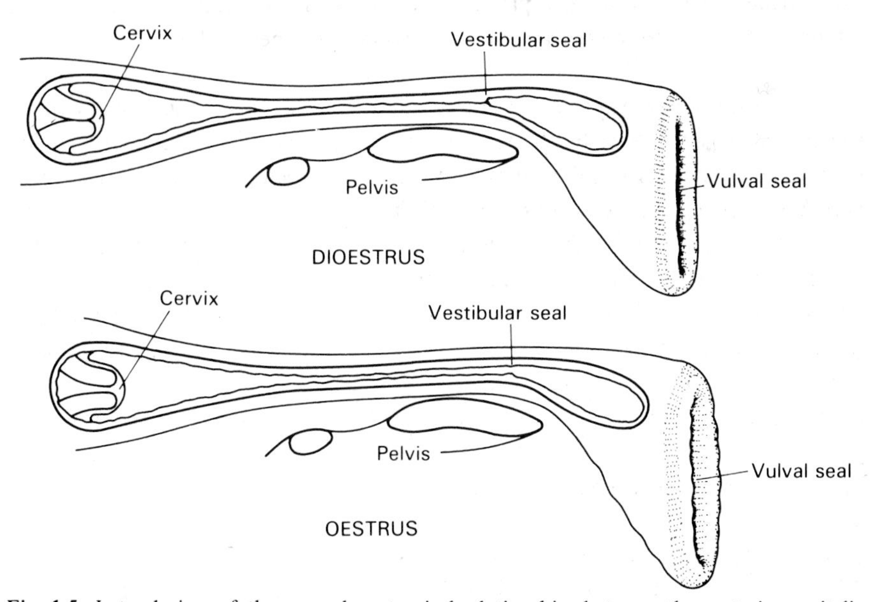

Fig. 1.5. Lateral view of the normal anatomical relationships between the posterior genitalia and the ischium, showing three functional seals between the uterus and the environment. *Above*, Dioestrus: cervix closed, vulval and vestibular seals effective. *Below*, Oestrus: cervix and vulva relaxed, vestibular seal penetrated at coitus. The natural immunological defence mechansims of the genital organs are now vital to maintain genital health. (*By kind permission of Professor R.M. Butterfield*)

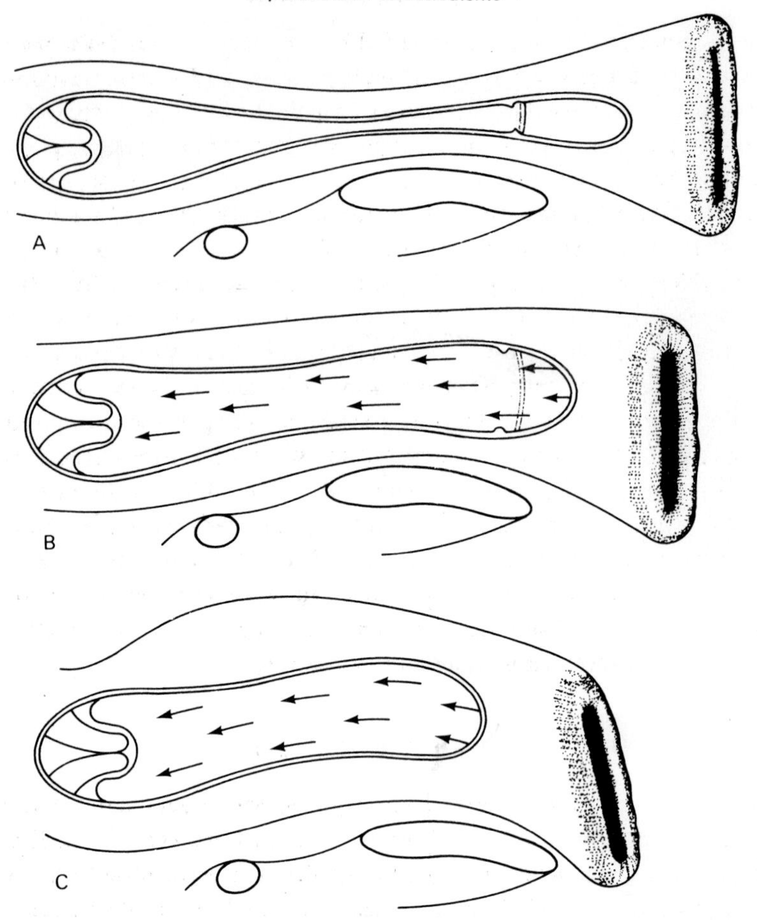

Fig. 1.6. As in Fig. 1.5, but in a mare with poor conformation, in dioestrus. A, Ischium low in relation to vagina, so vestibular seal is ineffective, but in this case the vulva is competent so that the cervix is not challenged. B, As for A, but with incompetent vulva, so that pneumovagina occurs and the cervix is directly challenged by environmental micro-organisms. C, As in B, further aggravated by sloping vulva which allows faecal contamination.

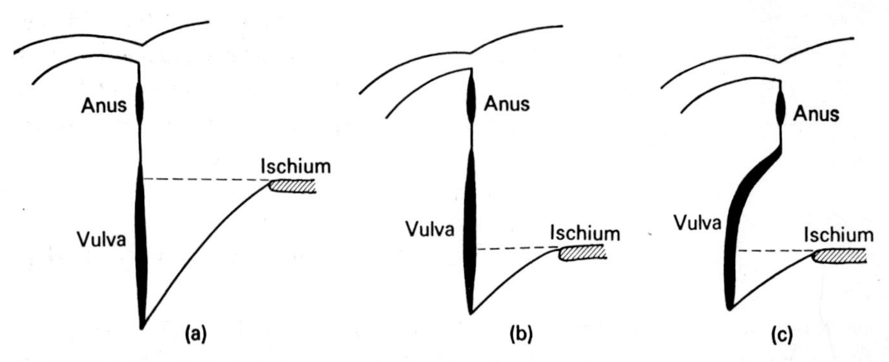

Fig. 1.7. A lateral view of the anatomical relationship between the anus, vulva and ischium. (*a*) Good conformation. (*b*) Poor conformation, predisposing to (*c*) in which the labia are in the horizontal plane.

The entrance to the vagina is protected by the vulval and vestibular seals (Fig. 1.5), the cervix acting as a further seal against the entry of air into the uterus. The vulval seal is formed by the perineum and vulva, the vestibular is formed by the posterior vagina, the pillars of the hymen and the floor of the pelvic girdle. The valves may be defective because of malconformation (Fig. 1.6) or breached by introducing a speculum into the anterior vagina. The optimal conformation is one in which the vulval labiae are in the vertical plane and 80% below the pelvic floor, i.e. the ischium (Figs 1.7, 1.8). If the pelvic floor is low relative to the labiae there is a tendency for the anus to retract anteriorly and the upper part of the vulva to 'fall' into the horizontal plane. The conformation of this region changes with the oestrous cycle and the seals are more likely to be breached when the tissues are relaxed in oestrus than when they are constricted during dioestrus or pregnancy.

Pascoe (1979) designed an instrument to measure the effective length (in cm) (l) and angle of declination (a) of the mare's vulva. From this he deduced a 'Caslick index' for determining the necessity for suturing the vulvas in mares exhibiting the classic signs associated with pneumovagina. The index was obtained from the product of $l \times a$ and less than 150 was found to be associated with a significantly higher pregnancy rate than mares with similar age and with an index greater than 150. The value l showed a significant increase with age.

THE OESTROUS CYCLE

The oestrous cycle is a pattern of physiological and behavioural events under hormonal control, forming the basis of sexual activity and conception. The cycle has two components: *oestrus* (heat) in which the mare is receptive to the stallion and the ovum is shed and *dioestrus* which is a period of sexual quiescence. The cycle typically lasts 21 days (five days of oestrus and 16 of dioestrus) and may recur throughout the year, although in equidae sexual activity is characteristically confined to a restricted breeding season and outside this period the cycles cease (anoestrus). There is considerable individual variation in cycle length and character. Oestrous periods are longer and less intense in behavioural terms at the start and end of the season than in the middle. The cycles start at puberty (about one and a half years) and continue throughout the mare's lifetime. It is convenient to discuss the cycle under the separate headings of its endocrinological and behavioural components.

Endocrinology

The classic view of the hormonal changes associated with the oestrous cycle (Fig. 1.9) is as follows:

1. Environmental factors, such as photoperiod (increasing daylight length) and to some extent warmth and improvements in available nutrients, stimulate hypothalamic secretion of gonadotrophin-releasing hormones (GnRH), which initiate the onset of oestrous cyclical activity in the spring.

2. FSH stimulates the development of ovarian follicles which secrete oestrogen. These hormones are responsible for oestrous signs and changes in the genital tract.

3. Rising blood levels of oestrogen stimulate the anterior pituitary to produce LH and reduce the secretion of FSH. Ovulation occurs and a corpus luteum forms which produces progesterone.

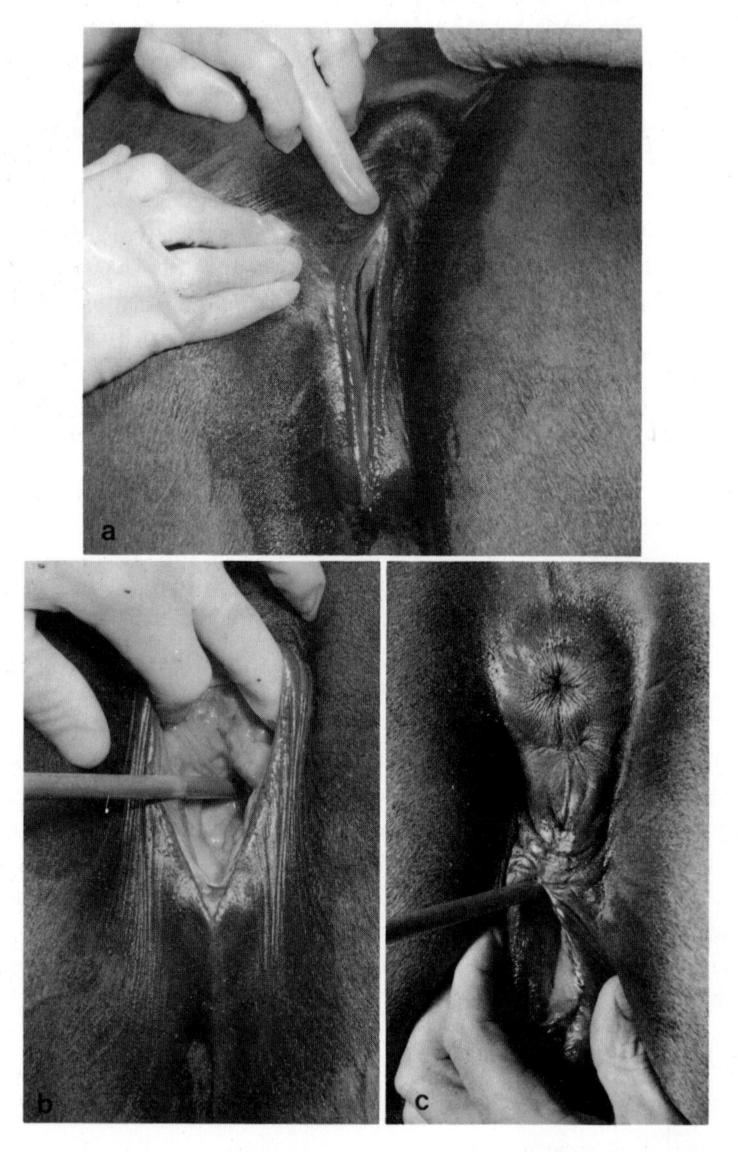

Fig. 1.8. (*a*) Normal vertical conformation of the vulva. (*b*) The metal tube is resting on the pelvic floor, illustrating the position relative to the vulva. (*c*) The position of the tube shows the point at which it is necessary to suture the vulva (Caslick operation). (*facing page*) (*d*) The metal tube indicates the floor of the pelvis (see text). (*e*) Vulva and perineum sloping towards the horizontal. Note the crinkled effect of vulval labiae, a sign that Caslick surgery is required.

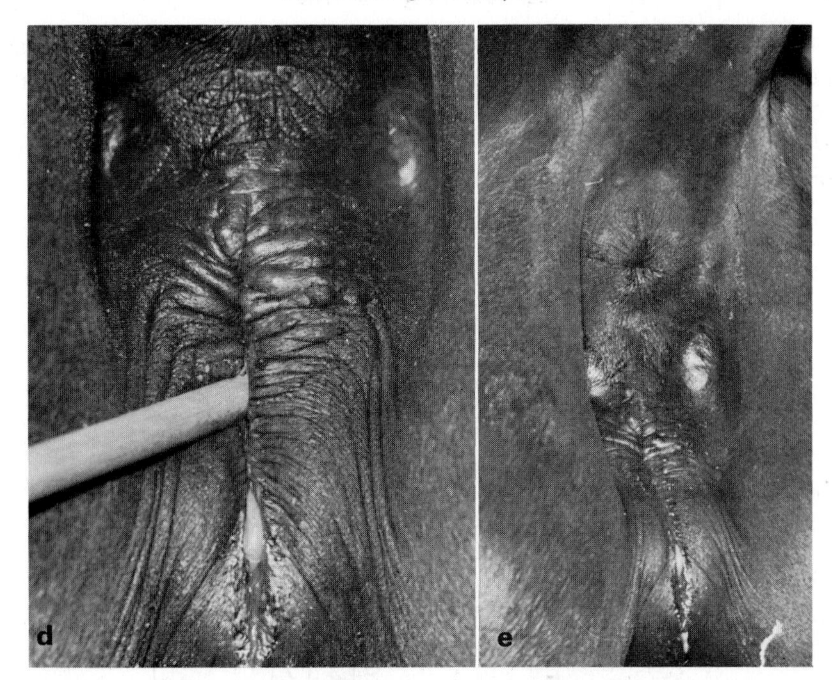

4. Falling oestrogen and rising progesterone levels in the blood are responsible for dioestrous signs and changes in the genital tract.

5. The secretion of a luteolytic hormone (now identified as prostaglandin) from the uterus ends dioestrus by arresting the functional life of the CL and causing blood progesterone levels to fall to zero.

6. Falling progesterone levels stimulate the anterior pituitary to secrete FSH and restart the cycle.

This account is a simplified one for ease of understanding and, as with all simplifications, it represents but part of the truth. There are many facets to the interaction of hormones on their target organs and it is usually the net effect of a balance which determines the resultant effect at any given instance. For example, oestrus represents a dominance of, rather than an absolute status of, FSH and oestrogen relative to LH and progesterone. The activation of endocrine glands may also be based on their sensitivity to changing levels and the rapidity with which these occur. Finally it should be emphasized that many hormones leave the endocrine gland in an inert form which becomes potentiated by the target cells.

This view of the cycle is based on observations from many mammalian species, but there are areas in which evidence is incomplete or facts not fully understood.

Initiation of oestrous cyclical activity

It has long been known that oestrous cycles are promoted by extrinsic factors such as daylight (Nishikawa et al. 1952). A long daily photoperiod artificially applied during the anovulatory season may advance the onset of the ovulatory season (the first ovulation) by at least two months in pony (Kooistra & Ginther 1975) and larger breeds (Oxender et al. 1977). Levels of LH follow a seasonal pattern and are minimal during the anovulatory season (Garcia & Ginther 1976). During the ovulatory season, the concentrations are maximal only during oestrus and they are minimal during dioestrus (Whitmore et al. 1973). However, in the absence of the

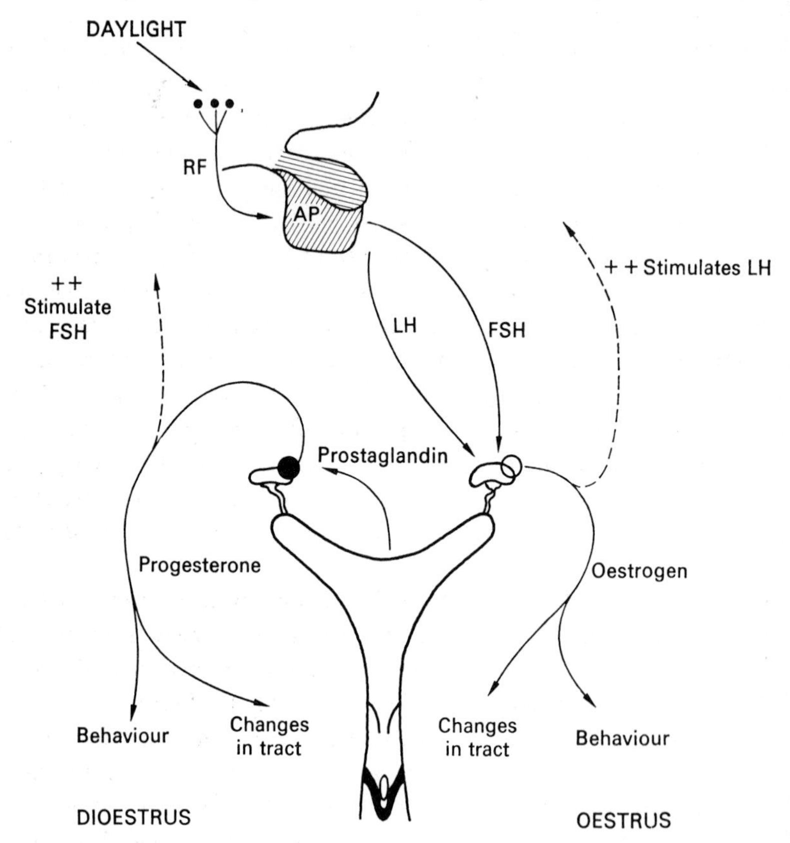

Fig. 1.9. Summary of the endocrinology of the oestrous cycle. RF = releasing factor from cells in the hypothalamus; FSH = follicle-stimulating hormone; LH = luteinizing hormone; AP = anterior pituitary.

influence of the ovaries, LH levels follow a seasonal pattern in ovariectomized mares and they are minimal during the anovulatory and maximal during the ovulatory season. Freedman et al. (1979) found that the changes of FSH and LH concentrations in ovariectomized mares were influenced by photoperiod. Thus there appears to be a primary central nervous system–pituitary component responsible for a basal circannual LH rhythm influenced by an environmental (photoperiod) factor and independent of ovarian influences (Garcia et al. 1979). A secondary ovarian (steroidal) component exists which modifies the primary rhythm during the ovulatory season. This hypothesis, put forward by Garcia et al., does not seem to apply in its entirety to FSH secretion and there may be other factors besides the ovarian and steroidal component which affect the basal rhythm.

Strauss et al. (1979) observed that total hypothalamic GnRH concentrations were not significantly different between seasons, although there was a trend towards increasing concentrations in the summer seasons. The distribution of the hormone activity was, however, significantly different between seasons and was highest at the most ventral locality during the summer when the demands on the hormone were, presumably, at their highest.

Sharp et al. (1979) reported the oestrous behaviour, ovarian follicular development, ovulation and changes in hair coat in two groups of pony mares, one of which had been subjected to bilateral superior cervical ganglionectomy. This operation, in effect, removed the light-mediated pathways between the eye and the pituitary. Surgery was performed during winter anoestrus in one year and reproductive patterns in all groups were similar during the next breeding season. But in the ganglionectomized mares there were significant differences between the members of this group and the sham-ganglionectomized control group. The pattern of follicular development, date of first oestrus and pattern of coat changes were all significantly delayed, indicating that the pineal–hypothalamopituitary axis may regulate or moderate annual reproductive rhythms at some time interval prior to their 'clinical' appearance. These findings could have a profound influence on our understanding of ovarian and oestrous activity under field conditions. For example, a mare suffering anoestrus in the normal breeding months may have been affected by treatment or management in the preceding winter or even during the previous 12 months.

The idea that physiological events in the oestrous cycle are predetermined by previous endocrine changes presents a challenging new dimension to our understanding of the oestrous cycle. If this is so, our concept of control of the oestrous cycle (see pp. 31–42) may have to be radically altered in the future.

Van Niekerk and Van Heerden (1972) found a significant correlation between high levels of nutrition and ovarian activity early in the breeding season. Of two groups, mares which received a supplementary diet of concentrate and lucerne hay came into oestrus and ovulated within 43 days compared with only 25% ovulation in mares which received no supplementary feeding.

Gonadotrophic hormones and the control of ovarian function

FSH concentration in mares' plasma has been found to rise five-fold by surges occuring at 10–11-day intervals during the oestrous cycle and early pregnancy (Evans & Irvine 1975). The late oestrous/early dioestrous surge of FSH appears to initiate development of up to ten follicles and the mid-dioestrous surge may be important for the further development of follicles destined to ovulate 10–13 days later. These same workers found that levels of LH increased at the onset of oestrus and reached their maximum one to two days after ovulation. They suggested that this rise in LH may stimulate maturation of the follicle throughout oestrus. They found an inverse relationship between progesterone and LH values but not between FSH and progesterone concentrations. It seems, therefore, that progesterone acts in a negative feed-back system with LH but not with FSH. The importance of these findings is that they throw considerable doubt on the rationale of many forms of hormone therapy practised in the past; the question is now of when administration should occur rather than what drug should be employed and how much should be administered. These last two considerations had been given priority in the past.

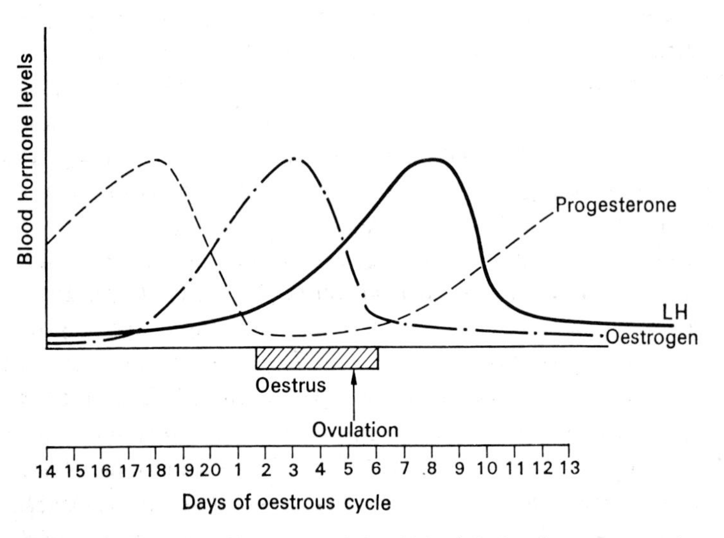

Fig. 1.10. Hormonal changes in peripheral blood during the oestrous cycle.

In equidae, progestagen and oestrogen levels follow the typical pattern (Fig. 1.10) but LH rises gradually to reach a peak after ovulation, in contrast to sheep in which levels rise steeply to a peak before ovulation. The dioestrous surge of FSH has already been discussed and, in addition, it seems that there may be rises in LH levels in mid-cycle (Vandeplassche et al. 1979).

Although the pituitary hormones LH and FSH play a predominant role in the endocrine mechanism of the oestrous cycle, the role of prolactin may also be significant (Short 1972).

Pregnant mares' serum gonadotrophin (PMSG) which contains FSH and LH does not cause follicular development when administered intramuscularly or intravenously as it does in some other species. The reason for this refractory state of the ovaries is incompletely understood, but Stewart and Allen (1979) have shown that PMSG does not bind to equine FSH receptors and only binds to equine LH receptors with one-tenth of the affinity observed with LH receptors of other species.

Stabenfeldt et al. (1972*a*) found that mares ovulate despite plasma progestagen levels greater than 5 ng/ml, which they suggest may indicate that in the mare ovulation control mechanisms are influenced by progestagens less than in other domestic animals. (The term progestagen is used to describe compounds which have a similar action to that of progesterone.)

Evans et al. (1979) reported LH levels in jugular blood samples obtained from eight mares at 5–20-minute intervals for two to five days during various phases of the oestrous cycle. An episodic release pattern was observed in one of three mares sampled during the ovulatory period. One mare had one secretory burst and the other mare had several periods of fluctuating plasma LH concentration. During dioestrus, episodic secretions were observed in two mares sampled 11–13 days before and, in one mare, nine days after ovulation. Dioestrous ovulations were accompanied by small increases in plasma LH (1–4 ng/ml) but many similar increases in LH were not accompanied by ovulation. In one mare, four ovulations occurred in the presence of a prolonged luteal phase; three were accompanied by increasing LH concentrations and one by LH at a low level. During oestrus the oestradiol curve precedes the LH curve by about two days (Pattison et al. 1974) and might, therefore, be responsible for the pre-ovulatory LH rise.

The life-span of the corpus luteum in the non-pregnant mare ranges from five to 18 days with a mean of 12 days (Stabenfeldt et al. 1972*a*). A significant increase in plasma progestagen levels occurs within 24 hours after ovulation and maximal levels (10 ng/ml) are reached about six days later. Oestrus does not occur until levels are less than 1 ng/ml (Stabenfeldt et al. 1972*a*; Allen & Rowson 1973).

It appears that the pituitary gland of mares contains a substance, possibly LH, which is necessary for the maintenance of the CL during dioestrus (Pineda et al. 1972) and the presence of the uterus is essential to CL regression (Stabenfeldt et al. 1972*b*). Catecholamines have been implicated in the maintenance of the CL in man and cow (Fylling 1971; Condon & Black 1976). However, in vitro studies of the CL by Condon et al. (1979) suggest that the equine CL is more refractory to exogenous stimulation by ovine LH and sympathomimetic compounds than is the bovine CL.

Ovarian control of oestrous behaviour

Equine follicular fluid contains the sex hormone steroids, their precursors and metabolites. The levels fluctuate during the cycle and tend to be lower in atretic than in viable follicles (Kenney et al. 1979). Equine follicular fluid contains progesterone, 17α-hydroxyprogesterone, androstenedione, epitestosterone, 19-nor-androstenedione, oestrone, oestradiol-17β and 6α-hydroxyoestradiol-17β; and luteal tissue progesterone, 20α-hydroxypregn-4-en-3-one and 17α-hydroxyprogesterone. Short (1962) suggests that these findings support a two-cell-type theory of steroid formation in the ovary. One type, possibly the theca interna cell, can convert progesterone into oestrogens. The other type, possibly the luteinized granulosa cell, has a diminished capacity to alter progesterone. Hay et al. (1975) examined the distribution of 3β-hydroxysteroid dehydrogenase (3β-HSD) in graafian follicles obtained from mares at different stages of the oestrous cycle. They found that 3β-HSD activity did not occur in the theca interna but was present in the membrana granulosa in the late luteal phase of the cycle and at oestrus, indicating that pregnenolone cannot be converted into progesterone in the theca. The authors suggest that this conversion occurs in the membrana granulosa and the progesterone then passes into the theca interna where it is converted into oestrogen. But Channing (1966), using tissue culture, found that granulosa cells are capable of androgen and oestrogen biosynthesis when gonadotrophin is present.

During oestrus, levels of oestrone and oestradiol-17β in follicular fluid increased significantly (Knudsen & Velle 1961) and mean levels were 3.75 μg oestradiol-17β and 0.3 μg oestrone/litre follicular fluid. A surge in plasma oestradiol-17β has been found to coincide with or just precede ovulation (Pattison et al. 1972). Hillman and Loy (1969) studied the relationship of urinary oestrogens to sexual behaviour and ovarian activity. They found that urinary oestrogen levels rose from 15–20 μg/litre a week before ovulation to 60 μg/litre the day before ovulation. A significant drop occurred on the day of ovulation and continued for two days. The urinary oestradiol-17β level accurately paralleled that of oestrone, and oestrous behaviour preceded rises in oestrogen levels and continued for about two days after their decline. Ovariectomy caused urinary oestrogen to fall from maximal to minimal levels within 24 hours of surgery. Injections of 5 mg oestradiol-17β resulted in peak excretion levels within three hours. No oestrus was observed and urinary levels dropped to a minimum during ovarian inactivity in autumn and winter. However, Munro et al. (1979) found no consistent relationship between circulating concentrations of oestrogens or androgens and the intensity of the behavioral signs exhibited by the mare during oestrus.

Luteolysis

Prostaglandin (PG) $F_2\alpha$ is produced in the uterus and has a luteolytic action on the corpus luteum. The route by which it reaches the target organ is unknown, but Ginther and First (1971) have shown by partial hysterectomy that removal of the uterine horn adjacent to the ovary containing the CL does not prolong the latter's life as it does in some other species. PG must therefore be systemically blood-borne rather than transferred locally through arteriovenous transfer or in lymph. Clinical trials of $PGF_2\alpha$ have been reported by Douglas and Ginther (1972), Allen and Rowson (1973) and Allen and Rossdale (1973).

Allen and Rowson (1973) showed that as little as 100 μg of a synthetic analogue of $PGF_2\alpha$ (ICI-79939) given to normal, cycling pony mares on two consecutive days, between Days 4 and 13 of dioestrus, induced a return to oestrus in two to four days. Further discussion of the use of exogenous PGF and other hormones can be found on pp. 31–42.

Normal cyclical changes in the ovaries and genital tract

Several follicles develop in the ovaries just before and during oestrus, but one usually outgrows the others which subsequently regress in size (see p. 2). However, various reports (Arthur 1958; Osborne 1966; Hughes et al. 1972*b*; Warszawsky et al. 1972) indicate that twin ovulations occur in 14.5–42.8% of cases. Ovulations may also occur in dioestrus (Stabenfeldt et al. 1972*a*; Vandeplassche et al. 1979). Follicles ovulate when they reach 2–6 cm in diameter (with an average of 4 cm) and their walls are thin and highly vascular. After ovulation, the follicular cavity is filled by blood and, after 24–48 hours, may project from the ovarian surface as a smooth, firm swelling. Atretic follicles may persist through dioestrus and in some cases through several cycles (see p. 2).

Uterine weight and the diameters of the horns vary during the cycle; the diameters of the horns also differ. During oestrus the uterine wall is relatively thin and oedematous, but in dioestrus the wall increases in thickness and tone.

The normal cyclical histological changes seen in the endometrium of the mare have been described by Seaborn (1925), Hammond and Wodzicki (1941) and Knudsen and Velle (1961) in necropsy material and by Andrews and McKenzie (1941), Ressang (1954), Brandt and Manning (1969) and Kenney (1978) in biopsy material. These authors described an increase in activity of the luminal epithelium and glands during oestrus. Andrews and McKenzie (1941) reported that luminal epithelial cells were cuboidal during dioestrus (20.0 μm in height), but became tall columnar during oestrus (23.3 μm in height). Mitotic activity increased in the luminal epithelial cells during early oestrus according to Seaborn (1925) who described 'epithelial degeneration' during mid-oestrus. Some pseudostratification of the luminal epithelium was reported after ovulation (Andrews & McKenzie 1941). During oestrus the epithelial nuclei were large, oval and basally situated but became more crowded and elongated during dioestrus.

Andrews and McKenzie (1941) reported similar increases in glandular activity during oestrus and early dioestrus (average gland diameter on the fifth day of dioestrus was 50.4 μm) in contrast to later in dioestrus (average gland diameter on the fifteenth day of dioestrus was 40.6 μm). Maximal activity of the luminal epithelium and glands was seen at the time of ovulation (Ressang 1954). Brandt and Manning (1969) reported numerous branched tubular glands during pro-oestrus, simple straight glands during oestrus and branched, lengthened, tortuous and sacculated glands during dioestrus. Knudsen and Velle (1961) suggested that the formation of gland 'nests' was a characteristic feature of pro-oestrus. These were numerous circumscribed groups of glandular lumens with marked boundaries. The epithelium in these groups was high columnar with markedly paler nuclei than that of the surrounding epithelium. The glands were often highly dilated and contained homogeneous eosinophilic material.

All authors reported increases in stromal oedema, vascular congestion and leucocytic infiltration during oestrus. Seaborn (1925) described collagenous stromal 'degeneration' during pro-oestrus and Brandt and Manning (1969) described an increase in stromal reticular fibres during oestrus.

Ricketts (1978) studied endometrial histological and histochemical cyclical changes using biopsy techniques. The normal histological architecture of the dioestrous endometrium of the mare is shown in Fig. 1.11. The changes in histological architecture during the oestrous cycle are shown in Table 1.1 and changes in

TABLE 1.1 Endometrial cyclical changes in histological architecture during the oestrous cycle

	Pro- or early oestrus	*Mid-oestrus*	*Post-ovulation*	*Early dioestrus*	*Mid-dioestrus*	*Late dioestrus*
Luminal epithelium						
Type	Columnar	Columnar	Columnar	Low columnar	Cuboidal	Cuboidal
Cytoplasm	Vacuoles throughout cytoplasm	Apical vacuoles	Vacuoles empty	No vacuoles	No vacuoles	No vacuoles
Cytoplasmic staining	Pale	Pale	Pale	Dark	Dark	Dark
Glands						
Configuration	Spaced out, somewhat straight	Packed, straight	Packed, straight	Spaced out, somewhat straight	Spaced out, tortuous	Spaced out, tortuous
Epithelial type	Columnar	Columnar	Columnar	Cuboidal	Cuboidal	Cuboidal
Epithelial cytoplasm	Vacuoles throughout cytoplasm, pale staining	Apical vacuoles, pale staining	Empty vacuoles	Dark staining	Dark staining	Dark staining
Lumens	Slightly open	Open, amorphous contents	Ducts open, basal glands closed	Closed	Closed	Closed
Stroma						
Oedema	++	+	+	±	–	±
Vascular congestion	++	+	+	–	–	–
Leucocytes	+	++	+	–	–	–

TABLE 1.2 Endometrial cyclical changes in histochemical staining affinity of endometrial sites during the oestrous cycle

	Pro- or early oestrus	*Mid-oestrus*	*Post-ovulation*	*Early-dioestrus*	*Mid-dioestrus*	*Late dioestrus*
Luminal epithelium						
PAS	+++	+++	++	++	++	+++
PAS (after diastase)	++	++	++	++	+	++
Alcian blue	+++	+++	+++	++	+	+
Alkaline phosphatase	±	++	++	±	–	–
Acid phosphatase	++	+	++	+++	+++	+++
Stroma						
PAS	L+	L+	L+	–	–	–
PAS (after diastase)	L+	L+	L+	–	–	–
Alcian blue	L+	L+	L+	–	–	–
Alkaline phosphatase	L/C+	L/C+	L/C+	C+	C+	C+
Acid phosphatase	–	–	–	–	–	–
Glands						
Duct cells						
PAS	+++	+++	+	–	–	–
PAS (after diastase)	++	++	+	–	–	–
Alcian blue	+++	++	+	–	–	–
Alkaline phosphatase	+	++	++	+	–	–
Acid phosphatase	++	+	++	+++	+++	+++
Basal gland cells						
PAS	++	++	+	–	–	+
PAS (after diastase)	+	++	+	–	–	±
Alcian blue	–	±	±	–	–	–
Alkaline phosphatase	+	++	±	–	–	–
Acid phosphatase	++	+	+	++	+++	+++
Luminal contents						
PAS	+++	+++	++	–	–	–
PAS (after diastase)	++	+++	++	–	–	–
Alcian blue	–	±	±	–	–	–
Alkaline phosphatase	–	–	–	–	–	–
Acid phosphatase	–	–	–	–	–	–

L = leucocytes; C = collagen.

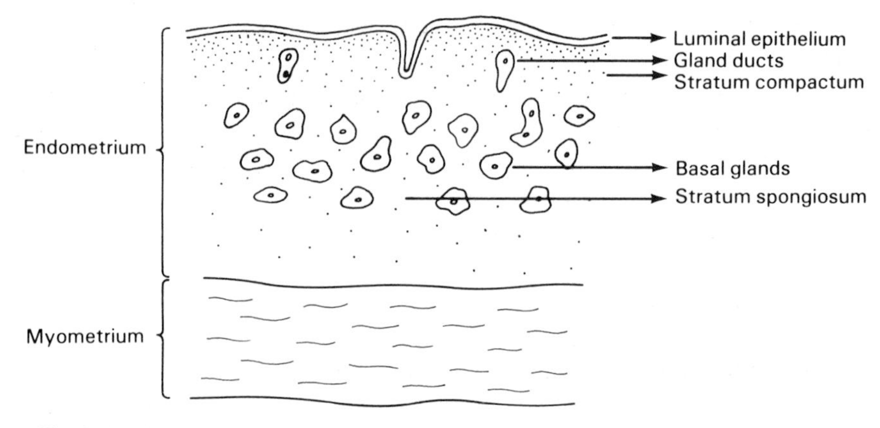

Fig. 1.11. The normal histological architecture of the dioestrous endometrium of the mare.

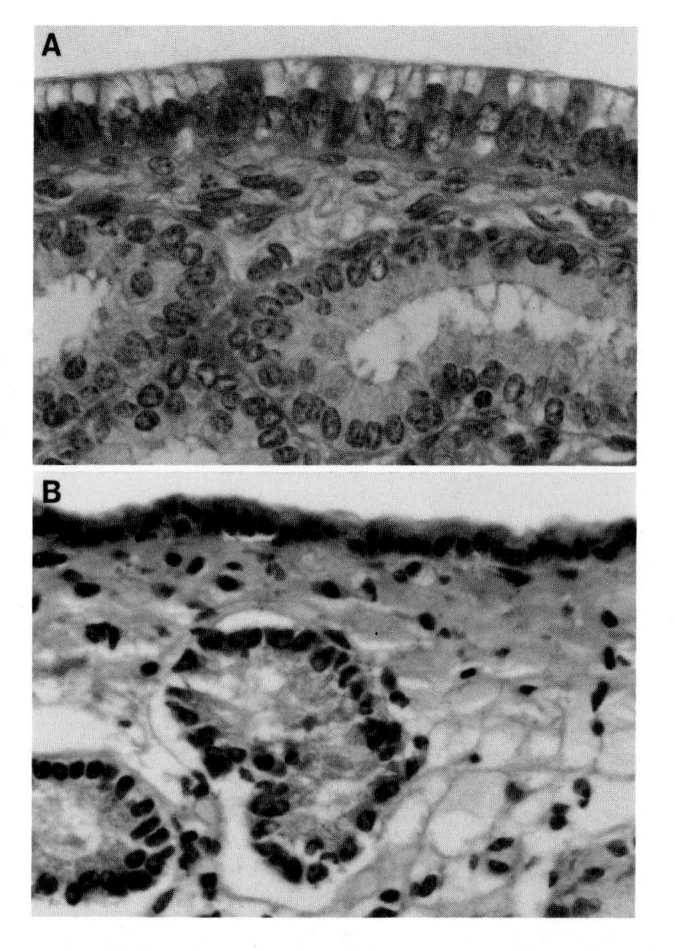

Fig. 1.12. Endometrial biopsies. A, Oestrus. Tall columnar epithelial cells with vacuolated apical cytoplasm. Some darker ciliated cells may be seen. B, Dioestrus. Cuboidal luminal epithelial cells. H & E × 450.

histochemical staining affinity of endometrial sites during the oestrous cycle are shown in Table 1.2.

The luminal epithelium was tall and columnar during oestrus (Fig. 1.12A), sometimes appearing pseudostratified, and became cuboidal during mid-dioestrus (Fig. 1.12B). Cytoplasmic activity started during early oestrus, with the presence of small vacuoles throughout the cytoplasm. These coalesced to form a large apical vacuole as the time of ovulation approached. The apical vacuoles had discharged their contents by early dioestrus, cytoplasmic activity disappeared and the cytoplasm stained darkly.

Histochemical staining affinity suggested that glycogen production in the luminal epithelium occurred during late dioestrus but was no longer detectable at the time of ovulation. Sections stained with Best's carmine gave similar results to those stained with PAS before and after diastase incubation. PAS-positive material, resistant to diastase, was present in the cytoplasm of the luminal epithelium throughout the cycle showing continual production of neutral mucopolysaccharides. Staining with Alcian blue suggested that acid mucopolysaccharide production by the luminal epithelium was maximal during oestrus and minimal during dioestrus. The luminal epithelial cytoplasm showed maximal alkaline phosphatase activity during mid-oestrus, and minimal activity during dioestrus. The luminal epithelial cytoplasm showed some acid phosphatase activity throughout the cycle and the highest intensity during dioestrus.

During dioestrus when the endometrium was quiescent the glands appeared spaced out and tortuous in configuration. During oestrus, glandular epithelial activity made the glands appear packed together and stromal oedema and vascular congestion made the ducts appear straight in configuration. The gland lumens were closed during the inactive dioestrus phase but during oestrus they showed activity with open lumens which contained amorphous material.

Glycogen production in the glandular epithelium became significant during early oestrus, maximal during mid-oestrus and decreased immediately after ovulation. PAS staining, resistant to diastase, showed significant production of neutral mucopolysaccharides throughout oestrus. Significant PAS activity was absent during dioestrus. A little acid mucopolysaccharide production was detectable during oestrus but not through dioestrus. Alkaline phosphatase activity was intense at the luminal borders of glandular epithelial cells during oestrus and absent during mid-dioestrus. Some acid phosphatase activity was associated with glandular epithelial cells throughout the cycle. This, however, was maximal during the dioestrous period.

Leucocytic infiltration of the superficial stroma started during early oestrus, reaching maximal levels at mid-oestrus and disappearing by late oestrus. Leucocytes showed significant staining for neutral and acid mucopolysaccharides and significant alkaline phosphatase activity. Stromal collagen stained intensely for alkaline phosphatase activity throughout the cycle. There was no significant stromal acid phosphatase activity throughout the cycle.

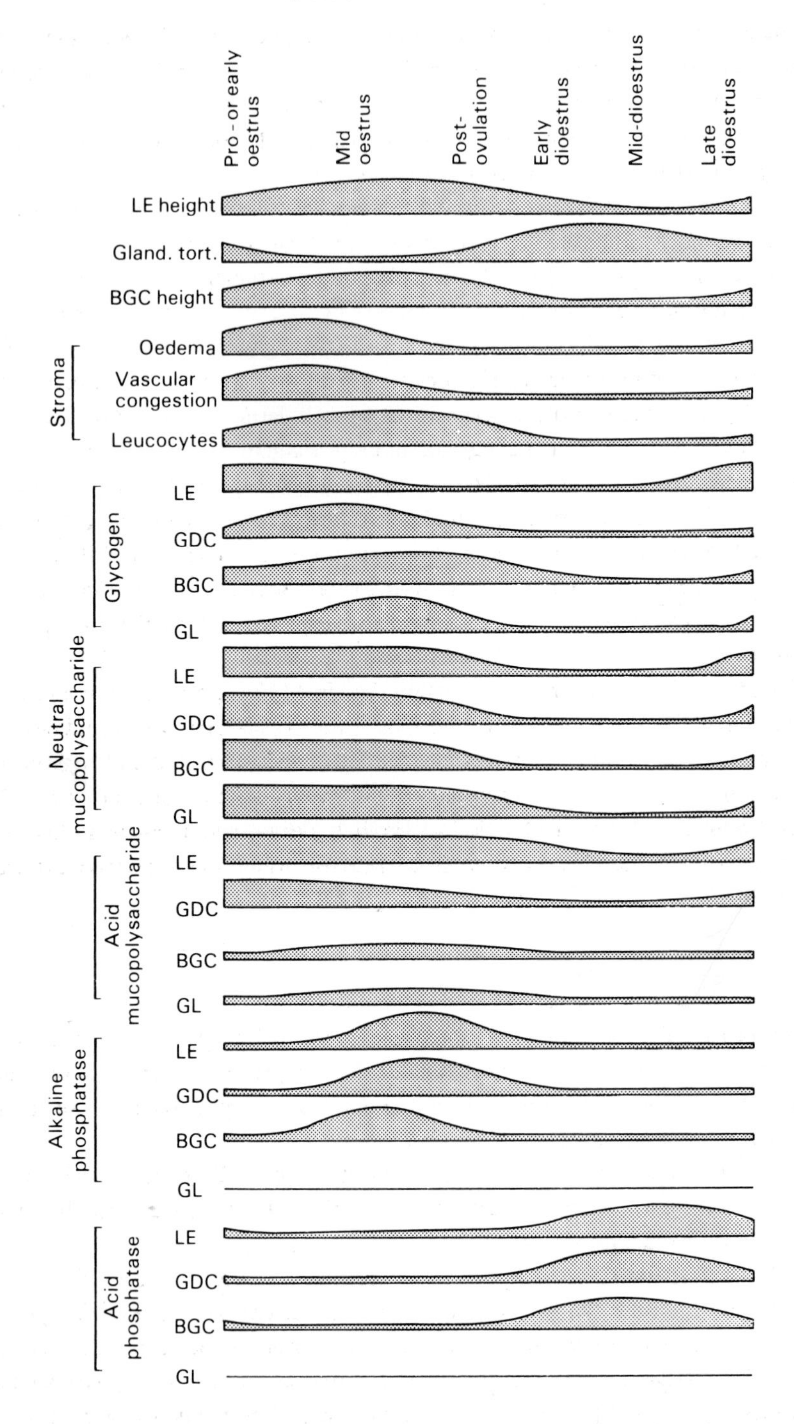

Fig. 1.13. Summary of endometrial histological and histochemical changes through the oestrous cycle. LE = luminal epithelium; GDC = gland duct cell; BCG = basal gland cell; GL = gland lumen.

There was good correlation between all the biopsies studied, when they were assessed critically for stage of cycle rather than day of cycle. Marked variations in cycle length and timing were found from mare to mare and from cycle to cycle.

A summary of the endometrial histological and histochemical changes seen through the oestrous cycle is shown in Fig. 1.13.

Samuel et al. (1979) have described scanning electron microscopical studies of the endometrium of the normal cyclic mare. During oestrus, ciliated and prociliated cells were distributed throughout the main 'carpet' of microvillous cells. At mid-oestrus, large numbers of secretory cells were present around the openings of the glands and along the ridges formed by the folding of the endometrial surface. The apical smooth-surfaced blebs of the secretory cells were occasionally pedunculated and, apparently, budding off into the uterine lumen. These findings correlated with the evidence of increased mucopolysaccharide production in the luminal epithelial cells by histochemical studies (Ricketts 1978) (see above). During dioestrus, secretory cells declined rapidly in number and few could be identified. The ciliated cells reached maximum density during mid-dioestrus and declined slightly towards the end of the period. Despite this decline the numbers of ciliated cells were still greater than during oestrus. Prociliated cells were present during the early part of mid-dioestrus.

The cervix changes during oestrus from the closed, firm, dry and white state of dioestrus to a dilated, oedematous, moist and red to red-pink state of mid-oestrus. Some authors recognize pro-oestrus in which the cervix is dilated and slightly red but still firm, and metoestrus in which the cervix has definite tone but is red and moist. Considerable individual variations occur in oestrus and dioestrus so that fine distinctions are not significant in clinical terms. We will discuss this aspect further when considering clinical examinations (see p. 51).

Variations in the oestrous cycle

So far we have described the physiological changes of the 'typical' oestrous cycle. However, a number of variations occur which have particular clinical importance with regard to the difference between pathological and physiological conditions responsible for infertility (see p. 58). Thus:

1. Individual oestrus lengths vary from one to 50 days. Extended length usually coincides with early spring months and low planes of nutrition, and shortened periods with late spring and summer.

2. Individual dioestrous lengths vary from about ten days to several months. The terms *prolonged dioestrus* and *anoestrus* are matters of definition. Hughes et al. (1972*b*) observed three types of anoestrus in a group of mares studied over two years: (*a*) ovulation on a regular cyclic interval but failure to show signs of oestrus; (*b*) persistent CL; and (*c*) inactive ovaries. For clinical purposes we define the last category as anoestrus (Fig. 1.14) and the first two categories as prolonged dioestrus (Figs 1.15, 1.16).

Dioestrus ovulations may occur between Days 2 and 15 of the luteal phase. Hughes et al. (1972*a*) found that these ovulations did not prolong dioestrus in their series. This requires explanation because the CL is refractory to the luteolytic action of prostaglandin for five days after ovulation.

Oestrus may occur without ovulation, especially outside the natural breeding season. Most of the variations from the physiological norm of the oestrous cycle

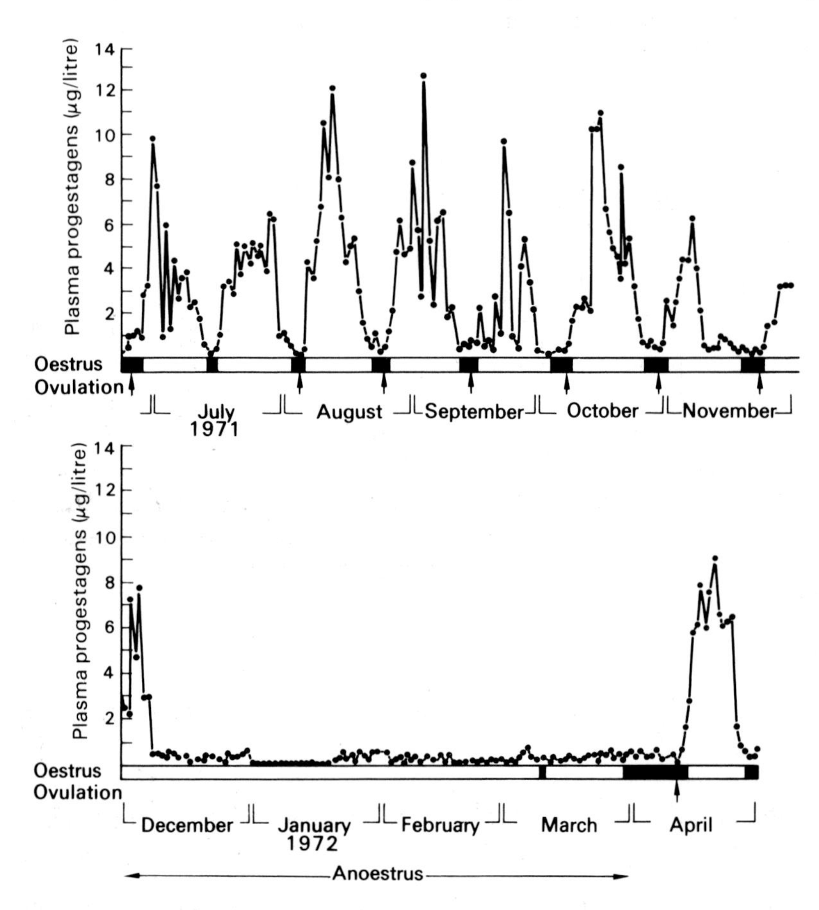

Fig. 1.14. Blood progesterone levels indicating true anoestrus occurring from December to early April. (*After Hughes et al. 1972b*).

are related to climatic and managerial factors, e.g. reduced daylight hours, low planes of nutrition and cold. But in some instances early embryonic death, lactation and genetic factors may be responsible.

Mares are essentially polyoestrous and breeding activity is restricted to a limited period of the year. Hughes et al. (1972*a, b*) found an average of 15 cycles each year and 22 ovulations. The number of ovulations was greater in March to November, as compared to December to February, and multiple ovulations were most frequent in March, April and May.

The follicular and gonadotrophic changes have been studied during transition from the ovulatory to anovulatory seasons in an effort to elucidate the causes of ovulatory failure. Snyder et al. (1979) concluded that failure may be due to a lack of an adequate ovulatory LH surge and final growth of the pre-ovulatory follicle. Vandeplassche et al. (1979) reported that mature follicles occur at all stages of the cycle (see p. 19) and concluded that lower levels of LH together with a high level of progesterone were responsible for failure of ovulation and regression of most mid-cycle mature follicles.

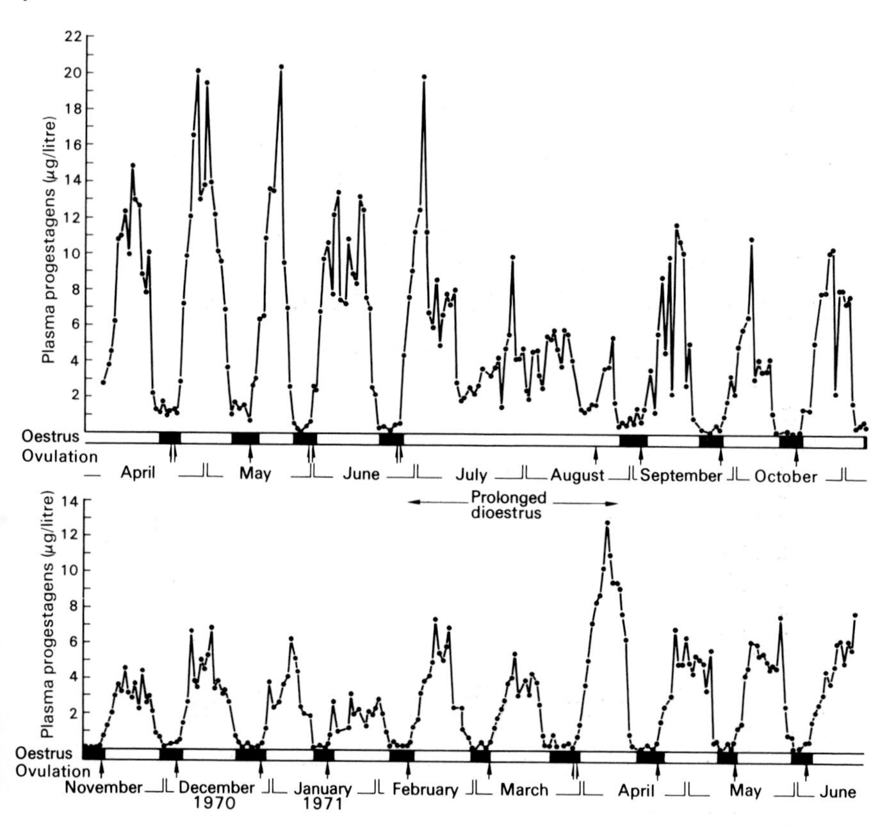

Fig. 1.15. Blood progesterone levels indicating prolonged dioestrus in July and August. (*After Hughes et al. 1972a*).

In summary, the variations in the oestrous cycle are based on a wide range of interrelated endocrine events and, therefore, a correspondingly high incidence of 'atypical' cycles is encountered in practice. This is reflected in the mare's behaviour at the trying board, the results of rectal and vaginal examinations and the ability of individuals to conceive in an arbitrarily selected seasonal period.

Foal heat

The first post-partum oestrus is commonly called foal heat. Matthews et al. (1967) reported that the mean day of onset was the eighth after foaling, with no difference

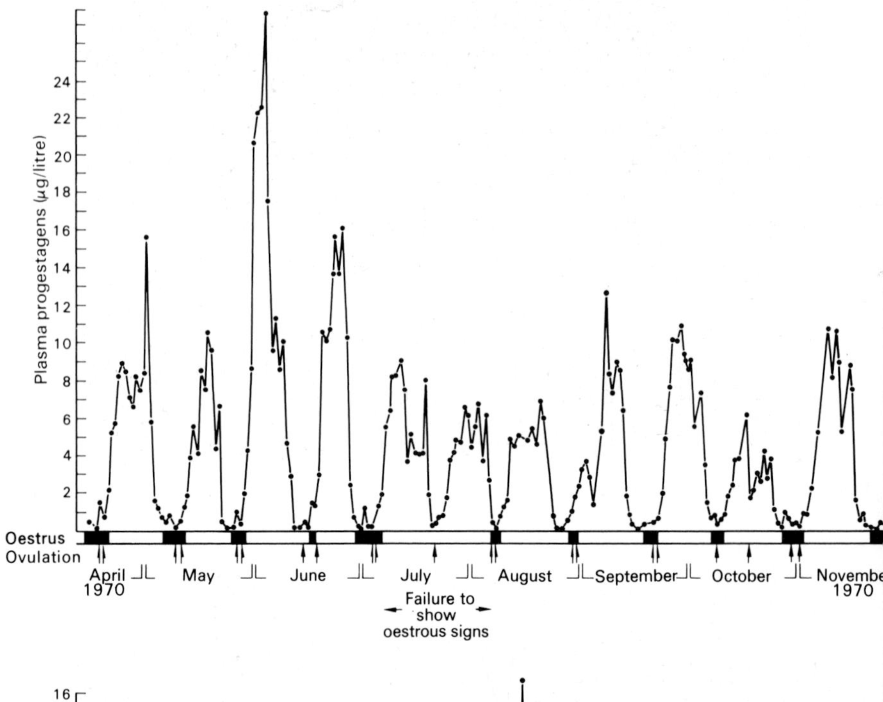

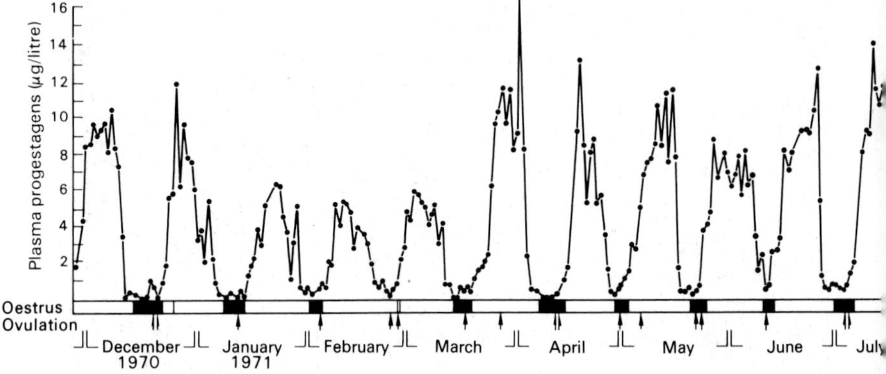

Fig. 1.16. Blood progesterone levels indicating missed oestrus in July due to failure to show signs. (*After Hughes et al. 1972a*).

within the months of the breeding season. Ovulation may occur from Day 4 to Day 18 post-partum.

Behaviour

Before describing behavioural signs, it must be emphasized that: (*a*) there is a wide range of variation in character and intensity of signs in any particular individual; (*b*) managerial influences may mask some signs and exaggerate others; and (*c*) the interpretation of signs is subjective, because the mare–stallion relationship appears to be based on smell and taste rather than sight.

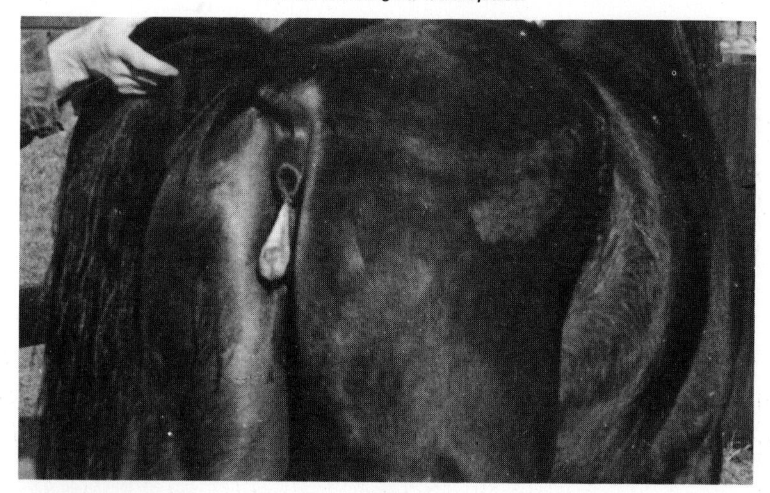

Fig. 1.17. Oestrous behaviour includes eversion of the vulva and exposure of the clitoris (winking).

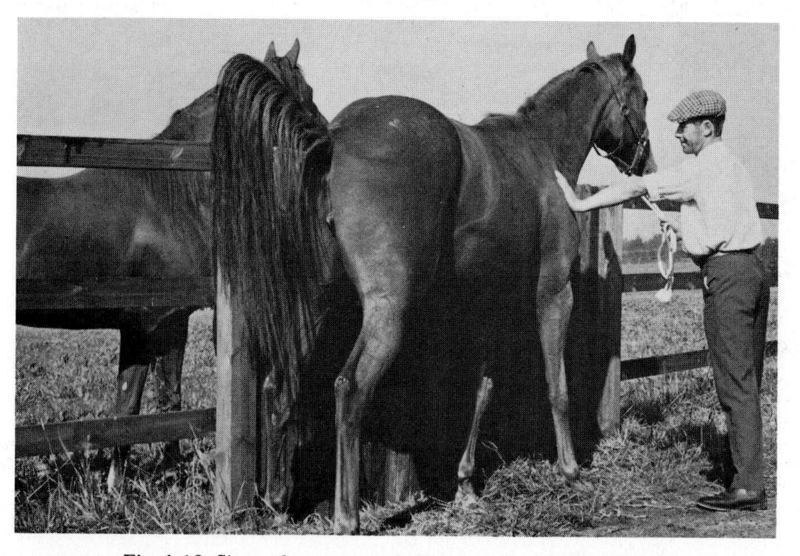

Fig. 1.18. Signs of acceptance in the presence of a male horse.

Oestrous behaviour (Figs 1.17, 1.18) is defined as acceptance of the male. It is associated with docility – a stance similar to that adopted for urination, but held repeatedly and for long periods – lengthening and eversion of the vulva and exposure of the clitoris (winking). The tail is raised and the mare often passes bright yellow urine with a characteristic odour. The urine contains pheromones which stimulate male sexual behaviour. For a further description of sexual signs, see Teasing (p. 42).

Dioestrous behaviour (Fig. 1.19) is seen when the mare rejects the stallion and is associated with attitudes of hostility, such as kicking, biting, flattening the ears, swishing the tail and resenting attendants' handling. Some mares show idiosyncratic behaviour such as squealing and squirting out urine when in dioestrus or oestrus.

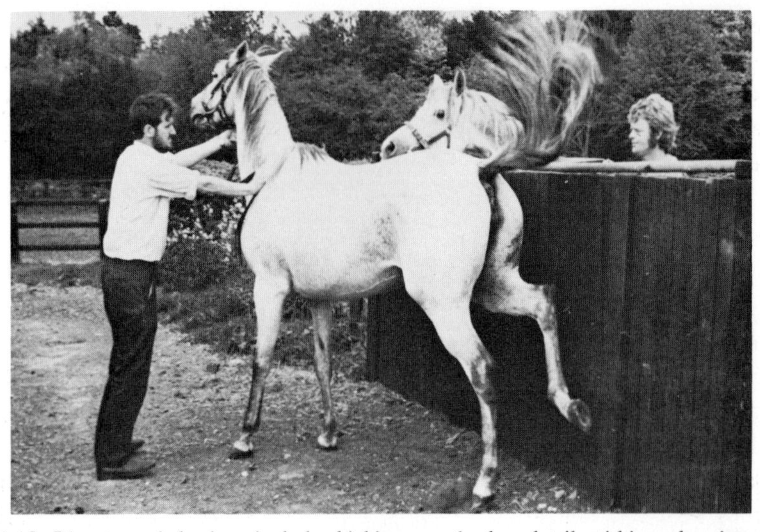

Fig. 1.19. Diœstrous behaviour includes kicking, ears back and tail-swishing when in contact with a male horse.

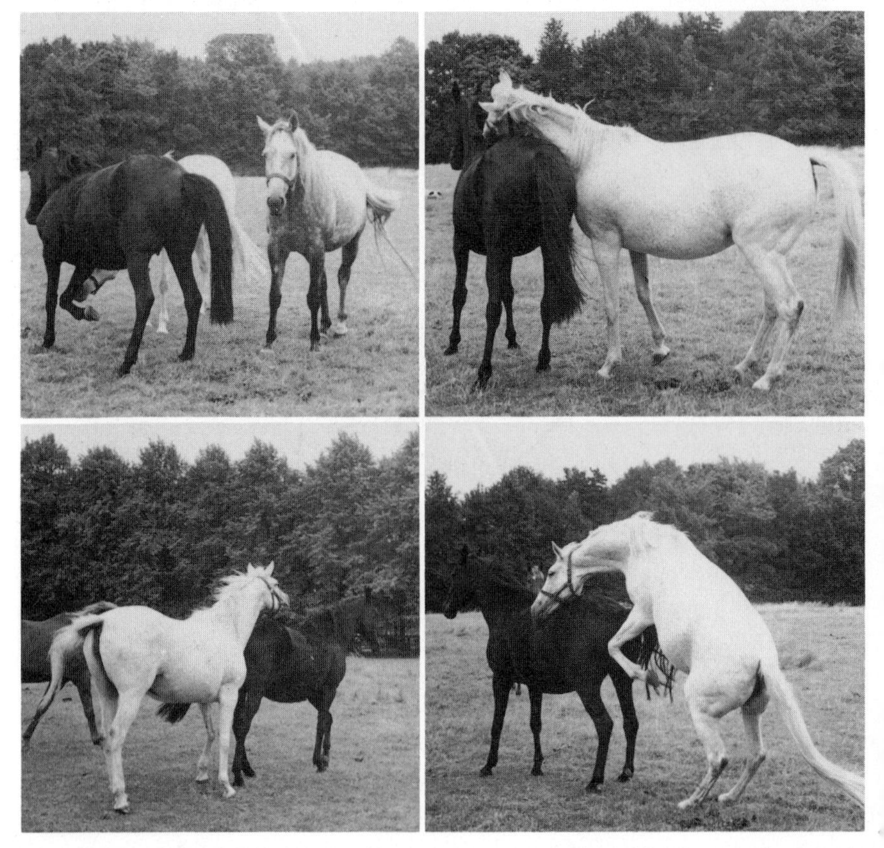

Fig. 1.20. The grey Thoroughbred mare is three months in foal. She shows male mounting behaviour towards a mare in oestrus at Cheveley Park Stud, Newmarket.

Mares rarely mount one another, but Thoroughbreds have been observed to do so (Fig. 1.20). One of us (P.D.R.) photographed a three-month pregnant mare who showed male behaviour and repeatedly mounted a mare in oestrus. The mounting mare foaled normally the following year and did not subsequently exhibit this type of behaviour.

Correlation of physiology and behaviour of the oestrous cycle

The physiological events of the cycle are usually correlated with those of behaviour, but individuals may exhibit signs of increasing intensity 24–48 hours prior to ovulation; the signs gradually diminish thereafter until dioestrus begins 24–48 hours after ovulation. Some mares apparently have silent heat, i.e. physiological oestrus including ovulation without the behavioural signs of oestrus. In most cases this is an error of interpretation and the mare will, if presented, accept the stallion. Ovulation may occur as the mare starts behavioural oestrus and the ensuing oestrous period is limited to 24–48 hours. Follicle development and ovulation during dioestrus is not rare (see p. 19). The relationship between the circulating levels of oestrogens and androgens and the intensity of behaviour is not consistent (Munro et al. 1979) (see p. 18).

Control of the oestrous cycle

It is often necessary for management to attempt to control the cycle, e.g. to facilitate breeding outside the natural season or to limit the number of services required of a stallion on a particular day or during the whole stud season. The synchronization of oestrus has received increasing attention as an aid to the management of herds for commercial purposes such as on farms producing pregnant mares' urine (Hyland & Bristol 1979) or to ensure maximal use of the stallion and labour while shortening the breeding season and thereby reducing costs (Voss et al. 1979) (see pp. 41–42).

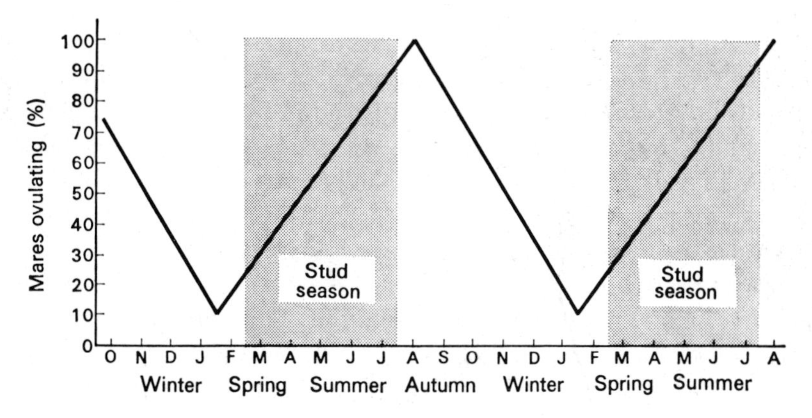

Fig. 1.21. The peak incidence of ovulation is outside the stud season in the northern hemisphere. (*After Osborne 1966*)

Ovulation is the critical factor on which conception is based. Several workers (Osborne 1966; Hughes et al. 1972*a*) have shown that the chances of ovulation occurring are greater in spring and summer months (Fig. 1.21). Since the arbitrarily defined limits of the Thoroughbred breeding season are outside the 'ideal' period and because the limited length of the breeding season restricts the number of ova available for fertilization, there is a corresponding limit to the chances of conception. A number of therapeutic measures have been used to control the cycle and the timing of ovulation.

Anoestrus

Anoestrus denotes ovarian inactivity, levels of progestagens less than 1 ng/ml and a cervical mucosa which may be sticky and pale or moist, pale and slightly relaxed. The condition is normally associated with winter and early spring conditions or in the case of lactating mares. Measures to counteract this condition come under the following headings.

Extended daylight. The effect of artificial light in inducing oestrus among anoestrous mares is well known (Burkhardt 1947). Nishikawa et al. (1952) used 200 and 400 W lamps and found that mares came into oestrus 65–80 days earlier than in the previous year. Merkt (1966) used 15 W bulbs and brought mares in five minutes earlier each day from 1 January. By the end of February, the mares were in light for 12 hours and in darkness for 12 hours. Conception in the test group occurred earlier than in a control group. A 16-hour daily photoperiod applied during the anovulatory season hastened the onset of the ovulatory season by two months in pony (Kooistra & Ginther 1975) and larger mares (Oxender et al. 1977) (see p. 13).

Cooper and Wert (1975) described a system to aid in the breeding of Standardbred mares during the winter period. After five years, 50% of foalings occurred during November, December and January, as opposed to 66% during April, May and June in the previous five years. Using a single 200 W (non-frosted incandescent) bulb in each stall, at a height of 7–8 ft (2–2.5 m) they replaced the natural light curve by increasing daylight length from 1 October in a step-wise manner, until a peak of 16 hours total was reached by 15 January, and this was maintained for the rest of the winter. Clear glass protective covers were used over the bulbs and they were routinely cleaned. The lights were controlled by automatic timers, going on at 16.00 and off at the designated times. The timers were changed once each week to add 30 minutes of light. The mares were housed individually in boxed stalls during the lighting period. During favorable autumn weather, barren and maiden mares were turned out at night after the lights went off. They were also out during the day except during unfavorable weather. Mares with foals at foot were turned out during the day for varying periods determined by weather and age of foal. The barren and maiden mares were in medium to thin condition prior to the onset of the breeding season. In mares with an obesity problem, weight reduction was accomplished by placing them in a grassless paddock for exercise and bedding them with wood shavings when inside. Three weeks before the beginning of the breeding season, the rations were increased for all barren and maiden mares. These mares were teased from 20 September, three times weekly, and an artificial insemination system, using washed and extended semen, was commenced on 15 December. This programme relates to horses with a birth date of 1 November. A similar system, however, arranged for an annual birth date on 1 January would be applicable to the Thoroughbred, using natural cover.

The long-term effects of regimens to control the oestrous cycle through extended daylight require further study. We have already discussed the manner in which ovarian activity was influenced by cervical ganglionectomy by Sharp et al. (1979) (see p. 15). The influence of one therapeutic measure to control the oestrous cycle in terms of its possible effects on future reproductive performance must always concern the clinician. There are two possibilities which must be taken into account. present measures may affect future performance adversely and the success of present measures may depend on some previous or preliminary factor that, if not introduced into the protocol of therapy, may prevent the current measures being successful. The mid-cycle administration of GnRH (see below) is an example of the latter situation.

The termination of the ovulatory season appears to be independent of the time when the ovulatory season begins (Ginther 1974) and therefore the use of an extended photoperiod does not appear to endanger the chances of successful fertilization occurring in the later part of the breeding season should these artificial means be applied.

FSH and releasing factors. Pregnant mares' serum gonadotrophin (PMSG), which has strong follicle-stimulating properties in other species, does not appear to affect equine ovarian activity, even in large and repeated doses. The reason for this refractory state is largely unknown but it has been suggested that it may be due to failure to bind to FSH receptor sites (Stewart & Allen 1979) (see p. 16). Follicular development and ovulation in seasonally anovulatory mares was induced by a treatment protocol of gonadotrophin-releasing hormone (GnRH) and progesterone (Evans & Irvine 1977, 1979). The courses of GnRH comprising four intramuscular injections of 1.2 mg were administered at about ten-day intervals to simulate the gonadotrophin surges normally preceding ovulation in a cyclic mare. The injections were given over three days and repeated at intervals of ten days on three subsequent occasions. Some mares were also injected with 150 mg progesterone in oil daily on Days 6 to 17 following the initial treatment with GnRH. This regimen did not result in normal luteal function because the mares developed follicles and appeared to ovulate but did not establish CLs. A second group of mares was treated with four courses of GnRH analogue at dose rates ranging from 10 to 20 μg on Days 1, 3 and 4, Days 10, 12 and 13, Days 17, 19 and 20 and Days 29 to 33. Progesterone (150 mg intramuscularly) was injected daily from Days 6 to 23. Nine of 10 mares treated in this manner developed follicles during the final treatment course, as did mares treated with progesterone only, while only one of five untreated control mares showed any ovarian development. The authors suggested that failure to induce final follicular maturation and CL development by this treatment may have been due to inadequate LH surge at the time of the expected ovulation associated with the low pre-ovulatory oestradiol-17β surge possibly being caused by the preceding FSH levels being inadequate or inappropriate. The progesterone treatment was found to increase base-line FSH concentrations and also to stimulate follicular development in mares not treated with GnRH, thus indicating a possible role for progesterone in folliculogenesis and, indirectly, ovulation.

The results and conclusions of Evans and Irvine (1979) demonstrate clearly the problems faced by clinicians in attempts to prevent anoestrous periods occurring during the months of the arbitrarily selected breeding season. The pressure for some type of therapy increases, of course, should these anoestrous periods extend into the natural breeding season, as may be the case in some individuals because they are lactating or for less readily understood reasons. Early field trials have been recently conducted with a gonadotrophin-releasing hormone in an attempt to stimulate pituitary and ovarian activity in anoestrus mares in early spring. In our experience, some mares appeared to respond but failed to produce a progesterone rise following apparent ovulation, at the induced oestrus period. Subsequent oestrus periods were quite normal. Further investigation of this drug is necessary but it may be practically useful in the future.

Exogenous progesterone. Van Niekerk et al. (1973) found that 100 mg of progesterone injected daily for seven days abolished prolonged oestrus early in the breeding season and that oestrus (seven to eight days ovulation) occurred within three days of the last injection. This treatment succeeded in anoestrous mares provided there was some ovarian activity but was not effective in mares with small, inactive ovaries. Daily injections of 100 mg of progesterone are necessary to produce plasma progestagen concentrations of greater that 1 ng/ml but these levels may not be maintained for 24 hours and 200 mg doses are preferable for this purpose (Hawkins et al. 1979). The mid-cycle administration of progesterone has been studied by Loy and Swan (1966). An oily solution given at a dosage rate of 100 mg/day intramuscularly blocked oestrus and ovulation and 50 mg/day prevented oestrus but not ovulation. Treatment starting on the first day of oestrus failed to stop behavioural oestrus or block ovulation, but daily administration before the foal heat effectively delayed onset. The interval from the end of treatment to oestrus appeared to be related to dosage and subsequent cyclic patterns to season of the year. Loy et al. (1975) found that the injection of 100 mg of progesterone per day from Days 5 to 14 after foaling blocked or delayed oestrus and ovulation in six out of nine mares; the other three mares ovulated during treatment without showing oestrus. Conception occurred in eight of 12 progesterone-treated mares as the result of mating at oestrous periods which were delayed until Days 15–28 after foaling.

Allen et al. (1980) describe the daily oral administration of 30 mg allyl trenbelone for 10–15 days to 61 barren, maiden and lactating Thoroughbred mares which were exhibiting deep anoestrus, shallow anoestrus (no oestrus behaviour but non-progressive follicular activity palpable on the ovaries), prolonged spring oestrus or lactation anoestrus. 54 mares (88%) showed oestrous behaviour within eight days, and 61 mares (84%) ovulated within 18 days after the last dose. The response rate was lowest in mares in deep anoestrus. Of the 38 treated mares which were covered during the induced oestrus, 21 (55%) conceived.

Nutritional supplements

Attempts have been made to determine whether there is an inherent stimulatory agent ('Dr Green', Owen 1978). Trials with oral and parenteral treatment with beta-carotene appear to have been a failure. Osborne (1979) has suggested that mares fed self-feed silage start normal oestrous cyclic activity early in the spring.

Prolonged dioestrus

The term prolonged dioestrus is used to denote a situation in which there is a functional CL persisting after the usual life-span of 15 days. The condition is confirmed by the finding of levels of plasma progestagen greater than 1 ng/ml. Prolonged dioestrus may occur in dry and lactating mares and in any month of the year. Treatment may be with uterine infusions or administration of prostaglandins.

Uterine infusion. Arthur (1970) studied seven Welsh mountain pony mares over a three-year period and found that 250 ml of normal saline at body temperature infused into the uterus through a Nielsen's catheter returned mares into oestrus on the fifth to ninth days of dioestrus, on average three to eight days earlier than expected. Clinical experience differs on the efficacy of this method. Burkhardt (1954) advocated uterine irrigation with normal saline where follicular development was present in the ovaries and Day (1957) observed oestrus within three to five days of treatment in mares that had follicles in their ovaries but a dry cervix.

In more recent years the influence of intrauterine saline infusion on the oestrous cycle has been studied by Arthur (1975) and Neely et al. (1975). The latter reported that plasma progestagen levels began to decrease approximately one day after infusion and declined to less than 1 ng/ml within four days. They concluded that the CL formed at the previous ovulation must be at least four to five days old before intrauterine saline will induce luteolysis.

In our experience in Thoroughbred mares infusion is regarded as being less reliable than prostaglandins and is more likely to cause endometritis. We prefer, therefore, to use prostaglandins to induce oestrus.

Prostaglandin (PG). Although prostaglandins (PG) were first discovered in 1930 it is only recently that their therapeutic properties have been recognized. There is now evidence that prostaglandin $F_2\alpha$ ($PGF_2\alpha$) is the uterine luteolysin which terminates the life of the cyclical corpus luteum (McCracken 1972). Exogenous $PGF_2\alpha$ induces luteolysis in the mare (Douglas & Ginther 1972) and is a powerful weapon in the practitioner's armoury of oestrus-inducing substances. Allen and Rowson (1973) showed that ICI-79939 (a synthetic prostaglandin analogue structurally related to $PGF_2\alpha$) is an effective luteolytic agent in normal cycling mares when administered on or after the fourth day of dioestrus. Allen and Rossdale (1973) described field trials with ICI-79939; 100 μg of the analogue administered intramuscularly or into the uterine body caused regression of the CL after Day 5 after ovulation, but not before. An immediate fall in the blood plasma progesterone levels occurred and mares returned to oestrus within four days after administration (Figs 1.22, 1.23). Allen et al. (1974) described field trials in mares

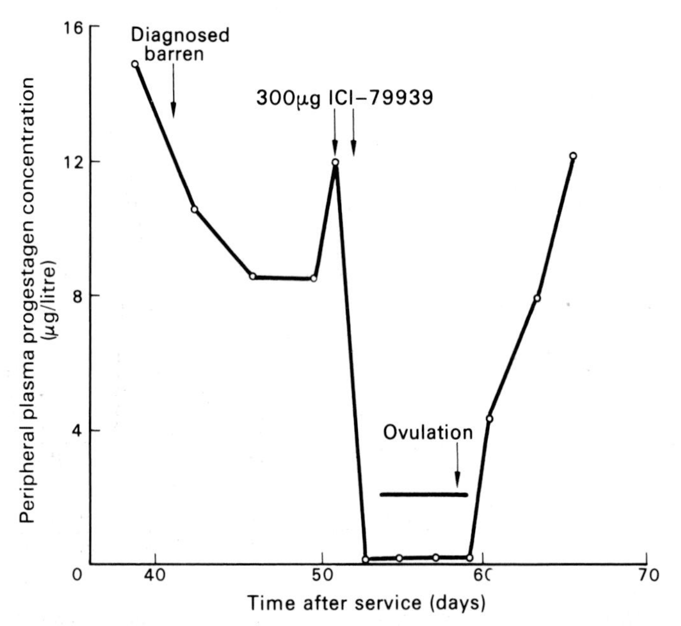

Fig. 1.22. Peripheral plasma progestagen concentrations in a Thoroughbred mare which resorbed its conceptus between 35 and 42 days after service. Intrauterine infusion of 300 μg 1C1-79939 on two successive days caused a rapid fall in progestagen levels. This was followed by oestrus with subsequent ovulation. (*After Allen & Rowson 1973*)

injected with a less toxic analogue ICI-81008 (Equimate) and found that a single dose of not less than 125 μg in Welsh pony mares and 250 μg in Thoroughbred mares consistently induced luteolysis and oestrus.

PG may be used to reduce the length of a normal dioestrous period or to end anoestrus caused by a persistent corpus luteum. It should be used only on mares in which a functional CL is present. The clinical application of prostaglandin therapy is to eliminate a functional corpus luteum, provided this is more than four days old.

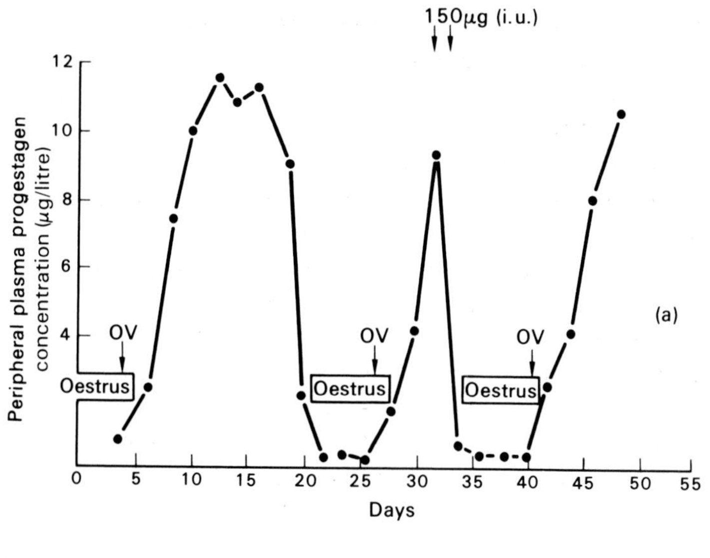

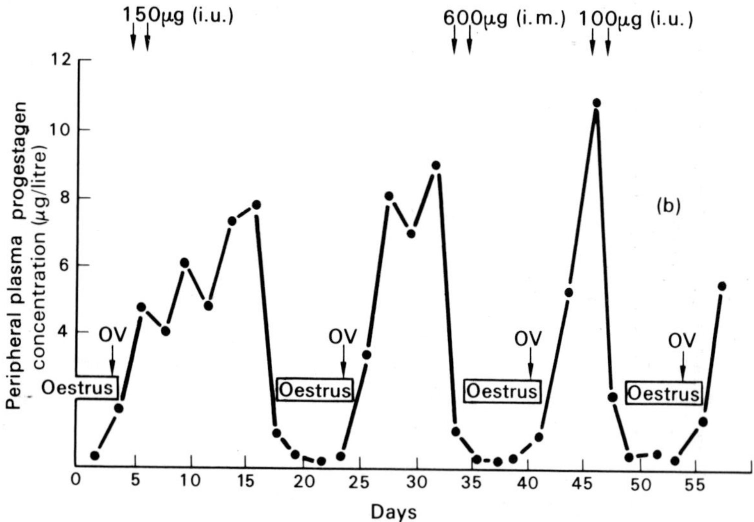

Fig. 1.23. Changes in oestrous cycle length and peripheral plasma progestagen concentrations in mares treated with 1C1-79939. (*a*) A mare given 150 μg on the sixth and seventh days of dioestrus. (*b*) A mare given 150 μg i.u. on the second and third days of dioestrus, then 600 μg i.m. on the ninth and tenth days of dioestrus and 100 μg i.u. on the fourth and fifth days of dioestrus. (*After Allen & Rowson 1973*)

Plasma progesterone levels greater than 1 ng/ml are evidence of a functional corpus luteum. Plasma levels of about 4 ng/ml are often found in cases of persistent CL function causing prolonged dioestrus.

Prostglandin can be used to induce oestrus in the following situations:

1. When a mare has been 'missed' and ovulation has occurred without coitus she can be returned into oestrus some ten days before her next anticipated oestrous period.

2. To terminate prolonged dioestrus due to a persistent corpus luteum.

3. To return into oestrus a mare that has undergone foal heat but has not been covered for veterinary or managerial reasons. For example, if ovulation has occurred on the seventh day after foaling, oestrus may be induced by Day 15 instead of by Day 24 as expected.

4. Out of the breeding season, oestrus may be induced for purposes of diagnosis or therapy.

5. Successive oestrous periods at relatively short intervals may be induced in mares suffering from infective endometritis or delayed post-parturient uterine involution to gain the therapeutic effect of oestrus.

6. In misalliance or cases of coitus followed by twin ovulations, early abortion can be induced five days after the last ovulation.

7. As an abortifacient in cases where twin fetuses are diagnosed at an early pregnancy diagnosis. This may be at any time after Day 19 but, in practice, the diagnosis is usually made after 30 days. PG, if used after the endometrial cups become active and in the presence of PMSG, may fail to achieve oestrus although causing abortion. Once high levels of PMSG are present (after about Day 42) increased doses of PG may be necessary to cause abortion, but used two or three times on successive days the method is usually successful. However, the aborted mare may show no oestrus or only shallow oestrus with no follicular development and ovulation until PMSG levels have diminished, which may not occur until Day 100 or more.

Our clinical experience suggests that the most successful use of PG is on cases where there is prolonged dioestrus over periods in excess of 20 days. In particular, the method is useful for mares examined 35 and 42 days after coitus and found not to be in foal. These individuals, when treated, usually exhibit oestrus within two days, although it may be necessary to make a vaginal and rectal examination on the second day after treatment to determine that the individual is in oestrus because the mare may not exhibit overt signs on these occasions. Furthermore, the time between treatment and ovulation varies and may depend on the follicular development present at the time of treatment.

Experiences with natural $F_2\alpha$ and prostaglandin analogues have been reported by Kenney et al. (1975*b*), Oxender et al. (1975), Douglas and Ginther (1975), Spincemaille et al. (1975) and Palmer and Jousset (1975).

Loy et al. (1979), using Prostalene, reported that although oestrus occurred in only 77% of mares, 98% ovulated at an average of six to eight days after treatment. The greatest variance of interval to ovulation was observed in mares having follicles greater than 4 cm diameter at the time of treatment due to regression of these follicles and late ovulation of a succeeding follicle. This resulted in the greatest uncertainty of prediction of ovulation time based on ovarian palpation. A further study using Prostalene has been reported by Kiefer et al. (1979), who found that progestagen patterns following administration of Prostalene suggested the following responses of the CL:

1. Luteolysis.
2. Incomplete luteolysis.
3. Incomplete luteolysis with subsequent recovery.
4. No luteolysis.

The number of Prostalene injections appeared not to have any subsequent effect on luteal responses and it seems, therefore, that repeated use is not associated with any carry-over effect from one cycle to another.

The release patterns of prostaglandin in the mare have been studied by Neely et al. (1979), who found that the prostaglandin metabolite, PGFM, was elevated between Days 14 and 17 after ovulation but that plasma progestagen, used to monitor luteal activity, decreased rapidly at the time of the first minor elevation in PGFM. Significant concentrations of PGFM were observed from one to four days following the initial elevation, both during normal oestrous cycles and in oestrous cycles in which luteal functions terminated with an analogue of $PGF_2\alpha$. These authors concluded that three mechanisms were involved in the development of the prolonged luteal phase:

1. The formation of the CL following ovulation during dioestrus which was unresponsive, due to immaturity, to the luteolytic effect of the $PGF_2\alpha$ released at the expected time.

2. The failure of the endometrial release of $PGF_2\alpha$ at the proper time.

3. The insignificant release of $PGF_2\alpha$ resulting in incomplete luteolysis in mares with degenerative endometritis (see p. 82).

Intrauterine saline infusion caused a similar release of $PGF_2\alpha$ to that found with the administration of prostaglandin. However, infusion of mares with severe degenerative endometritis frequently failed to stimulate the release of uterine $PGF_2\alpha$.

Inducing ovulation

Clinicians wish to induce ovulation so as to correlate the event with coitus and to ensure that semen is deposited in the uterus within 12–24 hours prior to the ovum entering the fallopian tube. In other circumstances it may be necessary to aid the ovulatory process in cases where failure to ovulate is anticipated by rectal examination or from the history of the case.

Human chorionic gonadotrophin (HCG), luteinizing hormone (LH). The use of LH to induce ovulation is a routine procedure on many stud farms. It is generally accepted that giving the hormone intravenously in dosage rates of 2000–10 000 units (Hancock 1948; Nishikawa 1959) causes ovulation within 20–60 hours (Berliner 1959), depending on the size of the follicle. It is important to ensure that the follicle in question is sufficiently mature to ovulate, otherwise giving LH may cause the luteinization of an immature follicle. The size and maturity of follicles depends largely on individual variation but, in practice, LH should not be used on follicles under 2.5 cm in diameter. We recommend that 4500 units should be administered intravenously about six hours before or immediately after coitus. The injection of HCG has been shown to shorten oestrus (Mirskaja & Petropavlovskii 1937; Day 1940; Loy & Hughes 1966) but Voss et al. (1975) found that mares injected with 2000 IU HCG on Day 2 of oestrus had a shorter oestrus and ovulated sooner than untreated control mares, but in the third cycle the treated mares had a longer oestrus and ovulated longer after the onset of oestrus than controls.

The possibility of antibody formation against the HCG should be considered. Roser et al. (1979) detected significant levels of antibodies in mares after two to five injections in mares injected with HCG on the day of appearance of a palpable 3.5 cm follicle during oestrus, the mares being injected throughout the 1977 breeding season. The half-life of the antibodies in individual mares ranged from 30 days to several months. However, cross-reactivity of anti-HCG antibodies with endogenous LH was thought by these authors to be improbable because no significant ovulatory refractoriness was observed in any of the treated mares and no cross-reactivity of equine LH with antibodies to HCG was observed when eight times the amount of serum that gave significant antibody binding to ^{125}I-labelled HCG was used.

HCG is used extensively in Thoroughbred practice and the experience of most clinicians is that it is helpful in shortening oestrus and that its repeated use does not appear to be contraindicated. The experiments on which Voss et al. (1975) based their conclusions involved the injection of mares on Day 2 of oestrus when the follicular development may not have been sufficiently mature and in a second series of experiments they used one intramuscular injection of 3300 IU HCG 24 hours before insemination and found that the conception rate in treated mares was higher than in controls. The number of inseminations per cycle to achieve fertility was also significantly less over three cycles in the treated mares. These findings seem to confirm our own clinical experience.

Gonadotrophin-releasing hormone (GnRH). Plasma luteinizing hormone (LH) concentrations have been measured in acyclic mares following single (Ginther & Wentworth 1974) and multiple (Evans & Irvine 1977) injections of GnRH. The LH increases following these GnRH injections were found to be of much shorter duration than the periovulatory surge of the normal cycle (Evans & Irvine 1975). Further studies have shown that the timing of the oestradiol surge is critical to inducing the prolonged periovulatory surge in the mare. Vivrette and Irvine (1979) found that injections of oestradiol on Days 1 to 3 had no effect on GnRH-induced LH increase when given concurrently but were more effective when the GnRH was administered on Days 4 to 7 following oestradiol treatment on Days 1 to 3. It is doubtful whether this regimen has practical application for routine use but may be helpful in cases where mares do not normally ovulate, e.g. in the early part of the breeding season or in individuals that have some idiopathic problem. Trials using the drug in anoestrus mares have been reported on p. 34.

Idiosyncratic behaviour patterns

Ovarian activity, including the presence of an apparently mature follicle, in the absence of behavioural oestrous signs, is a fairly common clinical experience during routine rectal examination. The effects of giving oestrogens are variable and their use may promote a uterine discharge, but claims have been made as to their efficacy in practice. In our experience, stilboestrol 5 mg intramuscularly can be used as an adjunct to prostaglandin to induce behavioural oestrus, but oestrogen therapy is not reliable and may be associated with ovulation before behavioural oestrus appears, if used when a mature follicle is present in the ovary.

The interaction of the oestradiol and GnRH on LH release in the mare has already been considered (see p. 40). Woodley et al. (1979) found that exogenous oestrogen treatment (10 mg oestradiol-17β) used daily from the time of ovulation did not prevent luteolysis nor did it alter oestrous behaviour, although it prevented follicular growth and inhibited ovulation.

Intrauterine and cervical manipulation

Hurtgen (1975) showed that uterine biopsy during the luteal phase resulted in decreased serum progesterone levels and a shorter dioestrous period. Further studies (Hurtgen & Ganjam 1979) showed that endometrial biopsy collected on Day 4 after oestrus induced lysis of the CL and shortened the interoestrous interval in eight of 12 cases. Cervical dilatation also shortened the interoestrous interval and these authors suggest that intracervical or intrauterine manipulations during the luteal phase of the oestrous cycle may directly or indirectly stimulate the release of endogenous luteolysin (prostaglandin). These and other findings demonstrate the care with which clinicians must assess the necessity for routine examinations and the need to consider possible side effects that they may have on the oestrous cycle.

Synchronized matings

The reasons for synchronizing oestrus are largely to allow mares to be inseminated at predetermined times without having to detect oestrus and/or to ensure that pregnancy and foaling occur within a limited time span. The object of these programmes is usually to facilitate commercial undertakings for example the collection of pregnant mares' urine. Synchronized mating in circumstances where artificial insemination can be practised enables maximal use of the stallion and labour, shortens the breeding season and thereby reduces costs. Hyland and Bristol (1979) synchronized oestrus in 116 mares by a protocol consisting of an intramuscular injection of prostaglandin $PGF_2\alpha$ (Day 0) and of fluprostenol on Day 15. The mares were further divided into three groups, group A being given 2500 IU HCG intramuscularly on Day 20 and artificially inseminated on Day 21 without detection of oestrus. Group B were injected intramuscularly with 2500 IU HCG on Day 20 and inseminated on Days 21 and 23 without oestrus detection. Group C were teased on Days 18, 19, 21, 23 and 25 and inseminated on Days 19, 21, 23 and 25 while they were in oestrus. A high rate of synchronization of oestrus (80%) was achieved within 48 hours of treatment with fluprostenol and 43 of 54 mares in group C showed in oestrus within four days following fluprostenol administration and by ten days only two mares had failed to come into oestrus. The combined pregnancy rate in the three groups was 64% and a further 34% of the experimental group became pregnant to natural breeding at the first oestrus after the insemination programme. Thus, a total of 114 of the 116 (98%) of the experimental mares became pregnant and the overall time taken to obtain this result was five weeks. If this method were to be applied to Thoroughbred stud farms it would provide a challenging basis for changes in management and provide enormous financial savings to the industry. We do not, however, anticipate its implementation for a considerable period.

Voss et al. (1979) made similar observations using two injections of $PGF_2\alpha$ 14 days apart without regard to the stage of the oestrous cycle with particular reference to the effect of frequency of insemination on fertility. They found that fewer treated mares became pregnant compared to controls (mares receiving saline injections in Days 0 and 14) but after three cycles the pregnancy rates for mares inseminated every other day or daily were higher than mares inseminated only once during oestrus.

MANAGEMENT OF THE MARE'S SEXUAL FUNCTIONS

Segregation of the stallion from his mares and the habit of breeding in hand has made it necessary for management to interpret the mare's sexual signs. The usual method is that of teasing, in which the mare is brought into contact with the male horse under varying conditions. Veterinarians confirm the diagnosis by internal examinations.

Lay responsibilities—teasing (trying)

The object of teasing is to cause the mare to display sexual behaviour. The advantage of this system compared with free-range breeding lies in the ability to control the number of services per stallion and concentrate them in the latter part of the oestrus when ovulation is most likely. Teasing also allows management to protect the stallion from injury by presenting for service only those mares showing oestrous behaviour.

The disadvantage of the teasing ritual is that it exaggerates the sexual response by concentrating it into a short time (often only a few minutes each day) and subjects the mare to the attention of the male in an arbitrarily selected manner. The majority of mares conform to the process by exhibiting true oestrous or dioestrous behaviour when in the presence of the male. However, a substantial number mask the signs of oestrus and exhibit dioestrous behaviour throughout the cycle. It is not clear to what extent this is the result of repeated unnatural stimulation while in true dioestrus, rather than an individual characteristic. It is well recognized that some individuals conform to similar behavioural patterns in succeeding seasons, for example by showing excessively strong or very weak signs of oestrus. A mare with foal at foot does not always display signs of oestrous behaviour, especially when separated from her foal. The time of teasing relative to the daily routine is important. Teasing before turning out or feeding can cause erroneous signs of dioestrus, as can teasing in high wind, rain or extreme cold.

The interval during which the mare is in contact with the male is of varying importance. Some individuals readily show signs of their sexual state, letting down and 'showing' as they approach the horse, while others need coaxing and respond only after many minutes. The influence of habit is reflected in those individuals who may show signs of sexual behaviour to the trying board in the absence of a horse. Other times when mares 'show' are in the covering yard and when handled in a manner associated with mating, e.g. washing the perineum, bandaging the tail or applying felt boots to the hind-feet.

Some mares show signs of oestrus only when a twitch is applied. Others become more tractable, allow themselves to be caught and handled more easily when in oestrus, without showing other outward signs. These mares may show typical dioestrous behaviour at the trying board, even though in oestrus, but often 'show' in the covering yard just before and at the time of mating.

The following description is of current methods used to stimulate signs of sexual state at different breeding centres. The teaser may be a male horse retained for the purpose, or the stallion.

The mare led in hand to the teaser. The mare and the male are introduced by allowing muzzles to meet and the teaser is allowed to stretch his head alongside the mare's neck (Fig. 1.24). This approach mimics the natural approach of two herd members or strangers. The teaser is allowed to nip the mare with his teeth, but too rough an attitude is discouraged by a sharp tug at the bridle. The attitude of the mare is noted: ears back, squealing and biting the teaser indicates dioestrus, although some individuals may show this attitude as a preliminary to oestrous behaviour. A mare in oestrous shows signs by raising the tail and leaning towards the trying board.

The mare should, after a few minutes, be turned so that her flank is parallel to the board (Fig. 1.25) and at right angles to the teaser. In view of the risk of spread of venereal disease (see pp. 75–81) the teaser should not be allowed to contact the mare's genitalia. This is not always easy to control, of course, but the teaser should be taught to remain at a safe distance. If a number of mares are teased one after the other in a short space of time, one cannot guarantee that the teaser may not transfer vulval discharges, containing potential veneral-disease-producing bacteria, on his nose. Most mares in oestrus will, after a minute or two, show obvious signs, although some may take several minutes. Those in dioestrus display marked hostility and kicking, but some individuals remain quite and sullen.

Applying a twitch may cause some individuals in oestrus to show, although it may make dioestrous mares exhibit apparent signs of oestrus. In some individuals interpretation is therefore difficult and signs should be confirmed by veterinary examination.

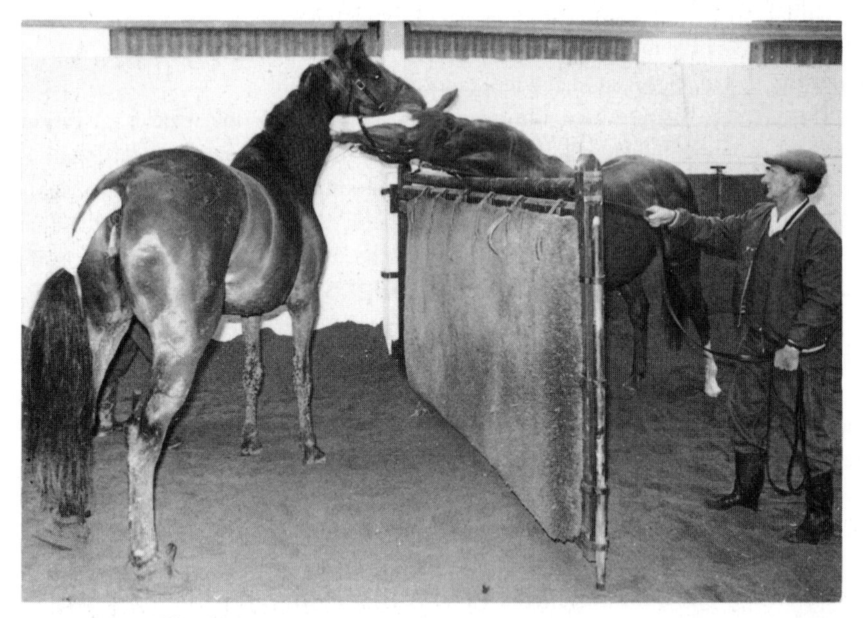

Fig. 1.24. The mare and 'teaser' are introduced head to head.

In the southern hemisphere, it is customary to have shutes or crushes through which mares are driven and held, one at a time, for attention by the teaser on the outside. This method gives convenient handling and reduces the amount of labour required to tease a large number of mares, but it should be used only where mares are accustomed to this handling.

The teaser led in hand to the paddock rail. Mares are teased across the paddock fence or, preferably, across a permanent trying board, or one that is moveable and slotted in position for the purpose. The reaction of the mares in the paddock is noted. Most come towards the teaser and some may show marked signs of oestrus; others show obvious hostility. However, a number remain neutral and these should be brought, by hand, to the board and tried by the method described first. The second method is useful because a group of mares can be tried at any time of the day after they have had their preliminary exercise following the night's confinement in a loose box. This method, used in the evening or early morning, is particularly useful for mares that are turned out night and day, because it enables management to tease them under optimal conditions away from midday heat and noxious interference from biting insects.

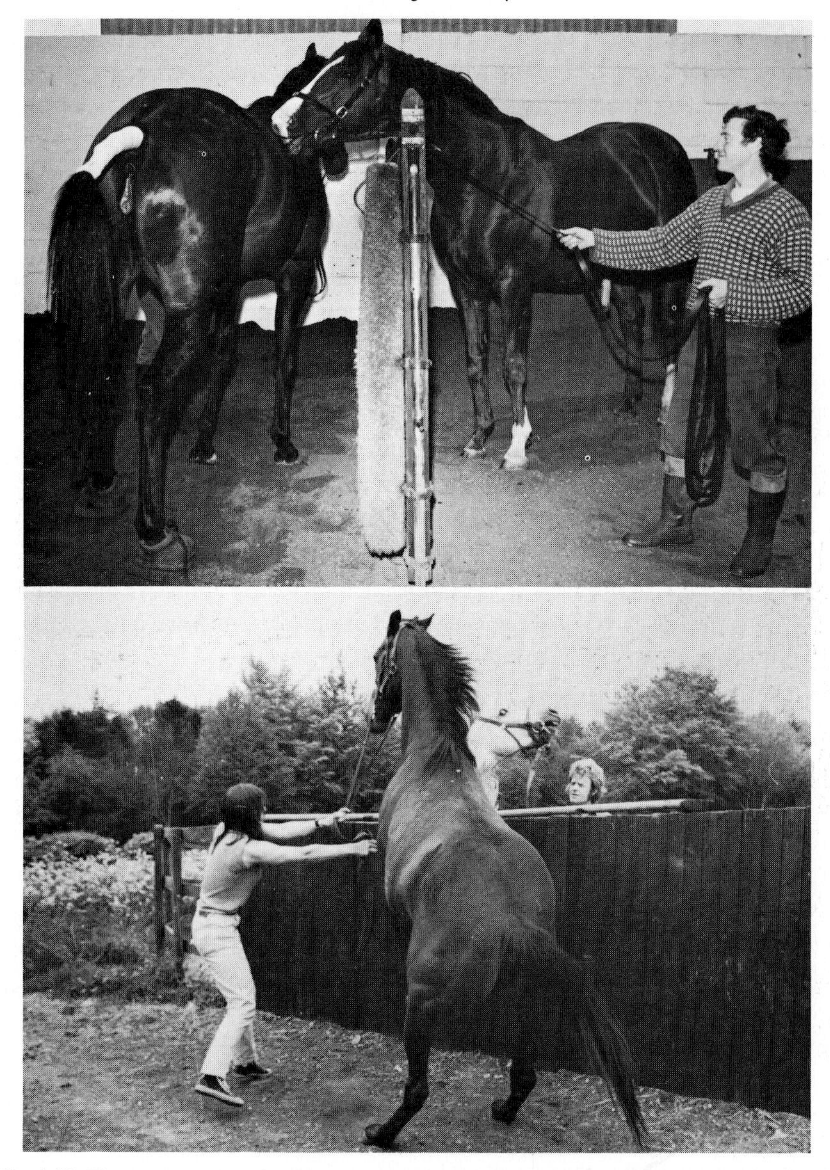

Fig. 1.25. The mare is induced to stand parallel to the trying board and shows oestrus behaviour (*above*) or dioestrus behaviour (*below*).

The method may be unsuitable for large numbers of mares with foal at foot because of the danger of accident. Teasing across a fence may also invite damage due to a mare kicking through the rails. In these circumstances, the process should be used with discretion.

The teaser led past the paddock. This method is useful where stallions are exercised by walking them through the stud farm. It also applies where teasers are ridden. The advantage of the method is that it may be performed readily at any time of day and repeated frequently with little or no disruption of routine. Mares will often show signs of oestrus when they see or hear horses moving past the paddock perimeter; they are unlikely to show dioestrous behaviour and the method cannot therefore replace but only supplement the first two methods.

The teaser led through the paddock. This method is not recommended as it may be dangerous.

The teaser confined to a railed or boarded area. There are a number of variations of this method, which is much favoured in the southern hemisphere. For instance the boarding may be high with small iron grilles or with openings through which the teaser can put his head. The teaser may be a pony or miniature breed restrained by a stout fence. If he escapes no harm can occur because his size precludes successful coitus with members of the group. The method is ideal for mares turned out day and night, although they must be carefully watched for signs of oestrus.

The method can be varied by confining the teaser to a box with a grille or opening into an adjacent box where a difficult mare is placed.

When the teaser is unsupervised in this manner there may always be the risk that infected vulval discharges may be transferred from mare to mare on the teaser's nose.

A vasectomized teaser. This animal may also be used to mount maiden mares or others in which the state of receptivity is doubtful. Although seldom used on Thoroughbred stud farms, the vasectomized teaser may run loose with his mares. There are obvious advantages in this method although intromission may expose mares to the risk of venereal infections. To overcome this, surgical retroversion of the penis has been practised. After this procedure, the penis extrudes caudally between the hind-legs, making intromission impossible. One of us (S.W.R.) has seen a hermaphrodite horse running with a group of mares. This was an especially useful technique to detect mares with low-intensity oestrous behaviour. Again, with unsupervised teasing, the risk of spread of venereal disease by muzzle to genital contact is present.

Aids to teasing

We have mentioned the need to allow time for a mare to respond to the teaser and that the hour of teasing in relation to the daily routine is important in avoiding false signs of dioestrus. The following measures may also be helpful:

1. Mares with foal at foot may sometimes show only if the foal is present at the trying board. Special pens may be built so that the foal can be confined close to the trying board, allowing the mare to see and touch the foal at the same time as she is in contact with the teaser across the trying board.

2. Raising the mare's tail and gently rubbing the perineum may cause the mare to 'let down' at the trying board or when not in the presence of the male. If this is done a separate pair of plastic disposable gloves should be used for each mare.

3. Careful observation of mares at all times may reveal indications of oestrus: lengthening of the vulva, staling on return to the loose box after visiting the teaser, showing to the foal in the paddock or loose box, showing to other mares in the paddock, frequent whinnying or restlessness (especially in response to the movement of other mares outside the paddock).

The results of teasing cannot be conclusive in every case. Individual variations in response and the limited time available give rise to erroneous interpretation. For this reason veterinarians have been drawn into management to confirm diagnosis of the sexual state.

Veterinary responsibilities

Gynaecological examinations fall into two categories: per rectum by which the ovaries and uterus are palpated and per vaginam in which the cervix is inspected and cervical or uterine material obtained for diagnostic purposes. The techniques involved will be described in Chapter 8. The purposes of these examinations are:

1. To confirm the sexual state, i.e. oestrus, dioestrus or pregnancy.
2. To correlate coitus within the period 48 hours before ovulation.
3. To diagnose the presence of venereal infection.
4. To diagnose pathological conditions and treat infertility.
5. To perform prophylactic procedures in 'susceptible' mares prior to coitus.

There is no clear demarcation between these various functions because any approach to the subject rests largely on the definition of infertility, an aspect discussed later. For example, a clinician's responsibility to determine the optimum time for mating relative to ovulation is, in itself, helpful in mares with pathological conditions of the genital tract. The methods of examination can not be considered in practice as a separate entity; the rectal and vaginal examinations complement each other, but, for our purposes, it is convenient to discuss them under separate headings.

Rectal palpation

The ovaries and uterus are carefully palpated by the technique described on p. 509. All findings should be noted and it is helpful to develop some system for recording. Ideally, results should be made according to a defined standard but at present clinicians vary in their methods. It is not claimed that the method described here has special merit but it serves as an illustration.

Measurements are determined by a knowledge of the operator's hand. Useful indices are the length of the end of the thumb, the breadth of the index finger, the combined breadth of the first two fingers, the breadth of the thumb and the distance between the thumb and the first finger when spread as far as possible apart. Greenhof and Kenney (1975) found the diameter of the lumen formed with the tip of the index or middle finger opposed to the tip of each thumb a useful callibration. This diameter may be callibrated at three positions, i.e. index finger to tip of thumb, index finger to second joint of thumb and index finger to first joint of thumb.

Each ovary should be taken between thumb and finger, its total size estimated and its length and breadth recorded in centimetres. The presence of follicles and their consistency (tense or soft) should be noted and their diameter estimated. A convenient method for recording the position of the follicles is to label the poles of the left ovary A and B and of the right, C and D. A follicle of 3 cm on the left hand pole of the left ovary is designated 3A, one placed between the two poles A3B. Similarly a follicle 4 cm in diameter on the right ovary would be 4C, C4D or D4 (Fig. 1.26).

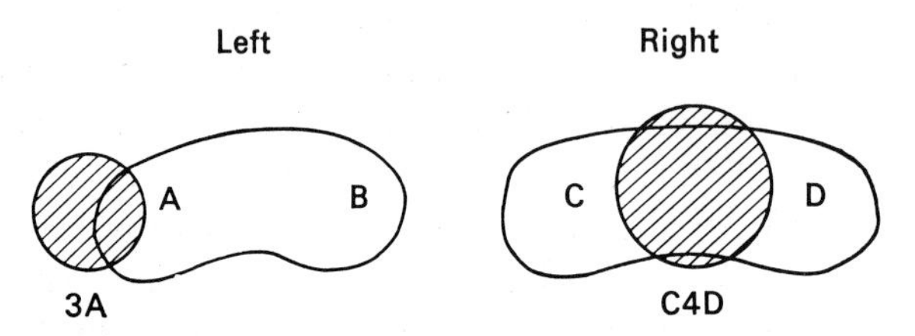

Fig. 1.26. The left and right ovaries with follicles 3 and 4 cm in diameter (shaded) identified by their position relative to the ovarian poles (A, B, C and D).

The advantage of this method is that a follicle found at one examination may be more readily identified at subsequent examinations and distinguished from others that develop later. Follicles in the centre of the ovary are closer to the ovulation fossa than those at the poles and can be expected to ovulate sooner. The total size of the ovary must also be considered. If the stroma is much larger than the follicle the significance of the actual size of the follicle is diminished. Conversely, a relatively small follicle on an ovary of small stromal size can be expected to ovulate sooner than one of equal size in other circumstances. If the ovary is spherical the follicle can be described only according to its presence in the left or right organ.

Estimating the time at which ovulation will occur depends on follicular size, consistency and position. Most follicles do not ovulate until they are 3 cm or more in diameter although this varies with ovarian size and other factors. Follicles about to ovulate become thin-walled and their contents are under reduced pressure. On palpation they can be felt as soft fluctuating swellings on the surface of the ovary. The size of mature follicles is extremely variable and the occasional follicle may be as much as 10 cm in diameter at ovulation (Greenhof & Kenney 1975). A follicle, when palpated in the process of ovulation, may appear deceptively small and thus apparently immature, because some of its contents is in passage through the ovulation fossa. Atretic or regressing follicles are tense and thick-walled (see p. 3).

For practical purposes, if a follicle greater than 3 cm is detected, it can be expected to ovulate within three days but, if soft, this time is reduced to 24 hours. Greenhof and Kenney (1975) recommend that follicular maturity may be estimated by size, amount of protrusion, sharpness of shoulder, wall thickness and tenseness.

A mature follicle is at least 2.5 cm in diameter, has a sharp (almost 90°) shoulder with the ovarian surface and protrudes above the surface an amount equal to its radius, while its wall is getting much thinner. They estimate tenseness by comparison with the web of skin between an operator's thumb and forefinger. When the thumb and forefinger are stretched apart the web blanches and a follicle this tense is three or more days away from ovulation. It should be emphasized that the estimated ovulation time is subjective and will vary according to the operator's experience. In addition there are seasonal and individual variations related to changes in hormone levels which cannot be anticipated by rectal palpation. At the beginning and end of the natural breeding season, follicles may take much longer than anticipated to reach maturity.

Recent ovulations can be recognized by the soft, friable mass which occupies the cavity of the ruptured follicle. After about 24 hours the area becomes firm and a pit can be felt. Later the area is palpated as a firm, plum-like swelling rather similar to a tense follicle. Two or three days after ovulation it may be difficult to distinguish between an ovulation and a follicle of about 2–3 cm in diameter. There are considerable variations in results obtained by palpation of ovaries after ovulation. In many cases it is possible to diagnose an ovulation only on the basis that the follicle palpated at a previous examination (say two days) has been replaced by a firm mass. In other instances the site of ovulation is obvious and the mare may show signs of pain when the site is palpated. Occasionally, there may be very little palpable difference between the mature follicle, palpated two days previously, and the recent ovulation cavity filled, presumably, with blood. Ovulation can sometimes be confirmed by visual inspection of the cervix (see below) but the most accurate confirmation of successful ovulation and luteinization is by the measurement of blood progesterone levels.

Truly anoestrous mares have small (2–5 cm long) ovaries which are firm and have no evidence of follicular development. During dioestrus mares often have some follicular development (less than 3 cm in diameter).

Twin ovulations are of concern to all clinicians. It is customary to withold service if the results of rectal examination indicate that two follicles may ovulate. If there is a discrepancy in size some clinicians advise mating after one and before the other has ovulated. Another approach is to rupture one follicle by inserting a needle through the vaginal fornix. The risk of haemorrhage or ovarian adhesions restricts this method. In Chapter 3 twin conceptions are discussed further; here we shall say only that in Thoroughbreds, about 1.5% of all pregnancies recorded annually in the General Stud Book are twins, yet several workers (Arthur 1958; Osborne 1966; Hughes et al. 1972*b*) have shown by post-mortem examination and clinical investigation that the incidence of twin ovulations is much higher. It is an impression held by many clinicians experienced in this field that the incidence of twin conception following mating in the presence of palpable twin follicles may not be higher than that following mating with only one palpable follicle. Ginther (1979) reports that twin ovulations are associated with a high rate of fertilization failure or pregnancy loss. There is obviously a need for further research into this subject.

Cysts sometimes develop in the ovarian ligament and may be palpated close to the ovaries. They should not be mistaken for follicles and, with care, can be distinguished as they are usually separate. Abnormal ovaries are discussed under Infertility and include the very small (less than 2 cm diameter) and the very large (greater than 15 cm). Failure to find one ovary at examination indicates a previous ovariectomy.

The uterus should be felt for size, tone and thickness of its walls. An estimate of uterine contents can be made on the presence of discreet or diffuse swellings. Pregnancy diagnosis is described on p. 206 and here we are concerned with the non-pregnant state.

The uterine horns may be felt between thumb and first finger or gently grasped with the whole hand. The body can be appreciated by palpation using the finger-tips. It may be helpful to press the horns and body against the pelvis or to allow air to enter the vagina by introducing a speculum so that the organ is pushed in front of the pubic brim. Greenhof and Kenney (1975) suggest that after determining that the mare is not pregnant, the uterus is grasped and palpated deeply for evidence of local thickenings, such as cysts or fibrotic areas. This is accomplished with the tip of one uterine horn lying on the palm side of the fingers of the hand and thumb on top. The entire uterus is then massaged or 'threaded' between the fingers and thumb. The diameter of each horn may be estimated by a system of calibration of the diameter of the lumen formed with the tip of the index finger and the thumb as described above.

During oestrus, when progesterone levels are minimal, the uterus is enlarged, has little or no tone and feels flaccid. In dioestrus during the luteal phase the uterine wall has tone and feels turgid.

The uterus returns to the non-pregnant size about four weeks after birth. Older mares and those that have had problems of chronic infertility may have a dilatation or ventral enlargement that can be palpated at the junction of uterine horn and body (see p. 97). Haemorrhages in the broad ligament may be felt as a hard or firm swelling varying from a few to 30 or 40 cm in diameter. The cervix may be palpated per rectum (Solomon 1971; Greenhof & Kenney 1975). This has been suggested as preferable to vaginoscopy, because air and possibly contaminant organisms are not introduced to the same extent. The cervix is palpated as a tense tight tube when in dioestrus or pregnancy. Gradual softening and broadening occur until the cervix is very diffuse, open and almost unpalpable. With experience, this method correlates well with vaginoscopy, but in our opinion cannot adequately replace a visual examination.

Voss et al. (1973) and Voss and Pickett (1975) conducted a trial with experimental mares palpated daily during oestrus. Palpations were performed by both an experienced and an inexperienced operator. Throughout the three years of the study, first cycle conception rates following insemination with undiluted semen were higher in non-palpated mares than in palpated mares. Although the figures presented are indisputable, the experimental design may have been such that the results bear little resemblance to the system as practised on most modern stud farms. Firstly, domesticated brood mares are so 'habituated' to rectal palpation that very little or no stress is involved with the handling and administration of this technique. Secondly, an experienced operator uses careful genital techniques deliberately to avoid damage to the rectum and genital organs. Kaufman (1975) surveyed 1373 mare-years at Claiborne Farm, Kentucky, during 1964, 1973, 1974 and 1975. The year 1964 differed from the other years in that routine ovarian palpation was not practised and artificial lighting programmes were not in operation. The results of this survey suggested that there was a beneficial effect on reducing the average number of oestrous periods per pregnancy and increasing the overall fertility percentage by using routine ovarian palpation and a lighting programme. Kaufman points out that rectal palpation is only one part, but a very necessary part, of a carefully formulated controlled breeding programme designed to increase reproductive efficiency.

It is our opinion that routine rectal palpation, if performed carefully, is essential to modern intensive stud farm management, using natural coitus. Without such a programme, one can diagnose a mare as being abnormal only after she has demonstrated this by a series of unsuccessful matings. By that time, valuable time has been lost in relation to the breeding season and in terms of response to treatments that might have been performed. Further damage, which might have been avoided, may have been caused to the genital organs.

Vaginal examination

A speculum is used to illuminate the vagina and cervix. There are several types in common use but those most favoured are tubular and of comparatively small size (about 6 cm), made of plastic which will withstand boiling in distilled water. For vaginal and other gynaecological techniques see Chapter 8.

The normal state of the cervix and vaginal mucous membranes changes during the oestrous cycle (Lieux 1970) and in pregnancy. In oestrus the appearance is red or pink, the cervix is relaxed and its lining oedematous. The mucus secretions are fluid and have a high chloride content, which reaches its peak just before ovulation.

Shortly after ovulation the cervix begins to constrict, is paler and the mucous secretion thinner.

In dioestrus the cervix is closed and pale and the mucous membrane dry. The cervix projects into the vagina as a clearly delineated structure. The mucosal secretions are sticky and may cause the vaginal walls to adhere to one another.

In pregnancy the cervix is usually closed and its surface white or pinkish in colour and covered by sticky mucus which may form a plug. The contours of the cervix become obliterated and in late pregnancy the mucosa of the vaginal wall is covered by a thick sticky exudate which prevents the usual ballooning effect caused by introducing a speculum.

During the vaginal examination abnormalities such as cervicitis, pneumovagina, vaginitis, depression of the vaginal floor and pooling of urine and other secretions should be noted. These conditions are discussed below (see Infertility, p. 99).

The results of a vaginal examination should be recorded in some standard form. The one recorded here categorizes the state of the cervix and is presented for guidance. For convenience of recording, abbreviations should be used. A system we find useful is suggested here: C refers to cervix, R = relaxed, and T = tight. The minus signs refer to degrees of relaxation.

1. *Oestrus:* the cervix is pink, oedematous and relaxed. The folds of the cervix appear wet, oedematous and drooping onto the vaginal floor. In some cases the endometrial surface may be visible through the cervical os: CR– pink.

2. *Early oestrus or early dioestrus:* the cervix is moist and reddened but has tone so that it projects, finger-like, into the vagina: CR– – pink.

3. *Dioestrus:* the cervix is pale, moist and with definite tone that causes it to project into the vagina: CT pale.

The pregnant cervix is often characterized by its intense whiteness and tightness and the entrance to the cervical os is often obscured by a sticky glazed mucus covering. In contrast, the anoestrous cervix is often quite relaxed although pale and dry. It must be emphasized that the condition of the cervix, while reflecting hormonal levels and sexual behaviour, may vary considerably between individuals. For instance, it is common in the early stages of oestrus for the cervix to be red and fairly relaxed, yet the cervical and vaginal mucus is sticky. In other cases the cervix may be relaxed and moist, yet pale. The sexual state should be interpreted with the results of uterine and ovarian palpation and, where necessary, with measurement of blood plasma progesterone levels.

Vulva and perineal region

This area should be inspected and note made of conformation, length of vulva, vesicles or ulcers due to herpesvirus or other infections, previous Caslick operation, length and slackness of the vulval labiae, catarrhal or mucopurulent exudates issuing from the vagina. These exudates dry and adhere to the tail, perineal region, thighs and vulval lips, especially round the lower commissure. (See Infertility, p. 102.)

Pascoe (1978) has described the use of a 'vulvometer' for the objective estimation of vulval length and degree of inclination (see p. 11).

Bacteriology of the genital tract

Techniques for collection of material for bacteriological culture from the cervix and uterus are described on p. 531. When collecting material via a vaginal speculum, the mare should be in oestrus, with a relaxed cervix, otherwise the results may bear little relation to the bacteriological flora of the uterus. If a gloved hand technique is used, guarding the swab, with manual dilatation of the cervix there would appear to be no reason why such swabs should not be valid when taken in dioestrus.

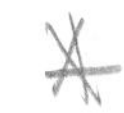

Bacteriological examinations of the mare's genital tract are taken, on a routine basis, for the following reasons:

1. To protect the stallion from infection with known venereal-disease-producing organisms, e.g. *Haemophilus equigenitalis, Klebsiella aerogenes* and *Pseudomonas aeruginosa.* Swabs are taken from the mare's cervix or uterus, urethral opening and clitoral area and cultured under aerobic and micro-aerophilic conditions. If these organisms are grown from any site, whether the mare is in oestrus or not, the mare may not be fit for natural cover. For further discussion of these organisms see p. 75.

2. To give the mare the best possible chance for conception and successful gestation by avoiding mating when genital infection and/or inflammation is present. Mating a mare when an acute endometritis is present is usually a waste of time. There is a lower chance of successful conception and, if this does occur, there is a higher incidence of gestational failure. In addition, there is a good possibility that endometrial inflammation may be made worse by natural cover and it has been postulated that exposing a damaged endometrium to sperm antigen may result in local immunological reactions which may cause infertility in other species (Katsh & Katsh 1968; Hartigan 1970). It would seem logical that a similar mechanism might apply in the mare. There is no doubt that endometritis is a major cause of infertility in mares (Peterson et al. 1969; Rooney 1970) and characterized by leucocytic infiltration; it appears to provide a hostile environment to sperm and fertilized ova (Roark & Herman 1950; Vickery & Bennett 1968). Leucocytes have been observed to ingest live spermatozoa (Mattner 1969). Cervicouterine bacteriological swabs have traditionally been used as an indirect indicator of the presence of acute endometritis. Unfortunately, the value of this assumption is highly questionable. Ricketts (1978) showed that of 114 mares with histopathological signs of acute endometritis, 44 mares (39%) showed significant cervicouterine bacteriological findings, whereas 70 mares (61%) did not. It would thus appear that the test is less than 50% accurate. A much better test for the presence of an acute endometritis is cervical cytology (Wingfield-Digby 1978) (see p. 537). When used in conjunction with cervicouterine bacteriological examinations, this test has the added advantage that it simplifies the interpretation of some aerobic bacterial growths (see p. 70).

There is no doubt that the veterinary surgeon's responsibility in the management of the mare's sexual function primarily involves preventive medicine (see Chapter 8) and the maintenance of acceptable reproductive efficiency and productivity in an industry that is highly intensive and 'unphysiological'. Many of the problems encountered could be overcome if intensification was reduced and the imposed breeding season was changed to coincide with the natural one.

INFERTILITY/SUBFERTILITY IN THE MARE

It has long been recognized that horses bred under intensive systems of management suffer from disappointingly low fertility. Andrews and McKenzie (1941) stated that low fertility was a more serious problem in mares than in any other class of livestock. Surveys of fertility from all over the world suggest that the percentage of mares producing live foals lies within the limits of 50–80% (Anderson 1922; Day 1939; Dimock 1939; Bain 1948; Mahaffey 1950*a*, *b*; Butterfield et al. 1964; Ensminger 1966; Bergin & Shipley 1968; Hutton & Meacham 1968; Rossdale 1968; Dewes 1973; Laing & Leech 1975; von Lepel 1975; Osborne 1975; Sullivan et al. 1975). Discrepancies between figures reflect varying populations of horses, systems of management and statistical methods. Jeffcott (1979), in a preliminary report of the British Equine Veterinary Association survey of wastage in Thoroughbred racing, suggests that over 20% of the overall 80% of losses from covering to training is due to failure to produce live progeny. This appears to be closely related to the mare's age (Fig. 1.27). For the years 1973 to 1977, fertility fell more or less linearly from about 75% at four years of age to less than 50% by 20 years of age. There is no doubt that the overall low fertility figures are an important source of economic loss, frustration and disappointment to the horse breeding industry.

Fertility is considered at two levels: firstly on a population basis, i.e. mares in a geographical area, on a given stud farm or visiting a given stallion, and secondly in relation to a given mare. Managemental inadequancies in relation to artificially imposed breeding seasons and human interference play a major role in the depression of population fertility figures. Day (1939) found the following fertility rates in England: heavy horses 59%, light horses 52%, Thoroughbreds at stud 68%, ponies running wild 95%. Under certain circumstances, however, the fertility rate

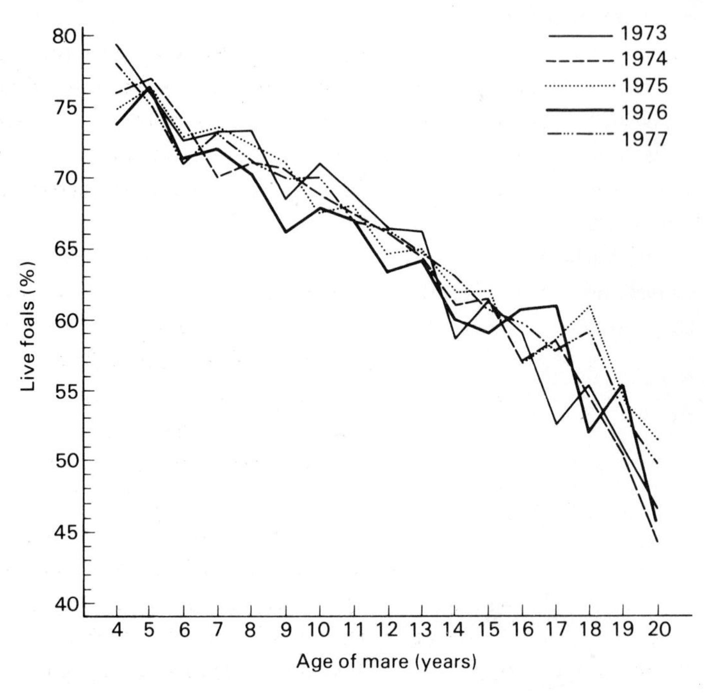

Fig. 1.27. Fertility of mares according to age. (*By permission of L.B. Jeffcott and the BEVA*)

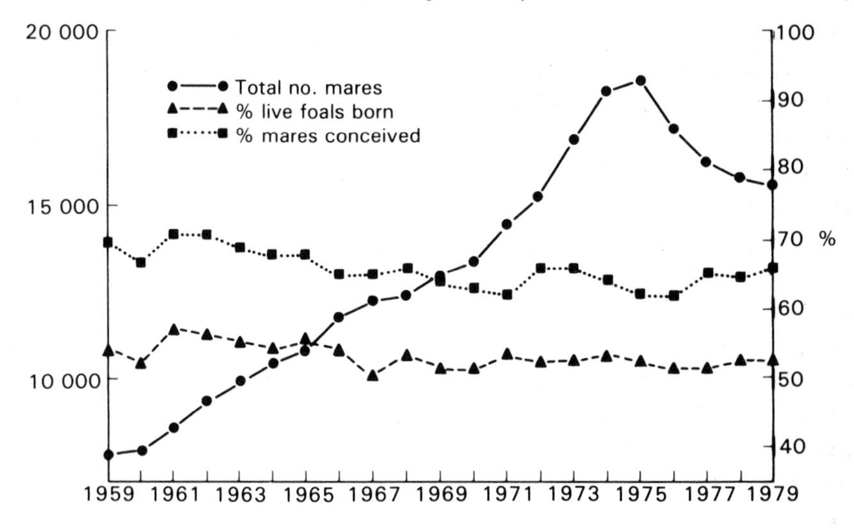

Fig. 1.28. An analysis of the Thoroughbred stud book returns from 1959 to 1979.

of a particular group of mares may be excellent. During the 1979 covering season we were supervising a young Thoroughbred stallion with a gynaecologically healthy 'book of mares'. Of 47 mares covered by this stallion, all were in foal. Problems are not always those of conception failure, however, and in the case of this particular stallion, at the time of writing, three of the mares are already known to have suffered a gestational failure.

The probability of conception from any given service is not a useful parameter because of the large number of variables involved, such as the time of coitus in relation to ovulation, the month in which mating takes place and the quality of semen deposited in the uterus. Bowen (1979) calculated from a controlled artificial insemination programme that the probability of conception at one insemination is 30–40%. This appears to be less than that expected of other species.

The probability of an individual conceiving in the four or five months of an arbitrarily defined breeding season also depends on many variables. Managerial and climatic factors often determine the chance of conception; mares who end the season barren are not necessarily suffering from pathological infertility.

Barrenness in successive seasons or a subnormal breeding record are more reliable indicators of pathological infertility. It is instructive to examine a mare's breeding record. Patterns develop, breeding performance usually deteriorating with age, as illustrated by the performance of Epsom Oaks winners at stud (Fig. 1.29). Many mares successfully carry foals in successive years and then become relatively infertile, while others may have periods early in life in which they fail to conceive but subsequently breed normally. These patterns are illustrated in the records of certain mares at Derisley Wood Stud, Newmarket, in 1972 (Table 1.3). Some authorities favour the definition of 'infertility' as failure to conceive in three consecutive breeding seasons.

The search for an objective definition of infertility is complicated further by fetal death after a pregnancy is established. It is customary to describe fetal death as an abortion and it is an arbitrary decision whether loss of the conceptus before age 19 days (or before a visual or known abortion) is classified as barrenness or abortion. A conceptus in the uterus may cause prolonged dioestrus for weeks or months after its death and some individuals suffer from early fetal death in successive breeding seasons.

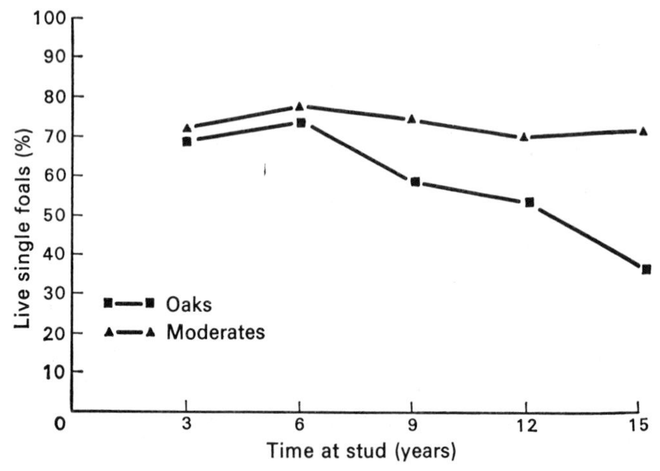

Fig. 1.29. The breeding performance of 26 Epsom Oaks winners at stud, judged by a single live foal produced annually. Results from the stud book mares which won the race in the period 1917 to 1949 grouped in three-year means are compared with 52 mares which had never won a race and which were selected at random from the General Stud Book over the same period. Oaks winners not registered in the General Stud Book were not included.

It is important to define some terms frequently used. A *fertile* mare is one that is capable of conceiving and producing a healthy newborn foal, following cover by a healthy fertile stallion. A *sterile* mare is one that is not capable of conceiving and producing a healthy newborn foal, following cover by a healthy fertile stallion. An *infertile* mare is, by correct definition, a sterile mare. A *barren* mare is a commonly used term and means that a mare is not pregnant at the end of the breeding season. This may be due to intrinisic factors, i.e. abnormalities or pathological conditions involving the mare's genital organs, or extrinsic factors, i.e. stallion or managemental factors, or a combination of these. Many barren mares may become pregnant the following season and subsequently produce a healthy newborn foal. Infertility in these cases is not absolute and may be more correctly referred to as *subfertility*.

Aetiology

The clinician must steer a reasonable path through the maze of inter-related factors which contribute to the problem (Fig. 1.30). A mare may be barren at the end of the imposed, unphysiological breeding season for:

1. Extrinsic, i.e. managerial, factors.
2. Intrinsic, i.e. pathological, factors.

TABLE 1.3 Breeding record (1960–71) of 6 mares resident at Derisley Wood Stud, Newmarket, in 1972

Name of mare	*Year of birth*	*1960*	*1961*	*1962*	*1963*	*1964*	*1965*	*1966*	*1967*	*1968*	*1969*	*1970*	*1971*	*Percentage live foals*	*Comments*
Greensward	1956	f	f	f	b	f*	f	b	s	st	b	b	b	41	Relatively fertile in first half of stud life then barren or failed to carry
Grey Sister	1957		b	s	b	s	b	f	f	f	f*	f	f	55	Unusual case. Infertile for first half of stud life and then bred consistently
Heavenly View	1957	b	b	f	f	s	f	f	f	b	b	f	f*	58	Infertile years alternating with fertile years
Holdfast	1951	f	f	f	f*	f	f	f	f	f	s	f	f	92	Consistent record of fertility
Mistafa	1955	f	f	f	f	f	b	b	b	f*	f	b	f	66	Good record for first 5 years, then 3 years barren followed by good record
Patience III	1952	f*	b	f	f	f	f	b	st	b	f	b	st	50	Good record for 6 years then infertile or failed to carry

b, barren; f, live single foal; s, aborted single fetus; st, aborted twin fetuses.
*Year in which mare first arrived at Derisley Wood Stud.
Reproduced by kind permission of Mr Irving Allen.

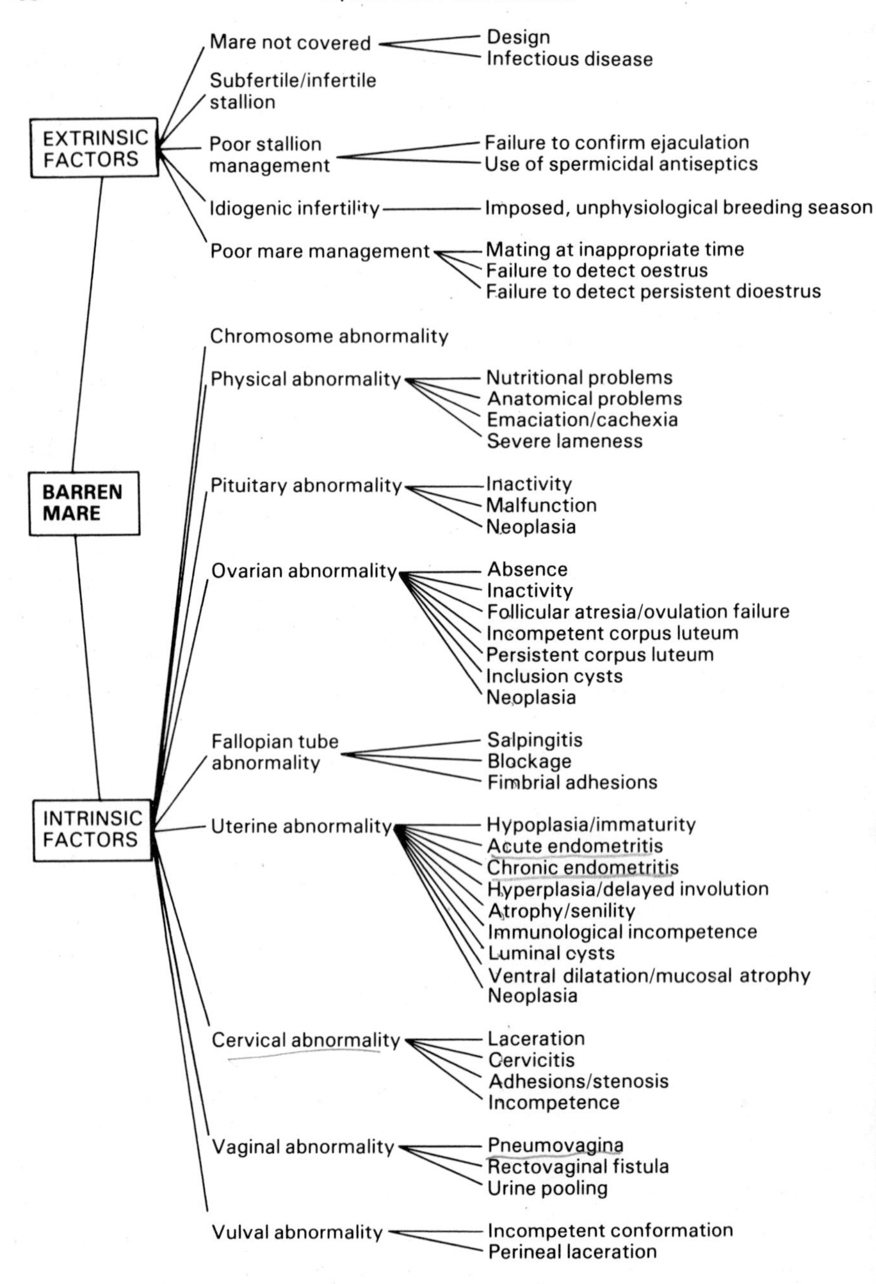

Fig. 1.30. Aetiological factors contributing to infertility.

Mare not covered

This may be by design or may be imposed. Foals born late in the breeding season are commercially at a disadvantage and thus when a mare foals towards the end of the season, she may be left barren so that an early start may be made the following season. Some owners, possibly for anthropomorphic reasons, will give a mare a 'rest' following a successful series of pregnancies. Paradoxically, these mares, for reasons not completely understood, often prove difficult to get in foal when mating is resumed, and thus unless there is a particular reason to do so, it is probably best to mate mares anually.

Infectious and contagious disease may present a situation where mating or movement of horses must stop on a particular stud farm and this may result in a particular mare not being covered. The conditions involved may be the venereal diseases, caused by *Haemophilus equigenitalis* (see p. 75), *Klebsiella aerogenes* (see p. 78) and *Pseudomonas aeruginosa* (see p. 80). Other contagious diseases that may be involved are equine coital exanthema (see p. 103), equid herpesvirus I abortion or neurological disease (see p. 425), equine influenza (see p. 424), salmonellosis (see p. 435) and strangles (see p. 430). It is fair to say that most of the managerial problems associated with these diseases are due to the failure of the industry to make use of artificial insemination (see p. 158), which, in such circumstances, could be used to abolish direct contact between mare and stallion and thus to control spread of disease.

Subfertile/infertile stallion

See Chapter 2.

Poor stallion management

This particulary concerns failure to confirm ejaculation and the over-zealous use of spermicidal anticeptics prior to cover. For more details see Chapter 2.

Idiogenic infertility

This concerns the statistical chances of successful conception from one mating of a normal fertile stallion and a normal fertile mare, where ejaculation of good quality semen occurs and the ovulation of a fertile ovum occurs soon afterwards. This percentage has not been accurately assessed for the horse, owing to the many uncontrolled and complicating factors involved with natural cover. Bowen (1979) has estimated that with a carefully controlled artificial insemination system the conception ratio at one insemination may be as low as 30–40%. This appears to be considerably lower than that expected of some other species and means that to obtain 100% conception in a group of 40–50 mares visiting one stallion, one would expect, by statistical chance factors alone, to have to mate several mares on two or three consecutive oestrous periods. It is the measurement of these figures in cattle that has resulted in the practical definition of a 'repeat-breeder cow', i.e. one that is still not pregnant after three consecutive potentially fertile matings. It may be that if idiogenic fertility ratios in mares are as low as suggested, one might have to accept more than three consecutive oestrous periods. Practical experience, in fact, suggests that the majority of normal fertile mares do conceive within three oestrous periods.

Poor mare management

In this context, the factors particularly involved are mating at an inappropriate stage of the oestrous cycle (see p. 48), failure to detect oestrus following unsuccessful mating and failure to detect a state of persistent dioestrus following unsuccessful mating. Failure to detect oestrus may involve inadequate teasing (see p. 42) and both latter factors may involve a failure of management to take advantage of veterinary services. There is no doubt that a significant proportion of the wastage in horse breeding is associated with poor management. Where management is good and veterinary services are used sensibly, wastage may be much reduced, especially when 'problem' mares are being dealt with.

Chromosome abnormality

Chandley et al. (1975) detected chromosomal abnormalities in seven mares who had a history of poor reproductive performance. All had small or rudimentary gonads and absent or irregular oestrous cycles. Two mares had an XO genotype (Turner's syndrome), one was a 65,XXX female and another a 64,XY sex-reversed female. Two other mares were sex chromsome mosaics of the 63,X/64,XX type. The seventh mare showed a normal female karyotype but a small extra autosomal fragment was found in a few cells. Trommershausen-Smith et al. (1979) reported similar findings and in addition 63,X/64,XY, the normal male complement (64,XY) and autosomal deletion (64,XX? del 2Q–). These authors found that the 63,XO genotype (Turner's syndrome) was the most common abnormality found and that cases with XY or autosomal deletion may be inherited defects or of spontaneous origin.

Diagnosis of this condition rests with a history of persistant anoestrus or irregular oestrous cycles. In some cases, the diagnosis is suspected where the ovaries are extremely small (less than 0.5 cm in diameter) or unpalpable. Endometrial biopsy is of great value in these cases, as the endometrium is extremely hypoplastic (Ricketts 1975*a, b*, 1978) (see p. 91). Definitive diagnosis is performed by specialized laboratories using leucocyte culture techniques from peripheral blood.

The intersex state is rare in the horse. In a series of 17 cases reported by Bornstein (1967) all had a penis-like clitoris and a pair of hypoplastic testes. Cases showed male libido although some showed oestrus every three weeks. Bouters et al. (1972) described male behaviour in an intersex horse with 64,XX/65,XXY mosaicism. Gerneke and Coubrough (1970) reported the case of an Arabian filly which was a genetic female with male gonads.

In two cases of chromosome abnormality we were able to remove the 'ovaries' and found that they consisted mostly of connective or adrenal tissue (unpublished data).

Physical abnormality

Mares that are severely lame with limb problems such as fracture of the pelvis may not be fit for natural cover. This may not be due solely to physical problems, since severe pain may result in oestrous cycle irregularities.

Oestrous cycle irregularities may be seen in mares that are thin and debilitated due to nutritional inadequacies or infectious or metabolic debilitating disease (Roberts 1971). To avoid this problem Roberts suggests that balanced nutritious rations should be fed in proper amounts. Exercise, sunlight and green pasture are helpful. Disease conditions should be corrected or alleviated. Van Niekerk (1964) reported a high incidence of early embryonic deaths from 25 to 31 days of gestation in mares that were malnourished.

Conversely, obesity may be a cause of oestrous cycle irregularities and possibly early fetal death. Clinicians recognize this in the occasional mare who becomes obese despite restricted rations. We are of the impression that there is a higher incidence of oestrous cycle irregularities and early fetal death in the Suffolk horse than in lighter horses. The Suffolk horse is renowned for its ability to 'do well' on a meagre diet. The problem is compounded by the fact that most Suffolk brood mares are kept in 'show condition' which can only be described objectively as obese. A traditional method of correcting this problem was by working the mare hard on the land. This is seldom practised today. It is considered beneficial to keep barren and maiden mares on a relatively low plane of nutrition, over the winter period, so that this may be increased as daylight length increases in the early spring. This may have beneficial effect on ovarian activity, in a similar manner to the 'flushing' of other species.

Pituitary abnormality

The way that the pituitary gland responds to external stimuli, via gonadotrophin-releasing hormone, to initiate cyclic ovarian inactivity by the production of the gonadotrophic hormones FSH and LH, has been described above (see pp. 13–15). Specific pituitary abnormality, e.g. neoplasia, is rare in the horse but apparent inactivity or malfunction may occur, usually as a temporary phenomenon, in the early breeding season. Owing to the enormous range of individual variation of oestrous cycle behaviour between and within mares it is very difficult to define where normal variation ends and abnormality starts. This is compounded by the fact that we expect mares to cycle normally in advance of their natural breeding season (see p. 31). Mares at the beginning and end of the natural breeding season may show a wide variety of 'abnormal' behaviour. Some may show persistent anoestrus. Others may show prolonged oestrus, frequently without palpable, on-going ovarian follicular activity. Other mares may have a very long oestrous phase in the presence of a large palpable ovarian follicle which appears slow to mature. In the absence of more specific data one must assume that this is part of normal variation and is associated with transitional phases into and out of the natural breeding season.

Foals born early in the year are at a commercial advantage and thus veterinary surgeons are asked to do all they can to promote early pituitary activity and normal oestrous cycle behaviour usually with oral or injectable hormone treatments (see pp. 33–35). Artificial environment control, with light, heat and nutritional programmes, may be the best approach (see p. 32).

Pituitary adenomas have been reported in the horse (Gribble 1972; Bostock & Owen 1975), most commonly in the pars intermedia and only rarely in the anterior hypophysis. Clinical signs include muscle wasting, polydipsia, polyuria, hyperglycaemia, glucosuria, hirsutism and docility. There is bilateral enlargement of the adrenal glands. A real or relative neutrophilia, lymphopenia and eosinopenia are frequently observed. Alopecia, hyperhidrosis, blindness and locomotor difficulties are occasionally present. Affected horses appear to be more susceptible to bacterial and fungal infections and wound healing may be delayed. Many of these clinical signs are associated with hyperadrenalism, i.e. Cushing's syndrome. Following dexamethasone injection, the plasma cortisol levels remain unchanged or are only slightly reduced. The diagnosis may be confirmed and distinguished from primary hyperadrenalism by finding elevated plasma levels of MSH or ACTH in addition to elevated plasma cortisol.

Ovarian abnormality

The ovaries may be absent in cases of chromosome abnormality (see p. 60). Ovarian inactivity or 'malfunction' during the early spring is an extension of the problem of seasonal transition discussed above under pituitary abnormality.

Follicular atresia with ovulation failure is not uncommonly encountered in mares (Van Rensburg & Van Heerden 1953; Arthur 1969; Roberts 1971; Kenney et al. 1979) (see p. 2). This process may occur at any stage of the breeding season and the reason why follicles become atretic is not understood. Kenney et al. (1979) found that a 3 cm diameter was a major turning point in follicular maturation since at that stage there was a three-fold increase in oestrogens and androgens. These authors concluded that follicular atresia in the mare appeared to be a gradual process, the initiating cause of which remained unknown. As a clinician, one has the impression that many apparent ovulations, as diagnosed by rectal palpation, may not be satisfactory and the measurement of plasma progestagen levels, following apparent ovulation, may be indicated in some cases.

Whether malfunction or incompetence of the formed corpus luteum does occur in the mare is unknown, but clinicians who believe in the exogenous supplementation of early pregnant mares with progesterone must believe that it does. There are a number of experienced veterinary surgeons in practice, and many more mare owners, who believe strongly, on the basis of past experience (which may be circumstantial), that progesterone supplementation may prevent early fetal loss. There appears to be no scientific evidence to support this (see p. 189). Ganjam et al. (1975) found that the dose of 250–500 mg of progesterone which is normally given every 10, 14 or 30 days during pregnancy, in an effort to supplement ovarian progesterone and so prevent abortion, is not capable, by itself, of providing sustained physiological progesterone levels. The subject of the function and integrity of the corpus luteum is one that obviously needs greater study.

Persistence of the corpus luteum longer than the normal 15 or so days, resulting in a state of prolonged dioestrus, has been discussed on pp. 27 and 35. Presumably this is caused by a failure of the endometrium to release natural prostaglandins at the usual time, but the reason why this should occur is not clear. Diagnosis of the condition rests on the mating and teasing history, the results of gynaecological examinations and peripheral progesterone levels. Once diagnosis has been made, and pregnancy has been ruled out, treatment with exogenous prostaglandin is usually highly successful.

Paraovarian cysts may occur quite frequently in the tissues surrounding the ovary (Arthur 1968) but are of no clinical significance. True follicular cysts, as commonly occur in other species such as the cow and the woman, are extremely rare in the mare. Follicular size is extremely variable in the mare and we have encountered cases with soft fluctuant ovarian structures up to 20 cm in diameter. These cases were showing behavioural signs of oestrus and endometrial biopsy studies showed a histological architecture indistinguishable from normal oestrus. Ovulation appeared to occur normally. Unless such cases are presented for post mortem examination, one cannot be sure whether these structures are large but normal follicles or cystic structures. In the occasional mare, large tense 'follicles' up to 10 cm in diameter appear to remain static for some considerable time, i.e. weeks. These cases are often seen during the early spring and may be part of normal variation during the transitional period into the breeding season. Prickett (1966) describes the condition of ovulation fossa cysts which are found in mares of all ages, but are more common in older mares. These cysts are located just beneath the epithelium of the ovulation fossa and grossly are of a variable size, never more than a few millimetres in diameter, and contain a clear serous fluid and have a tough white fibrous capsule. Clinically, these mares may show irregular oestrous cycles and rectal palpation reveals enlarged, relatively hard, 'bunch of grapes' ovaries. Even when cyclical behaviour is occurring, it is frequently impossible to palpate significant changes in follicular activity and thus prediction of the optimal time for covering is difficult. Prickett reports that these cysts are lined by a low cuboidal or flattened endothelial-type epithelium and are surrounded by connective tissue indistinguishable from the normal ovarian stroma. The cuboidal epithelial cells are usually ciliated, which suggests that the cysts originate from the epithelium of the fimbria. He postulates that pieces of fimbrial epithelium are entrapped in the corpora haemorrhagica and drawn back into the ovulation fossa as the corpora lutea form. These cysts thus fulfil the general requirements

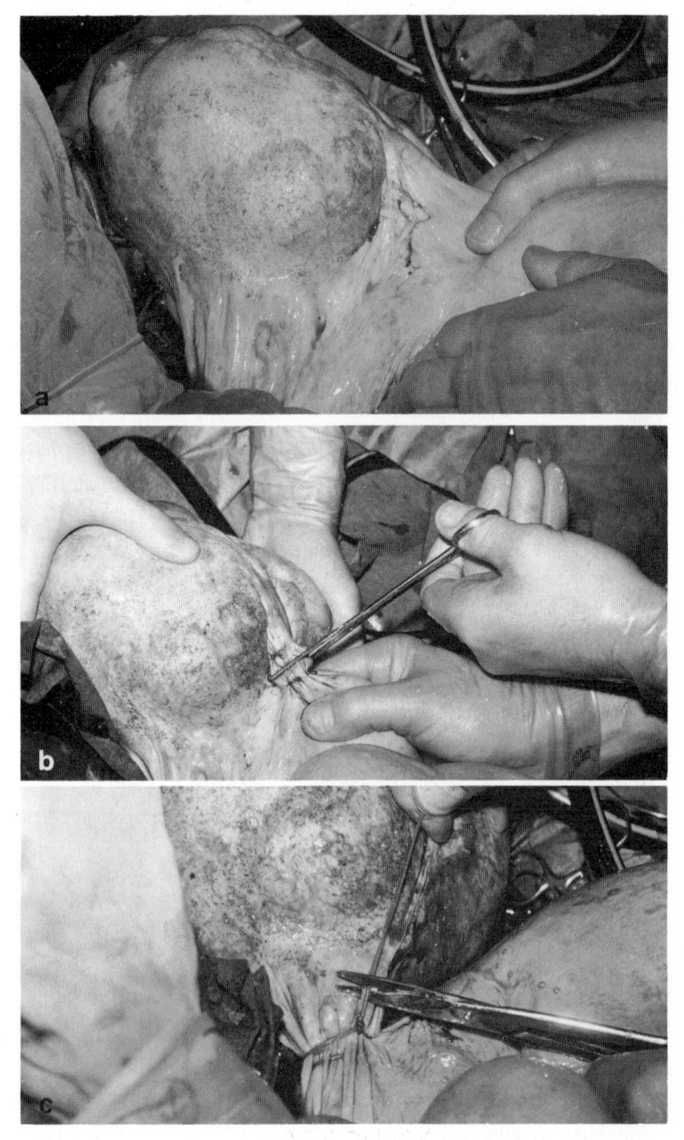

Fig. 1.31. (*a*) A granulosa cell tumour being brought through a midline incision. (*b*) Ligating the utero-ovarian artery and veins, which are then cut. (*c*) Ligating the ovarian ligament. (*facing page*) (*d*) The ovary is removed. (*e*) A section of the granulosa cell tumour showing many cysts containing blood-stained fluid and two cavities (top and bottom) with friable blood clots.

for germinal inclusion cysts. Prickett suggests that in some cases the cysts cause a mechanical obstruction of the ovulation fossa and may thus cause infertility in some older mares. In some species, wedge resection of the ovary is a surgical treatment. We have tried, in some mares who appear to fit the defined criteria, a rather empirical treatment of 9000 IU of chorionic gonadotrophin followed two days later by a further 9000 IU. Five to seven days later this is followed by 500 μg

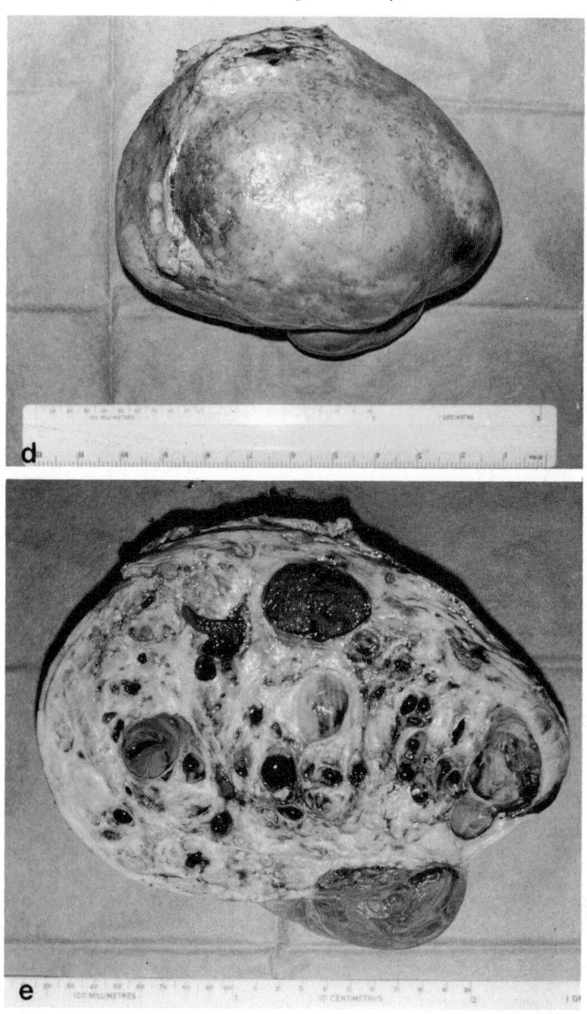

fluprostenol. In some cases, this treatment appears to have worked, in that ovarian size is reduced, normal cyclic behaviour resumes and ongoing ovarian follicular activity could be palpated.

Granulosa cell tumours (Fig. 1.31e) are the most common neoplastic lesion affecting the equine ovary (Norris et al. 1968; Bostock & Owen 1975; Stickle et al. 1975; Meagher et al. 1977). In the series of Norris et al. (1968) the affected ovaries weighed 1–8 kg. They were yellowish, multicystic and haemorrhagic. Microscopically they were characterized by prominent microcysts and tubules with cells at the periphery of the cysts in a double paired layer. The cells were elongated, had abundant lightly-stained cytoplasm and were similar to cells at the periphery of the developing follicle, as well as to Sertoli cells of the testes and testicular tumours in other species. A prominent supporting stroma of spindle cells was present. Cases may present with a variety of different behavioural features. Some may be diagnosed at routine examination following normal foaling. Some mares may appear nymphomaniac, others stallion-like and others anoestrous. The difference in presenting behaviour is presumably due to the fact that granulosa cell tumours are capable of producing or concentrating progesterone, oestrogen and/or testosterone (Stickle et al. 1975). These authors found that the concentration of these hormones in the tumour fluid was several times higher than the preoperative plasma concentration. Correspondingly, endometrial biopsy of affected cases may reveal endometrial histological architecture suggestive of oestrogen or progesterone domination. Diagnosis is based upon the palpation, per rectum, of an enlarged hard 'knobbly' ovary on one side with a small hard inactive ovary on the other.

Treatment is by surgical removal of the affected ovary under general anaesthesia, via laparotomy (Fig. 1.31). Depending on the position, size and mobility of the affected ovary per rectum, a midline or flank incision may be used. Careful ligation of the blood supply to the affected ovary is essential prior to removal and wound closure by standard methods. The technique of ovariectomy, by ecraseur, via the vaginal fornix, has been described with the mare standing (Scott & Kunge 1977). On grounds of basic principles and safety, most clinicians prefer a laparotomy technique under general anaesthesia. Once the affected ovary has been removed, the remaining ovary usually becomes functional, normal oestrous cycles resume and conception and normal pregnancy may follow. We have encountered one mare who has shown no signs of oestrus or activity in the remaining ovary, two years after granulosa cell tumour removal.

Ovarian teratomas, containing hair and sometimes teeth, occur rarely and were possibly seen more commonly in the heavy breeds of mares.

Ovarian adenocarcinoma is also rare and, in contrast to the granulosa cell tumour and terotoma, may be highly malignant. Affected cases may show abdominal pain and ascites with metastasis throughout the peritoneal cavity. In one such case, we were able to demonstrate exfoliate cells, suggestive of neoplasia, in a peritoneal fluid sample prior to exploratory laporotomy. Such cases are inoperable.

Fallopian tube abnormality

Fallopian tube abnormality in the mare, as judged by an English slaughter-house survey, was rare (Arthur 1958). Vandeplassche and Henry (1977) studied, in detail the genital organs of 700 Belgian mares of different breeds (Trotters, Cross-breds, saddle horses, draught horses and ponies) of ages varying from six to 20 years. They found a surprisingly high incidence of fallopian tube abnormality. More than 40% of the infundibula had adhesions to the uterus, mesovarium and/or ovary. The incidence of adhesions was markedly higher on the right than on the left side. Almost 100% of the ampullae were patent for fluid under pressure. Histologically, a marked diffuse or focal lymphocytic infiltration of the epithelium and lamina propria was seen, in some cases, and occasionally neutrophils and eosinophils were seen. Epithelial damage was marked in some cases. In addition to cellular infiltrations, an accumulation of fluid and leucocytes was sometimes found adhering to the epithelium or filling the lumen of the oviduct. Complete luminal block, or string-like occlusion of the isthmus or ampullae, was rare. This led the authors to conclude that salpingitis in the mare is a non-occlusive infiltrative or less often exudative infundibulitis, isthmitis and ampullitis. The incidence of these conditions in this series was infundibulitis 37%, ampullitis 20.8% and isthmitis 8.7%. Not one case of hydrosalpinx was seen. The incidence of endometritis was 31% and, as a rule, this degree of inflammation was more severe than in the oviduct. The authors conclude that endometritis could be an important cause of salpingitis. Whereas the overall incidence of endometritis was 31%, it was 80% in those associated with isthmitis. There may be some relationship between infundibular adhesions and ampullitis and isthmitis because all three conditions are more commonly seen on the right than on the left side. Why this is so is not clear. It has always been thought that the strong valvular occlusion at the uterotubal junction prevents extension of material and infection from the uterine lumen to the fallopian tube. This may explain why ampullitis is much more common than isthmitis but this would suggest that the source of inflammation originates from the peritoneum. Kenney (1977) suggests that follicular fluid and blood released at ovulation may contribute to the formation of infundibular adhesions. Blood clots may become organized into adhesions which could then become secondarily infected by haematogenously derived organisms. He postulates that follicular fluid could induce a hypersensitivity reaction in the infundibulum, or that the migrating larval form of *Strongylus edentatus,* which migrates over serosal surfaces, may be a cause of infundibulitis. Vandeplassche and Henry found that whereas 50% of ovulations occur in the left ovary, infundibular adhesions and salpingitis are more common on the right ovary. Vandeplassche and Henry (1977) and Kenny (1977) conclude that, contrary to previous belief, non-occlusive salpingitis really does occur in mares but its role in infertility or subfertility has yet to be defined. Kenney concludes that clinicians need an in vivo diagnostic method for the presence or absence of salpingitis in individual mares.

Allen et al. (1979) examined two procedures for the evaluation of fallopian tube function in mares. The phenol-sulphonphthalein (PSP) test was not reliable. The starch grain test was, however, successful; 1 g of sterile soluble starch powder is thoroughly mixed in 10 ml of sterile water. The mare is restrained in the standing position and an area of about 100 cm^2, in the middle of the sublumbar fossa, is clipped and prepared for surgical interference. The ovary on the side of the fallopian tube under investigation is held per rectum and pushed towards the sub-lumbar fossa so that the optimum site for injection may be determined. Local anaesthetic is injected subcutaneously and deep into the muscle of the flank after which the skin is punctured with a 5 cm 14 gauge hypodermic needle. This is then withdrawn and a sterile 18 gauge 12 cm needle is carefully inserted through the puncture hole in the skin and the muscle of the flank to penetrate the peritoneum. The ovary is manually positioned adjacent to the needle tip and 5 ml of starch solution are quickly injected onto its surface. The needle is completely evacuated by injecting 5 ml of air. Care is taken not to penetrate the ovary with the end of the needle. Washings are collected from the anterior vagina and cervix from 24 hours after the injection of the starch. This is performed after cleansing of the perineal area via a sterile self-iluminating speculum (see Chapter 8). 10 ml of sterile saline are flushed over the cervix and anterior vagina from a 20 ml disposable syringe attached to a 60 cm long (5 mm internal diameter) sterile glass tube. As much as possible of the saline is aspirated back into the syringe. Approximately 1 ml of the washings is placed on a clean dry microscope slide and a few drops of 2% Lugol's iodine are added and mixed in by rocking the slide. A coverslip is placed over the solution and the slide is examined microscopically (X 10) for the presence of dark blue granules. Starch grains are recovered from the cervical area 24 hours after injection over a non-ovulating ovary. In ovulating ovaries, however, starch grains are not recovered for at least four days, and are not recovered in all mares until the seventh day. Allen et al. (1979) suggest that this delay may be involved in the tube's ability to retain non-fertilized ova or may be a mechanism ensuring that the zygote does not reach the uterus until it is mature enough. This test may be very useful in proving that the fallopian tubes are patent.

Uterine abnormality

The continual cycle of natural cover, infection, pregnancy and involution in the mare results in repeated damage and progressive deterioration in the integrity of the uterus (Kenney et al. 1975; Ricketts 1978). A much better understanding of uterine abnormality in the mare has followed the use of endometrial biopsy as a diagnostic aid over recent years (Kenney 1978; Ricketts 1978) (see p. 541).

Acute endometritis

Acute endometritis is characterized by a significant polymorphonuclear cell infiltration (Fig. 1.32). Significance must be judged by the knowledge of the normal cellular infiltrations expected during different stages of the oestrous cycle (see p. 19).

Polymorphonuclear leucocytes are seen migrating between cells of the luminal epithelium and sometimes they are retained in an amorphous layer over the surface of the epithelium. Severe cases may constitute pyometra. Luminal epithelial cells show varying degrees of degenerative change from virtually none to marked degeneration of the apical cytoplasm and ulceration in some cases. Marked degenerative change with vacuolation is seen in cases of *Haemophilus equigenitalis* infection (see p. 77) (Ricketts et al. 1978; Ricketts & Rossdale 1979). In cases where acute endometritis has been long-standing, the luminal epithelium may be pseudostratified to an extent considered to be greater than normally seen during oestrus. Occasionally, in sections stained with Gram twort, bacteria may be associated with the luminal epithelial cells, often phagocytosed by polymorphonuclear leucocytes. Congested superficial blood vessels and a polymorphonuclear cell infiltration may be seen in the stratum compactum, but the density of the infiltration and the stromal depths to which it extends is very variable. In the majority of cases, the infiltration is extremely superficial and is confined to the stratum compactum and luminal epithelium only. In some cases, examination of the deeper stromal blood vessels reveals congestion and margination with polymorphonuclear leucocytes, which are sometimes seen to have just left a deep

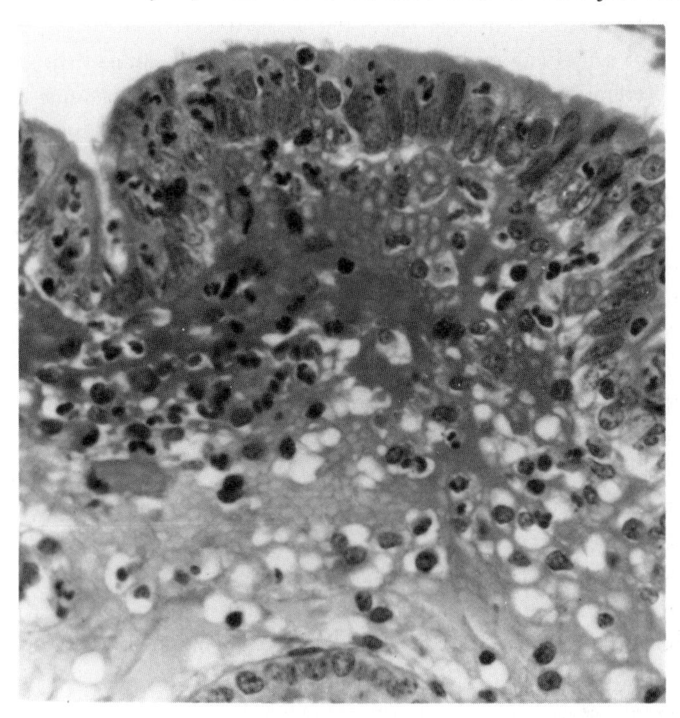

Fig. 1.32. Endometrial biopsy of acute endometritis. Polymorphonuclear leucocytes may be seen in the stratum compactum and migrating through the luminal epithelium. H & E × 450.

stromal blood vessel, into the surrounding tissue, on their way to the superficial areas.

Acute endometritis is a major cause of infertility in mares (Peterson et al. 1969; Rooney 1970) and appears to provide a hostile environment to sperm and fertilized ova (Roark & Herman 1950; Vickery & Bennett 1968). Leucocytes have been observed to ingest live spermatozoa (Mattner 1969).

Acute endometritis is usually associated with, or the result of, uterine infection. Active demonstrable infection, as judged by cervicouterine bacteriological swab results, may not always be present, however. Ricketts (1978) found that of 114 mares showing histopathological signs of acute endometritis, only 44 (39%) had significant bacteriological findings. Thus bacteriological examinations are not sufficiently accurate as an indirect indicator of the presence of an acute endometritis and clinicians must use the additional techniques of cervical cytology and/or endometrial biopsy.

The stallion's penis is normally covered with a varied bacterial flora (see p. 157). The horse is unusual in that natural cover involves ejaculation of semen contaminated with this microflora through the cervix directly into the uterus (Kenney et al. 1975). This normally results in an acute endometritis at natural cover (Hughes & Loy 1969; Peterson et al. 1969). This normal acute endometritis is usually resolved by the mare's natural defence mechanisms by 72 hours after mating, so that the endometrium is back to normal condition when the fertilized ovum arrives. The persistence of acute endometritis signifies either that the endometritis is associated with a bacterium which is capable of primarily infecting the endometrium and is difficult to clear or that there has been a breach of the mare's natural endometrial defence mechanisms. Successful treatment and management of mares with persistent acute endometritis depends on a good fundamental understanding of these basic principles.

A large variety of bacterial organisms may be cultured from cervicouterine swabs. They may be broadly classified into three types:

1. Contaminant organisms.
2. Potential acute endometritis producers.
3. Primary acute endometritis producers.

Contaminant organisms are usually grown as a result of a technical problem, especially when unguarded swabs or faulty technique are used. They include *Streptococccus faecalis, Staphylococcus albus,* coliforms, diphtheroids, *Alcaligenes faecalis* and others. These organisms are rarely, if ever, incriminated as a cause of acute endometritis, as judged by cervical cytology and endometrial biopsy.

Potential acute endometritis producers are naturally found in the mare's environment and in the microflora of the mare's perineum and stallion's penis. These include *Streptococcus zoeepidemicus* (β-haemolytic streptococcus), haemolytic *E. coli, Klebsiella aerogenes* capsule type 7, *Staphylococcus aureus* (coagulase-positive) and some *Proteus* species. These organisms may cause, or be associated with, a demonstrable acute endometritis where the natural defence mechanisms of the mare have been breached.

Incompetence of the vulva (see p. 11) is an important factor resulting in pneumovagina, vaginitis, cervicitis and endometritis, with these environmental organisms. This condition responds well to adequate vulval suturing following early diagnosis (Caslick 1937) (see p. 99).

Cervical incompetence may follow traumatic parturition and this is another very significant breach of the mare's natural defence mechanisms. This condition is far more difficult, if not in many cases impossible, to correct adequately (see p. 99).

In the absence of these obvious specific problems, it appears that more basic, as yet undefined, local immunological defects may occur. Kenney and Khaleel (1975) obtained uterine flushings and biopsy samples for analysis by immunodiffusion and indirect immunofluorescence. The globulins IgA, IgGa, IgGb and IgGc were detected in the uterine flushings but IgT, IgG(B) and IgM were absent. IgA was detected in the biopsy samples in randomly distributed cells in a lamina propria and particularly in the stratum compactum, in the lumina of some glands, in the cytoplasm of some glandular epithelial cells and on the distal surface of luminal epithelial cells. These authors concluded that the mare can produce IgA and possibly also IgGa, IgGb and IgGc. Unfortunately, there is as yet no published investigation of findings in mares who appear to be 'susceptible' to endometrial infection. We hope that this work will be done in the near future.

Valuable results might also be obtained by studies on equine leucocyte antigens (ELA) (Bright et al. 1977). These authors suggest that an established leucocyte antigen system might be used as a marker for those animals likely to be susceptible to various diseases, as is the case with a variety of human diseases. Diseases of an infective nature can show HLA association, but this is never absolute and is probably observed because of closely linked immune response genes. The association between antigens and disease may be more pronounced in the horse because of its high degree of in-breeding. If such an association could be demonstrated, the ELA system might be a useful guide to the use of prophylactic breeding measures in horses.

The treatment of acute endometritis caused by or associated with one of the potential acute endometritis-producing bacteria is based on a course of local treatment by intrauterine infusion with antibiotic or antiseptic drugs to which the organism is sensitive. It is based on the use of in vitro antibiotic sensitivity tests. The drugs used should be water-soluble, since those produced in oily bases, and particularly those produced in chalky pessaries, may cause acute endometritis in their own right. A particularly convenient and useful drug, containing antibiotics to which most of the isolated bacteria are sensitive, is a water-soluble intramammary preparation containing 250 mg neomycin sulphate, 125 mg nitrofurazone and 10 000 units polymixin B sulphate (Vagifurin). For each infusion, we dissolve four to six 'tubes' in 100 ml of sterile water.

Infusions may be made, after hygenic preparation of the perineum and vulva, via a Neilson catheter inserted per vaginam with a gloved hand. The catheter is inserted through the cervix into the uterus along the index finger. Infusion may be made through the catheter via a 'flutter valve'. A very convenient method of treating the mare's uterus is via an indwelling uterine infuser (Fig. 1.33) (Kortum 1979). Infusers are sterile and disposable and will remain in place provided they are used during dioestrus. The plastic 'ram's horn' device, which is used to maintain the position of the infuser anterior to the cervix, is first straightened into the outer tube. This is then introduced through the cervix with a gloved arm, per vaginam, along the index finger. The middle tube is then pushed forwards to extrude the ram's horn device, attached to the inner catheter, into the body of the uterus. The outer and middle tubes are then carefully removed leaving the inner catheter in place. We have found it convenient to suture the catheter to the side of the vulva to maintain its position (Fig. 1.33). Two blebs of local anaesthetic are placed at the junction of the vulva and the buttock, approximately 5 cm apart. Nylon sutures are first placed loosely on the skin and the catheter is then tied on top of this so that

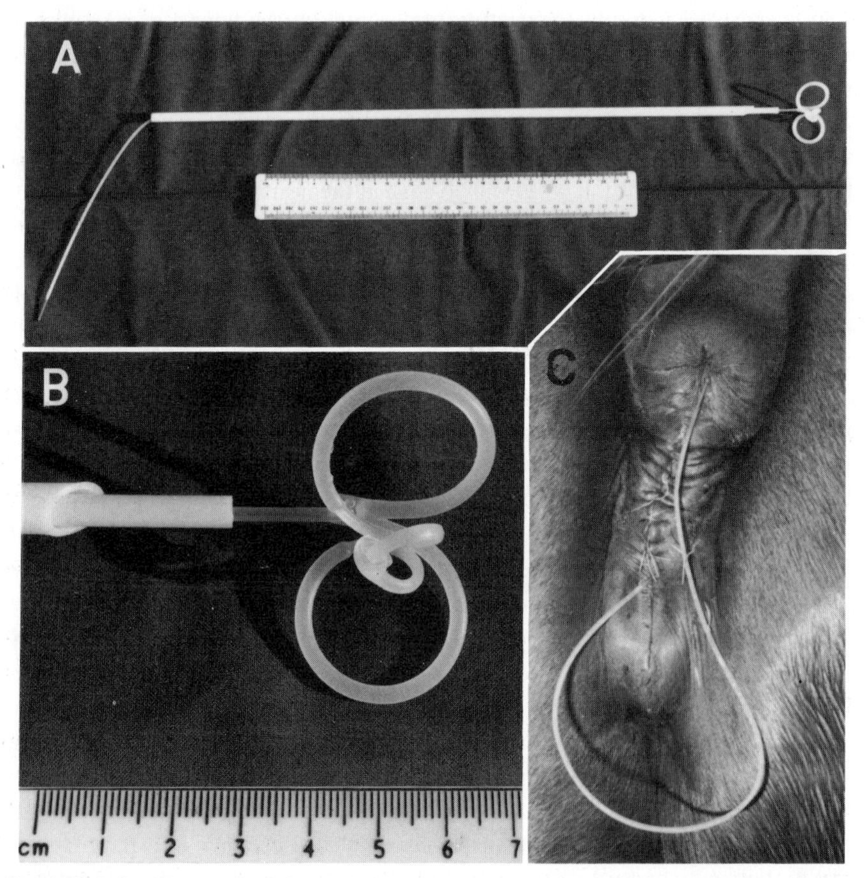

Fig. 1.33. Indwelling uterine infuser. A, Complete apparatus removed from its sterile packaging. The infuser is pulled back inside the outer tube before insertion. B, The infuser with the attached catheter extended from the tip of the inner and outer placement tubes. C, Cather in place and 'stay' sutured to perineum.

it does not pull tight to the skin. Infusions may be made regularly, through the catheter, using a 60 or 100 ml syringe with a 16 gauge needle attached. The 16 gauge needle fits snuggly into the indwelling catheter. The plastic plug should be replaced after infusion and treatment may be daily for seven to ten days. The catheter is then removed, by removing the sutures and gently pulling the tube. Kortum suggests that there may be some beneficial 'foreign body' reaction in the uterus when the infuser is left in place for up to a month or more. There appears to be no evidence, from endometrial biopsy studies, that this is so, and in our opinion, even if it were so, a true granulomatous endometritis might be a disadvantage. In our opinion leaving the infuser in place in the absence of concurrent antibiotic treatment may be hazardous.

In addition to local treatment with antibiotics, systemic treatment may, on occasion, be indicated. In our experience and, we believe, in the experience of most clinicians involved in this type of practice, systemic antibiotic treatment alone is of little value in the treatment of uterine infection in the mare. O'Driscoll et al. (1977) have criticized the use of local antibiotic treatment in this manner and suggest that only systemic treatment is indicated.

In addition to specific antibiotic treatment, mares with acute endometritis should be carefully checked for cervical damage (see p. 99) and pneumovagina (see p. 11). Vulval surgery should be performed if indicated (see p. 99).

The success or otherwise of treatment may be monitored by 'follow-up' endometrial biopsy, taken approximately four weeks after the end of treatment.

In mares where there is evidence that the natural defence mechanisms against infection are defective or absent, prophylactic measures at the time of covering are essential, if recurrence of the same condition is to be avoided. Treatment with antibiotics is not the end of the matter and can only be looked upon as a starting point for a programme of careful management and prophylactic measures. With such a programme, in this type of mare, successful conceptions and gestations may be obtained. It is only worth starting if done properly and not in a half-hearted manner. It may involve the mare owner in considerable patience and expense and the stud farm management and veterinary surgeon in considerable effort and expertise.

Kenney et al. (1975*a*) have described the technique and preliminary findings for minimal contamination techniques for mating mares. In horses where artificial insemination is applicable, the technique is as follows:

The stallion is trained to mount a phantom and to ejaculate into a carefully presterilized artificial vagina. The collection is performed in a dust-free area. Before collection the stallion's penis and prepuce are thoroughly washed with warm soapy water (not detergent) using either absorbent cotton, disposable paper towels or a freshly laundered wash cloth. A soapy residue is then removed by multiple warm water rinses. Following ejaculation, the semen is poured through a sterile in-line milk filter into a sterile disposable plastic beaker and the semen is evaluated for quality (see p. 142). In order to reduce the contaminating organisms to an absolute minimum, sperm was 'washed' (see p. 158) by centrifuging at 500 rpm for three minutes, so as to produce a soft pellet. The resulting supernatant is removed by rapid decantation or aspiration with a sterile pipette or syringe and the pellet gently resuspended in the appropriate amount of warm water extender for the number of mares to be inseminated. The compositon of semen extenders has been discussed by Kenney et al. (1975*a*) and by Pickett and Voss (1975). The resuspended sperm are aspirated into sterile, disposable, pre-warmed 100 ml syringes and the tip is capped. The full syringe is then insulated by wrapping in two or more paper towels and sealed in a large plastic bag. The bag has the name of the stallion (and the mare if desired) written on it, using a felt-tip pen with indelible ink. The packaged syringe is then placed in a refrigerator or pre-cooled portable icebox held at 4°C. The semen is held under these conditions for at least one hour before insemination. The mare's perineum is rigorously cleansed and disinfected with a surgical scrub and the inseminator uses a plastic sleeve on top of which he wears a sterile disposable rubber glove. The pipette is taken into the vagina enclosed in a sterile gloved hand, with the tip closed by a sterile index finger. The pipette is then passed through the cervix and insemination is performed.

For the Thoroughbred mare, artificial insemination is not as yet applicable, and thus Kenney et al. (1975*a*) have described minimal contamination techniques for natural service. They suggest that the mare and stallion are prepared as described for artificial insemination but just before natural cover is permitted, the uterus of the mare is filled to overflowing with antibiotic-containing semen extender warmed to body temperature. The amount of extender required varies from 100 to 300 ml depending on the size of the uterus and vagina. These authors consider that it is desirable to deposit sufficient extender in the uterus so that it will flow out and coat the cervix and vagina but not remarkably pool or distend the uterus. As soon as the extender is deposited in sufficient quantity, the horse is allowed to cover the mare. In doing so he will ejaculate directly into the antibiotic-containing extender.

TABLE 1.4 Pre-breeding semen extender for use with natural coitus

Instant, dried, low fat skimmed milk (Marvel)	2.5 g
Gelatin, BP	0.5 g
Glucose	5 g
Penicillin, crystalline	300 mg
Streptomycin, crystalline	300 mg
Water, sterile, for injection	100 ml

Adapted from Kenney et al. (1975*a*).

For the past seven years, we have used this method for natural cover with, we believe, very satisfactory results. The semen extender that we have used is based on a penicillin and streptomycin recipe (Table 1.4) described by Kenney et al. (1975*a*). The recommended extenders containing gentamicin sulphate have not been used because of the high cost of this drug. The mixture is made up in powder form in individual plastic sachets, and deep frozen. A new tin of 'Marvel' is opened for each batch of manufacture. Immediately before use, one sachet is dissolved in 100 ml of sterile water and warmed to body temperature. The mixture is then instilled into the uterus of the mare, in an aseptic manner, as soon before natural cover as is possible. In addition to this procedure, the mares are allowed one cover per oestrous period only, as close to ovulation as possible, as judged by careful ovarian palpation. In addition, human chorionic gonadatrophin is given to try to hasten ovulation. This type of mare should not be mated during the early spring when normal oestrous cycle patterns may not have been established and there is a higher chance of follicular atresia and failure of ovulation. Natural cover may be regarded as a 'necessary evil' as far as the endometrial 'health' of the mare is concerned. In the absence of acute information on the specific immunological lesion present (see p. 71) in 'susceptible' mares, immunoglobulin sources, such as mare's plasma or colostrum (a rich source of immunoglobulins), have been used with intrauterine pre-breeding prophylactic programmes.

Primary acute endometritis producers are organisms which have been associated with outbreaks of venereal disease in groups of mares mated by the same stallion. They appear to be capable of infecting not only those mares that have their natural defence mechanisms breached but other apparently healthy mares.

Haemophilus equigenitalis. A number of cases of an unusual genital infection, characterized by a vaginal discharge varying from frank pus to a glary mucopurulent fluid of variable quantity, was first described, in Newmarket, by Crowhurst (1977). The spread of the disease was mainly venereal and symptoms appeared from two days after covering. The infection was described as being extremely contagious and Crowhurst warned that veterinary examinations of mares must be carried out with extreme care. Routine aerobic bacteriological culturing methods had not revealed significant findings. O'Driscoll et al. (1977) explained that the condition had been seen previously in Ireland and he believed the causal organism to be *Proteus mirabilis.* This turned out to be incorrect, as a Gram-negative micro-aerophillic coccobacillus was eventually isolated at the regional Public Health Laboratories, Cambridge, and transmission studies demonstrated that this was the organism responsible (Platt et al. 1977; Ricketts et al. 1977; Timoney et al. 1977). This organism was eventually described and characterized by Taylor et al. (1978) as a previously undescribed organism and proposed that its name should be *Haemophilus equigenitalis.* The technical conditions needed for the growth of this particular organism have been described in Chapter 8.

Owing to the problems of identifying this organism and the reluctance of some stud farm managers to cease breeding operations in the presence of infection, the disease reached epidemic proportions and serious disruption and financial loss occurred. The Horserace Betting Levy Board in Great Britain set up a scientific committee of enquiry to control the disease for the 1978 breeding season (David et al. 1977). The committee described, for the benefit of veterinary surgeons and stud farm managers alike, the nature of the infection and highlighted the need for careful hygiene especially when teasing, covering and examining mares (see p. 502). They emphasized the need for open frank communication between stud farm managers and veterinary surgeons and suggested that the practice of 'walking in' mares to a stud farm during the covering season should be actively discouraged as it facilitated the spread of infectious disease. The committee recommended that mares should be carefully swabbed by the correct technique (see p. 532), using suitable transport medium, and examined under the correct micro-aerophilic conditions by an experienced laboratory. A register of 'approved' laboratories was set up to identify those that were experienced and competent in the technique. It was appreciated that the organism could remain in a 'carrier' state and one examination might give a false-negative result. A series of three sets of bacteriological examinations were recommended.

In most cases, the organism responded well to local and systemic treatment with penicillin (Platt et al. 1977; Taylor et al. 1978). It became clear, however, that symptomless carriers occasionally remained. Areas of the posterior genital tract, including the urethral opening, the clitoral fossa and sinuses were incriminated (Ricketts et al. 1977; Simpson & Eaton-Evans 1978*a*, *b*). It became clear that mares could be clinically symptomless and cure themselves of endometritis rapidly enough to become pregnant. Ricketts et al. (1977) described one mare that first showed signs at 80 days of pregnancy and despite a copious discharge, which was refactory to treatment with antibiotics, produced a normal live healthy foal. She remained as a chronic symptomless carrier for the following breeding season.

H. equigenitalis is highly sensitive to chlorhexidine gluconate in vitro (Platt et al. 1977; Taylor et al. 1978). The response in vivo appears to be less successful and Jackson et al. (1979) warned that untoward local reactions, with severe irritation, may result if excessively concentrated solutions are used. Swerczek (1979*a*) has suggested that the prophylactic use of chlorhexidine gluconate as a general 'disinfectant' may be contraindicated as it is very good at removing the useful contaminant organisms of the genital microflora and allowing venereal-disease-producers such as *H. equigenitalis, Kl. aerogenes* and *Ps. aeruginosa* to proliferate.

The enthusiastic application of the 'code of practice' by Thoroughbred and non-Thoroughbred horse breeders, and the lessons learned after the initial outbreak, resulted in a dramatic reduction in acute cases during the 1978 breeding season.

Meanwhile, cases were reported in other parts of the world (Bryans & Hendrick 1979; Hazard et al. 1979; Swerczek 1979*a*). Reports of disease in non-Thoroughbred horses have been made in North America and parts of Europe.

Swerczek (1979*a*) described *H. equigenitalis* infection in Kentucky with the previously described streptomycin-resistant strain and a streptomycin-sensitive strain. The latter provided particular problems with diagnosis in stallions, as the streptomycin-containing 'selective' medium was of no value. This author also described the inhibition of *H. equigenitalis* by other aerobic bacterial organisms in the normal microflora of the stallion's reproductive tract. These findings led him to criticize the 'prophylactic' treatment of uninfected stallions by scrubbing the penis with antibacterial agents. Unless a known pathogenic venereal-disease-producing organism is cultured from the genital organs of a stallion, it is highly dangerous, from the bacteriological point of view, to use antibacterial drugs for this purpose (see p. 158). Up to the present time, the streptomycin-sensitive strain of *H. equigenitalis* has not, to our knowledge, been isolated from clinical cases in Great Britain.

Serological reactions for CEM-infected mares were reported using the serum agglutination test (SAT), Coombs's antiglobulin test (AGT) and the complement-fixation test (CFT) (Benson et al. 1978; Croxton-Smith et al. 1978). Fernie et al. (1979) described a passive haemagglutination test (PHT) which appeared to be a more rapid and sensitive test. There is no doubt that serological tests are invaluable in terms of epidemiological surveys and may be a piece of extra evidence to comfort veterinary surgeons attending Thoroughbred stud farms, but they cannot be relied upon to identify chronic symptomless carriers in 100% of cases, any more than bacteriological examinations can (Bowen 1979; Crowhurst et al. 1979). The latter authors described a 'prophylactic' treatment for the clitoral area in 'high risk' mares which would appear to be no more fool-proof than the diagnostic test. Swerczek (1979*b*) described a surgical procedure for the removal of the clitoral sinuses from mares harbouring *H. equigenitalis.* The procedure involved a simple technique where the sinuses were excised from the clitoris under local anaesthesia. He concluded that

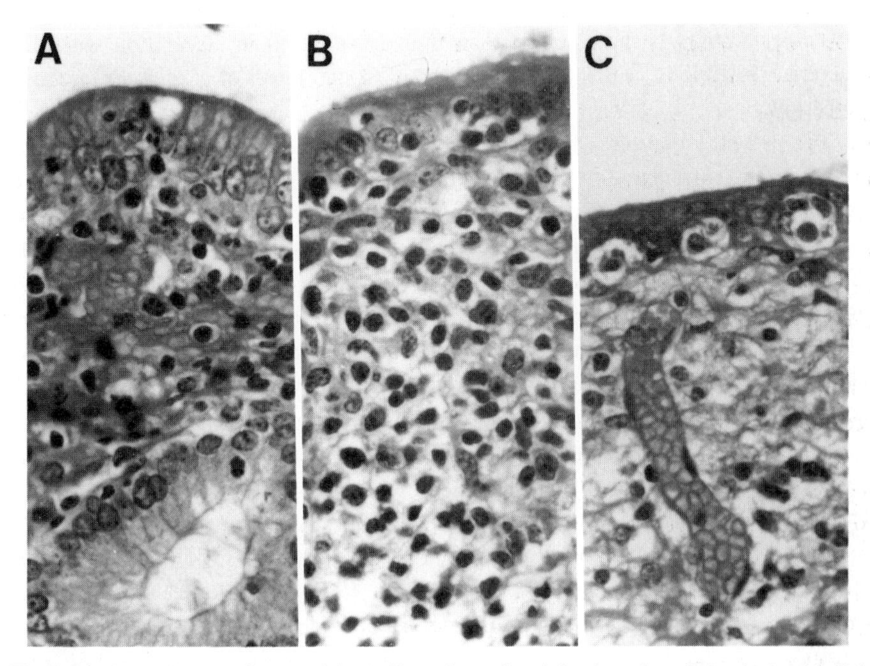

Fig. 1.34. Contagious equine metritis. A, Four days after infection, there is luminal epithelial proliferation and polymorphonuclear leucocyte infiltration. B, Six days after infection marked mononuclear infiltration of the stroma is seen. C, 47 days after infection, basal vacuolation of the luminal epithelium. H & E × 450.

surgical removal of these sinuses was the only positive method of treatment to make sure that a suspect mare is free of infection. It is extremely frustrating that despite the disruption and financial loss to the industry in the face of infection, and the financial involvement with diagnostic and preventive measures, the industry has not formulated a practical artificial insemination programme to be used under carefully controlled circumstances (Rossdale et al. 1979). This would appear to be the most logical method of control (see p. 159).

The pathological features of the disease have been described in post mortem specimens by Platt et al. (1978) and endometrial biopsy specimens by Ricketts et al. (1978) and Ricketts and Rossdale (1979). The features were a very marked initial acute endometritis accompanied by luminal epithelial proliferation (Fig. 1.34A) which gave a very marked pseudostratified appearance. The acute endometritis rapidly resolved and was replaced by a very marked mononuclear cell infiltration of the stroma (Fig. 1.34B) containing many plasma cells. Basal vacuolation of the luminal epithelium (Fig. 1.34C) was noted, to a degree that had not been previously seen in cases of acute endometritis associated with more commonly isolated aerobic organisms, and these vacuoles contained amorphous debris and degenerate leucocytes. Transmission and scanning electron micrographs confirmed the histological findings and identified damage and degenerative change in epithelial cells, especially the ciliated ones, and those surrounding the mouths of the luminal openings of the endometrial glands. It was concluded that the response of the endometrium to *H. equigenitalis* was more severe than that usually seen in association with other bacterial infections, with the exception of some cases of *Klebsiella aerogenes* infection.

The present situation is that the incidence of disease in the British Isles is, as far as we know, extremely low. The diagnosis of chronic symptomless carriers is still a problem, especially now that the diagnosis of 'high-risk' status, on historical grounds, is more difficult. The occasional acute case will almost certainly continue to appear but the greater awareness, stricter hygiene, immediate cessation of natural cover and better knowledge of treatment make control of the disease now relatively simple. Extirpation of the clitoris would appear to be a sensible measure to avoid the production of chronic symptomless carriers with this and other venereal diseases. We hope that the industry will give serious thought to the provision of a carefully controlled artificial insemination system for use in the face of disease outbreaks.

Klebsiella aerogenes. Pathogenic strains of this species have been incriminated as a cause of venereal disease in horses (Dimock & Edwards 1926; Hunt & Rossdale 1963; Farrely & Mullaney 1964; Crouch et al. 1972). Infection causes acute endometritis which may vary in degree and persistence. Clinical signs vary from none to a profuse mucopurulent vulval discharge, two to seven days after infection. Infection is usually venereally transmitted, but the organism may also be transmitted at teasing or during routine veterinary examinations, if adequate safeguards are not made, as is the case for *H. equigenitalis* (see above). Growth of the organism from infected mares, using standard aerobic techniques, is simple. The organism grows readily and is usually characteristic in appearance. The disease is endemic and fairly widespread, partly because its significance was ignored for many years but mainly because some types of the organism are normally found on the external genital skin of healthy male and female horses.

It is the identification of venereal-disease-producing strains which is the major difficulty. *Klebsiella* species are classified according to cultural, biochemical and serological characteristics (Ørskov 1954, 1955*a*, *b*, *c*, *d*, 1956). Of the several hundred known strains only a small number are pathogenic for horses. Forty-five different strains of *Klebsiella* species were identified from pathogenic cases (Marca et al. 1972), 43 of which belonged to the K_1 *pneumoniae* group serotype 1 and one to serotype 30 in accordance with the classification of Kauffman and Ørskov (Marca et al. 1972). The only strain identified as *Kl. aerogenes* belonged to serotype 5 and appeared identical to the strain reported by Crouch et al. (1972) from a stallion responsible for numerous cases of metritis. More recently, problems with venereal disease outbreaks associated with *Kl. aerogenes* capsule type 1 have been seen (Greenwood & Ellis 1976; Ricketts 1976). These reports found that, as is the case with *H. equigenitalis,* a reservoir of infection may occur at the urethral opening and the clitoral area, and that cervicouterine swabs alone are not a sufficiently accurate screening test. *Kl. aerogenes* capsule type 7 appears to be a non-pathogenic contaminant of the genital skin of the mare and stallion (Atherton 1975).

To the clinician, the major problem is the confirmation of the capsule type involved and, in some cases, its relation to pathogenicity. The most meaningful test is test mating. If the organism is found to be transmitted from mare to stallion to mare, and to cause acute endometritis, pathogenicity has been proved. This may be readily seen, under natural conditions, if an acute outbreak suddenly occurs, but if such an organism is found in a screening test, for either a mare or a stallion, the problems of setting up a test mating programme may be enormous. Nevertheless, in some cases, one finds that this is the only definitive test. Atherton (1975) described the identification of equine genital strains of *Klebsiella* and *Enterobacter* species using the laboratory tests of gas production from glucose, fermentation of dulcitol and sorbitol, urease production, citrate utilization, decarboxylation of ornithine, motility and cultural characteristics. We have found these methods to be extremely useful but not definitive. A readily available, rapid, accurate and definitive serological capsule typing service is essential.

When unusual serotypes are identified, the pathogenicity is generally unknown and there is no alternative but to attempt some form of test mating. It must be remembered that, even with those strains considered to be non-pathogenic, e.g. capsule type 7, severe acute endometritis may occur in those mares with damaged or absent natural uterine defence mechanisms.

The response to infection with *Kl. aerogenes* varies in degree from mild to severe. In some cases, marked degeneration of the luminal epithelium is seen, including subepithelial vacuolation. In an experiment involving three mares, one infected with *H. equigenitalis,* one infected with *Kl. aerogenes* capsule type 1 and the other challenged with phosphate-buffered saline, the degree of acute endometritis seen with *Kl. aerogenes* was much more low-grade and insidious than that with *H. equigenitalis.* Whereas the uterus reacted violently to *H. equigenitalis* and appeared to clear itself readily, it appeared to clear itself of *Kl. aerogenes* capsule type 1, only to reappear some time later. This very limited study confirmed the clinical impression that it is very difficult to be sure that a mare is free from *Kl. aerogenes* infection once she has been infected. A series of negative bacteriological swabs may be obtained from various sites in the genital tract only to find that reinfection occurs at a later stage. It may be that the severity of the inflammation in some cases is insufficient to remove all sources of the organism and/or in view of the organisms known predilection for the urinary tract, a reservoir of infection may be established in the urethra and/or bladder.

Treatment with antibiotics is sometimes extremely difficult. In vitro sensitivities are frequently extremely 'narrow' and neomycin or gentamicin are sometimes the only useful drugs. Despite intensive local and systemic treatment with these drugs, which can be very expensive in the case of gentamicin, clearance of the organism does not always follow. There is no doubt that, because of its capsule and apparent insensitivity to antibiotics, the indiscriminate use of antibiotic and antiseptic agents on the genital organs of mares and stallions encourages the establishment of *Kl. aerogenes.* We have found that a clean bucket containing the manufacturer's recommended concentration of chlorhexidine solution will not kill some strains of *Kl. aerogenes* after one or two hours immersion. It was for this reason that portable washing systems (see p. 504) were first used. Chemical sterilization of gynaecological instruments cannot be relied upon (see p. 504).

The control of *Kl. aerogenes* infection relies upon rapid diagnosis and cessation of natural cover. Again, it is hoped that the breeding industry eventually makes provisions for the controlled use of artificial insemination in the face of venereal disease.

Pseudomonas aeruginosa. This organism appears to have some primary infecting capacity and may occur in mares after mating with an infected stallion. Hughes et al. (1966) studied 70 mares harbouring *Ps. pyocyanea* and in 42 mares they found clinical evidence of cervical inflammation. Cases were mainly older mares and those treated with antibiotics to control other bacteria. These findings suggest that some predisposing factor may be necessary before the organism can become established in the genital tract. Hughes and Loy (1975) found that the majority of stallions that harboured *Pseudomonas* in their genital tracts had conception rates that compared favourably with stallions not harbouring the organism. They also found that certain strains of *Pseudomonas* may have a greater effect on the survival of sperm, or the establishment of infection, than others and these might affect fertility. Diagnostic criteria for the identification of different strains have not been reported for this organism and one can only rely on test matings.

The clinical signs and diagnostic problems are almost identical to those described above for *Kl. aerogenes.* The organism is readily grown using standard aerobic techniques and is culturally very characteristic. Although, as with *Kl. aerogenes* and *H. equigenitalis*, not all exposed mares become infected, the organism does not infect only those mares that have defective or absent uterine defence mechanisms. When a stallion is contaminated, it is thus impossible to predict which and how many of his mares will become infected during natural cover. This makes it impossible for an attending veterinary surgeon to recommend that natural cover continues, despite the knowledge that many of the mares covered would probably become pregnant and not become infected.

Treatment is again a major problem as in vitro antibiotic sensitivity tests are usually extremely 'narrow' and the in vivo response is frequently disappointing. Treatment with inadequate antibiotic or antibacterial medication may make the situation worse by killing the competing microflora. Polymixin B sulphate and gentamicin appear to be of most value. Recently we have heard that local treatment with 1% water-miscible silver sulphadiazine cream has had some success. This drug is used in man in the treatment of chronic granulating burn wounds infected with *Pseudomonas.*

Control of the disease depends upon early diagnosis and the cessation of natural cover. Again, it is hoped that the breeding industry will develop some form of controlled artificial insemination programme for use in the face of venereal disease.

There is no doubt that the culturing and isolation of potential venereal-disease-producing organisms from apparently healthy stallions and mares provides a number of problems for stud farm management and veterinary surgeons. The ultimate decision on the course of action must lie with the manager, in consultation with his veterinary surgeon, on the basis of risk assessment. The breeding industry must decide upon what degree of risk is acceptable, if any. The situation at present is that these diseases occur sporadically and may either be dealt with easily or, in some cases, may cause fairly major disruption. If the industry wishes to irradicate these diseases, or render them of no significance, artificial insemination is the only answer.

Pyometra

Sixteen cases ofpyometra of spontaneous development and long-standing duration were studied by Hughes et al. (1979). The condition was not associated with clinical signs of systemic disease. Pus varied in quantity and character between mares, and within the same mare, over long periods of time. Single or multiple isolations of bacteria were usually obtained on culture of the pus, but occasional negative culture results were noted. *Str. zooepidemicus* was most commonly found and other organisms included *E. coli, Actinomyces, Pasteurella* spp., *Pseudomonas* and *Propionibacterium* species. Total leucocyte counts were usually within, but occasionally below, the low normal range as a result of a neutropenia and sometimes lymphopenia.

At autopsy, the uteri contained various amounts of pus. When large amounts were present, it was thin and watery and usually grey in colour. With small amounts of pus, it was sometimes inspissated and cheesy. The endometrial surface was smooth and glistening but in a few cases, where the endometrium was eroded and the epithelial layer had degenerated, the surface was rough and finely granular. In all cases, the damage was most severe in the body of the uterus. A mosaic appearance was sometimes given by islands of relatively normal endometrium surrounded by areas of atrophy. All mares had endometritis, but the type and severity varied not only within the group but also from area to area within each uterus. The damage was usually superficial with involvement of myometrium and serosa. In three cases, the entire endometrium was replaced by inflamed granulation tissue. Focal areas of granulation tissue occurred in other uteri. Atrophy and fibrosis were common findings. In general, the least endometrial damage was observed in mares that had shortened oestrous cycles, involving the premature release of prostaglandins and consequent regression of the corpus luteum. More severe endometrial damage was associated with lengthening of the oestrous cycle, resulting from prolonged luteal activity due to delayed or inadequate prostaglandin release. These findings were monitored by the measurement of progesterone and 15-keto-13,14-dihydro-$PGF_2\alpha$ (PGFM) (the principle plasma metabolite of $PGF_2\alpha$) by a radio-immunoassay method. In a few animals, there was complete loss of

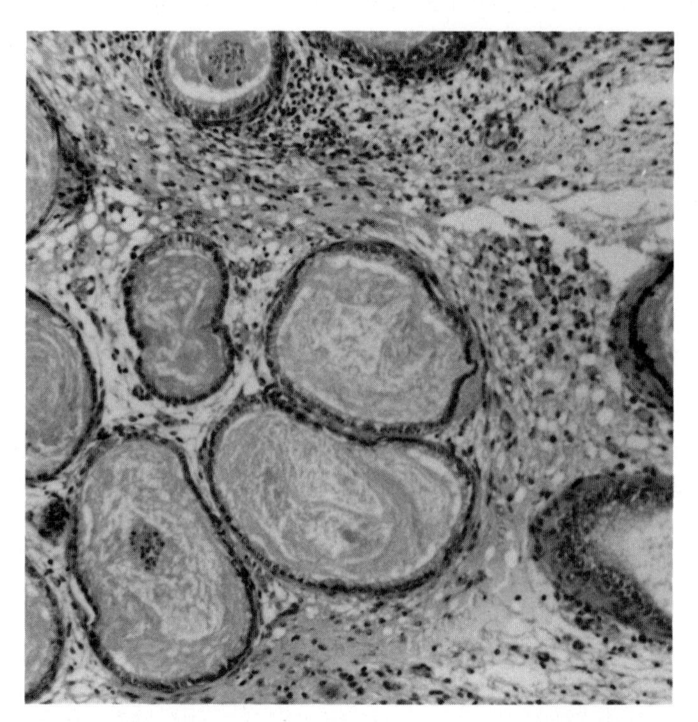

Fig. 1.35. Pyometra. Endometrial biopsy specimen showing cystic glandular change. Glands are distended by hyaline secretion. H & E × 100.

cyclic luteal function, the longest continuous luteal phase observed being 613 days; no cyclic $PGF_2\alpha$ release patterns were observed in these animals.

Pyometra in mares is more common in California than in some other parts of the world. We have seen very few cases of true pyometra and those have usually been associated with short cycling mares with a severe acute endometritis and endometrial hyperplasia (Ricketts 1978) (Fig. 1.35).

The cause of pyometra in the mare remains obscure. Hughes et al. (1979) suggest that interference with natural drainage of normal or abnormal fluids from the uterus, due to cervical adhesions and closure, may lead to pyometra but in other instances, the purulent material collects without demonstrable occlusion of the cervix. The condition can occur as a consequence of the trauma and accompanying bacterial infection associated with some dystocias, but most do not have such a history. An excess of progesterone does not appear to have the singificance that it does in a bitch. Mares with lowered endometrial resistance to disease may develop pyometra with or without a closed cervix. In the few cases that we have seen it appeared that the prognosis was extremely poor, if not hopeless. Treatment has been attempted by the daily passage of two stomach tubes through the cervix into the uterus and the passage of large volumes of water containing mild antiseptics through one tube and draining out of the other. Temporary improvement has often occurred but recurrence usually occurs either spontaneously or following mating. If such cases are improved to the state that they are considered fit for mating, then minimal contamination techniques are essential.

Mycotic endometritis

Mycotic infection of the uterus may cause abortion (Mahaffey & Adam 1964; Mahaffey & Rossdale 1965) but does not appear to interfere with conception unless

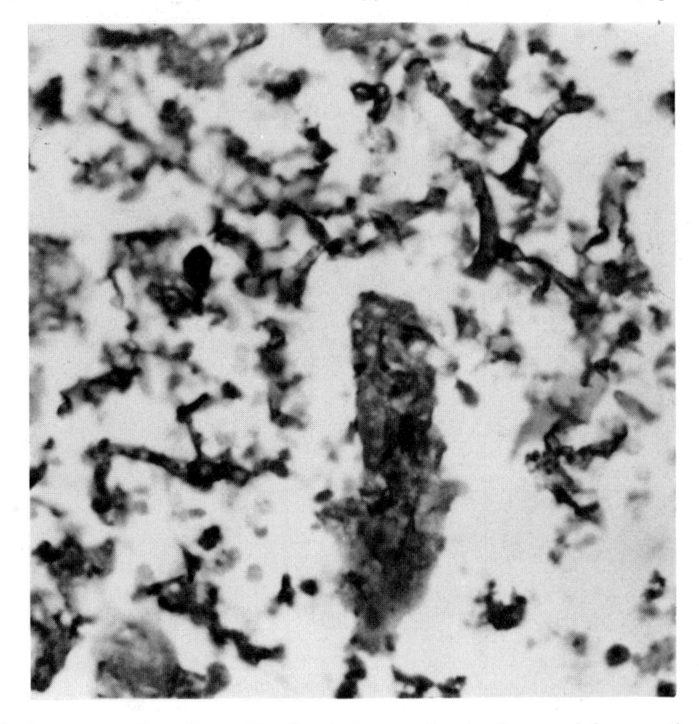

Fig. 1.36. Acute mycotic endometritis. Cervical smear showing fungi and degenerative material. PAS × 450.

a true acute endometritis is present. The significance of fungal organisms grown from cervical swabs, even in the presence of visible signs of inflammation, must be supported by the evidence of cervical cytology (Fig. 1.36) and endometrial biopsy.

Fungal contamination or infection may appear after prolonged intrauterine antibiotic treatment. Zafracas (1975) described 16 cases of *Candida* infection of the genital tract in Thoroughbred mares. It was significant that pneumovagina was observed in 12 of the 16 mares although a Caslick's operation had been performed. Uterine biopsy was performed in eight of the infected mares and histological examinations showed various degrees of endometrial oedema and round cell infiltration, especially around the endometrial glands and blood vessels. From these findings it would appear that these cases were probably contaminated with *Candida* but not infected in the true sense of the word. The fact that these mares were subfertile does not imply that the fungus was significant. Zafracas (1975) tried treatment with Lugol's iodine and nystatin but his results appeared variable.

Chronic infiltrative endometritis

Chronic infiltrative endometritis is characterized by a mononuclear cell infiltration of the superficial stromal layers (Fig. 1.37A). These cells are of the mononuclear

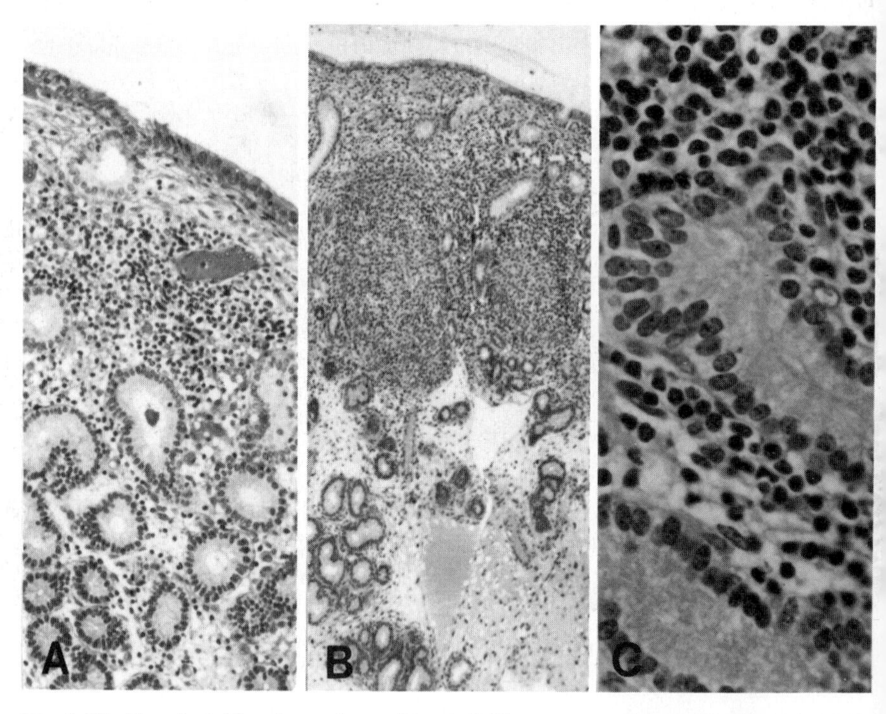

Fig. 1.37. Chronic infiltrative endometritis. A, Diffuse mononuclear cell infiltration of the stroma. B, Similar infiltration giving the appearance of lymphoid follicules. C, Infiltration in periglandular aggregations. H & E. A × 200; B × 100; C × 450.

phagocyte system (van Furth et al. 1972) mostly histiocytes. Plasma cells are seen in some cases, sometimes in large numbers. Eosinophils and mast cells are seen in varying numbers. Sometimes cells resembling lymphocytes are seen but in most cases these are thought to be histiocytes. Aggregations in the form of 'lymphoid follicles' do occur (Fig. 1.37B). Mononuclear cell infiltrations are seen either diffusely or in perivascular or periglandular aggregations (Fig. 1.37C).

This condition is not associated, by itself, with infertility (Ricketts 1978) but appears to be a manifestation of the normal cell-mediated immunological defence mechanisms of the endometrium in response to challenge by infection and pregnancy. A degree of chronic infiltrative endometritis is probably a 'healthy' sign but severe cases usually denote either persistent infection or a very 'busy' breeding career (see p. 110).

Chronic degenerative endometritis

Chronic degenerative endometritis is characterized by the presence of glandular degenerative changes and stromal fibrosis (Fig. 1.38A). Glandular degenerative changes are of two basic appearances (Fig. 1.38B). (*a*) Gland 'nests' where an area of glandular tissue becomes well circumscribed, often surrounded by variable thickness of fibrous tissue lamellae. The luminal epithelium appears low cuboidal and inactive and in most cases histochemical staining affinity is low (Ricketts 1978) suggesting inactivity. (*b*) Gland 'cysts' (Kenney & Ganjam 1975) where the

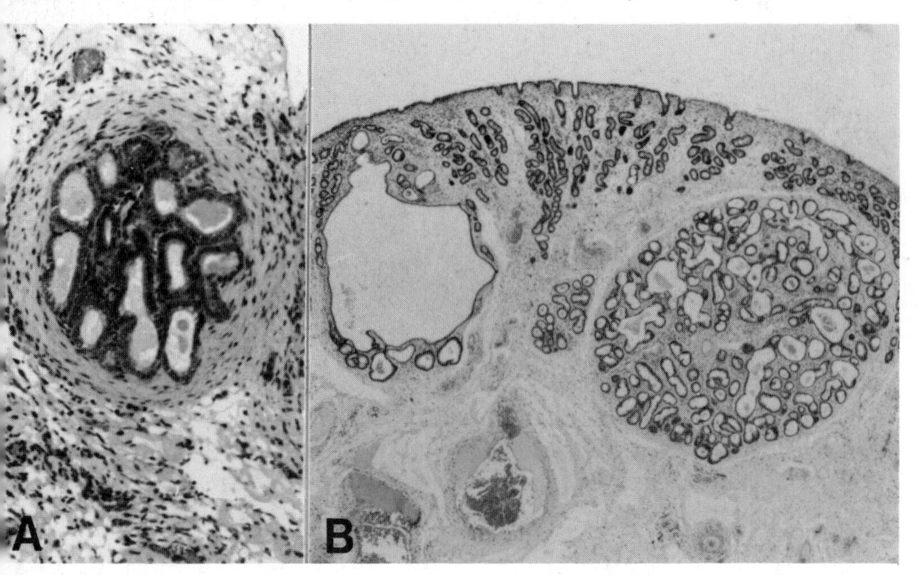

Fig. 1.38. Chronic degenerative endometritis. A, Marked periglandular fibrosis. H & E × 200. B, Gland cyst (*left*) and gland nest (*right*). H & E × 30.

glandular lumen has significantly enlarged. The cyst is often surrounded by a variable thickness of fibrous tissue lamellae. In some cases, the lumen appears full of amorphous PAS-positive material and in others appears empty. The epithelium varies from appearing hyperactive to appearing atrophic on histological and histochemical grounds. Sometimes gland nests appear in the process of degeneration into a gland cyst. Stromal fibrosis is either diffuse (Fig. 1.39A) or arranged around the glands. In some cases, stromal oedema is very marked between the endometrial glands and between the glands and the myometrium. Pools of tissue fluid or 'lymphatic lacunae' (Fig. 1.39B) may occur (Kenney & Ganjam 1975) (see also pp. 87 and 97).

It appears that chronic degenerative endometritis is a manifestation of endometrial 'wear and tear', in response to repeated infection and gestation. Repeated

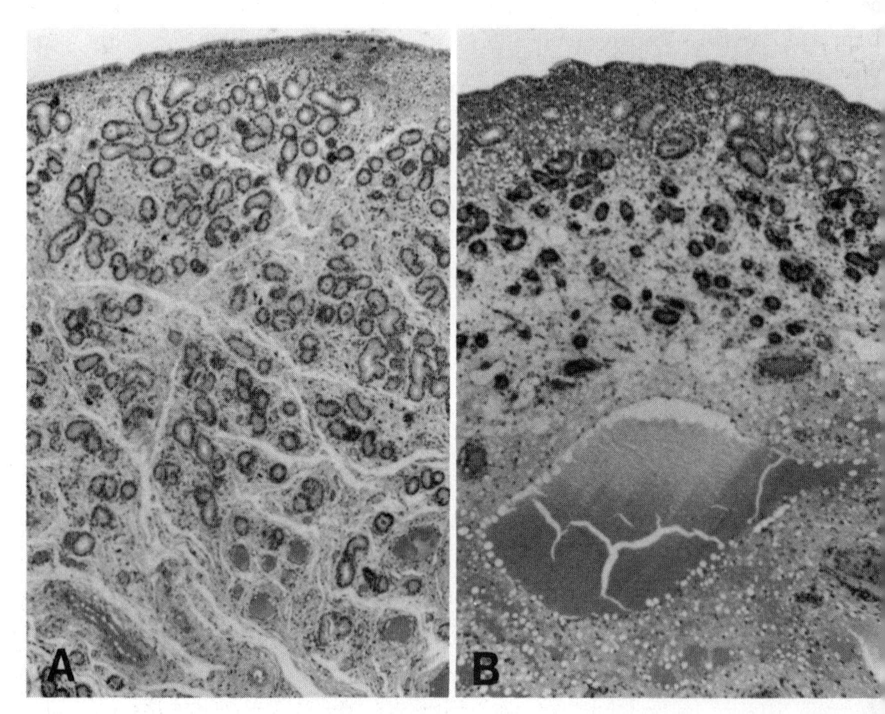

Fig. 1.39. Chronic degenerative endometritis. A, Diffuse stromal fibrosis. B, Pool of stromal oedema ('lymphatic lacuna'). H & E × 100.

acute endometritis followed by immobilization of cell-mediated defence mechanisms results in chronic infiltrative endometritis. Repeated tissue damage results in fibrous tissue proliferation. Diffuse stromal fibrosis may embarrass the blood supply to the endometrium, which is an important factor limiting endometrial cell-mediated defence mechanisms, and the nutrition of the fetus via placental perfusion. Stromal fibrosis develops around the glands and ducts resulting in chronic degenerative glandular change. Although this may be a major factor associated with glandular degenerative change, other causes cannot be ruled out:

1. Massive glandular hyperplasia, with widening of gland lumens, occurs normally during pregnancy (Kenney & Ganjam 1975). After repeated pregnancies some glands do not return to normal size, appear cystic and may become atrophic.

2. Glandular degenerative change occurs in tubular gland structures, progressing to atrophy, associated with endometrial senility and/or ovarian inactivity (Dallenbach-Hellweg 1971). As far as we know primary ovarian malfunction and hormonal imbalance is not as common in the mare as it is in other species.

It is thought that superficial stromal fibrosis and/or tissue damage may cause stenosis or obliteration of gland ducts. This leads to progressive glandular degenerative change. Firstly, as glandular function continues a degree of hyperplasia occurs and the gland stands out in the tissue as a 'nest' formation. Gland function may continue and cyst formation occurs until the 'back-pressure' of luminal secretions becomes great enough to halt production from the glandular luminal epithelium. Depending on the stage at which the biopsy is taken the luminal epithelium appears very tall columnar and possibly hyperactive or low cuboidal, degenerate and inactive. In other cases cyst formation does not occur, luminal epithelial secretion ceases at an earlier stage and the 'nest' shows signs of degeneration and becomes atrophic.

Stromal fibrosis itself may in some cases be produced by hormonal imbalance and is a common feature of hyperoestrogenism in women (Dallenbach-Hellweg 1971). This may be an additional causal factor in mares where the repetitive three-week oestrous cycle is not interrupted by normal pregnancy, and in 'short cycling' mares.

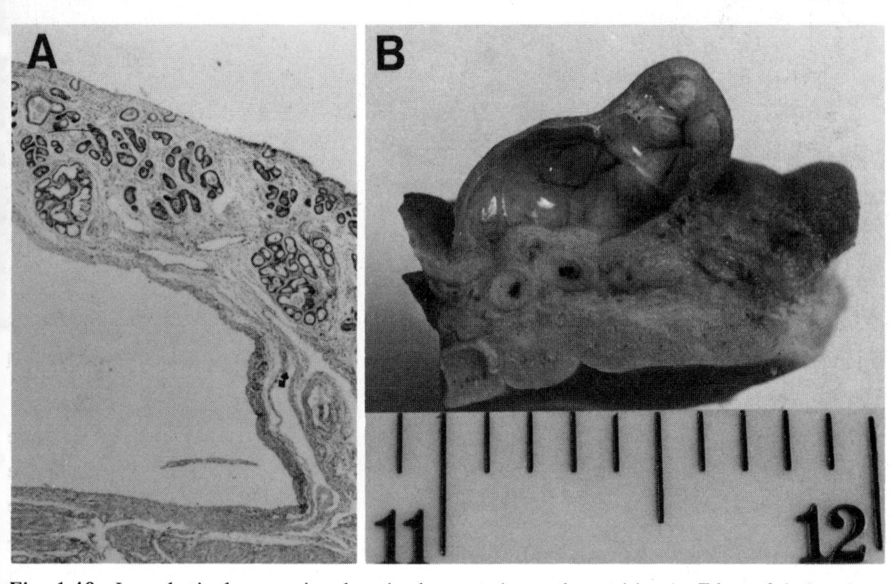

Fig. 1.40. Lymphatic lacunae in chronic degenerative endometritis. A, Edge of lesion in necropsy section. H & E × 30. B, Transverse section after fixation.

Another response to endometrial 'wear and tear' in chronic degenerative endometritis cases is pooling of tissue fluid and lymph producing lymphatic lacunae (Bergman & Kenney 1975; Kenney & Ganjam 1975) (Fig. 1.40). These may be seen in the stroma in biopsy specimens or large cysts may be formed, projecting into the uterine lumen, which may vary from a few millimetres to several centimetres in diameter. These large cysts are not diagnosed by endometrial biopsy.

When considering the significance of a degree of chronic degenerative endometritis in a biopsy specimen of a subfertile mare, one must take into consideration the mare's age and previous breeding history. One cannot expect an aged mare, who has produced several foals, to have a 'normal' endometrium. Nevertheless, chronic degenerative endometritis of this kind is, in our opinion, a major cause of subfertility in the mare and is one of the most common histopathological features in biopsy specimens (see Fig. 1.47).

Treatment of chronic degenerative endometritis is based upon an attempt to stimulate the growth of healthier endometrial tissue. Endometrial curettage

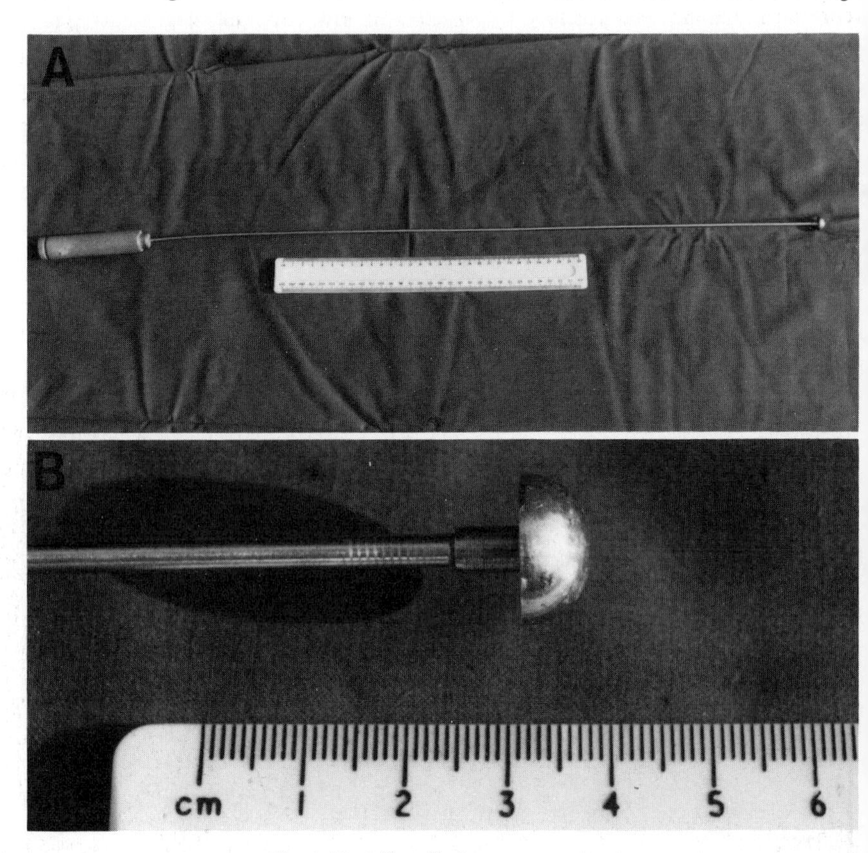

Fig. 1.41. A Fort Dodge mare curette.

(Morrow 1967; Lanfenstein-Duffy 1968; Solomon et al. 1970; Witherspoon 1972) has been described for use in the mare but we were extremely sceptical of this technique, considering the physiology and anatomy of the mare's uterus. In women, curettage is successful because of the smooth, pear-shaped menstrual uterus. The endometrium of the mare is highly folded and non-menstrual, making curettage, in the true sense of the word, impossible. Nevertheless, for the lack of better ideas, we have tried mechanical endometrial curettage, performed with a Fort Dodge mare curette (Fig. 1.41) followed by a course of seven daily intra-uterine infusions of saline and antibiotics via an indwelling catheter as described on p. 71. Endometrial biopsy studies before and approximately four weeks after curettage showed, in most cases, a significant improvement in the degree of chronic degenerative endometritis seen. Following this treatment, stringent minimal contamination techniques are used when the mare is next to be mated.

Using this procedure we have now treated a large number of mares, some of whom have had extremely poor pre-treatment breeding histories, with apparently successful results. It may be that curettage had nothing to do with the result but it is our opinion that the technique is worth while. If it does work, endometrial curettage must just stimulate local hyperaemia and inflammatory processes. The amount of endometrial damage done by the curette is minimal. It is for that reason that we prefer to use mechanical curettage rather than chemical curettage, e.g. with Lugol's iodine, as this is completely uncontrollable and sometimes very severe (Mather et al. 1979) (see p. 107). Using this method, we have never encountered transluminal adhesions or cervical damage after treatment.

Endometrial atrophy

Endometrial atrophy is characterized by atrophy and disappearance of significant numbers of endometrial glands (Fig. 1.42). The luminal epithelium often appears

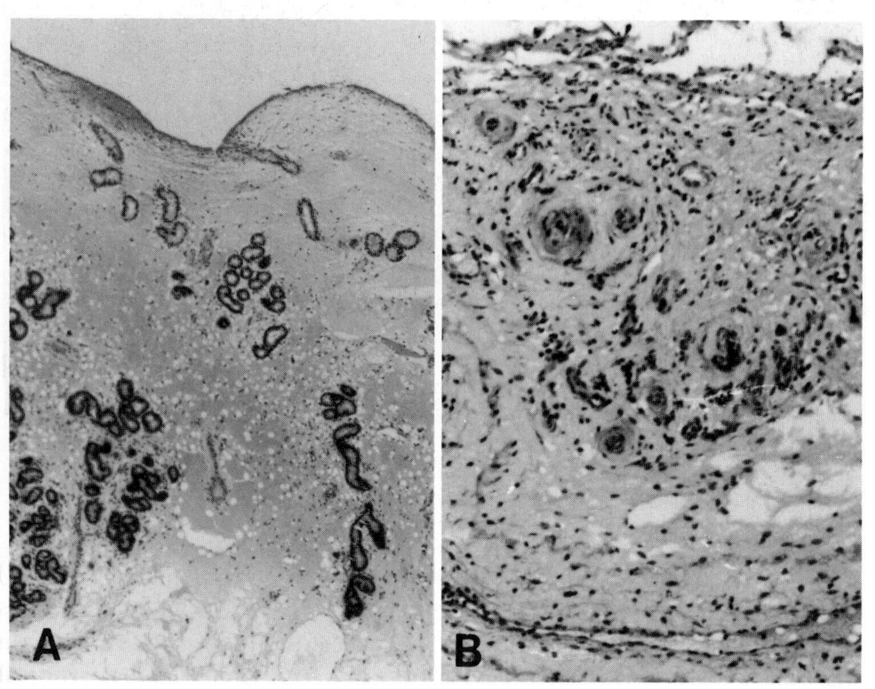

Fig. 1.42. Endometrial atrophy. A, Few, widely spread, atrophic glands. H & E × 40. B, Extreme glandular atrophy. H & E × 100.

cuboidal despite the presence of ovarian follicular structures and behavioural signs of oestrous. The luminal epithelium and glandular epithelium show very little or no histochemical staining affinity. Signs of chronic infiltrative or degenerative endometritis are usually present.

True endometrial atrophy, which persists throughout the breeding season, must be differentiated from that which occurs during deep winter anoestrus (Fig. 1.43) (Kenney 1975). If this condition is diagnosed by endometrial biopsy during anoestrus, a repeat biopsy should be taken during the breeding season, before the mare is condemned.

Significant endometrial atrophy is thought to be a progression of extreme chronic degenerative endometrial change or to reflect ovarian inactivity or primary endometrial senility. No obvious menopause is recognized in the mare, but some mares, late in their breeding careers, start to cycle irregularly and their ovaries appear small, hard and inactive on rectal palpation. Post mortem examinations

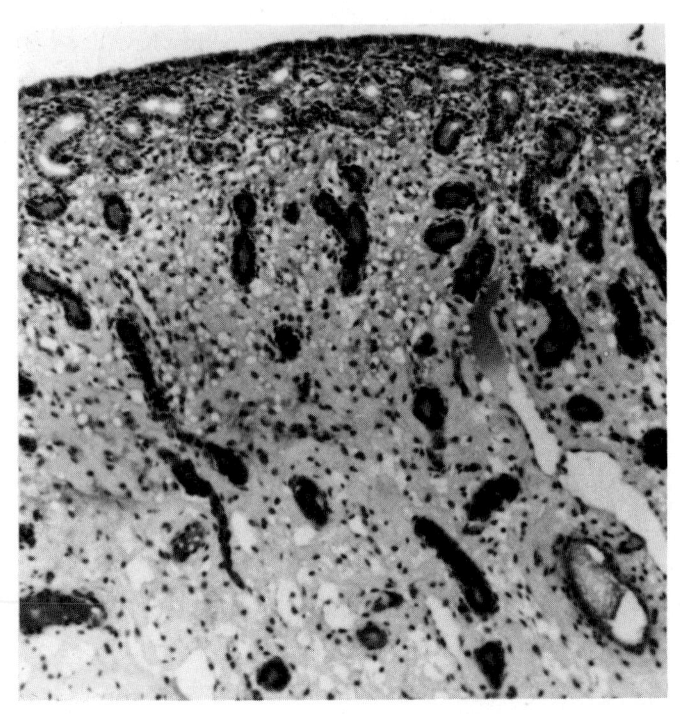

Fig. 1.43. Endometrial 'atrophy' of winter anoestrus, showing 'atrophy' of glands which contain amorphous inspissated secretion. H & E × 100.

reveal the ovaries to be small, fibrotic and scarred. The fact that endometrial atrophy occurs in young mares during periods of deep anoestrus confirms that prolonged ovarian inactivity may result in endometrial atrophy. In other mares, who appear to be cycling normally during the breeding season and have palpable ovarian follicles, endometrial atrophy is usually complicated by advanced chronic degenerative endometritis and one can only postulate that this is a progression of the endometrial 'wear and tear' process.

In cases of true endometrial atrophy associated with senility, no treatment could be expected to be of value. Ricketts (1978) found that despite careful attempts at breeding such mares, the prognosis was extremely poor. Of 16 mares showing signs of true endometrial atrophy, only two produced a live foal to a mating in the breeding season following the biopsy (see Fig. 1.55).

Endometrial hypoplasia

Hypoplasia is characterized by a low cuboidal and inactive luminal epithelium which shows, in some cases, an indented appearance similar to that seen in the developing endometrium (Ricketts 1978). The endometrial glands are of the simple tubular type extending for only a short distance into the stratum spongiosum and giving an underdeveloped appearance rather than an atrophic one. The glandular

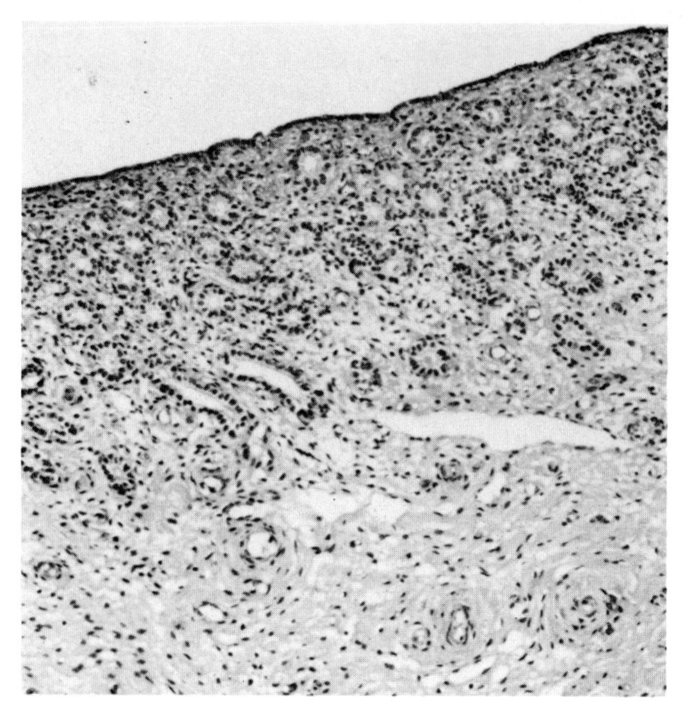

Fig. 1.44. Endometrial hypoplasia in a mare with XO chromosome abnormality (Turner's syndrome). H & E × 100.

epithelium appears low and cuboidal but not degenerate. There is no underlying evidence of chronic infiltrative or degenerative endometritis in these cases.

Studies of the development of the endometrium and the fact that this condition is usually seen in young maiden mares suggest that endometrial hypoplasia is a manifestation of endometrial immaturity. Why some mares appear mature at the age of four or five years, whereas the normal age of puberty is approximately 18 months, is not known. Genetic factors may be involved and in some cases one wonders if steroid hormone treatment given to fillies in training may be a factor. In mares with extreme endometrial hypoplasia (Fig. 1.44), coupled with cyclic irregularities and palpably small or absent ovaries, chromosome abnormalities may be suspected (see p. 60).

In mares unassociated with chromosome abnormality, one can give a fairly confident good prognosis because development of the endometrium and successful fertility is usually just a matter of time (see p. 110).

Endometrial hyperplasia

Hyperplasia is characterized by an overall hyperplasia of the endometrial glands, packed tightly together in the stroma and stretching deep into the stratum spongiosum (Fig. 1.45). The luminal epithelium is often highly pleomorphic and pseudostratified in areas. In some cases histochemical staining affinity is intense, indicating

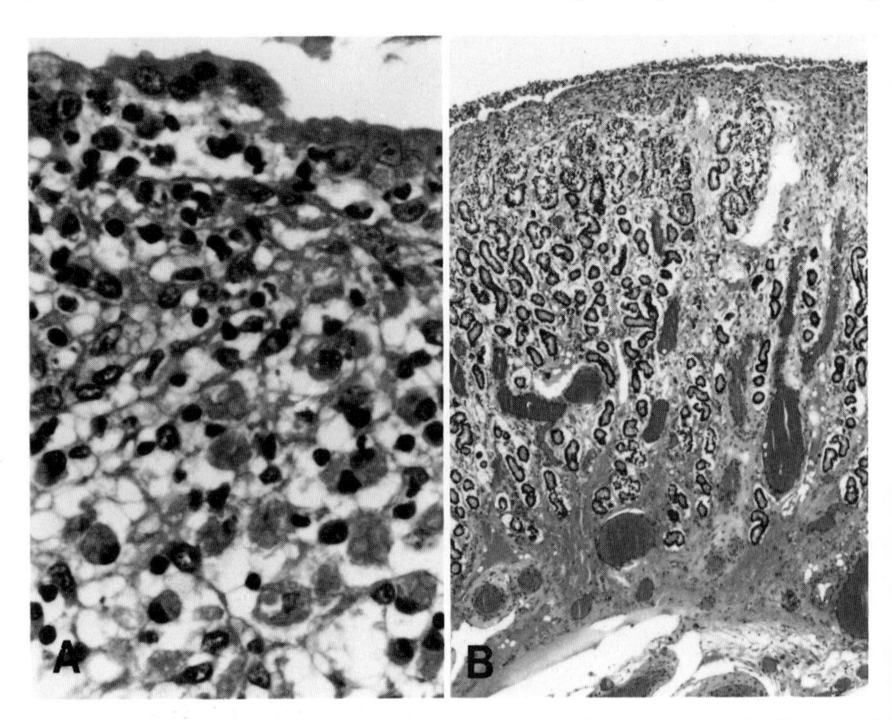

Fig. 1.45. Endometrial hyperplasia. A, Polymorphonuclear and mononuclear cell infiltration of the stratum compactum and many haemosiderin-laden macrophages. H & E × 100. B, Six weeks post-partum, showing diffuse glandular hyperplasia. A severe acute endometritis is also present. H & E × 40.

vigorous mucopolysaccharide production, but in other cases, histochemical staining affinities appear relatively normal as if glandular involution has become blocked at a particular stage. Acute endometritis is often associated with delayed endometrial post-partum involution (Fig. 1.45B). In these cases, haemosiderin-laden macrophages are often seen in large numbers.

Kenney (1978) states that glandular hyperplasia, as suggested by high gland density, is a physiological phenomenon and not a pathological one. He criticizes the use of this term (Ricketts 1975*b*). This disagreement may be a matter of terminology. Post-parturient endometrial hyperplasia is part of the normal physiological process of endometrial involution but in a small number of mares this process appears to be delayed in resolution to histological normality. In our opinion, endometrial hyperplasia, in cases of delayed endometrial involution, usually with acute endometritis and sometimes infection is 'pathological'.

Endometrial hyperplasia associated with long-standing acute endometritis (Fig. 1.46) is presumably a result of repeated oestrogenic stimulation. In addition, diffuse endometrial fibrosis is often found in these cases. Stromal fibrosis is a common feature of hyperoestrogenism in women (Dallenbach-Hellweg 1971). In such cases, if the acute endometritis and hyperplasia is removed and pregnancy occurs, the degree of diffuse stromal fibrosis appears to improve dramatically.

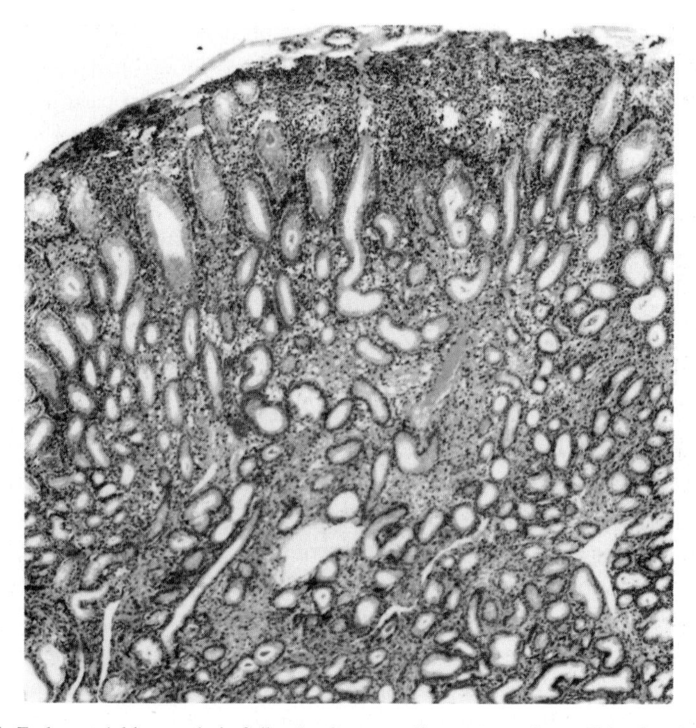

Fig. 1.46. Endometrial hyperplasia following long-standing acute endometritis, showing marked glandular hyperplasia. H & E × 100.

Treatment of endometrial hyperplasia is concerned with the removal of the acute endometritis and infection, if present, and completing endometrial involution. Mares may be given a five- or seven-day course of intrauterine antibiotic irrigation via an indwelling catheter as described before (see p. 71). On the second or third day of treatment, the mare is given an intravenous drip containing 60 IU oxytocin in 500 ml of sterile saline solution (Vandeplassche et al. 1972). By this time, the manipulative procedures associated with treating the mare's uterus have usually stimulated an oestrogenic phase (Hurtgen 1975) and the endometrium is in a 'primed' state for the action of oxytocin. In addition to the effects on the myometrium, there is evidence in other species that oxytocin has a direct action on endometrial blood vessels which may have the effect of reducing glandular hyperplasia (Porter, D.G., personal communication).

Clinicians involved in equine practice recognize the very important part played by a delay in endometrial involution in triggering reproductive problems. It is the duty of the clinician to screen mares at the first post-partum oestrus period (foal heat) for evidence of delayed involution and to warn the mare owner that natural cover may result in serious damage. The exact mechanism of this process is incompletely understood but a logical hypothesis may be made. Hartigan (1970) noted that the normal involutionary period of the cow varied considerably, often depending on milk yield. He studied alkaline and acid phosphatase activity in the involuting endometrium and noted an absence of alkaline phosphatase activity in the incompletely recovered endometrium. Ricketts (1978) made limited studies of endometrial phosphatase activity in mares at the first post-partum oestrus but failed to show any significant correlation between activities in mares with normal or abnormal foaling, involution or subsequent breeding histories. The fact still remains, however, that delayed endometrial involution, as confirmed by acute endometritis and endometrial hyperplasia, is often followed by a poor breeding history if the mare is covered. It seems logical that pathological changes may alter the anatomical, physiological and immunological integrity of the endometrium resulting in an impaired response to the challenge of semen and micro-organisms at natural cover. The details of events that follow have yet to be elucidated but sensitization of the endometrium to sperm antigen in these cases cannot be ruled out (Katsh & Katsh 1968). One can posulate such a mechanism in a mare when her endometrium is incompletely involuted, and who becomes endometrially 'susceptible' to infection (see p. 70). Each time she is covered, an impairment of her natural defence mechanisms allows a persistent acute endometritis to follow.

There is no doubt that the uterus is often not histologically recovered until 12–14 days after parturition (Ricketts 1978; Gygax et al. 1979). Thus the endometrium may not be in a favourable state at the first post-partum oestrus. Gygax et al. (1979) point out that a higher rate of fetal loss occurs in mares that conceive during the foal heat. If conception and normal gestation do occur, it is an advantage not only to the owner of the mare, in the production of an early foal, but also the stud farm, by reducing the number of mares to be covered later in the season. Generally speaking, to some extent depending on the time of the year, we recommend that mares are mated at the first post-partum oestrus only if their uterus appears palpably to be within acceptable normal size limits, and the results of cervicouterine bacteriological and cytological examinations are satisfactory. Further studies are needed on the effects of prophylactic management measures and hormonal treatments of mares during the post-partum period.

In cases where involution is considered to be unsatisfactory, mating is not recommended and the mare is treated by intravenous drip with 60 IU of oxytocin in 500 ml of sterile saline (Vandeplassche et al. 1972). Where the results of cervico-uterine bacteriological and cytological examinations are unsatisfactory, a minimum of three daily intrauterine infusions are made with suitable antibiotic solutions (see p. 71).

In endometrial biopsy specimens of most mares sampled for reasons of subfertility, a combination of histopathological findings are invariably seen (see Table 1.5, p. 110). Rickets (1978) described 15 combinations of histopathological findings in 323 subfertile or infertile mares (Fig. 1.47). Combinations of chronic infiltrative and degenerative endometritis were most common. The average age of the population sample was 11.5 years and there was a trend to increasing age from

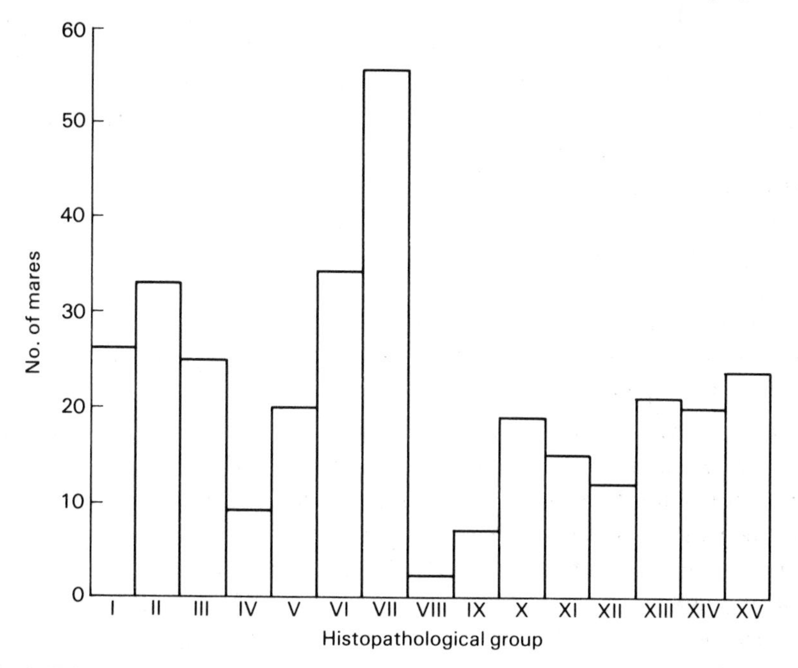

Fig. 1.47. Number of mares classified in each histopathological group (see Table 1.5, p. 110).

those with no significant endometrial histopathological findings to acute endometritis to chronic infiltrative endometritis to chronic degenerative endometritis and then to endometrial atrophy. Those mares with endometrial atrophy were statistically older and those with endometrial hyperplasia were statistically younger than the population mean (Fig. 1.48). This trend tends to support the hypothesis that these changes are a 'wear and tear' process (see pp. 86 and 105). The average number of foals produced prior to biopsy in the population sampled was four. Mares with endometrial atrophy were on the limit of statistical significance of having produced more foals than the population mean (Fig. 1.49) and mares with endometrial hyperplasia were all maidens. The general trend in the other groups was similar to that seen with age, i.e. an increasing number of foals previously born from those with no significant endometrial findings to acute endometritis to chronic infiltrative and degenerative endometritis to endometrial atrophy. These findings also tend to support the 'wear and tear' hypothesis.

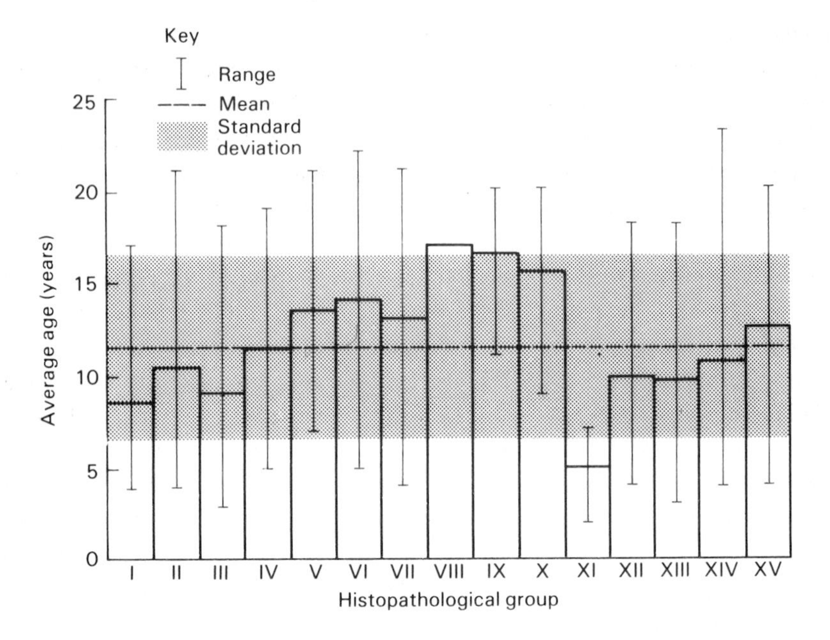

Fig. 1.48. Age of mares in each histopathological group (see Table 1.5, p. 110).

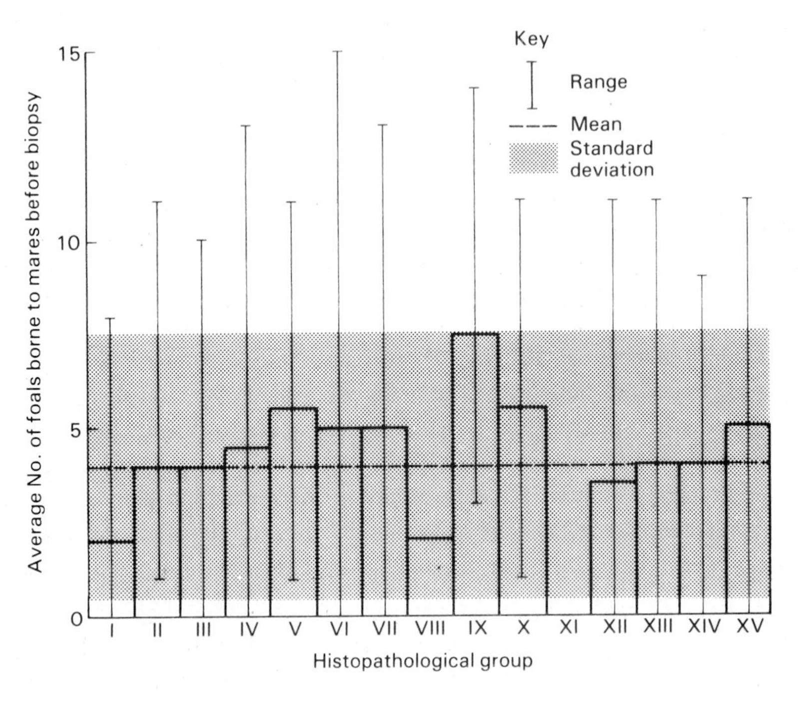

Fig. 1.49. Pre-biopsy foaling histories of mares in each histopathological group (see Table 1.5 p. 110).

Luminal (lymphatic) cysts

Large thin-walled cysts (more than 3 cm in diameter), filled with lymph and projecting into the lumen of the uterus, have been described by Kenney and Ganjam (1975) and Ricketts (1978) (see Fig. 1.40). They are quite distinct from the microscopic cystic glands (see p. 85). These large cysts have been called 'lymphatic lacunae' and are seen in mares aged over 10 years and may be associated with chronically inflamed or a normal endometrium (Kenney & Ganjam 1975). In a series of 50 necropsy uteri examined (Ricketts 1978), lymphatic cysts were seen in 28 mares. The average age of these mares was 18.9 years with a range of 14–28 years. Kenney and Ganjam report that they have been found in uteri containing endometrial cups but no conceptus and also in subfertile mares. These authors conclude that they may interfere with the ability of a mare to become pregnant and may be a cause of abortion. If these cysts are large enough and present in sufficient numbers, they may reduce the functional area of the endometrium available for placental perfusion and could be a cause of habitual abortion. These large cysts are not diagnosed by endometrial biopsy. Very large ones may sometimes be palpated per rectum (Greenhoff & Kenney 1975) or they may be observed by hysteroscopy (Mather et al. 1979).

Where treatment is considered necessary, because of the size or number of cysts which are present, and the history of subfertility and habitual abortion, removal may be attempted by endometrial curettage (see p. 88), by puncturing the cysts with the biopsy attachment of a fibreoptic endoscope, viewed directly, or by intrauterine surgery, via laparotomy under general anaesthesia.

Ventral dilatation/mucosal atrophy

Knudsen (1964) described the condition of partial dilatation of the uterus. When the genital tract is suspended by the cervix and ovaries, at necropsy examination, the dilated segment can be readily appreciated as a pendulous area with poor tone. When transilluminated, the wall appears extremely thin in the abnormal area. On opening the uterus, the endometrial folds appear obliterated in the affected areas, which may contain few, if any, glandular structures.

Kenney and Ganjam (1975) examined the genital tracts of 128 mares at necropsy. They described ventral uterine enlargements in mares between nine and 24 years of age, similar to those described by Knudsen (1964). These enlargements occurred in the area of implantation, i.e. at the junction of the uterine horn and body following repeated pregnancies. The enlargements may have been associated with cysts or atrophy in the endometrium or atonia or fluid accumulations (lymphatic lacunae) in the myometrium. Areas of endometrial atrophy had a reduced number of glands and an increased collagen and inflammatory cell content.

There is no information on the specific effect on subfertility or infertility of these ventral dilatations but they tend to occur in subfertile mares that have other evidence of chronic degenerative endometritis and/or endometrial atrophy. They may be diagnosed by uterine palpation per rectum (Greenhoff & Kenney 1975) (see p. 50) and the histopathological features may be defined by endometrial biopsy of the area of dilatation and other palpably more normal areas.

In view of the loss of endometrial structure in the dilated areas, treatment is unlikely to succeed but uterine irrigations and intravenous oxytocin drips, as for the treatment of endometrial hyperplasia and delayed involution (see p. 93), may be attempted as possibly the most logical approach. Treatment with hot saline irrigations has been suggested as being useful.

Neoplasia

Neoplasia of the equine endometrium is rare. The most commonly seen appears to be the leiomyoma (Fig. 1.50) which is usually small, 2.5–5 cm in diameter, and sometimes multiple (Jubb & Kennedy 1967; Rooney 1970; Roberts 1971; Bostock

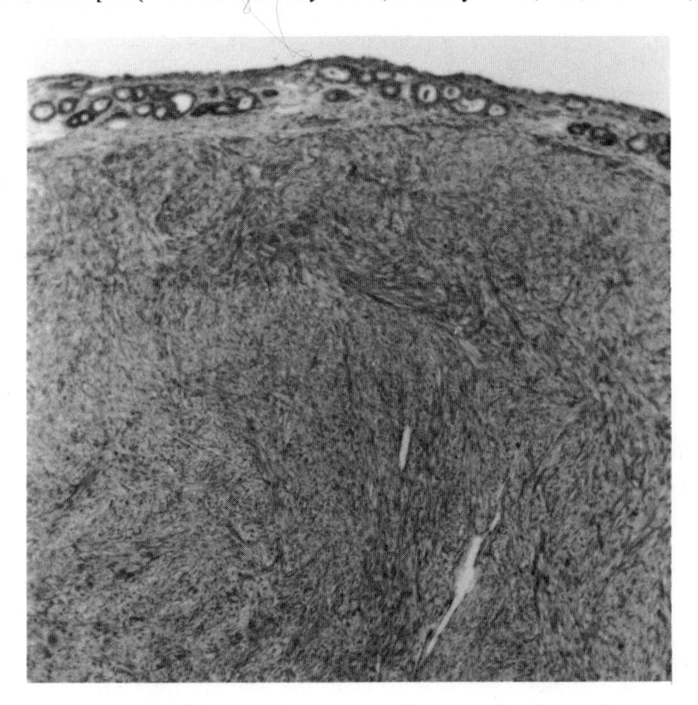

Fig. 1.50. Endometrial leiomyoma. H & E × 30.

& Owen 1975). Even rarer tumours of the equine endometrium are fibromas, fibroadenomas and adenosarcomas (Jubb & Kennedy 1967; Roberts 1971; Bostock & Owen 1975). Kenney (1978) reports that when he examined several hundred pathological uterine biopsies, as well as dozens at necropsy, evidence of neoplasia involving the endometrium was never seen.

Diagnosis of endometrial neoplasms may be made by rectal palpation, direct palpation of the endometrium through the cervix (Greenhoff & Kenney 1975), and by hysteroscopy (Mather et al. 1979). Endometrial neoplasia must be considered in all cases of persistant vulval haemorrhage. Some leiomyomas may be pedunculated and easily removed surgically. Some may impinge on the cervix and cause incompetence and secondary endometrial infection.

Cervical abnormality

Cervicitis usually accompanies endometritis as it is involved in the same pathogenesis, especially in cases of pneumovagina (see p. 8). The cervix appears inflamed and moist and sometimes frank pus is seen on a vaginoscopic examination. The diagnosis is confirmed by cytological and bacteriological examinations. Cervicitis and endometritis are major causes of subfertility in mares (see p. 69) and the treatment is as for acute endometritis (see p. 71). Correction of pneumovagina, where it occurs, is essential (see below).

Injury and laceration to the cervix may occur at traumatic parturition. This is an extremely serious problem. Healing usually results in cervical incompetence and adhesions and stenosis may occur. In our experience, damage to the cervix is one of the most serious breeding problems that may occur and invariably the prognosis is hopeless. A recurrent acute cervicitis and endometritis usually occurs and, despite minimal contamination techniques at the time of covering, conception is unusual. Even if it does occur, gestation failure invariably follows. Various surgical treatments have been reported, including the use of intracervical implants to prevent stenosis during healing (McGee 1962, see Lieux 1972).

In some pony mares, some degree of cervical incompetence appears to occur. Their cervix never seems to relax to the extent normally expected, despite normal oestrous behaviour throughout the breeding season. One imagines that conception failure occurs because the stallion is unable to ejaculate any or sufficient quantities of semen into the uterus. Treatment has been attempted by injection of oestrogens, with apparently variable success.

Vaginal abnormality

Pneumovagina is a common cause of subfertility in Thoroughbred mares and invariably caused by incompetence of the vulva associated with poor conformation (see p. 8). The condition is diagnosed vaginoscopically by the presence of inflammation, bubbles at the cervix and cervical cytological and bacteriological examinations (see pp. 531 and 537). The condition may be suspected by the sound of air entering the genital tract as the mare moves (wind-sucking).

The diagnosis and treatment of this condition was first described by Caslick (1937) (Figs 1.51, 1.52). The vulval labiae are infiltrated with local anaesthetic from the upper commissure to the level of the pelvic floor. A narrow strip of mucosa is then cut away on each side with straight scissors. The wounds are sutured together with soft nylon thread and healing occurs within about a week. In mares treated in this manner, for the first time, a continuous interlocking suture is found both practical and successful. In mares that are being resutured, that have been opened or that have torn at foaling, single interrupted sutures are recommended.

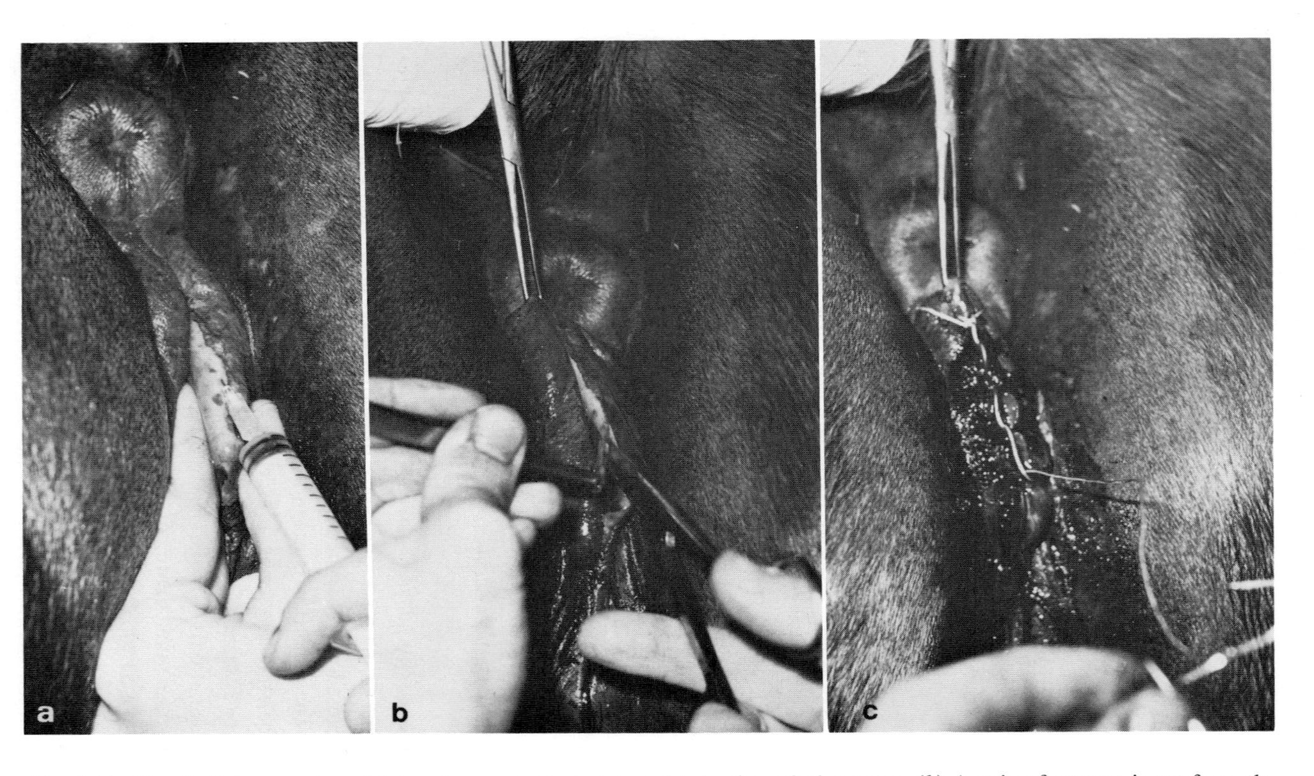

Fig. 1.51. The Caslick operation. (*a*) Local anaesthetic is injected into the vulval mucosa. (*b*) A strip of mucosa is cut from the vulval labia. (*c*) The wounds are brought together by a continuous or interrupted suture.

Perineal lacerations and rectovaginal fistulae may occur at parturition (see p. 269). This condition results in a severe acute endometritis and infertility, until the damage is corrected and the endometritis is treated. Treatment of the condition has been discussed on p. 270 using either the technique of Aanes (1964) or that of Geering (1979). The latter described the use of a temporary colostomy, so that

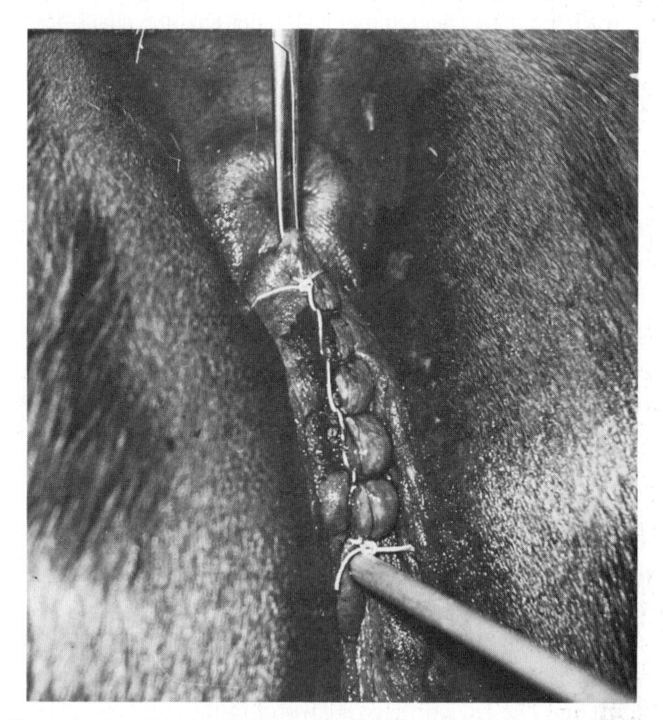

Fig. 1.52. The vulva should be sutured to the level of the pelvic floor, indicated here by a metal rod inserted into the vagina.

repair of the vaginal and perineal damage could be made almost immediately, without the complication of faecal contamination. This method also reduces the risk of faecal contamination of the uterus.

Some mares show a condition referred to as 'urine pooling' where vaginoscopic examination reveals a pool of urine sometimes partially covering the cervix. The condition results in an acute vaginitis, cervicitis and endometritis and usually prevents conception. This condition usually occurs in older mares whose uteri are enlarged and pendulous into the abdomen. The condition is also seen temporarily in some mares, at the first post-partum oestrus, and appears to resolve itself naturally, by the second post-partum oestrus. The uterus is then considerably smaller in size. Presumably the condition is caused by a 'dragging forward' of the posterior vagina and urethral opening and the forward and downward angle of the anterior vagina and cervix.

Mares showing evidence of this condition at the first post-partum oestrus should not be mated. In those where the condition does not resolve naturally, treatment should first be attempted by trying to reduce the size of the uterus. This may be achieved using uterine irrigation and intravenous oxytocin drips similar to that described before for the treatment of endometrial hyperplasia (see p. 93). Monin (1972) described a vaginoplasty operation for the correction of this condition. A transverse fold lies dorsal to the urethral orifice and runs horizontally across the vaginal floor. With the mare tranquillized and under epidural anaesthesia, the transverse fold is retracted posteriorly for approximately 5 cm and sutured, along its side, to the vaginal floor. This has the effect of extending the urethra caudally by 5 cm which allows complete evacuation of urine.

Vulval abnormality

Faulty vulval conformation, leading to incompetence and pneumovagina, has already been discussed (see above).

Perineal lacerations may occur at traumatic foaling (see p. 269) or by injury on sharp objects. Mares in oestrus, in a paddock with others, are sometimes prone to kicks in the vulval area resulting in bruising or laceration. Any damage to the vulva should be treated as carefully and as quickly as possible to try to prevent vulval incompetence, which may jeopardize her future breeding career. Episiotomy wounds made at foaling should be repaired as soon as convenient. There is no doubt that the immediate suturing of these wounds, without local anaesthetic, soon after expulsion of the foal often results in better healing and less scarring. This, of course, is not always practical.

Intermittent vulval bleeding is sometimes seen in mares with very prominent and probably varicosed veins at the dorsal aspect of the vulvovaginal area. These haemorrhaging veins may be diagnosed by parting the vaginal lips manually or by vaginoscopic examinations. The haemorrhage is a worry to the mare owner but appears to have no effect on the well-being of the mare or her fertility. On occasions, we have treated such mares with electrocautery.

The area of the clitoris, involving the clitoral fossa and sinuses (see p. 8) and the area of the urethral opening, may be sites for chronic 'infection' or 'contamination' with venereal-disease-producing bacteria, e.g. *H. equigenitalis, Kl. aerogenes* and *Ps. aeruginosa* (see pp. 75–81). These areas normally contain a varied micro-flora of contaminant organisms and bacteriological examination and the significance of the results obtained has already been discussed (see p. 70). If specific infection or contamination with a venereal-disease-producing organism is diagnosed, intensive local treatment is indicated with antibiotics suggested by the results of in vitro sensitivity tests. In some cases, surgical extirpation of the clitoris may be indicated (see p. 77). The injudicious use of prophylactic antibiotics and antiseptics on this area should be avoided, as the ease of removal of the normal contaminant micro-flora may encourage the establishment of the more resistant venereal-disease-producing organisms.

Persistent hymen can be recognized by resistance to the speculum about 12 cm inside the vulval labiae. An almost complete membrane with a series of pin-head-sized openings may be seen through the speculum. The presence of the membrane may cause apprehension that a congenital abnormality exists and that abdominal contents may be present on its anterior aspect. Such abnormalities are extremely rare but can be diagnosed by palpating the uterus per rectum and, if further evidence is required, by passing a laryngoscope through the centre of the membrane. Usually, if the genital organs are normal on the other side of the membrane, it may be broken down easily with a finger.

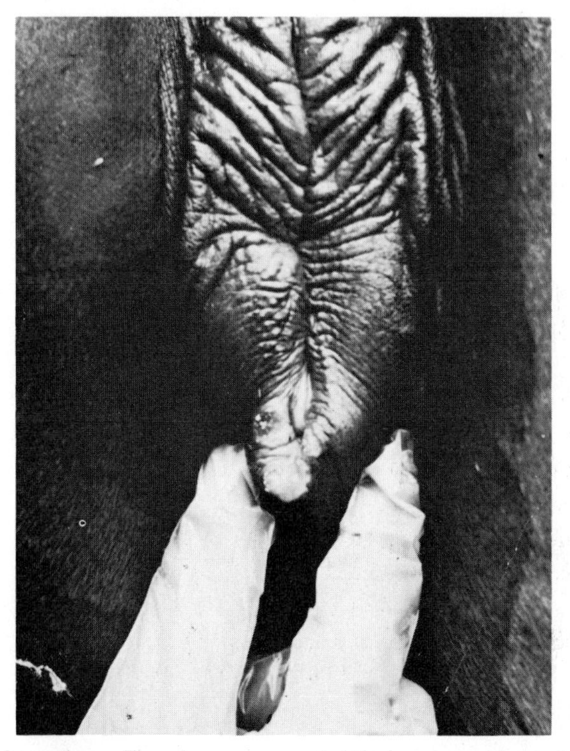

Fig. 1.53. Coital exanthema. Two ulcers are present at the lower commisure of the vulva labiae.

Equine coital exanthema is a specific herpesvirus infection causing vesiculation and ulceration of the mare's vulva (Fig. 1.53) and the stallion's penis (Pascoe et al. 1968, 1969 ; Gibbs et al. 1972). A symptomless carrier mare, or an overt but undiagnosed case, may infect the stallion, who may then infect the mares he mates until a diagnosis is made. The localized infection has no direct effect on fertility but mating must cease and this may cause managerial problems. The vesicles on the vulval labiae burst after two or three days, leaving ulcers which become secondarily infected with contaminant organisms and irritate the mare, who may appear in oestrus, repeatedly 'swishing' the tail or rubbing the hind-quarters. Mares usually appear free of clinical signs within 10–20 days but may be left with white scars in 'spot' form. Treatment is by local hygiene and antibacterial creams or powders to prevent secondary infection. Mares should always be examined for overt clinical signs before mating is allowed. For further discussion of the condition see p. 156.

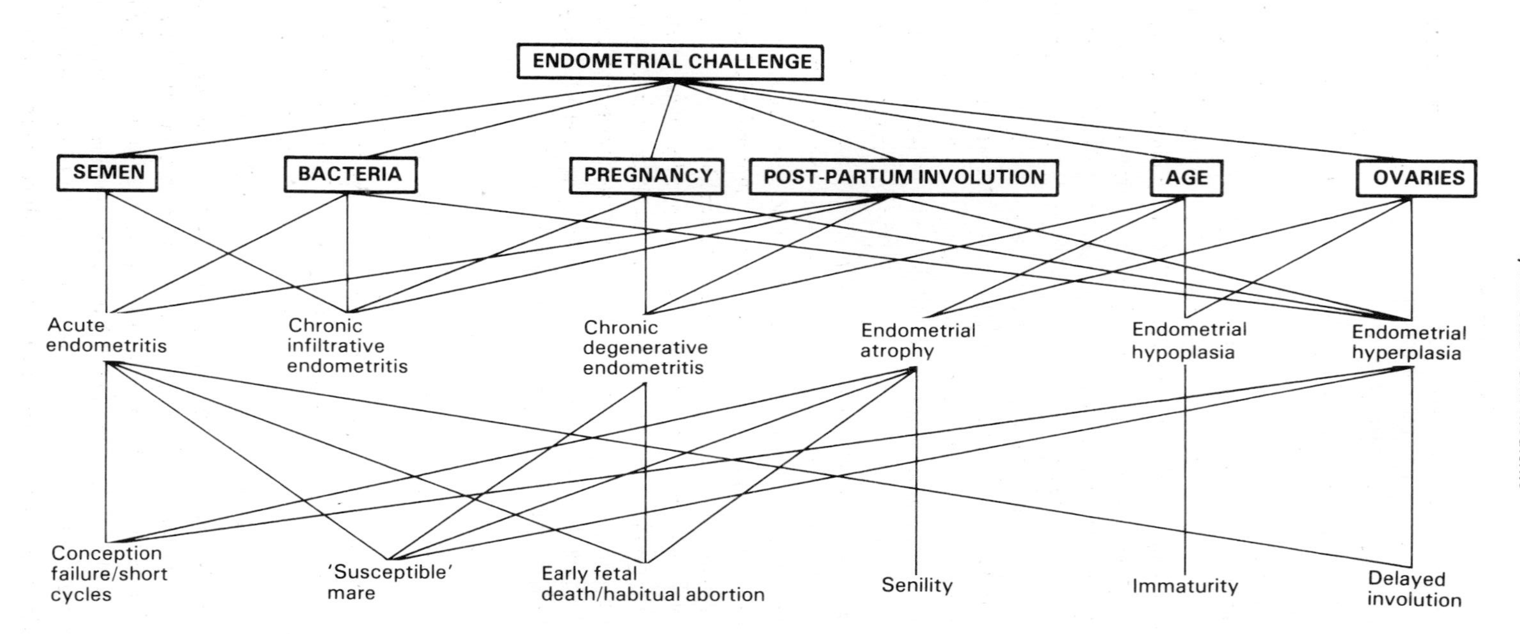

Fig. 1.54. Pathogenesis of endometrial abnormality leading to infertility or subfertility.

Pathogenesis

There is invariably a complex relationship and interaction between the various aetiological factors described above in the production of subfertility and infertility. It appears that endometrial abnormalities play a very important role in the subfertility syndrome in mares and a summary of the pathogenesis involved is represented in Fig. 1.54.

During her breeding career, a brood mare suffers 'challenge' to the endometrium by the repeated deposition of semen and bacteria into the uterus, the effects of repeated pregnancy and post-partum involution and the cyclic adaptations of the endometrium to changing hormonal patterns. The combination of these factors results in a progression of histopathological features, which form the endometrial 'wear and tear' syndrome. The endometrium responds to challenge by producing an acute endometritis which elicits a local immunological response demonstrated by the presence of a chronic infiltrative endometritis. The response to tissue damage and the glandular adaptations to pregnancy and hormonal changes result in a chronic degenerative endometritis. Advanced chronic degenerative endometritis and the affects of age and ovarian inactivity may lead to endometrial atrophy. Endometrial immaturity and chromosome or ovarian abnormality may manifest in endometrial hypoplasia. Delayed post-partum involution and repeated oestrogenic stimulation, seen in recurrent acute endometritis or cases of ovarian abnormality, may result in endometrial hyperplasia. Mares with a recurrent or persistent acute endometritis usually 'short cycle' and do not conceive. Many have a combination of endometrial histopathological lesions and are immunologically 'susceptible' to uterine infection. If conception does occur, or if the endometrium is chronically damaged and incompetent to maintain gestation, early fetal death and habitual abortion may occur. Some cases of true atrophy may reflect ovarian and endometrial senility. Most cases of endometrial hyperplasia, often associated with acute endometritis, may suggest delayed endometrial involution following parturition or abortion.

Diagnosis

The complex aetiology and pathogenesis of subfertility and infertility in the mare has already been discussed and the problems of diagnosis, as with many other aspects of veterinary medicine, may be compared to solving a jigsaw puzzle. The more diagnostic methods and aids that are used, the more pieces will be available to solve the puzzle. Most of these techniques have been discussed previously and brief reference only will be made here.

History. The individual's breeding record should be examined. A good chance of conception may be expected in maiden mares, those with a history of consecutive pregnancies or which have not been barren more than one year in four. Conversely, poor breeding performance can be expected in mares that have failed to conceive in two or more consecutive years, have produced fewer than three foals in four years, have aborted single or twin fetuses in the previous three years or have suffered abnormal gestation or birth in the previous year. Some mares breed only every other year and have reduced chances of conceiving or carrying a live foal to full term in two consecutive years.

A study of the individual's oestrous behaviour and clinical data from previous breeding seasons or in the preceding year may help diagnose infertility due to physiological or managerial factors. Silent heat and tendencies to undergo asynchrony between physiological events and behavioural patterns may be diagnosed in retrospect and confirmed by current rectal and vaginal examination.

The mare's previous bacteriological history of known contact with infected or contaminated stallions may be very important. A history of short cycling invariably indicates the presence of an acute endometritis whereas abnormally long dioestrous periods or erratic cycling may indicate ovarian malfunction, behavioural abnormalities, bad management, persistent corpus luteum or early fetal death.

Examination of the external genitalia. Visual examination of the vulva is important for signs of infection, damage and competence (see p. 102).

Vaginal examination. Vaginoscopic examination (see pp. 51 and 512) is valuable in diagnosis of infection, inflammation and damage to the vagina and cervix. In addition, it will give a useful indication of the stage of the mare's oestrous cycle, which may be compared with the findings of rectal palpation, teasing behaviour and endometrial histology.

Rectal palpation. Palpation of the ovaries and uterus per rectum (see p. 47) may reveal evidence of abnormality. Ovarian palpation may reveal the presence or absence of follicles which may be correlated with stage of cycle suggested by vaginoscopic examination and teasing behaviour.

Cervical cytological examinations. These examinations (see p. 537) may confirm or rule out the presence of an acute cervicitis or endometritis by the presence or absence of polymorphonuclear leucocytes.

Bacteriological examinations. Bacteriological examinations of the clitoral area, urethral opening and cervix/uterus may confirm or rule out the presence of potentially important bacterial organisms. The interpretation of bacteriological growths from these sites has been discussed previously (see pp. 70–81).

Endometrial biopsy. The technique has been discussed previously (see p. 54). Ricketts (1978) studied its use under practice conditions and found it to be safe and simple and a useful diagnostic and prognostic aid in subfertile and infertile mares. Bergman and Kenney (1975) and Ricketts (1978) found that one mid-horn biopsy was diagnostically representative of the whole uterus in the vast majority of cases. In those cases where palpable uterine abnormality was present, they recommended more than one site of biopsy. Hughes et al. (1979) suggested that, in mares with gross pyometra, one biopsy might not be representative of the whole endometrium.

The histopathological findings seen in cases of subfertility and infertility in mares have been previously described (see p. 95) and their significance has been discussed (see pp. 86 and 105). The technique gives more objective basis for logical treatment and may be used to monitor progress. There is no doubt that the widespread use of this technique has resulted in a much better understanding of the subfertility syndrome in mares and in particular its pathogenesis (see Fig. 1.54).

Assay of blood hormone levels. Hormonal 'imbalance' has long been a popular diagnosis for mares that fail to conceive and which undergo irregular oestrous cycles, fail to ovulate or remain in dioestrus or oestrus for prolonged periods. Hormonal therapy has also been practised in a wide variety of conditions associated with infertility. With the development of highly sensitive assay techniques which can measure changing blood hormone levels it should, in the future, be possible to verify diagnosis and create a rationale for therapy which up to now has been based on rather slender and subjective clinical impressions.

Normal endocrinological physiology in the mare has been discussed on pp. 11–18.

The influence of ovarian hormones on bacterial growth has been studied in a number of species (Black et al. 1953: Rowson et al. 1953; Hawk et al. 1960). Codazza and Nelli (1971) demonstrated that progesterone inhibited the growth of streptococci isolated from the equine uterus but oestradiol had a bacteriocidal action on this organism and inhibited *Staph. aureus* and *Klebsiella* spp.

The presence of a corpus luteum may be diagnosed by rising levels of blood progesterone from zero during oestrus to greater than 3 ng/ml three days after ovulation. Assay may therefore be used to confirm the diagnosis of failure to ovulate and provide a more accurate assessment than rectal examination.

Although better knowledge of the endocrinology of FSH, LH and oestrogens are now available (see p. 15), the value of these estimations in the face of subfertility still remains to be examined.

Hysteroscopy. Mather et al. (1979) have described the use of fibreoptic techniques for hysteroscopy in 40 subfertile mares. Transluminal adhesions, endometrial cysts, diffuse fibrosis, fluid accumulation and myometrial tumours were found in 26 mares. When compared to other techniques, hysteroscopy did not seem to be superior to uterine biopsy but had some advantage over rectal palpation as a single diagnostic technique. They studied the use of various antibiotics and disinfectants in the uteri of clinically normal dioestrous mares. Fibreoptic examinations were performed before and after infusion of three mares. No gross pathological changes were seen three days after the infusion of potassium, penicillin, chloramphenicol succinate or a soluble oxytetracyline powder in a dextrose base. Lugol's iodine caused severe inflammation, fibrin deposition and ulceration of the endometrium. Ampicillin resulted in a white precipitate which adhered to the endometrium for 10 days after treatment.

Fallopian tube patency test. The starch grain test has been described by Allen et al. (1979) (see p. 67).

Laparoscopy. A laparoscope introduced into the abdomen through a skin incision provides a means of visual examination of the internal genital organs (Heinze et al. 1972). This technique has use for research and for diagnosis in a limited number of clinical cases where adhesions, neoplasia or haemorrhage are causing infertility. It could be developed, where other routes are impractical, for biopsy, withdrawal of fluid samples and injection of therapeutic substances.

Laparotomy. In cases where fallopian tube abnormality is suspected (see p. 66), exploratory laparotomy under general anaesthesia may be indicated.

Chromosome analysis. In cases with ovarian cyclic irregularities and very small or absent ovaries, this technique may be indicated (see p. 60).

Treatment

Treatment of subfertility in mares is based first on the accurate diagnosis of abnormality and an accurate interpretation of the significance of that abnormality. Experience and knowledge of the pathogenesis of these conditions is essential. Logical treatment must be based on this overall appraisal. The success or otherwise of treatment must be assessed by follow-up diagnostic methods. Then a prophylactic programme with which to structure the future breeding management of the mare may be developed. Specific treatments have already been discussed.

Prognosis

On the basis of diagnostic techniques performed and in particular those of endometrial biopsy, Kenney (1978) classifies mares in terms of their ability to carry a foal to term, in the following way:

Category 1. Mares with no significant histopathological findings. These are given a good prognosis.

Category 2. Various combinations of moderate, widespread or scattered inflammatory or fibrotic lesions and any type of endometrial atrophy are classified in this group. These mares are given a reasonable prognosis with rational treatment and breeding using minimal contamination techniques.

Category 3. Widespread periglandular fibrosis, of any severity, and wisespread severe inflammatory changes are in this group. Mares are given a very poor prognosis even with treatment followed by breeding with minimal contamination techniques.

The post-biopsy breeding history of mares in his series support Kenny's classification.

Of the 323 mares examined for reasons of infertility or subfertility by Ricketts (1978) reliable post-biopsy breeding histories were available in 194 cases. The breeding histories for the covering season following endometrial biopsy were compared with endometrial histopathological changes (Fig. 1.55). Interpretation of these data is complicated by the fact that the mares, being clinical cases, were treated following the biopsy, if treatment was indicated. In many of the cases, follow-up biopsies suggested that the endometrial histopathological lesions previously noted had been removed or changed. Thus, the post-biopsy breeding statistics reflected the ability of different histopathological groups to respond to treatment and prophylactics.

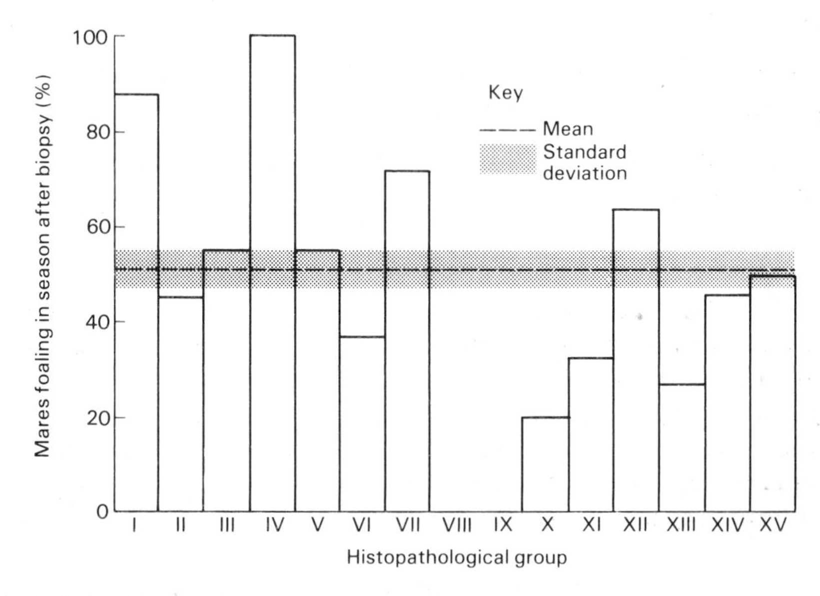

Fig. 1.55. Post-biopsy performance of mares in each pathological group (see Table 1.5, p. 110).

The standard error of the group was calculated at 4% and thus those groups with a foaling percentage of over 55% (Groups I, III, IV, V, VII and XII) were considered to have a reasonably good prognosis for response to treatment and future breeding. Those with a foaling percentage of less than 47% (Groups II, VI, IX, X, XI, XIII and XIV) were considered to have a relatively poor prognosis for response to treatment and future breeding. The figures for mares in Group XV were not statistically different from the overall foaling percentage and they were thought to have a future breeding prognosis of 50 : 50. There were insufficient mares in Group VIII to make meaningful comments. Similarly there were insufficient numbers of mares who aborted or were recorded as having early fetal deaths to make meaningful comment on this subject.

It would appear from these figures that endometrial atrophy is a very significant histopathological finding, suggesting an extremely poor response to treatment and future breeding prognosis and justifiable grounds for retiring the mare. This does not apply to mares with the endometrial atrophy of deep winter anoestrus which disappeared following ovarian activity.

TABLE 1.5 Endometrial histopathological findings: the combinations of histopathological findings associated with each histopathological group

Histopathological group	*Histopathological findings*
I	No significant endometrial histopathological findings
II	Acute endometritis (AE)
III	Chronic infiltrative endometritis (CIE)
IV	AE + CIE
V	Chronic degenerative endometritis (CDE)
VI	AE + CIE + CDE
VII	CIE + CDE
VIII	Endometrial atrophy (EA)
IX	AE + EA
X	CIE + CDE + EA
XI	Endometrial hypoplasia (E Hypo)
XII	Endometrial hyperplasia (E Hyper)
XIII	AE + E Hyper
XIV	CIE + CDE + E Hyper
XV	AE + CIE + CDE + E Hyper

Mares showing signs of endometrial hypoplasia appeared to have had a poor breeding prognosis. Closer examination of this group, however, suggested that except in cases of specific genital abnormality the reverse was in fact true. Of the eight mares who did not produce foals following the covering season after biopsy, three were associated with chromosome abnormalities and two were associated with ovarian granulosa cell tumours. If these five mares are removed from the series, the breeding prognosis for this histopathological lesion was good (57% of the mares produced a live foal after the covering season following the biopsy).

It is comforting to see that mares showing no signs of significant endometrial histopathological findings had an excellent post-biopsy breeding prognosis.

Mares with acute endometritis but also signs of a healthy cell-mediated response (Group IV) had an excellent response to treatment. This was not so, however, for those without chronic infiltrative endometritis (Group II) or for those complicated by chronic degenerative abnormalities (Group VI), endometrial atrophy (Group IX) and endometrial hyperplasia (Group XIII). This would appear logical as many of these latter groups contained cases of long-term infection, mares with 'wear and tear' lesions and 'susceptible mares'.

Uncomplicated cases of endometrial hyperplasia (Group XII) responded well to treatment. These mares were often cases of early fetal loss. Those complicated by acute endometritis (Group XIII) and by chronic infiltrative and degenerative endometritis (Group XIV), often long-standing infection or delayed post-parturient involution cases, did not respond so well to treatment. The better response to treatment of mares in Group XV is not easily explained.

By themselves, chronic degenerative endometritis ('wear and tear') lesions (Group VII) respond well to treatment but it must be emphasized that these mares were given intensive treatment prior to the breeding season and then very strict prophylactic measures, using minimal contamination methods (Kenney et al. 1975*a*) during the season. It is considered that the success rate for this type of mare is directly proportional to the effort of the clinician and the stud farm management and to the patience of the owner.

References and further reading

Aanes, W.A. (1964) Surgical repair of third-degree perineal laceration and rectovaginal fistula in the mare. *J. Am. vet. med. Ass.*, **144**, 485.

Allen, W.E., Kessey, B.M. & Noakes, D.E. (1979) Evaluation of uterine tube function in pony mares. *Vet. Rec.*, **105**, 364.

Allen, W.R. & Rossdale, P.D. (1973) Preliminary studies upon the use of prostaglandins for inducing and synchronizing oestrus in Thoroughbred mares. *Equine vet. J.*, **5**, 137.

Allen, W.R. & Rowson, L.E.A. (1973) Control of the mare's oestrus cycle by prostaglandins. *J. Reprod. Fert.*, **33**, 539.

Allen, W.R., Stewart, F., Cooper, M.J., Crowhurst, R.C., Simpson, D.J., McEnery, R.J., Greenwood, R.E.J., Rossdale, P.D. & Ricketts, S.W. (1974) Further studies into the use of synthetic prostaglandin analogues for inducing luteolysis in mares. *Equine vet. J.*, **6**, 31.

Allen, W.R. Urwin, V., Simpson, D.J., Greenwood, R.E.S., Crowhurst, R.C., Ellis, D.R., Ricketts, S.W., Hunt, M.D.N. & Wingfield-Digby, N.J. (1980) Preliminary studies on the use of an oral progestagen (Regumate) to induce oestrus and ovulation in seasonally anoestrous Thoroughbred mares. *Equine vet. J.*, **12**, 141.

Anderson, S.J. (1922) Sterility in relation to animal breeding. *Res. Bull. Ky agric. exp. Stn*, **244**, 203.

Andrews, F.N. & McKenzie, F.F. (1941) Estrus, ovulation and related phenomena in the mare. *Res. Bull. Mo. agric. Exp. Stn*, 329.

Atherton, J.G., (1975) The identification of equine genital strains of *Klebsiella* and *Enterobacter* species. *Equine vet. J.*, **7**, 207.

Arthur, G.H. (1958) An analysis of the reproductive function of mares based on post-mortem examination. *Vet. Rec.*, **70**, 682.

Arthur, G.H. (1969) The ovary of the mare in health and disease. *Equine vet. J.*, **4**, 153.

Arthur, G.H. (1970) The induction of oestrus in mares by uterine infusion of saline. *Vet. Rec.*, **86**, 584.

Arthur, G.H. (1975) Influence of intrauterine saline infusion upon the oestrous cycle of the mare. *J. Reprod. Fert.*, Suppl. **23**, 231

Bain, A.M. (1948) Problems associated with infertility in the brood mare. *Aust. vet. J.*, **24**, 152.

Benson, J.A., Dawson, F.L.M., Durrent, D.S., Edwards, P. & Powell, D.G. (1978) Serological response in mares affected by contagious equine metritis 1977. *Vet. Rec.*, **102**, 277.

Bergin, W.R. & Shipley, W.D. (1968) Genital health in the mare, II. The vulva. *Vet. Med. small Anim. Clin.*, **63**, 447.

Bergman, R.V., & Kenney, R.M., (1975) Representativesness of a uterine biopsy in the mare. *Proc. 21st ann. Conv. Am. Ass. equine Practnrs*, 355.

Berliner, V.R. (1959) The estrous cycle of the mare. In *Reproduction in Domestic Animals*, ed. H.H. Cole & P.T. Cupps, 4th ed., p. 267. New York and London: Academic Press.

Black, W.G., Ulberg, L.C., Kidder, H.E., Simon, J., McNutt, S.H. & Casida, L.E. (1953) Inflammatory response of the bovine endometrium. *Am. J. vet. Res.*, **14**, 179.

Bornstein, S. (1967) The genetic sex of two intersexual horses and some notes on the karyotype of normal horses. *Acta vet. scand.*, **8**, 291.

Bostock, D.E. & Owen, L.N. (1975) *Neoplasia in the Cat, Dog and Horse.* London: Wolfe Medical Publications.

Bowen, J.M. (1979) Problems that can affect some stallions in the breeding season and their management. Paper presented to 18th ann. Congr. BEVA, Exeter.

Bouters, R., Vandeplassche, M. & De Moor, A. (1972) An intersex (male pseudo-hermaphrodite) horse with 64 XX/65 XXY mosaicism. *Equine vet. J.*, **4**, 150.

Brandt, G.W. & Manning, J.P. (1969) Improved uterine biopsy techniques for diagnosing infertility in the mare. *Vet. Med.*, **64**, 977.

Bright, S., Antczak, D. & Ricketts, S.W. (1976) Studies on equine leucocyte antigens. *Proc. 4th int. Conf. equine infect. Dis.*, 229.

Bryans, J.T. & Hendrick, J.B. (1979) Epidemiological observations on contagious equine metritis in Kentucky 1978. *J. Reprod. Fert.*, Suppl. **27**, 343.

Burkhardt, J. (1947) Transition from anoestrus in the mare and the effects of artificial lighting. *J. agric. Sci., Camb.*, **37**, 64.

Burkhardt, J. (1954) Treatment of anoestrus in the mare by uterine irrigation. *Vet. Rec.*, **66**, 375.

Butterfield, R.M., Matthews, R.G. & Ropiha, R.T. (1964) Observations on the fertility of Thoroughbred mares. *Aust. vet. J.*, **40**, 415.

Caslick, E.A. (1937) The vulva and vulvo-vaginal orifice and its relation to genital tracts of the Thoroughbred mare. *Cornell Vet.*, **27**, 178.

Chandley, A.N., Fletcher, J., Rossdale, P.D., Peace, C.K., Ricketts, S.W., McEnery, R.J., Thorne, J.P., Short, R.V. & Allen, W.R. (1975) Chromosome abnormalities as a cause of infertility in mares. *J. Reprod. Fert.*, Suppl. **23**, 377.

Channing, C.P. (1966) Progesterone biosynthesis by equine granulosa cells growing in tissue culture. *Nature, Lond.*, **210**, 1266.

Codazza, D. & Nelli, A. (1971) Research into equine infertility of bacterial origin. 1. Effects of hormonally active substances on bacteria, often associated with 'non-specific' metritis. *Folia vet.*, **1**, 268.

Condon, W.A. & Black, D.L. (1976) Catecholamine induced stimulation of progesterone by the bovine corpus luteum in vitro. *Biol. Reprod.*, **15**, 573.

Condon, W.A., Ganjam, V.K. & Kenney, R.M. (1979) Catecholamines and equine luteal progestagens. *J. Reprod. Fert.*, Suppl. **27**, 199.

Cooper, W.L. & Wert, N.E. (1975) Wintertime breeding of mares using artificial light and insemination: six year's experience. *Proc. 21st ann. Cong. Am. Ass. equine Practnrs,* 245.

Cross, B.A. (1972) The hypothalamus. In *Reproduction in Mammals. 3. Hormones in Reproduction,* ed. C.R. Austin & R.V. Short, p. 29. Cambridge: Cambridge University Press.

Crouch, J.R.F., Atherton, J.G. & Platt, H. (1972) Venereal transmission of *Klebsiella aerogenes* in a Thoroughbred stud from a persistently infected stallion. *Vet. Rec.*, **90**, 21.

Crowhurst, R.C. (1977) Genital infection in mares. *Vet. Rec.*, **100**, 476.

Crowhurst, R.C., Simpson, D.J., Greenwood, R.E.S. & Ellis, D.R. (1979) Contagious equine metritis. *Vet. Rec.*, **104**, 465.

Croxton-Smith, P., Benson, J.A., Dawson, F.L.M. & Powell, D.G. (1978) A complement fixation test for antibody to the contagious equine metritis organism. *Vet. Rec.*, **103**, 275.

Dallenbach-Hellweg, G. (1971) *Histopathology of the Endometrium.* Berlin: Springer.

David, J.S.E., Frank, C.J. & Powell, D.G. (1977) Contagious metritis 1977. *Vet. Rec.*, **101**, 189.

Day, F.T. (1939) Some observations on the causes of infertility in horse breeding. *Vet. Rec.*, **51**, 581.

Day, F.T. (1940) Clinical and experimental observations on reproduction in the mare. *J. agric. Sci., Camb.*, **30**, 244.

Day, F.T. (1957) The veterinary clinician's approach to breeding problems in mares. *Vet. Rec.*, **69**, 1258.

Dewes, H.F. (1973) Thoroughbred breeding in New Zealand. *Proc. 19th ann. Conv. Am. Ass. equine Practnrs,* 39.

Dimock, W.W. (1939) Equine breeding hygiene. *J. Am. vet. med. Ass.*, **94**, 469.

Dimock, W.W. & Edwards, P.R. (1928) Pathology and bacteriology of the reproductive organs of mares in relation to sterility. *Res. Bull. Ky agric. Exp. Stn,* 286

Douglas, R.H. & Ginther, O.J. (1972) Effect of prostaglandin $F_2\alpha$ on length of diestrus in mares. *Prostaglandins,* **2**, 265.

Douglas, R.H. & Ginther, O.J. (1975) Effects of prostaglandin $F_2\alpha$ on the oestrous cycle and pregnancy in mares. *J. Reprod. Fert.*, Suppl. **23**, 257.

Ensminger, E.M. (1966) Breeding horses in the United States. *Veterinarian, Oxford,* **4**, 47.

Evans, J.W., Hughes, J.P., Neely, D.P., Stabenfeldt, G.H. & Winget, C.M. (1979) Episodic LH secretion patterns in the mare during the oestrous cycle. *J. Reprod. Fert.*, Suppl. **27**, 143.

Evans, M.J. & Irvine, C.H.G. (1975) Serum concentrations of FSH, LH and progesterone during the oestrous cycle and early pregnancy in the mare. *J. Reprod. Fert.*, Suppl. **23**, 193.

Evans, M.J. & Irvine, C.H.G. (1977) Induction of follicular development, maturation and ovulation by gonadotrophin releasing hormone administration to acyclic mares. *Biol. Reprod.*, **16**, 452.

Evans, M.J. & Irvine, C.H.G. (1979) Induction of follicular development and ovulation in seasonally acyclic mares using gonadotrophin-releasing hormones and progesterone. *J. Reprod. Fert.*, Suppl. **27**, 113.

Farrely, B.T. & Mullaney, P.E. (1964) Cervical and uterine infection in Thoroughbred mares. *Ir. vet. J.*, **18**, 201.

Fernie, D.S., Cayzer, I. & Chalmers, S.R. (1979) A passive haemagglutination test for the detection of antibodies to the contagious equine metritis organism. *Vet. Rec.*, **104**, 260.

Freedman, L.J., Garcia, M.C. & Ginther, O.J. (1979) Influence of ovaries and photoperiod on reproductive function in the mare. *J. Reprod. Fert.*, Suppl. **27**, 79.

van Furth, R., Cohn, Z.A., Hirsch, J.G., Humphery, J.H., Spector, W.G. & Langevoort, H.L. (1972) The mononuclear phagocyte system: a new classification of macrophages, monocytes, and their precursor cells. *Bull. Wld Hlth Org.*, **46**, 845.

Fylling, P. (1971) Vasopressin-induced increase in peripheral plasma progesterone levels during early human pregnancy. *Acta endocr., Copenh.*, **66**, 273.

Ganjam, V.K., Kenney, R.M. & Flickinger, G. (1975) Plasma progestagens in cyclic, pregnant and post-partum mares. *J. Reprod. Fert.*, **23**, 441.

Garcia, M.C., Freedman, L.H. & Ginther, O.J. (1979) Interaction of seasonal and ovarian factors in the regulation of LH and FSH secretion in the mare. *J. Reprod. Fert.*, Suppl. **27**, 103.

Garcia, M.C. & Ginther, O.J. (1976) Effects of ovariectomy and season on plasma luteinizing hormones in mares. *Endocrinology*, **98**, 958.

Geering, R.R. (1979) An alternative approach to treatment of rectovaginal fistulae. Paper presented to 18th ann. Congr. BEVA, Exeter.

Gerneke, W.H. & Coubrough, R.I. (1970) Intersexuality in the horse. *Onderstepoort J. vet. Res.*, **37**, 211.

Gibbs, E.P.J., Roberts, M.C. & Morris, J.M. (1972) Equine coital exanthema in the United Kingdom. *Equine vet. J.*, **4**, 74.

Ginther, O.J. (1974) Occurrences of anestrus, diestrus and ovulation over a 12 month period in mares. *Am. J. vet. Res.*, **35**, 1173.

Ginther, O.J. (1979) *Reproductive Biology of the Mare*, p. 247. Cross Plains, Wis.: Ginther.

Ginther, O.J. & First, N.L. (1971) Maintenance of the corpus luteum in hysterectomized mares. *Am. J. vet. Res.*, **32**, 1687.

Ginther, O.J. & Wentworth, B.C. (1974) Effect of a synthetic gonadotrophin releasing hormone on plasma concentrations of luteinising hormone in ponies. *Am. J. vet. Res.*, **35**, 79.

Greenhof, G.R. & Kenney, R.M. (1975) Evaluation of reproductive status of non-pregnant mares. *J. Am. vet. med. Ass.*, **167**, 449.

Greenwood, R.E.S. & Ellis, D.R. (1976) *Klebsiella aerogenes* in mares. *Vet. Rec.*, **99**, 439.

Gribble, D.H. (1972) The endocrine system. In *Equine Medicine and Surgery*, ed. E.J. Catcott & J.F. Smithcors, p. 433. Wheaton, Ill.: American Veterinary Publications.

Gygax, A.P., Ganjam, V.K. & Kenney, R.M. (1979) Clinical microbiological and histological changes associated with uterine involution in the mare. *J. Reprod. Fert.*, Suppl. **27**, 571.

Hammond, J. & Wodzicki, K. (1941) Anatomical and histological changes during the oestrous cycle of the mare. *Proc. R. Soc. B*, **130**, 1.

Hancock, J.L. (1948) Notes on oestrus, ovulation and pregnancy in the mare. *Vet. Rec.*, **60**, 679.

Hartigan, P.J. (1970) A Study of the Histopathology and Histochemistry of the Endometrium in the Repeat Breeder Cow. PhD thesis, Trinity College, Dublin.

Hawk, H.W., Turner, G.D. & Sykes, J.F. (1960) The effect of ovarian hormones on the uterine defence mechanism during early stages of induced infection. *Am. J. vet. Res.*, **21**, 644.

Hawkins, D.L., Neely, D.P. & Stabenfeldt, G.H. (1979) Plasma progesterone concentrations derived from the administration of exogenous progesterone to ovariectomised mares. *J. Reprod. Fert.*, Suppl. **27**, 211.

Hay, M.F., Allen, W.R. & Lewis, I.M. (1975) The distribution of Δ^5-3β-hydroxysteroid dehydrogenase in the graafian follicle of the mare. *J. Reprod. Fert.*, Suppl. **23**, 323.

Hazard, G.H., Hughes, K.L. & Penson, P.J. (1979) Contagious equine metritis in Australia. *J. Reprod. Fert.*, Suppl. **27**, 337.

Heinze, H., Klug, E. & von Lepel, J.D.F. (1972) Visual examination of the internal genital organs of mares for diagnosis and treatment (preliminary report) (In German with English summary). *Dt. tierartzl. Wschr.*, **79**, 49.

Hillman, R.B. & Loy, R.G. (1969) Estrogen excretion in mares in relation to various reproductive states. *Proc. 15th ann. Conv. Am. Ass. equine Practnrs,* 111.

Hughes, J.P. & Loy, R.G. (1969) Investigations on the effect of intrauterine inoculations of *Streptococcus zooepidemicus* in the mare. *Proc. 15th ann. Conv. Am. Ass. equine Practnrs,* 289.

Hughes, J.P. & Loy, R.G. (1975) The relation of infection to infertility in the mare and stallion. *Equine vet. J.,* 7, 155.

Hughes, J.P., Loy, R.G., Atwood, C., Astbury, A.C. & Burd, H.E. (1966) The occurrence of *Pseudomonas* in the reproductive tract of mares and its effect on fertility. *Cornell Vet.,* **56**, 595.

Hughes, J.P., Stabenfeldt, G.H. & Evans, J.W. (1972*a*) Estrous cycle and ovulation in the mare. *J. Am. vet. med. Ass.,* **161**, 1367.

Hughes, J.P., Stabenfeldt, G.H. & Evans, J.W. (1972*b*) Clinical and endocrinological aspects of the estrus cycle of the mare. *Proc. 18th ann. Conv. Am Ass. equine Practnrs,* 119.

Hughes, J.P., Stabenfeldt, G.H., Kindall, H., Kennedy, P.C., Edquist, L.E., Neely, D.P. & Schalm, O.W. (1979) Pyometra in the mare. *J. Reprod. Fert.,* Suppl. **27**, 321.

Hunt, M. & Rossdale, P.D. (1963) A specific venereal diseas of Thoroughbred mares. *Vet. Rec.,* **75**, 1092.

Hurtgen, J.P. (1975) Alterations of the equine estrous cycle following uterine and/or cervical manipulations. *Proc. 21st ann. Conv. Am. Ass. equine Practnrs,* 368.

Hurtgen, J.P. & Ganjam, V.K. (1979) The effect of intrauterine and cervical manipulation on the equine oestrous cycle and hormone profiles. *J. Reprod. Fert.,* Suppl. **27**, 191.

Hutton, C.A. & Meacham, T.N. (1968) Reproductive efficiency on fourteen horse farms. *J. Anim. Sci.,* **27**, 434.

Hyland, J.H. & Bristol, F. (1979) Synchronization of oestrus and timed insemination of mares. *J. Reprod. Fert.,* Suppl. **27**, 251.

Jackson, P.S., Allen, W.R., Ricketts, S.W. & Hall, R. (1979) The irritancy of chlorhexidine gluconate in the genital tract of the mare. *Vet. Rec.,* **105**, 122.

Jeffcott, L.B. (1979) Report on the thoroughbred wastage survey. Paper presented to 18th ann. Cong. BEVA, Exeter.

Jubb, K.V.F. & Kennedy, P.C. (1968) *Pathology of Domestic Animals,* Vol 1. New York and London: Academic Press

Katsh, S. & Katsh, F. (1968) Immunology of sperm-induced in fertility. *Postgrad. Med.,* **43**, 230.

Kaufman, W.C. (1975) The effect of rectal palpation on reproduction in mares. *Proc. 21st. ann. Conv. Am. Ass. equine. Practnrs,* 229.

Kenney, R.M. (1975) Prognostic value of endometrial biopsy of the mare. *J. Reprod. Fert.,* Suppl. **23**, 347.

Kenney, R.M. (1977) Salpingitis in the mare. *Proc. 23rd ann. Conv. Am. Ass. equine Practnrs,* 127.

Kenney, R.M. (1978) Cyclic and pathologic changes of the mare endometrium as detected by biopsy with a note on early embryonic death. *J. Am. vet. med. Ass.,* **172**, 241.

Kenney, R.M., Bergman, R.V., Cooper, W.L. & Morse, G.W. (1975*a*) Minimal contamination techniques for breeding mares: technique and preliminary findings. *Proc. 21st ann. Conv. Am. Ass. equine Practnrs,* 327.

Kenney, R.M., Condon, W.A., Ganjam, J.K. & Channing, C. (1979) Morphological and biochemical correlates of equine ovarian follicles as a function of their state of viability or atresia. *J. Reprod. Fert.,* Suppl. **27**, 163.

Kenney, R.M. & Ganjam, V.K. (1975) Selected pathological changes of the mare uterus and ovary. *J. Reprod. Fert.,* Suppl. **23**, 335.

Kenney, R.M., Ganjam, V.K., Cooper, W.L. & Lauderdale, J.W. (1975*b*) The use of prostaglandin $F_2\alpha$-THAM salt in mares in clinical anoestrus. *J. Reprod. Fert.,* Suppl. **23**, 247.

Kenney, R.M. & Khaleel, S.A. (1975) Bacteriostatic activity of the mare uterus; a progress report on immunoglobulins. *J. Reprod. Fert.,* Suppl. **23**, 357.

Kiefer, B.L., Roser, J.F., Evans, J.W., Neely, D.P. & Pacheco, C.A. (1979) Progesterone patterns observed with multiple injections of a $PGF_2\alpha$ analogue in the cyclic mare. *J. Reprod. Fert.,* Suppl. **27**, 237.

Knudsen, O. (1964) Partial dilatation of the cervix as a cause of sterility in the mare. *Cornell Vet.,* **54**, 423.

Knudsen, O. & Velle, W. (1961) Ovarian oestrogen levels in the non-pregnant mare. Relationship to histological appearance of the uterus and its clinical status. *J. Reprod. Fert.,* **2**, 130.

Kooistra, L.H. & Ginther, O.J. (1975) Effect of photoperiod on reproductive activity and hair in mares. *Am. J. vet. Res.,* **36**, 1413.

Kortum, B. (1979) Use and significance of an indwelling uterine infusor (IUI) in the mare's uterus. Paper presented to 18th ann. Congr. BEVA, Exeter.

Laing, J.A. & Leech, F.B. (1975) The frequency of infertility in thoroughbred. *J. Reprod. Fert.,* Suppl. **23**, 307.

Lanfenstein-Duffy, H. (1968) Indications of surgical procedure for uterine curettage in the mare. *J. Am. vet. med. Ass.,* **153**, 1570.

Lieux, P. (1970) The relationship between the appearance of the cervix and the heat cycle in the mare. *Vet. Med.,* **65**, 879.

Lieux, P. (1972) Reproductive and genital disease. In *Equine Medicine and Surgery,* ed. E.J. Catcott & J.F. Smithcors, 2nd ed., p. 597. Wheaton, Ill.: American Veterinary Publications.

von Lepel, J. (1975) Control of fertility in thoroughbred horses in West Germany. *J. Reprod. Fert.,* Suppl. **23**, 311.

Loy, R.G., Buell, J.R. Stevenson, W. & Hamm, D. (1979) Sources of variation in response intervals after prostaglandin treatment in mares with functional corpora lutea. *J. Reprod. Fert.,* Suppl. **27**, 229.

Loy, R.G. & Hughes, J.P. (1966) The effects of human chorionic gonadotrophin on ovulation, length of estrus and fertility in the mare. *Cornell Vet.,* **56**, 41.

Loy, R.G., Hughes, J.P., Richards, W.P.C. & Swan, S.M. (1975) Effects of progesterone on reproductive function in mares after parturition. *J. Reprod. Fert.,* Suppl. **23**, 291.

Loy, R.G. & Swan, S.M. (1966) Effects of exogenous progestagens on reproductive phenomena in the mare. *J. Anim. Sci.,* **25**, 821.

McCracken, J.A. (1972) Prostaglandins and luteal regression. A review. *Res. Prostaglandins,* **1**, 1.

Mahaffey, L.W. (1950*a*) Studies of fertility in the Thoroughbred mare. 1. Introduction. *Aust. vet. J.,* **26**, 267.

Mahaffey, L.W. (1950*b*) Studies of fertility in the Thoroughbred mare. 2. Early post-partum oestrus ('foal heat'). *Aust. vet. J.,* **26**, 295.

Mahaffey, L.W. & Adam, N.M. (1964) Abortions associated with mycotic lesions of the placenta in mares. *J. Am. vet. med. Ass.,* **144**, 24.

Mahaffey, L.W. & Rossdale, P.D. (1965) An abortion due to *Allescheria boydii* and general observations concerning mycotic abortions of mares. *Vet. Rec.,* **77**, 541.

Marca, G. Codazza, D. & Lodola, F. (1972) Sulla caratterizzione della klebsiellae associate a infertilita equina da causa batteriche. *Folia vet.,* **2**, 369.

Mather, E.C., Refsal, K.R., Gustafsson, B.K., Seguin, B.E. & Whitmore, H.L. (1979) The use of fibre-optic techniques in clinical diagnosis and visual assessment of experimental intrauterine therapy in mares. *J. Reprod. Fert.,* Suppl. **27**, 293.

Mattner, P.E. (1969) Phagocytosis of spermatozoa by lecuocytes in bovine cervical mucus in vitro. *J. Reprod. Fert.,* **20**, 133.

Matthews, R.G., Ropiha, R.T. & Butterfield, R.M. (1967) The phenomenon of foal heat in mares. *Aust. vet. J.,* **43**, 579.

Meagher, D.M., Wheat, J.D., Hughes, J.P., Stabenfeldt, G.H. & Harris, B.A. (1977) Granulosa cell tumours in mares – a review of 78 cases. *Proc. 23rd ann. Conv. Am. Ass. equine Practnrs,* 133.

Merkt, H. (1966) Foal heat and fetal absorption (In German with English summary). *Zuchthyg. FortpflSto. Besam. Haustiere,* **1**, 102.

Mirskaja, L.M. & Petropavlovskii, V.V. (1937) The reduction of normal duration of heat in the mare by the administration of prolan. *Problemy Zhivot.,* **4**, 22 (*Anim. Breed. Abstr.,* **5**, 387).

Monin, T. (1972) Vaginoplasty: a surgical treatment for urine pooling in the mare. *Proc. 18th ann. Cong. Am. Ass. equine Practnrs,* 99.

Morrow, G.L. (1967) Uterine curettage. *J. Am. vet. med. Ass.,* **151**, 1615.

Munro, C.D., Renton, J.P. & Butcher, R.A. (1979) The control of oestrous behaviour in the mare. *J. Reprod. Fert.,* Suppl. **27**, 217.

Neely, D.P., Hughes, J.P., Stabenfeldt, G.H. & Evans, J.W. (1975) The influence of intrauterine saline infusion on luteal function and cyclical activity in the mare. *J. Reprod. Fert.,* Suppl. **23**, 235.

Neely, D.P., Kindahl, H., Stabenfeldt, G.H., Edqvist, L.E. & Hughes, J.P. (1979) Prostaglandin release patterns in the mare: Physiological, pathophysiological and therapeutic responses. *J. Reprod. Fert.*, Suppl. **27**, 181.

Nishikawa, Y. (1959) *Studies on Reproduction in Horses: Singularity and Artificial Organ Control in Reproductive Phenomena.* Tokyo: Japan Racing Association.

Nishikawa, Y., Sugie, T. & Harada, N. (1952) Studies on the effect of day length on reproductive functions in horses. I. Effect of day length on function of ovaries. *Bull. nat. Inst. agric. Sci.*, **3**, 35.

Norris, H.J., Taylor, H.B. & Garner, F.M. (1968) Equine ovarian granulosa tumours. *Vet. Rec.*, **82**, 419.

O'Driscoll, J.G., Troy, P.I. & Geoghegen, F.T. (1977) Contagious equine metritis. *Vet. Rec.*, **101**, 491.

Ørskov, I. (1954) O antigens in the *Klebsiella* group. *Acta path. microbiol. scand.*, **34**, 145.

Ørskov, I. (1955*a*) The biochemical properties of *Klebsiella (Klebsiella aerogenes)* strains. *Acta path. microbiol. scand.*, **37**, 353.

Ørskov, I. (1955*b*) Serological investigations in the *Klebsiella* group. 1 New capsule types. *Acta path. microbiol. scand.*, **36**, 449.

Ørskov, I. (1955*c*) Serological investigations in the *Klebsiella* group 2. Occurrence of *Klebsiella* in sputa. *Acta path. microbiol. scand.*, **36**, 454.

Ørskov, I. (1955*d*) Serological investigations in the *Klebsiella* group 3. Occurrence of *Klebsiella* strains in the faeces of normal infants. *Acta path. microbiol. scand.*, **36**, 461.

Ørskov, I. (1956) 'Immunological paralysis' induced in rabbits by heavily capsulated *Klebsiella* strain. *Acta path. microbiol. scand.*, **38**, 375.

Osborne, V.E. (1966) An analysis of the pattern of ovulation as it occurs in the reproductive cycle of the mare in Australia. *Aust. vet. J.*, **42**, 149.

Osborne, V.E. (1975) Factors influencing foaling percentages in Australian mares. *J. Reprod. Fert.*, Suppl. **23**, 477.

Osborne, M. (1979) Some new thoughts on nutrition and housing horses. Paper presented to 18th ann. Congr. BEVA, Exeter.

Owen, R. ap R. (1978) Selenium deficiency and grass sickness. *Vet. Rec.*, **103**, 222(C).

Oxender, W.D., Noden, P. & Hafs, H.D. (1975) Oestrus, ovulations and plasma hormones after prostaglandin $F_2\alpha$ in mares. *J. Reprod. Fert.*, Suppl. **23**, 251.

Oxender, W.D., Noden, P. & Hafs, H.D. (1977) Estrus, ovulation and serum progesterone, estradiol and LH concentrations in mares after an increased photoperiod during winter. *Am. J. vet. Res.*, **38**, 203.

Palmer, E. & Jousset, B. (1975) Synchronization of oestrus in mares with a prostaglandin analogue and HCG. *J. Reprod. Fert.*, Suppl. **23**, 269.

Pascoe, R.R. (1979) Observations on the length and angle of declination of the vulva and its relation to fertility of the mare. *J. Reprod. Fert.*, Suppl. **27**, 299.

Pascoe, R.R., Spradbrow, P.B. & Bagust, T.J. (1968) Equine coital exanthema. *Aust. vet. J.*, **44**, 485.

Pascoe, R.R., Spradbrow, P.B. & Bagust, T.J. (1969) An equine genital infection resembling coital exanthema associated with a virus. *Aust. vet. J.*, **45**, 166.

Pattison, M.L., Chen, C.L., Kelley, S.T. & Brandt, G.W. (1974) Luteinizing hormone and estradiol in peripheral blood of mares during the estrous cycle. *Biol. Reprod.*, **11**, 245.

Pattison, M.L., Chen, C.L. & King, S.L. (1972) Determination of LH and estradiol-17β surge with reference to the time of ovulation in mares. *Biol. Reprod.*, **7**, 136.

Peterson, F.B., McFeely, R.A. & David, J.S.E. (1969) Studies on the pathogenesis of endometritis in the mare. *Proc. 15th ann. Conv. Am. Ass. equine Practnrs*, 279.

Pickett, B.W. & Voss, J.L. (1975) The effect of semen extenders and sperm numbers on mare fertility. *J. Reprod. Fert.*, Suppl. **23**, 95.

Pineda, M.H., Ginther, O.J. & McShan, W.H. (1972) Regression of corpus luteum in mares treated with an antiserum against an equine pituitary fraction. *Am. J. vet. Res.*, **33**, 1767.

Platt, H., Atherton, J.G. & Simpson, D.J. (1978) The experimental infection of ponies with contagious equine metritis. *Equine vet. J.*, **10**, 153.

Platt, H., Atherton, J.G., Simpson, D.J., Taylor, C.E.D., Rosenthal, R.O., Brown, D.F.J. & Wreghitt, T.G. (1977) Genital infection in mares. *Vet. Rec.*, **101**, 20.

Powell, D.G., David, J.S.E. & Frank, C.J. (1978) Contagious equine metritis. The present situation reviewed and a revised code of practice for control. *Vet. Rec.*, **103**, 399.

Prickett, M.E. (1966) Pathology of the equine ovary. *Proc. 12th ann. Conv. Am. Ass. equine Practnrs*, 145.

Ressang, A. (1954) Infertility in mares. A clinical, bacterilogical and histopathological investigation. Thesis, University of Utrecht.

Ricketts, S.W. (1975*a*) Endometrial biopsy as a guide to diagnosis of endometrial pathology in the mare. *J. Reprod. Fert.*, Suppl. **23**, 341.

Ricketts, S.W. (1975*b*) The technique and clinical application of endometrial biopsy in the mare. *Equine vet. J.*, 7, 102.

Ricketts, S.W. (1976) *Klebsiella aerogenes* in mares. *Vet. Rec.*, **99**, 489

Ricketts, S.W. (1978) Histological and histopathological studies of the endometrium of the mare. Fellowship Thesis, Royal College of Veterinary Surgeons.

Ricketts, S.W. & Rossdale, P.D. (1979) Endometrial biopsy findings in mares with contagious equine metritis. *J. Reprod. Fert.*, Suppl. **27**, 355.

Ricketts, S.W., Rossdale, P.D. & Samuel, C.A. (1978) Endometrial biopsy studies of mares with contagious equine metritis 1977. *Equine vet. J.*, **10**, 160.

Ricketts, S.W., Rossdale, P.D., Wingfield-Digby, N.J., Falk, M.M., Hopes, R., Hunt, M.D.N. & Peace, C.K. (1977) Genital infection in mares. *Vet. Rec.*, **101**, 65.

Roark, D.B. & Herman, H.A. (1950) Physiological and histological phenomena of the bovine estrual cycle with special reference to vaginal-cervical secretions. *Bull. Mo. agric. Exp. Stn*, 455.

Roberts, S.J. (1971) *Veterinary Obstetrics and Genital Disease.* Ann Arbor, Michigan: Edwards.

Rooney, J.R. (1970) *Autopsy of the Horse. Technique and Interpretation.* Baltimore: Williams & Wilkins.

Roser, J.F., Kiefer, B.L., Evans, J.W., Neeley, D.P. & Pacheco, C.A. (1979) The development of antibodies to human chorionic gonadotrophin following its repeated injection in the cyclic mare. *J. Reprod. Fert.*, Suppl. **27**, 173.

Rossdale, P.D. (1968) Modern stud management and its relation to the oestrous cycle and fertility of Thoroughbred mares. *Equine vet. J.*, **1**, 65.

Rossdale, P.D., Hunt, M.D.N., Peace, C.K., Hopes, R., Ricketts, S.W. & Wingfield-Digby, N.J. (1979) CEM: The case for AI. *Vet. Rec.*, **104**, 536.

Rowson, L.E.A., Lamming, G.E. & Fry, R.M. (1953) The relationship between ovarian hormones and uterine infection. *Vet. Rec.*, **65**, 335.

Samuel, C.A., Ricketts, S.W., Rossdale, P.D., Steven, D.H. & Thurley, K.W. (1979) Scanning electron microscope studies of the endometrium of the cyclic mare. *J. Reprod. Fert.*, Suppl. **27**, 287.

Scott, E.A. & Kunge, D.J. (1977) Ovariectomy in the Mare: Presurgical, surgical and post-surgical considerations. *J. equine Med. Surg.*, **1**, 5.

Seaborn, E. (1925) The oestrous cycle in the mare and some associated phenomena. *Anat. Rec.*, **30**, 227.

Sharp, D.C., Vernon, M.W. & Zavy, M.T. (1979) Alteration of seasonal reproductive patterns in mares following superior cervical ganglionectomy. *J. Reprod. Fert.*, Suppl. **27**, 87.

Short, R.V. (1962) Steroids in the follicular fluid and the corpus luteum of the mare. A 'two-cell type' theory of ovarian steroid synthesis. *J. Endocr.*, **24**, 59.

Short, R.V. (1972) Role of hormones in sex cycles. In *Reproduction in Mammals. 3. Hormones in Reproduction,* ed. C.R. Austin & R.V. Short, p. 42. Cambridge: Cambridge University Press.

Simpson, D.J. & Eaton-Evans, W.E. (1978*a*) Developments in contagious equine metritis. *Vet. Rec.*, **102**, 19.

Simpson, D.J. & Eaton-Evans, W.E. (1978*b*) Sites of CEM. *Vet. Rec.*, **102**, 48(c).

Sisson, S. (1953) In *The Anatomy of the Domestic Animals,* ed. J.D. Grossman, 4th ed. Philadelphia and London: Saunders.

Snyder, D.A., Turner, D.D., Miller, K.F., Garcia, M.C. & Ginther, O.J. (1979) Follicular and gonadotrophic changes during transition from ovulatory to anovulatory seasons. *J. Reprod. Fert.*, Suppl. **27**, 95.

Solomon, W.J. (1971) Rectal examination of the cervix and its significance in early pregnancy evaluation in the mare. *Proc. 17th ann. Conv. Am. Ass. equine Practnrs,* 119.

Solomon, W.J., Raker, C.W., McFeely, R.A. & Peterson, F.B. (1970) Uterine curettage in the mare. *J. Am. vet. med. Ass.*, **156**, 333.

Spincemaille, J., Coryn, M., Vandekerchkhove, D. & Vandeplassche, M. (1975) The use of prostaglandin $F_2\alpha$ in controlling the oestrous cycle of the mare and steroid changes in the peripheral blood. *J. Reprod. Fert.*, Suppl. **23**, 263.

Stabenfeldt, G.H., Hughes, J.P. & Evans, J.W. (1972*a*) Ovarian activity during the oestrous cycle of the mare. *J. Endocr.*, **90**, 1397.

Stabenfeldt, G.H., Hughes, J.P., Wheat, J.D. & Evans, J.W. (1972*b*) The role of the uterus of the mare in cyclic ovarian activity. *Fedn Proc. Fedn Am. Socs exp. Biol.*, **31**, 292.

Stewart, F. & Allen, W.R. (1979) Binding of FSH, LH, and PMSG to equine gonadal tissue. *J. Reprod. Fert.*, Suppl. **27**, 431.

Stickle, R.L., Erb, R.E., Fessler, J.F. & Runnels, L.J. (1975) Equine granulosa cell tumours. *J. Am. vet. med. Ass.*, **167**, 148.

Strauss, S.S., Chen, C.L., Kalra, S.P. & Sharp, D.C. (1979) Localization of gonadotrophin-releasing hormone (GnRH) in the hypothalamus of ovariectomized pony mares by season. *J. Reprod. Fert.*, Suppl. **27**, 123.

Sullivan, J.J., Turner, P.C., Self, L.C., Gutteridge, H.B. & Barttell, D.E. (1975) Survey of reproductive efficiency in the Quarter-horse and Thoroughbred. *J. Reprod. Fert.*, Suppl. **23**, 315.

Swerczek, T.W. (1979*a*) Contagious equine metritis – outbreak of the disease in Kentucky and laboratory methods for diagnosing the disease. *J. Reprod. Fert.*, Suppl. **27**, 361.

Swerczek, T.W. (1979*b*) Elimination of CEM organism from mares by excision of clitoral sinuses. *Vet. Rec.*, **105**, 131.

Taylor, C.E.D., Rosenthal, R.O., Brown, D.F.J., Lapage, S.P., Hill, L.H. & Legross R.M. (1978) The causative organism of contagious equine metritis 1977 – proposal for a new species to be known as *Haemophilus equigenitalis. Equine vet. J.*, **10**, 136.

Timoney, P.J., Ward, J. & Kelly, P. (1977) A contagious genital infection of mares. *Vet. Rec.*, **101**, 103.

Towers-Clark, P. (1968) Fertility in mares. *Stud and Stable Veterinary Handbook*, London.

Trommershausen-Smith, A., Hughes, J.P. & Neely, D.P. (1979) Cytogenetic and clinical findings in mares with gonadal dysgenesis. *J. Reprod. Fert.*, Suppl. **27**, 271.

Vandeplassche, M. & Henry, M. (1977) Salpingitis in the mare. *Proc. 23rd ann. Conv. Am. Ass. equine Practnrs*, 123.

Vandeplassche, M., Henry, M. & Coryn, M. (1979) The mature mid-cycle follicle in the mare. *J. Reprod. Fert.*, Suppl. **27**, 157.

Vandeplassche, M., Spincemaille, J., Bouters, R. & Bonte, P. (1972) Some aspects of equine obstetrics. *Equine vet. J.*, **4**, 105.

Van Niekerk, C.H. (1964) Early embryonic resorption in mares. *J. S. Afr. med. Ass.*, **36**, 61.

Van Niekerk, C.H., Coughbrough, R.I. & Doms, H.W.H. (1973) Progesterone treatment of mares with abnormal oestrous cycle earlyin the breeding season. *J. S. Afr. vet. Ass.*, **44**, 37.

Van Niekerk, C.H., Morgenthal, J.C. & Gerneke, W.H. (1975) Relationship between the morphology of and progesterone production by the corpus luteum of the mare. *J. Reprod. Fert.*, Suppl. **23**, 171.

Van Niekerk, C.H. & Van Heerden, J.S. (1972) Nutritional and ovarian activity of mares early in the breeding season. *J. S. Afr. vet. Ass.*, **43**, 351.

Van Rensburg, S.W.J. & Van Heerden, J.S. (1953) Infertility in mares caused by ovarian dysfunction. *Onderstepoort J. vet. Res.*, **26**, 285.

Vickery, B.H. & Bennett, J.P. (1968) The cervix and its secretion in mammals. *Physiol. Rev.*, **48**, 135.

Vivrette, S.L. & Irvine, C.H.G. (1979) Interaction of oestradiol and gonadotrophin-releasing hormone on LH release in the mare. *J. Reprod. Fert.*, Suppl. **27**, 151.

Voss, J.L. & Pickett, B.W. (1975) The effect of rectal palpation on the fertility of cyclic mares. *J. Reprod. Fert.*, Suppl. **23**.

Voss, J.L., Pickett, B.W. & Back, D.G. (1973) The effect of rectal palpation on fertility in the mare. *Proc. 19th ann. Conv. Am. Ass. equine Practnrs*, 33.

Voss, J.L., Sullivan, J.J., Pickett, B.W., Parker, W.G., Burwash, L.D. & Larson, L.L. (1975) The effect of H.C.G. on duration of oestrus, ovulation time and fertility in mares. *J.Reprod. Fert.*, Suppl. **23**, 297.

Voss, J.L., Wallace, R.A., Squires, E.L., Pickett, B.W. & Shideler, R.K. (1979) Effects of synchronization and frequency of insemination on fertility. *J. Reprod. Fert.*, Suppl. **27**, 257.

Warszawsky, L.F., Parker, W.G., First, N.L. & Ginther, O.L. (1972) Gross changes of internal genitalia during the estrous cycle in the mare. *Am. J. vet. Res.*, **33**, 19.

Whitmore, H.L., Wentworth, B.C. & Ginther, O.J. (1973) Circulating concentrations of luteinizing hormone during estrous cycles of mares as determined by radio immunoassay. *Am. J. vet. Res.*, **34**, 631.

Wingfield-Digby, N.J. (1978) The technique and clinical application of endometrial cytology in mares. *Equine vet. J.*, **10**, 167.

Witherspoon, D.M. (1972) Technique and evaluation of uterine curettage. *Proc. 18th ann. Conv. Am. Ass. equine Practnrs,* 51.

Witherspoon, D.M. (1975) The site of ovulation in the mare. *J. Reprod. Fert.*, Suppl. **23**, 329.

Woodley, S.L., Burns, P.J., Douglas, R.H. & Oxender, W.D. (1979) Prolonged inter-ovulatory interval after oestradiol treatment in mares. *J. Reprod. Fert.*, Suppl. **27**, 205.

Zafracas, A.M. (1975) *Candida* infection of the genital tract in Thoroughbred mares. *J. Reprod. Fert.*, Suppl. **23**, 349.

The Stallion 2

A healthy, fertile stallion is an essential element of any breeding programme. The stallion provides 50% of the genetic material of the newly conceived individual and his fertility can thus be as important as that of the mare. Routine monitoring of the stallion is therefore just as important as the examinations of individual mares.

SELECTION OF STALLIONS

The selection of Thoroughbred stallions for stud purposes is based on racing ability, but the unwitting selection of unsound or infertile stallions reduces fecundity and perpetuates undesirable traits which may have a highly undesirable effect on the breed in general. The use of a few very successful but conformationally unsound racehorses for stud had led to the production of a large number of horses that will not stand up to hard training. A racehorse for stud should therefore be chosen for constitutional, conformational and reproductive soundness as well as for racing performance.

REPRODUCTIVE ANATOMY (FIG. 2.1)

The *scrotum* is situated between the thighs and, as in other animals, is capable of vascular and muscular adaptations to environmental temperature. The testes are usually descended into the scrotum at birth, or shortly afterwards. The *testes* in the horse, when relaxed, lie in the horizontal position. When retracted, they become nearly vertical. Normally they measure 6–12 cm long × 4–7 cm high × 5 cm wide. Testicular size increases with age (Thompson et al. 1979) up to maturity at five years (Table 2.2). The head of the *epididymis* lies cranial to the testis and continues dorsally as the body. The tail is caudal and loosely attached to the testis. The vas deferens lies dorsomedial to the testis and continues into the spermatic cord.

The *spermatic cord* contains the vas deferens, spermatic vasculature, nerves and cremaster muscle. It may be clearly palpated as it disappears into the external inguinal ring.

Testes and epididymis should be readily moveable within the *tunica vaginalis.*

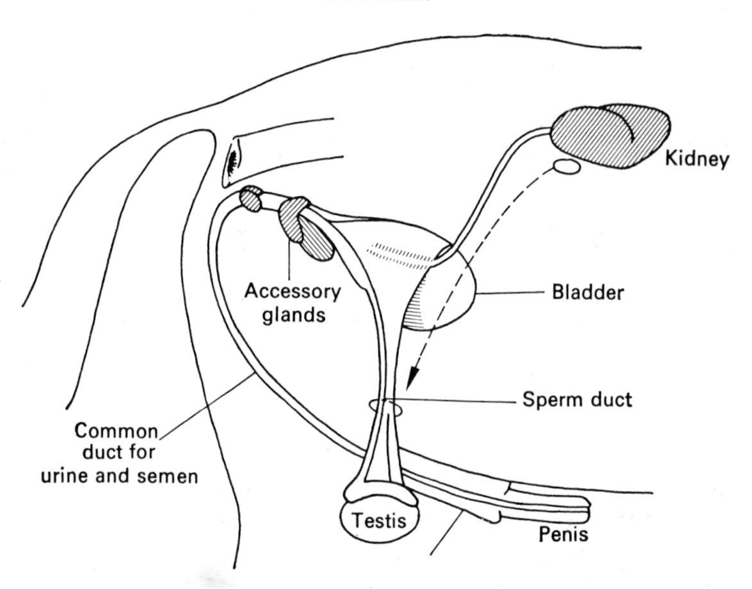

Fig. 2.1. The reproductive anatomy of the stallion. The dotted line indicates the route of descent of the testis.

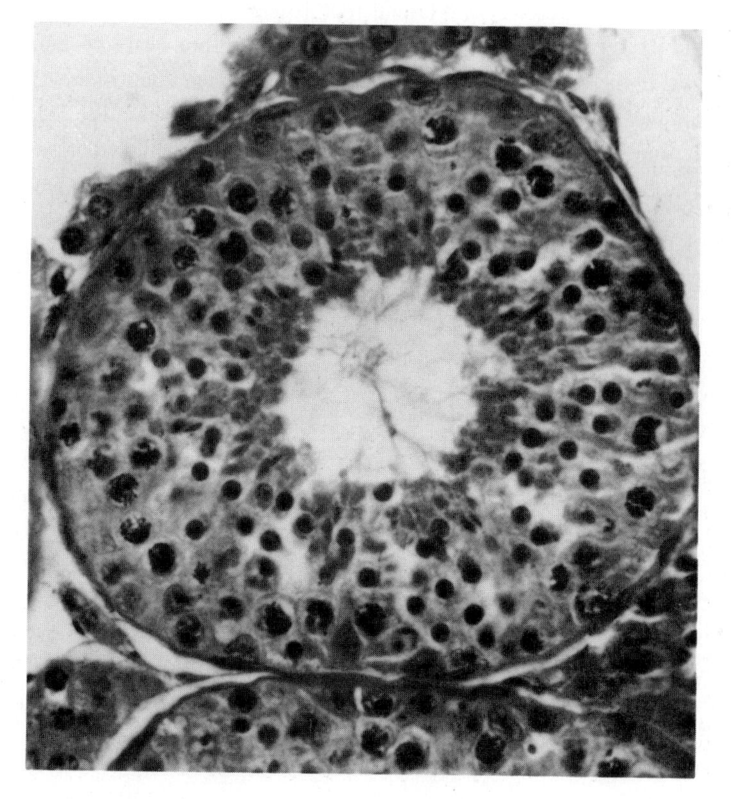

Fig. 2.2 Photomicrograph of a seminiferous tubule in transverse section in a two-year-old colt, showing cell types of spermatozoa. H & E × 450.

TABLE 2.1 Reproductive characteristics of stallions (n = 43)

Characteristic	*Value* (mean ± SD)
Measurement (mm)	
Scrotal width	102.1 ± 9.9
Left width	57.8 ± 5.2
Right width	55.8 ± 5.8
Left length	103.1 ± 8.2
Right length	107.5 ± 8.0
Parenchyma weight, paired (g)	328 ± 104
Daily sperm	
Production ($\times 10^9$)	4.55 ± 1.45
Output ($\times 10^9$)	3.35 ± 1.41

From Thompson et al. (1979).

The *accessory glands* comprise the seminal vesicles, ampullae, bulbourethral glands and prostate gland. The seminal vesicles are paired, bladder-like structures on the floor of the pelvis, cranial and lateral to the neck of the urinary bladder. Their six to eight excretory ducts open into the pelvic urethra near the ischial arch.

The *penis* of the stallion is haemodynamic, has a large amount of erectile tissue, measures an average of 44 × 5 cm and at rest is totally enclosed in the prepuce. On erection it doubles in length and thickness and the glans penis enlarges to three times its resting size. The urethra, which projects a few millimetres beyond the glans penis, is surrounded by the urethral fossa which contains a dorsal diverticum (Fig. 2.3). The urethral fossa and diverticulum are often filled with smegma and may

TABLE 2.2 Effect of age on testicular size in stallions

Characteristic	*Age* (years)		
	2–3 (n = 11)	4–6 (n = 14)	≥7 (n = 18)
Measurement (mm)			
Scrotal width			
Mean	96[a]	100[a]	109[b]
1 SD	88–103	93–107	102–117
2 SD	81–111	85–115	95–124
Left width			
Mean	55[a]	57[a]	61[b]
1 SD	50–59	53–62	57–65
2 SD	46–63	49–66	52–70
Right width			
Mean	53[a]	55[a]	60[b]
1 SD	48–58	50–60	55–64
2 SD	43–62	45–65	50–69

From Thompson et al. (1979).
Means with different superscripts differ significantly ($P < 0.05$).

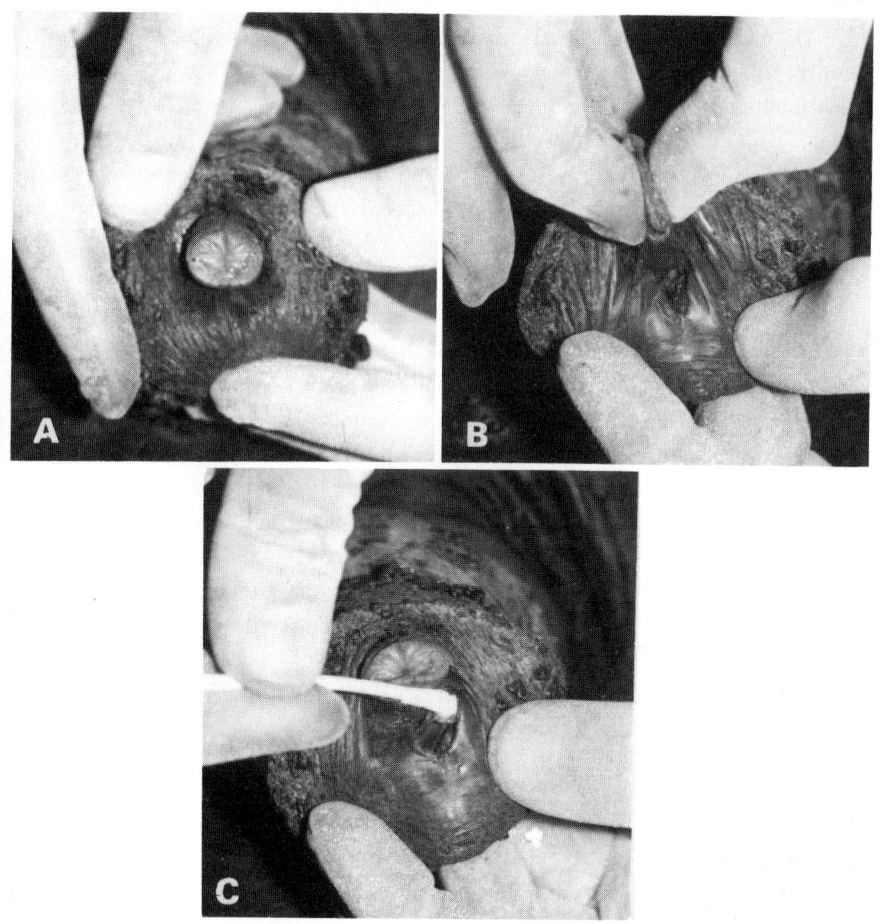

Fig. 2.3. Anterior view of the glans penis. A, Projecting terminal urethra. B, Terminal urethra pulled upwards to show the urethral fossa and diverticulum. C, Swab placed inside the diverticulum.

harbour potential venereal-disease-producing bacteria, e.g. *Haemophilus equigenitalis, Klebsiella aerogenes* or *Pseudomonas aeruginosa* (see p. 157).

The *prepuce* (sheath) is quite voluminous and movement of the penis at the trot frequently causes a sucking noise in geldings or stallions. Preputial glands secrete a substance which, with epithelial debris, forms the deep red-brown-coloured smegma.

ENDOCRINOLOGY

Environmental stimuli, especially increases in daylight length, stimulate the hypothalamus, via nervous pathways from the sense organs, to produce releasing factors (GnRF). The measurable effects of changing external stimuli throughout the year on semen quality and sexual behaviour have been described by Pickett et al. (1970,

1975*a*) and Pickett and Voss (1972). Significant changes in semen volume, sperm density, total sperm per ejaculate, semen pH, reaction time and average number of mounts required per ejaculation in and out of the breeding season were demonstrated. GnRF is carried by the hypophyseal portal blood stream to the basophilic delta cells of the anterior pituitary gland and causes them to release gonadotrophic hormones, i.e. follicle-stimulating hormone (FSH) and luteinizing hormone (LH). These hormones are identical to those secreted in the female (see p. 15). LH is sometimes referred to as interstitial-cell-stimulating hormone (ICSH). The hypophyseal mechanism initiates the reproductive process at the time of puberty, between one and two years.

The testes are the target organs for the gonadotrophic hormones. FSH stimulates spermatogenesis from the spermatogonia to secondary spermatocyte stages. ICSH stimulates the interstitial (Leydig) cells, between the seminiferous tubules, to secrete testosterone. Testosterone is a steroid hormone responsible for spermatogenesis from secondary spermatocyte to spermatozoa stages, development of male genitalia, descent of the testes in the fetus or neonate, the further growth and development of the male genitalia at puberty and the growth, maintenance and function of the accessory glands. It stimulates the central nervous system in producing libido, male sexual responses and secondary sexual characteristics, i.e. personality, muscular development and 'cresty' neck.

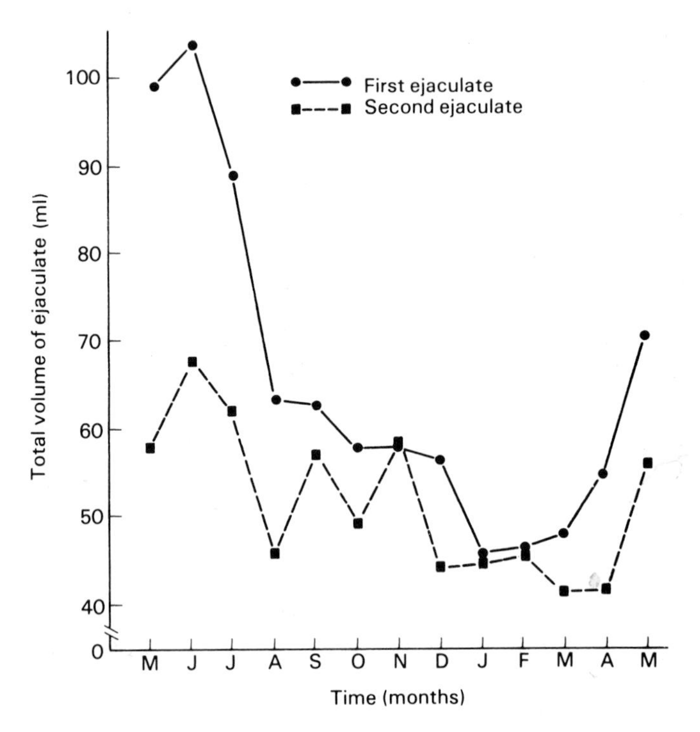

Fig. 2.4. Total seminal volume throughout the year. (*After Pickett & Voss 1972*)

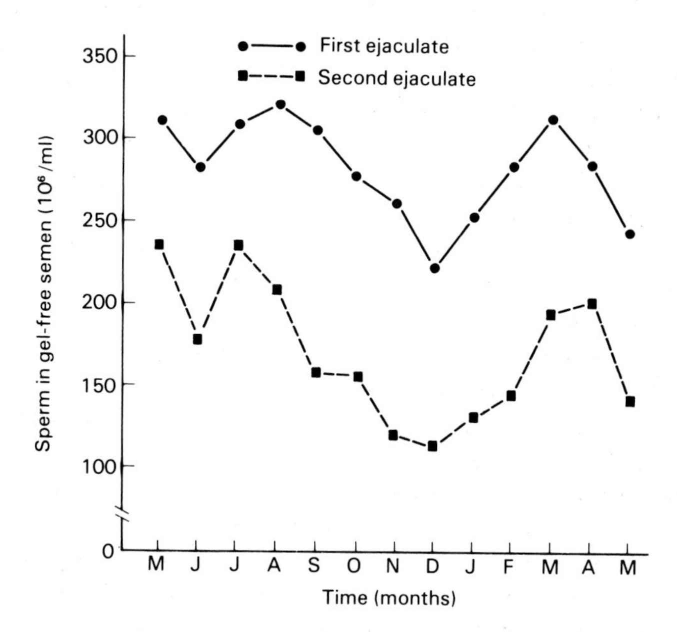

Fig. 2.5. Number of sperm in gel-free semen throghout the year. (*After Pickett & Voss 1972*)

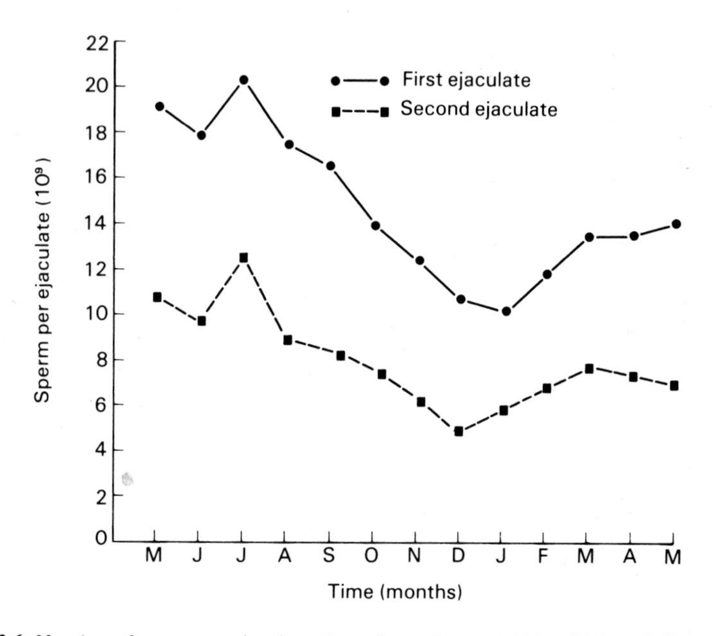

Fig. 2.6. Number of sperm per ejaculate throughout the year. (*After Pickett & Voss 1972*)

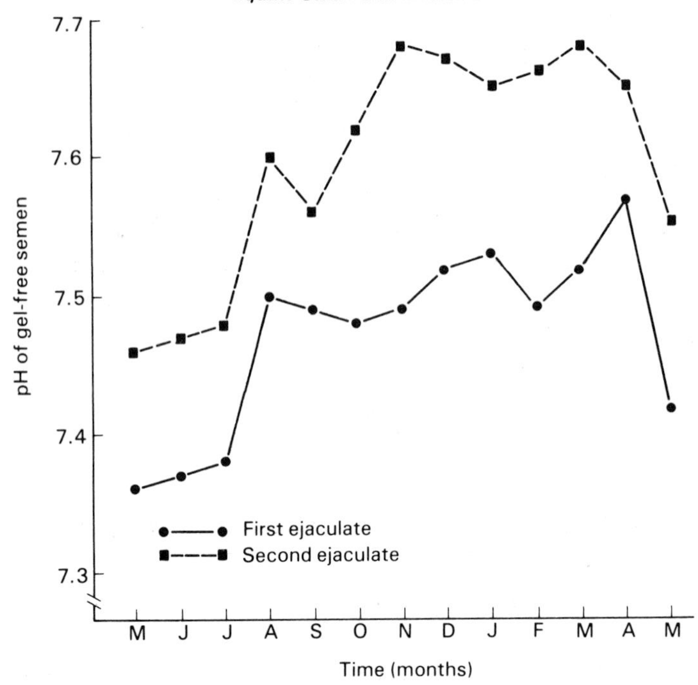

Fig. 2.7. pH of gel-free semen throughout the year. (*After Pickett & Voss 1972*)

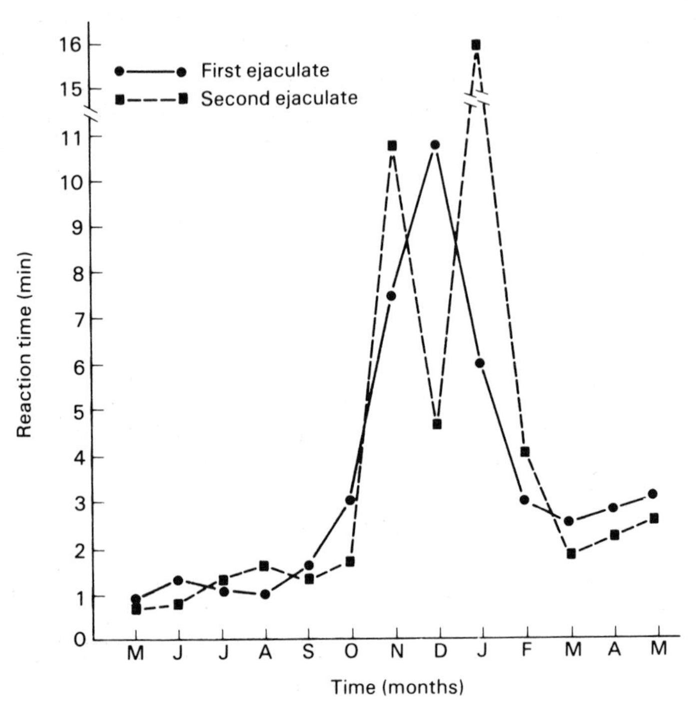

Fig. 2.8. Effect of season on sexual behaviour as measured by reaction time. (*After Pickett & Voss 1972*)

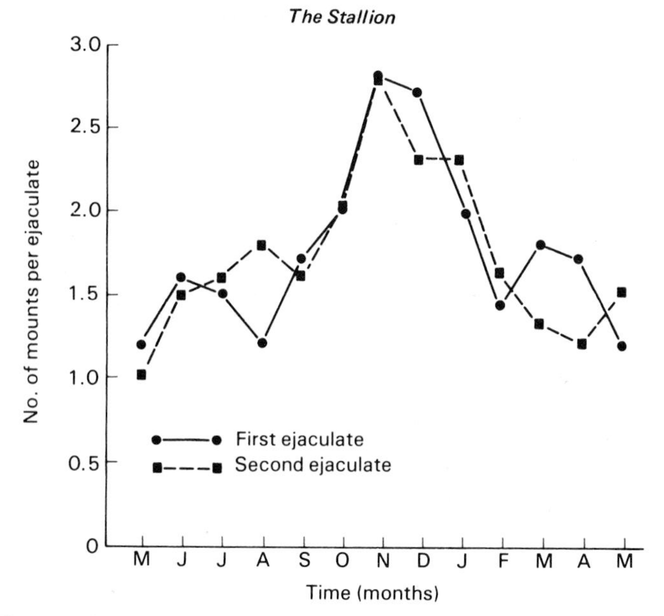

Fig. 2.9. Mean number of mounts required per ejaculation throughout the year. (*After Pickett & Voss 1972*)

Androgenic hormones (i.e. testosterone and closely related steroids with masculinizing properties) are produced by adrenal cells or tumours. Cells resembling testicular Leydig cells have been found in the spermatic cord of stallions (Bishop et al. 1966) and these may be responsible for continued 'rig' tendencies in geldings which have been adequately castrated as opposed to being 'cut proud'.

Berndstone et al. (1974) showed a significant seasonal change in plasma testosterone concentration (Fig. 2.10). They postulated that the high mean concentration

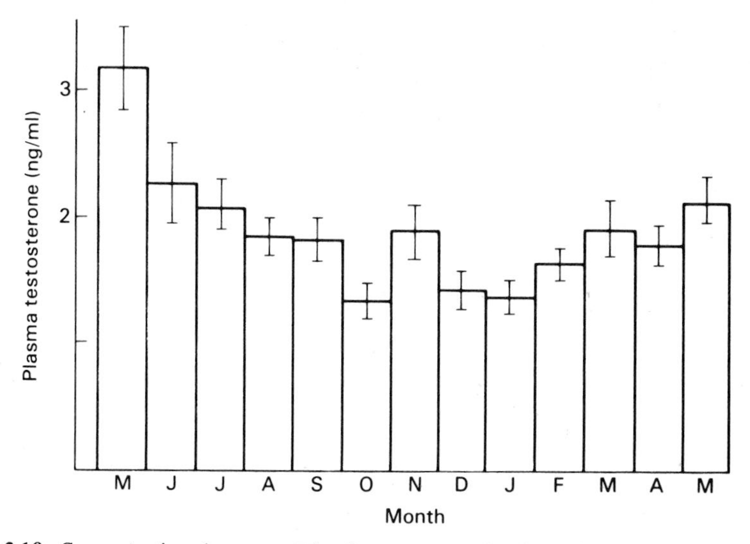

Fig. 2.10. Concentration (mean ± SE) of testosterone in the peripheral plasma of mature stallions over a 13-month period. (*After Berndstone et al. 1974*)

during May (3.2 ng/ml) was at least partly responsible for the high sperm output observed in July. A similar seasonal effect on the pattern of secretion was demonstrated by Cox and Williams (1975) and Ganjam and Kenney (1975). Both these latter papers demonstrated a diurnal rhythm for serum testosterone concentration with higher levels at 06.00 hours than at 18.00 hours. Sexual stimulation and the injection of exogenous luteinizing hormone significantly increased testosterone level. Berndstone et al. (1974) noted wide fluctuations in plasma testosterone level within and among stallions and postulated that pulsatile secretion may occur as in other animals. Ganjam (1978) confirmed the absence of a steady state and showed how single sample assays could be very misleading.

REPRODUCTIVE BEHAVIOUR

The stallion in courtship is an awesome spectacle; he is an animal of great presence and beauty. On first seeing the mare he fixes his eyes on her, arches his neck and becomes restless, pawing or stamping his feet and drawing himself to full height. He shows a marked '*Flehmen*' response (Fig. 2.11) (curling of the upper lip and usually

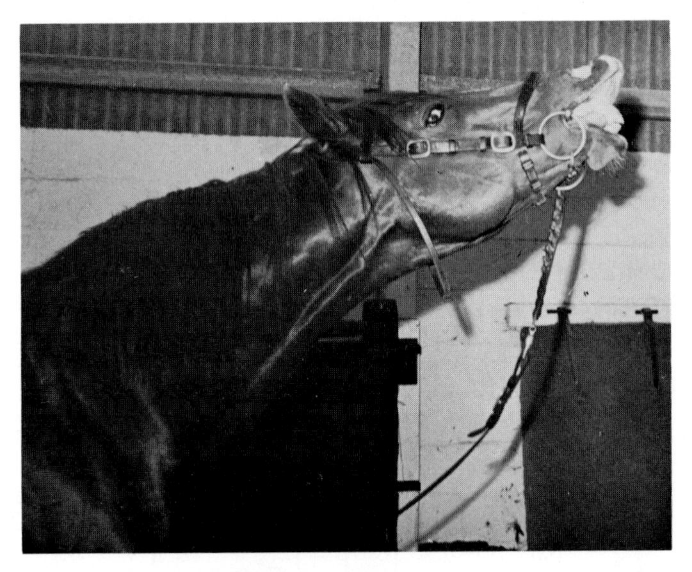

Fig. 2.11. The *Flehmen* stance.

raising of the head as if in response to olfactory stimuli) and may emit a roar to which the mare responds with a nicker. He approaches the mare at the head or neck, 'talking' to her, nudging her and sometimes biting her neck. He works down to the flanks, buttocks and perineum and nudges her vulva and clitoris. The mare truly in oestrus remains very still during this approach behaviour. After a relatively short period of genital stimulation, the stallion, by now with penis fully erect, mounts, usually from the left side. Some stallions mount directly, but others nudge the mare slightly off balance with the right shoulder before mounting or make repeated half-mounting movements. Presumably these actions give confidence to the horse that the mare will not kick him at the vulnerable moment of intromission.

Mounting behaviour is influenced by season and reaction time and the number of mounts per ejaculate is lower in spring and summer than in winter (Pickett et al. 1970, 1975; Pickett & Voss 1972) (Figs 2.8, 2.9).

Ejaculation follows a variable number of pelvic oscillations during which the stallion may 'dance' on his hind-feet. Ejaculation is signified by a rhythmic 'flagging' of the tail and followed by a terminally inactive phase in which the stallion remains on the mare and penile erection subsides. Tischner et al. (1974) have shown that, at the moment ejaculation begins, pelvic thrusts cease. Using a specially devised open-ended artificial vagina, Kosiniak (1975) has shown that ejaculation occurs in a

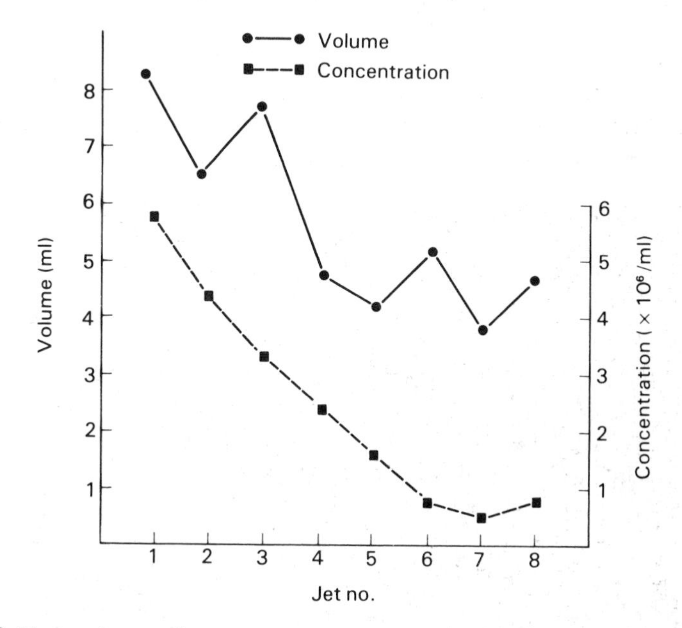

Fig. 2.12. Mean volume and sperm concentration of successive seminal jets. (*After Kosiniak 1975*)

series of six to nine jets resulting from the contractions of the urethra. There is a reduction in the volume of each succeeding jet and 70% or more of the spermatozoa and of the basic biochemical constituents are contained in the first three jets (Fig. 2.12).

Managerial influences

The transition from racing to stud life demands radical changes in management. During training, normal sexual behaviour will have been actively discouraged. When first presented with an in-oestrus mare, the young stallion may be severely inhibited by the anticipation of disciplinary measures. Managerial changes should be aimed at preparing the stallion physically and psychologically for his new tasks. He is no longer required to be an athlete, but must be prepared for short periods of physical exertion. Stallion boxes should be large, well ventilated, clean and without any sharp projections on which the stallion might injure himself. Each stallion should have his own well fenced or boarded paddock large enough for him to exercise adequately during the day.

Not all stallions show intense sexual or purposeful mounting behaviour. Young, overworked or physically or psychologically traumatized stallions may show little interest, weak libido and clumsy mounting behaviour. Modern systems of stud farm management may affect the stallion's sexual behaviour. The stallion covering two and sometimes three mares a day during the season may show reflexes to the sound, sight and smells of the covering area. Much of the initial courtship phase is curtailed as the stallion is presented with only those mares found to be in oestrus by teasing and veterinary examinations. The mare is restrained by hobbles; a front leg is held up and/or a twitch applied to prevent her showing any response to the advances of the stallion. An experienced stallion, after a momentary nudge of the perineum, mounts, achieves intromission and ejaculates. An example of conditioned sexual reflexes can sometimes be seen under systems of artificial insemination where the stallion does not become excited or show interest in the mare until an attendant appears with the artificial vagina. Conditioned sexual reflexes may be strong enough to allow the training of some stallions to ejaculate into an artificial vagina while mounted on a 'phantom mare' (Kenney & Cooper 1974) (see p. 151).

In the wild state, stallions cover mares many times during an oestrous period, but under modern systems of management they are seldom allowed to cover more than twice. Stallions are capable of covering eight to ten times in 24 hours (Wierzbowski 1966) depending on breed and other factors. Valuable stallions are usually restricted to two or three matings a day and 40–50 mares per breeding season.

There are variations in managerial methods applied to stallions and mares at mating, but most impose a degree of restraint, taking into account the value of the stallion. Figs 2.13 to 2.20 show examples of typical covering yard management.

The mare is bridled and restrained by an attendant at her head. Felt boots are usually fitted to the hind-feet (Fig. 2.13); care should be taken to ensure that these are firmly applied and that no loose strap ends project. Often a twitch is applied (Fig. 2.15) to the nose or ear and one fore-leg held in carpal flexion by a second attendant, sometimes using a knee strap with a quick release. The traditional hind-leg hobbles are seldom used in the UK but are still favoured in other countries, notably Australia and the USA. A third attendant stands to one side (usually the right) of the mare's hind-quarters. Blinkers, hood and blindfold are sometimes used on maiden mares or those which become frightened by the stallion's approach and mounting activity. The administration of tranquillizers, intramuscularly or intravenously, 15–30 minutes before mating, may be helpful in nervous or vicious mares that are not showing strong signs of oestrus.

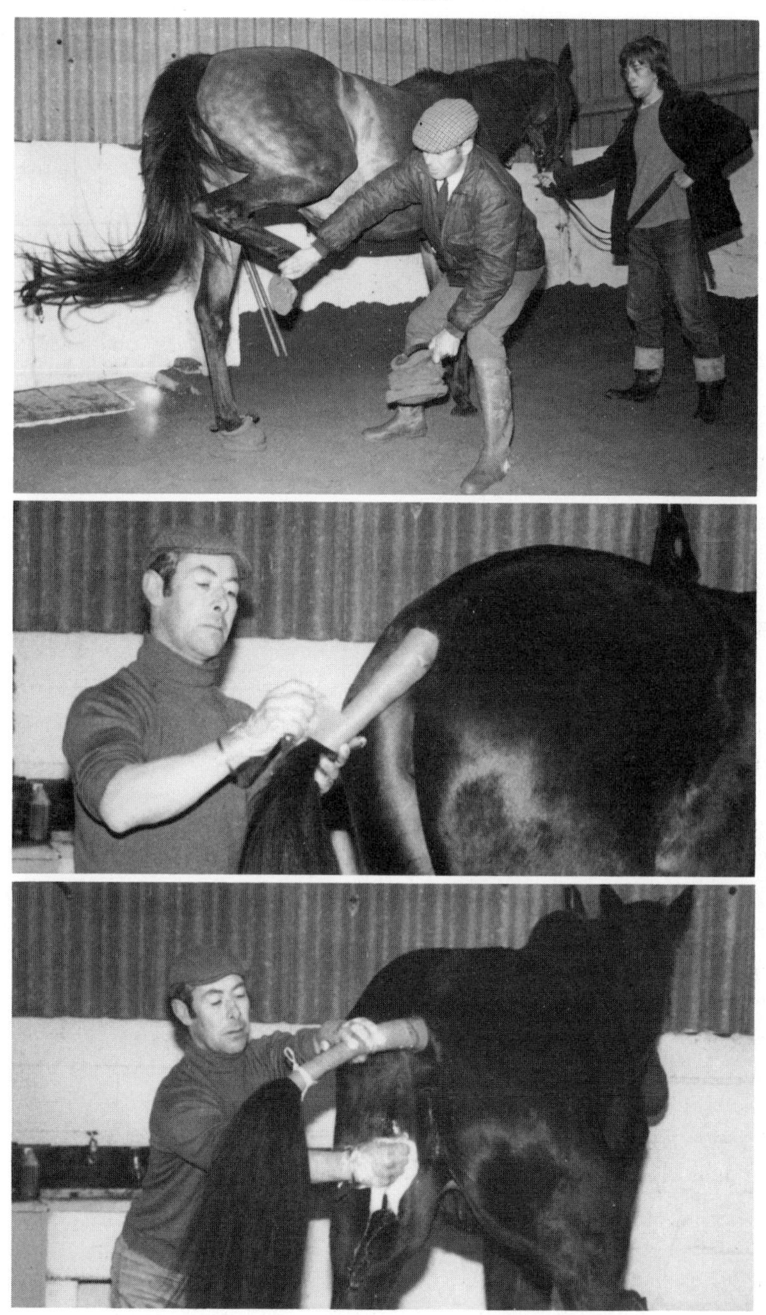

Fig. 2.13. The mare is prepared for covering.

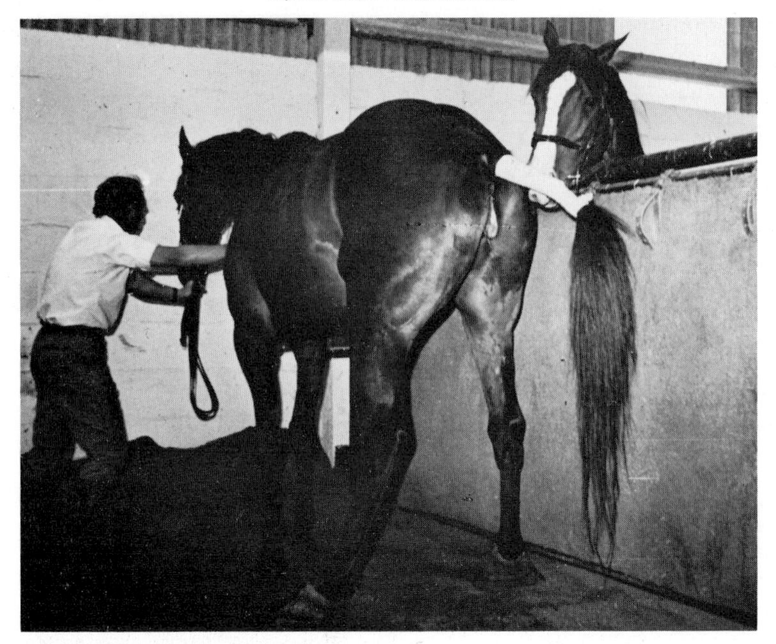

Fig. 2.14. A final check for oestrous signs.

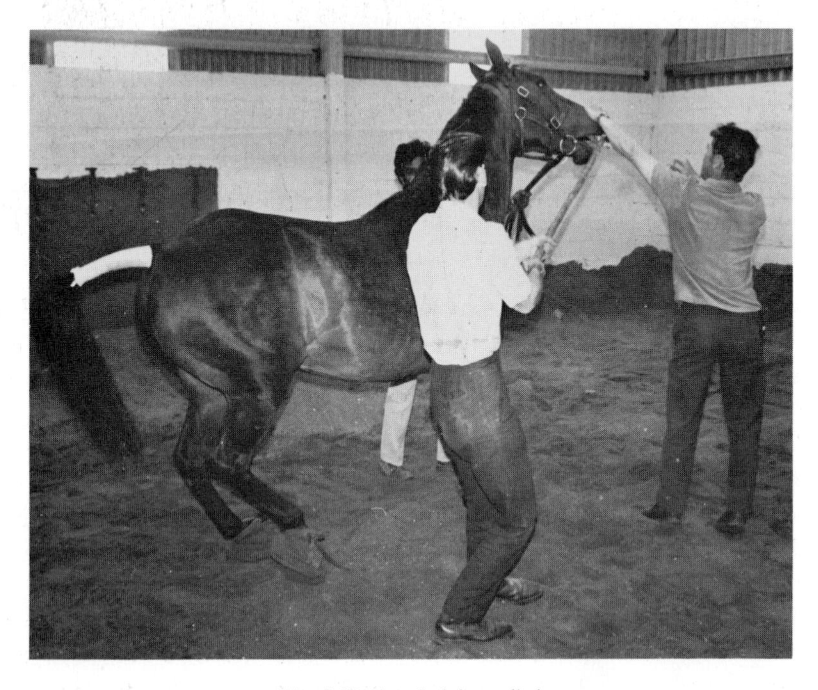

Fig. 2.15. A twitch is applied.

It is customary to prepare the mare for mating by washing the perineal region. Care must, however, be exercised to avoid leaving remnants of antiseptic soap or detergent that might have a contraceptive effect. In some countries it is customary to wash the stallion's penis thoroughly before covering. Again, it is extremely important to remove all traces of soap, detergent or antiseptic prior to covering. The use of antiseptics on the genital organs may be contraindicated, as they may adversely effect the normal bacterial microflora (see p. 157). The mare's tail is usually bandaged, preferably using disposable materials. In the interests of disease control, all persons handling the genital organs of either mare or stallion should wear disposable gloves and use disposable paper towels.

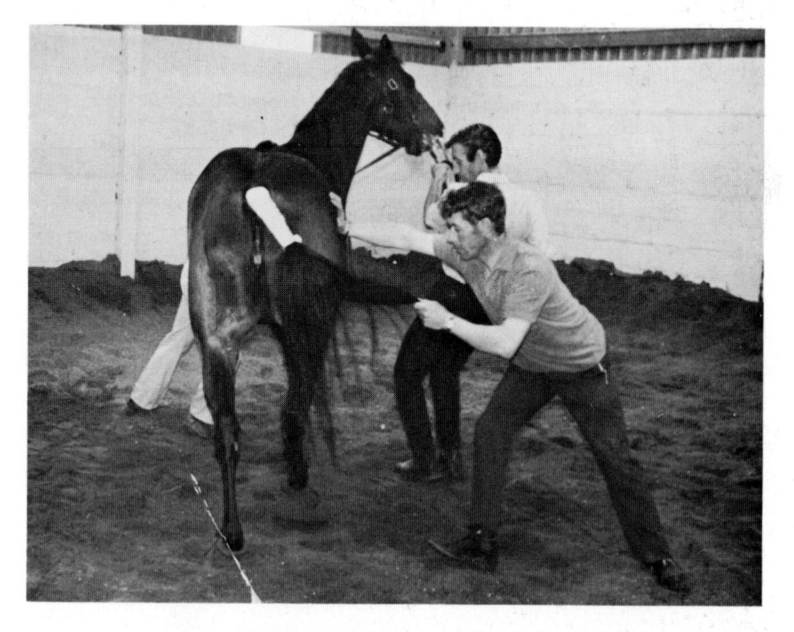

Fig. 2.16. The mare is positioned.

In exceptional cases it may be necessary to perform an episiotomy if the vulval commissures have been sutured to leave less than the minimal aperture for intromission. If this is not done, damage and haematoma to the penis may occur. Another measure to help the stallion is to stand the mare with her hind-legs in a hollow or on a mound, depending on the discrepancy in size of mare and stallion. Some stallions may slap the mare vigorously with the fore-feet as if attempting to obtain a more stable position and others may take vicious bites at her neck. A leather pad for the stallion to bite may be strapped to the mare's neck to prevent injury and help the stallion maintain his position.

The stallion is bridled and held on a long rein. He is allowed to approach from one side (usually the left) with the stallion man on his near side. He is brought to the mare's hind-quarters and is allowed to smell, taste and lightly bite the hocks or flanks. In the interest of venereal disease control, the stallion should not be allowed to nuzzle the mare's vulva directly. When an erection is achieved the stallion man encourages his charge to mount the mare by pulling him alongside the hind-quarters and turning the stallion's head over her hind-quarters (Figs 2.17, 2.18).

As the stallion mounts, the attendant lets go of the mare's tail. When the stallion has mounted, the attendant may again hold the tail and the stallion man may guide

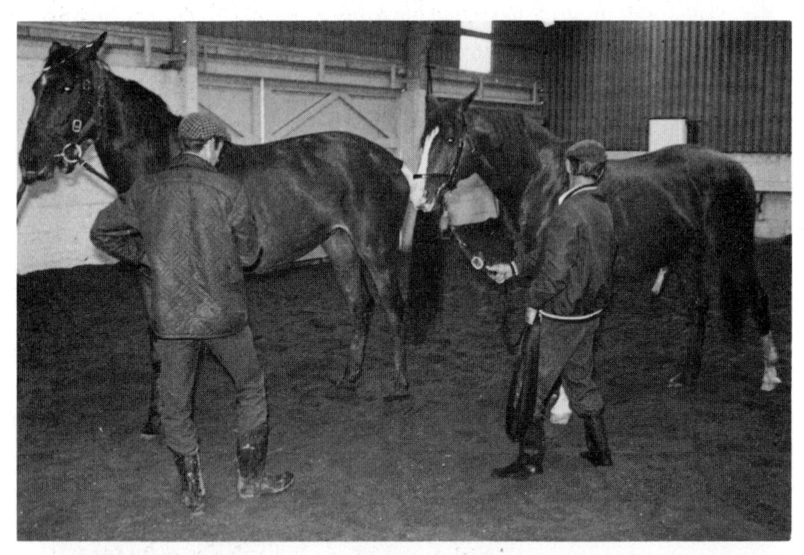

Fig. 2.17. The stallion is taken to the mare and when the penis is erect he is encouraged to mount.

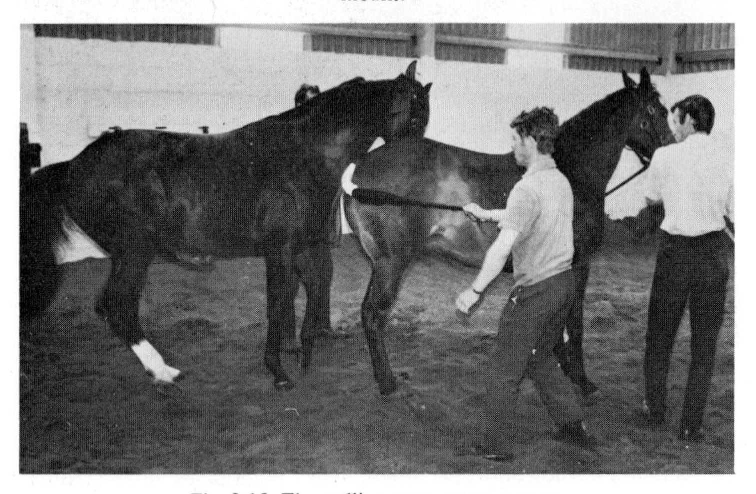

Fig. 2.18. The stallion prepares to mount.

the penis through the vulva (Fig. 2.19). Undue force should never be used when handling the stallion's penis as bruising can occur. Handling is thus not recommended unless essential. Some stallions may mount many times without gaining intromission unless assisted. Assisted intromission is sometimes necessary when a mare is

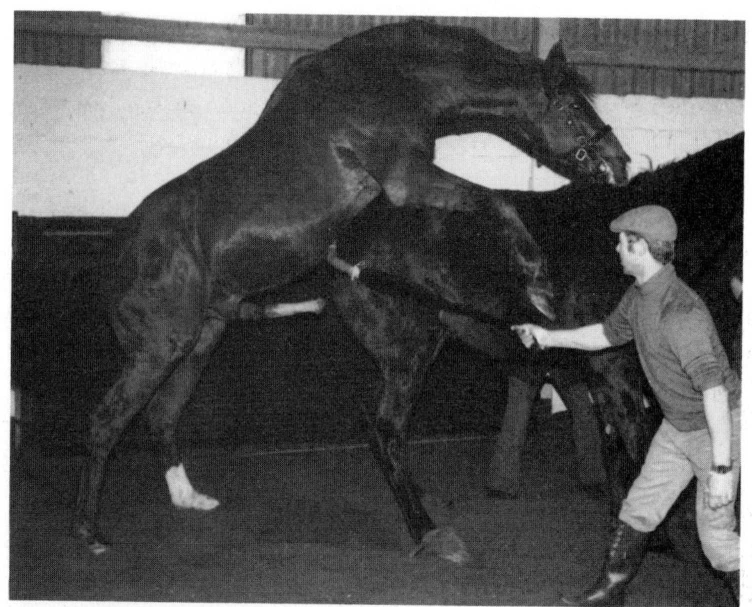

Fig. 2.19. The stallion has mounted and is about to gain intromission. The attendant should not assist directly unless essential, as some stallions resent it.

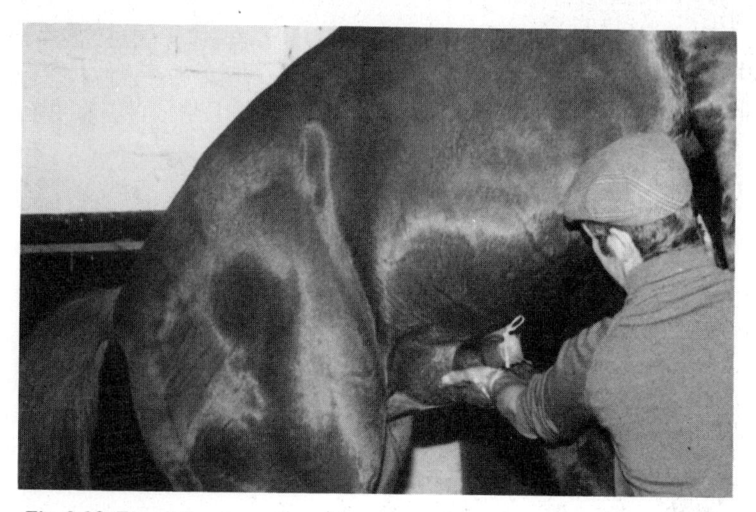

Fig. 2.20. Ejaculation is confirmed by placing a hand lightly under the urethra.

positioned awkwardly for the stallion or if her vulva has been sutured or has sloping conformation. In these cases an attendant should gently guide the penis into the vulva. Once intromission is gained, the stallion man may, with the attendant on the other side, pull the horse's fore-legs forward. Some stallions appear to have difficulty in maintaining their position during ejaculation. In these cases the handlers may hold the stallion's fore-legs firmly against the mare's thorax until ejaculation is complete.

Failure to maintain erection or gain intromission is a signal for the stallion man to 'rein' the horse off the mare. Following a suitable interval of stimulation the process is then repeated until intromission and ejaculation are achieved. Ejaculation is recognized by 'tail flagging' and by the urethral pulses, which the attendant holding the tail may feel with the hand held lightly on the underside of the penis (Fig. 2.20).

It is customary to wash the stallion's penis and sheath immediately on dismount (Fig. 2.21). It is more important to wash off the mare's genital secretion than to attempt the impossible task of trying to sterilize the penis bacteriologically.

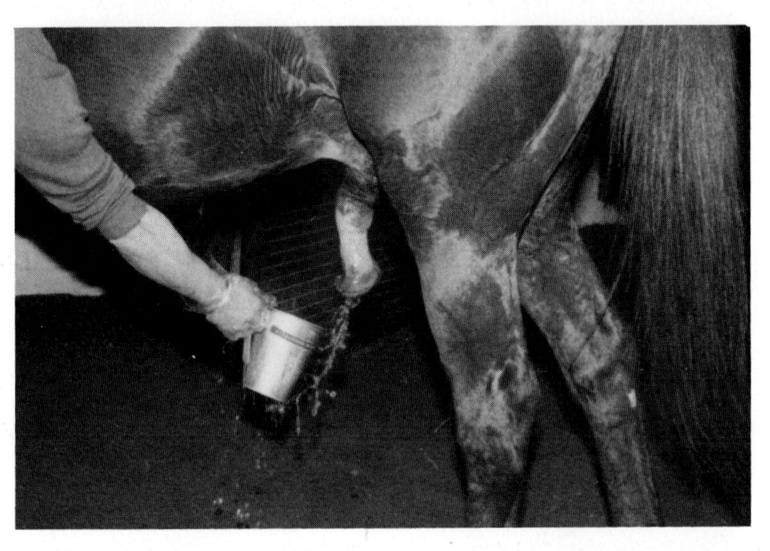

Fig. 2.21. After dismounting the stallion is washed with a mild antiseptic solution or just clean water.

Attempts at the latter, by using high concentration disinfectants, may be positively dangerous and may cause either severe irritation or an alteration of the normal bacteriological flora of the stallion's penis (see p. 157). The capsulated *Klebsiella* organisms are more resistant to disinfectants than non-capsulated organisms. The *Klebsiella* and *Pseudomonas* population may increase in the absence of competition from these other organisms.

Masturbation is a fairly common vice in working stallions (Pickett & Voss 1972). There is little evidence to suggest that it has any significant effect on fertility but many people believe it affects libido or sexual drive. It is unlikely that a stallion could deplete his normal extragonadal sperm reserves by masturbation as erection usually occurs without ejaculation. Well exercised and managed stallions, used regularly, seldom masturbate. In exceptional cases a plastic ring fitted behind the glans is used to prevent masturbation and must be removed before covering. An accumulation of smegma in the prepuce may irritate and encourage masturbation.

SEMEN

Stallion semen is a milky white to grey white gelatinous liquid. The liquid comprises spermatozoa and seminal plasma.

In the testis, the germinal cells or primary spermatogonia develop through the spermatocyte stage to spermatids and then to spermatozoa (see Fig 2.2, p. 121). This cycle takes approximately 49 days (Sweistra et al. 1975). These authors calculated the mean daily sperm production of the average mature stallion to be 8.0×10^9 sperm. Sexual maturity in the stallion, in terms of daily sperm production and testicular size, occurs by five years of age (Aman et al. 1978). Sperm production per gram of testis, with age, is constant (Aman et al. 1978) and thus as testicular size increases, sperm production increases (Table 2.3).

TABLE 2.3 Effect of age on seminal characteristics of stallions

Characteristics	*Age* (years)			
	2–3 (n = 7)	4–6 (n = 16)	9–16 (n = 21)	P*
Seminal volume (ml)				
Gel	2.1	5.1	13.3	N.S
Gel-free	14.2^a	26.2^b	29.8^b	<0.05
Total	16.2^a	31.4^{ab}	43.2	<0.01
Spermatozoa				
Concentration (10^6/ml)	120.4	160.9	161.3	N.S.
Total (10^9)	1.8^a	3.6^{ab}	4.5^b	<0.05
Motility (%)	55.0	63.1	59.9	N.S.
pH	7.68^a	7.64^{ab}	7.59^b	<0.05

From Squires et al. (1979).
Means in the same row with different superscripts differ.
*Based on F-ratio calculated in analysis of variance.

Gebauer et al. (1974*a*) found that the average time taken for sperm to travel from the testis through the extragonadal ducts to the exterior was between 7.5 and 11 days. These authors also found that the extragonadal sperm reserves of stallions, ejaculating daily, were 58.6×10^9 sperm of which 88% were located in the epididymis. Frequency of ejaculation obviously has a marked effect on the size of the extragonadal sperm reserves.

Dott (1975) described the normal morphological characteristics of stallion spermatozoa. The heads are elliptical, with a length of 6.62 ± 0.22 μm, width 3.62 ± 0.19 μm and area 16.28 ± 0.8 μm^2. The neck is inserted abaxially into the head. The mid-piece is on average 9.83 ± 0.33 μm long. A variable number of morphologically abnormal sperm are found in the semen from normal fertile stallions. These abnormalities are described as primary (failure of spermatogenesis), secondary (failure of maturation) or tertiary (damage occurring during or after ejaculation). Large heads may contain the diploid complement of chromosomes and may have two tails. Surveys of the morphology of sperm from normal fertile stallions, reported by Dott (1975), suggested that up to 1.1 or 1.8% abnormal heads and up to 6.4 or 11.4% proximal and distal cytoplasmic droplets on the mid-piece may be seen. During maturation, droplets normally move distally before disappearing and thus their presence in ejaculated sperm signifies a failure of maturation and such sperm may not be capable of fertilization. Primary tail abnormalities seen are double-headed sperm with tails attached along their length, absent mid-piece, rudimentary tails or extreme coiling. Such sperm are usually dead. Most morphologically abnormal sperm have secondary tail abnormalities, often an L-shaped bend of the tail at the distal aspect of the mid-piece. Most of these sperm are alive but cannot move progressively.

The seminal plasma contains energy sources and chemicals capable of maintaining sperm through their process of maturation (Mann 1975). The ampullae secrete ergothionine, which may protect sperm from the immobilizing action of oxidizing or peroxidizing agents.

The seminal vesicles secrete citrate (which may act as a buffer) and gel. Surgical removal of the seminal vesicles (Klug et al. 1979) results in a decreased semen volume and increased sperm concentration. The epididymis secretes glycerylphosphorylcholine and glycosidases which may be involved in sperm maturation and may be used as epididymal function tests. Fructose is virtually absent from stallion's semen but lactate concentration is relatively high.

Semen evaluation and prediction of fertility

Despite the publication of statistical surveys producing reference values for semen constituents in 'normal' fertile stallions, all authors report great variation from stallion to stallion, at different times of the year, with ejaculation frequency and between different methods of semen collection. This, and our lack of knowledge of the correlation between semen constituent measurements and fertility, makes the job of stallion 'fertility testing' very difficult. It requires specialized equipment, some degree of expertise and experience and often a great deal of time and patience. The procedure requires a methodical approach, fitting many pieces into the 'jigsaw' so that some useful interpretation may be made at the end. Some details of technique and interpretation vary from author to author, but three practical reviews on this subject are available (Pickett & Back 1973; Kenney 1975; Pickett 1979).

History

A detailed account of the stallion's past health and sexual history should be recorded. If the stallion has been standing at stud and is suspected of subfertility or infertility then the teasing, examination, covering and pregnancy records of the mares concerned should be examined carefully. Poor management and/or a book of 'problem' mares can give any normal stallion a low conception or foaling rate. Study of the mares' bacteriological examination records can give useful information with respect to venereal disease.

Physical examination

Age, general bodily condition and conformation, in particular the condition of the hooves and limbs, should be examined. The heart should be carefully auscultated and an electrocardiogram may be recorded. The reproductive organs should be examined carefully and systematically. The sheath, scrotum and testes should be palpated with particular regard to size and constituency of the testes and epididymes. Testicular and scrotal dimensions may be measured with calipers (Gebauer et al. 1974*b*) (see Tables 2.1 and 2.2). Each gram of normal testicular tissue produces 20×10^6 sperm daily and thus from testicular size one can predict daily sperm production (Thompson et al. 1979). Approximately 80% of the daily sperm production may be collected with an artificial vagina (daily sperm output), after the extragonadal sperm reserves have been depleted by daily ejaculations for five to seven days. Thus the daily sperm output, calculated from testicular measurements, may be compared with the actual semen sample collected, and if the latter is lower abnormal testicular tissue may be present.

Kenney (1975) suggests that the best time to palpate the testes is after ejaculation, when the scrotum is relaxed, the area seems less sensitive and the testes are less apt to be reflexly withdrawn. At this time it should be possible to slip the testes and epididymis up and down within the cavity of the tunica vaginalis; if not, adhesions are probably present. Any evidence of trauma to the scrotum should be carefully noted. The spermatic cord and associated structures may be palpated up to the external inguinal ring. A rectal examination may allow palpation of the accessory glands for signs of obvious abnormality, if the stallion is cooperative. Kenney (1975) describes the position of the isthmus of the prostate (a firm 2×4 cm structure a little over wrist depth in the rectum). Anteriorly and ventrally to the prostate, the ampullae may be palpated and if the seminal vesicles are easily detectable they are probably abnormal. The internal inguinal canals may be palpated approximately 10 cm anteroventrally from the pelvic inlet and just lateral to the midline. On presentation with an in-oestrus mare, the penis may be further examined for abnormalities or signs of trauma. With an excitable stallion, this procedure is best carried out with the mare on the opposite side of a teasing board.

Bacteriological examinations

Swabs, previously moistened with transport medium or sterile distilled water, should be carefully taken from the urethra, urethral fossa and prepuce and placed immediately into Amies' charcoal transport medium prior to transport to the laboratory for aerobic and micro-aerophilic bacteriological culture (David et al. 1977; Platt et al. 1977). The presence of organisms which have been associated with venereal disease (*Haemophilus equigenitalis,* some capsule types of *Klebsiella aerogenes* and *Pseudomonas aeruginosa*) must be distinguished from the large number of bacterial and fungal surface contaminants often isolated from these sites in normal healthy stallions (Burns et al. 1975; Kenney 1975; Kenney et al. 1975) (see p. 157).

Sexual behaviour

The stallion should be watched teasing and covering an in-oestrus mare. Libido may be estimated when the stallion is presented with the mare and his behaviour pattern observed. The stallion's ability to enter and ejaculate can also be observed. The number of mounts and time from intromission to ejaculation should be recorded, and any antagonistic behaviour noted.

Semen collection

Semen may be collected by several methods. The examination of dismount samples (semen drips) into a sterile jar is the easiest method but results are unreliable. The quality is very variable and samples often contain accessory fluid and urine. The

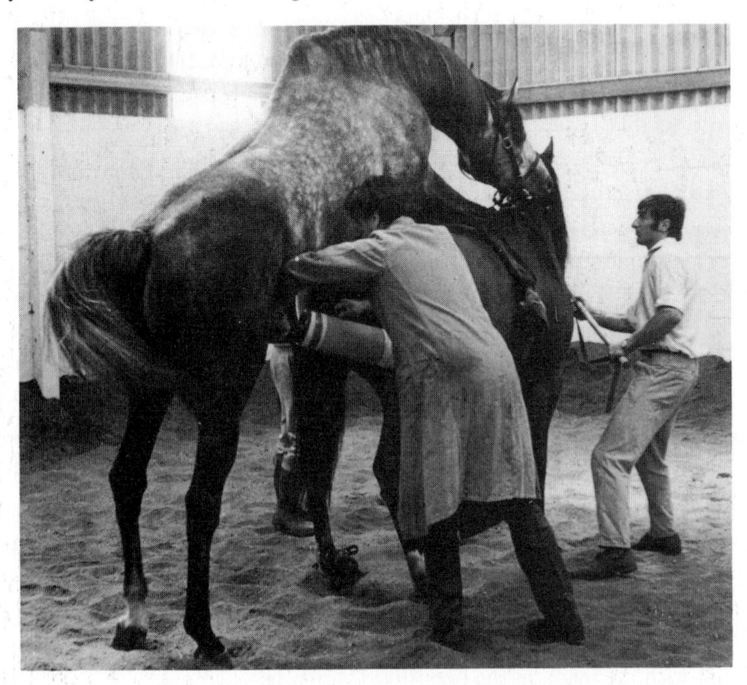

Fig. 2.22. Collecting semen into an artificial vagina.

presence of leucocytes, clots or potentially pathogenic bacteria may be significant, but it must be determined whether these materials come from the stallion or from the mare.

Semen may be recovered from the anterior vagina of the mare immediately after service. This method is inadequate because the assessment of seminal volume is impossible and after the specimen has been mixed with vaginal secretions, its pH, sperm motility, morphology and bacterial content are altered.

Semen may be collected in a condom. Sometimes technical difficulties are encountered with this method; the condom may burst or come off the penis during mating or dismounting and if this happens part or the whole of the semen sample may be lost.

The best way to collect semen is with an artificial vagina (Fig. 2.22). Various models have been designed, but we have found a light Japanese aluminium model, originally designed by Nishikawa (1959), to be convenient and easy to handle (Fig. 2.23). Most stallions can be persuaded to thrust and ejaculate into an artificial vagina and a satisfactory sample may be obtained. Before collecting a semen sample

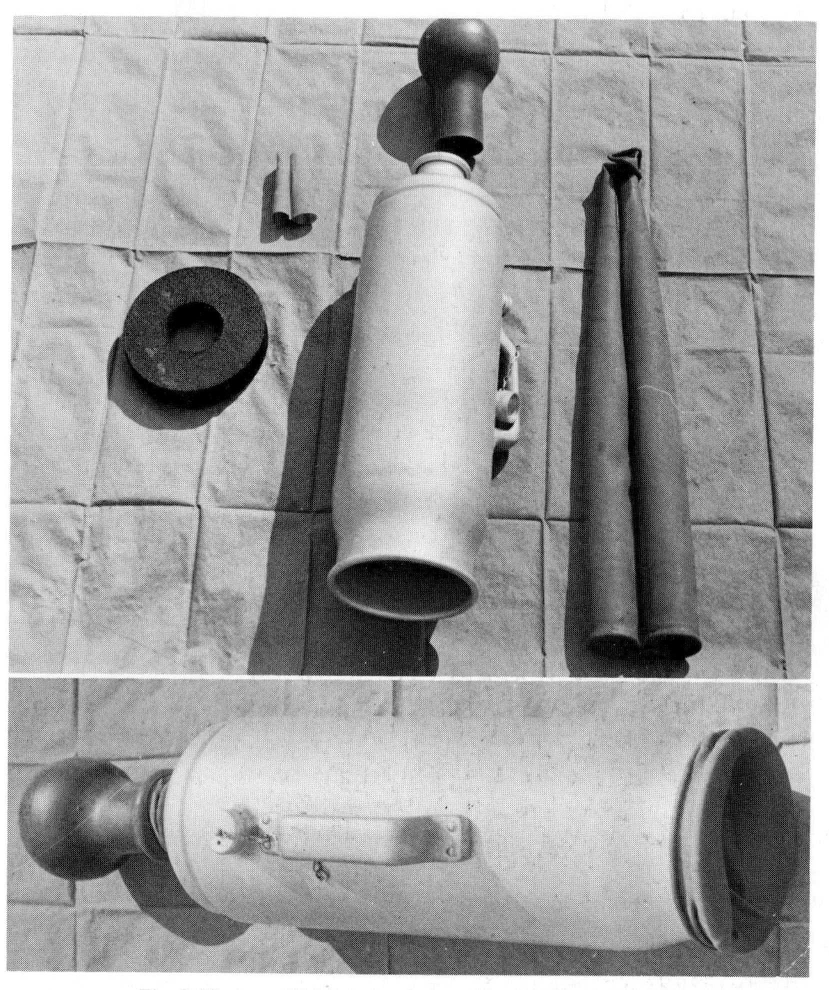

Fig. 2.23. An artificial vagina designed by Nishikawa (1959).

it is essential to check that all equipment is present and satisfactory, ready for the handling of the semen sample immediately after collection. It is also essential to make sure that all attendants are reliable and are briefed as to what is expected of them during the procedure; not only does this affect the success of the operation but it is essential for everyone's safety. It is considered sensible for the semen collector to wear a crash hat and strong boots with toe protectors. The in-oestrus mare should be one that can be relied upon to stand rigidly; she is prepared and restrained as for natural cover.

The water jacket in the artificial vagina should be filled with water at a temperature of 45–50°C. Stallions do not appear to be so sensitive to temperature as some other species; however, if the internal temperature of the artificial vagina exceeds 50°C there is a strong possibility of damaging the semen (Pickett & Back 1973). Approximately three-quarters of the length of the liner should be lubricated with sterile obstetrical lubricant; excessive quantities are likely to contaminate the semen.

The operator stands on the right side of the stallion and mare, near the mare's hind-quarters. When the stallion mounts, an attendant on the left side pulls the mare's tail to her left and the semen collector deflects the stallion's penis gently to the right side, guiding it towards the opening of the artificial vagina. This should be pushed against the hind-quarters of the mare, to gain stability, and the stallion should be allowed to gain intromission, rather than have the artificial vagina pushed onto the penis. Ejaculation may be monitored with a finger lightly held under the urethra, palpating the seminal jets and observing 'tail flagging'.

The collection bulb, bottle or bag should be pre-warmed and firmly insulated, especially in cold weather. After ejaculation the collection vessels should be carefully removed from the artificial vagina and the semen should be examined immediately in either a proper or a 'make-shift' laboratory as close to the collection area as possible. The gel fraction of the semen is a nuisance during both semen evaluation and artificial insemination. There are four main methods of dealing with the gel:

1. Careful aspiration with a sterile syringe (Cooper & Wert 1975).
2. Filtration through a sterile gauze in a pre-warmed sterile funnel.
3. An 'in-line' filter system incorporated into the artificial vagina (Pickett & Back 1973).
4. Carefully decanting the gel as if separating the yolk from the white of an egg.

Kenney (1975) recommends first aspirating the gel with a syringe and then filtration.

Semen examination

The semen sample should be examined as follows.

Gross appearance. The colour of the semen sample should be milky white, evenly turbid, without clots and there should be no unusual smell. Any pink or red colouring may suggest haemospermia, which is detrimental to fertility (Voss & Pickett 1975; Voss et al. 1976).

Volume. The volume of the semen sample should be measured in a pre-warmed, sterile measuring cylinder. The total volume of the ejaculate should be 60–120 ml and the gel-free volume 50–100 ml. These figures are highly variable between stallions and with season and pre-collection ejaculation frequency.

Motility. The motility of gel-free semen should be estimated immediately after collection on a pre-warmed microscope slide (Kenney 1975) or in a comparison chamber (Blom 1946). Both these methods are highly subjective and very dependent on the experience of the examiner. More objective methods which have been described, and which may be of use in the future, are a dark field photographic method (Elliott et al. 1973) and a cinematographic method (Plewinska-Wierzbowski & Bielanski 1970). Motility is classified, in percentage form, as oscilatory or progressive, i.e. those that are alive but are moving on the spot and those that are actively swimming across the field of observation. Stallion sperm have abaxial midpieces and they often move in a circle. Very tight circles, however, are considered abnormal. Sperm from a normal fertile stallion should have an immediate motility of 80% oscillatory and 60% progressive. Pickett and Voss (1972) note that stallion sperm tend to clump or agglutinate. To eliminate this, they suggest that semen is diluted with a dried skim milk extender prior to the estimation of motility. Kenney (1975) estimates motility in undiluted semen as extenders may have an enhancing effect. Motility estimates are more easily made under phase-contract illumination. A similar effect may be gained by lowering the condenser on a conventional microscope.

Longevity. Semen samples may be examined on warm microscope slides at five-minute intervals up to 30 minutes. If the semen sample is kept at body temperature, the progressive motility should fall off very little over the 30-minute period, but at room temperature, progressive motility starts to deteriorate after 15 minutes. Bielanski (1975) describes a method of estimating sperm survival time in vitro which closely correlates with survival time in the uterus. The semen sample is diluted 1 : 3 in 7% glucose solution at 0°C. A survival index is calculated by multiplying the percentage of motile sperm by the time interval between serial examinations under the microscope. A survival time of 24 hours is minimal, 24–36 hours good and greater than 36 hours very good. At room temperature (18°C) survival times of 18, 18–20 and greater than 20 hours were recorded. Kenney (1975) suggests that a sample is kept in the dark at 22°C and examined every hour until 10% or less of the sperm are motile. He also washes a sample by mixing equal parts with a non-fat dry skim milk, glucose and antibiotic extender and centrifuging for three minutes at 1500 rpm (300*g*). The pellet is then re-suspended in extender and kept at room temperature for 15 minutes, after which motility is again estimated. 15 minutes should be allowed for the sperm to recover from the effects of centrifugation.

pH. A standardized pH meter is preferable. A pH of between 7.3 and 7.7 is considered normal depending on seasonal effects (Pickett & Back 1972).

Sperm concentration. Sperm concentration may be measured using a haemocytometer or spectrophotometer. With the latter instrument, the semen is diluted 1 in 30 with 10% formalin in 0.9% saline (Pickett & Back 1972). Bielanski (1975) described the use of a principle, known as the 'wedge of Karras', using a spermiodensimeter with a scale from 1 to 0.1 which measures the transparency of the test sample, under contrast light, against a table of standards. This technique is simple for use in the field but has a high range of inaccuracy depending on the experience of the operator. Kenney et al. (1971) suggest that the concentration of sperm is unimportant if it exceeds 10×10^6/ml. Pickett and Voss (1972) have reported concentrations of between 100 and 350×10^6/ml depending on the seasonal influences and ejaculation frequency. Using our methods of semen collection and examination, sperm concentrations usually fall in the range of 50 to 100×10^6/ml.

Pickett and Voss (1972) and Kenney (1975) recommend a collection of two semen samples, one hour apart. Using this method Kenney (1975) describes his criteria of representativeness:

1. The volume of both ejaculates should be the same.
2. The total number of sperm in the second ejaculate should be half that of the first.
3. The pH should stay the same or increase slightly.
4. The motility should stay the same or increase.

If the ejaculate is proved not to be representative, the collections are repeated the next day.

Live/dead ratio. Smears are made using an equal volume of semen and nigrosin–eosin stain. The heads of live sperm remain unstained while the heads of dead ones are eosinophilic. The proportion of live and dead sperm is arrived at by a differential counting method. The live/dead ratio appears to be highly variable but one hopes to see a minimum of 50% live and usually more than 60%. Dott and Foster (1972) have described a refined staining method which allows more accurate examination and quantitation. A mixture of 0.67 g eosin and either 10 or 5 g nigrosin is added to 100 ml tap water and brought to the boil, then cooled. One drop of semen is added to at least eight drops of stain (pre-heated to 30°C). After incubation for five minutes at 30°C, smears are made on pre-heated slides so that it is easy to see through the smears when held over a light background. When dry, a portion of the smear is mounted and cover-slipped. When set, the slide is shaken in a mixture of equal volumes of 5% acetic acid and 0.6 N perchloric acid for 10–30 seconds and the excess is washed off in running tap water. After brief immersion in ethanol and then ether to remove water, another portion of the slide is mounted and cover-slipped. These authors describe eosinophilic spermatozoa as ones that were ‘past their best’.

Dott and Foster (1975) point out that the precise conditions required for obtaining comparable results with this method are best achieved in a properly equipped laboratory. They described the use of a formol citrate ‘suspended animation’ diluent, to make the time between collection and staining less critical. The diluent is made up of 2.9 g trisodium citrate dihydrate and 0.1 ml of a 40% solution of formaldehyde in 100 ml de-ionized water, and is added to an equal volume of semen. Samples may be stored for 48 hours at room temperature with no significant change in the proportion of eosinophilic spermatozoa counted, and very little change after storage for three weeks.

Morphology. The spermatozoa are examined after nigrosin–eosin stain. They may also be examined unstained, using phase-contrast or interference phase-contrast illumination or with the electron microscope after suitable preparation (Dott 1975).

The normal and abnormal morphology of stallion sperm has been described above (see p. 137). Bielanski (1975) reports an inverse correlation between percentage sperm with primary abnormalities and the fertility of the stallion. Greater than 10% primary abnormalities were associated with a depression of fertility whereas less than 30% secondary abnormalities need have no clinical significance. Dott concludes that fertility prediction should be based on two ejaculates collected four to six weeks apart, especially if the first ejaculate has more than 10% primary or secondary abnormalities. A high proportion of primary abnormalities suggests a testis defect, whereas a high proportion of secondary abnormalities suggests an epididymal defect. Changes in seminal plasma may affect sperm morphology and so render them more susceptible to damage from manipulation after ejaculation. Spermatogenesis and/or the passage of sperm through the epididymis may be affected by local increases in temperature, a generalized rise in body temperature, the action of some drugs and over-conditioning.

Normal live sperm per ejaculate. From the figures obtained from the above examinations it is possible to calculate the total number of morphologically normal, live sperm per ejaculate. Data reported by Pickett and Voss (1975) suggest that 500×10^6 normal live sperm are needed to obtain optimal conception rates with artificial insemination. Kenney (1975) reports that with individual stallions, under certain management conditions, acceptable conception rates have been achieved with extended semen using 100 and 300×10^6 normal motile sperm. Pickett and Voss (1972) report total numbers of sperm per ejaculate to vary between 600 and 2000×10^6 depending on seasonal effects and assuming 50% normal live sperm in the ejaculate. Most stallions are well in excess of these minimal requirements.

Cytology. A sample of semen should be mixed with an equal volume of 50% ethanol or 10% formol saline and stained by a rapid trichrome method (Sano 1949), haematoxylin and eosin or Wright's stain. Up to 1500 leucocytes per ml may be seen in normal semen samples. No erythrocytes should be seen. The occasional primary spermatogenic cell may be seen in normal semen samples (Roberts 1971; Swerczek 1975).

Bacteriology. A swab from the semen sample should be placed in Amies' charcoal transport medium prior to aerobic and micro-aerophilic culture (see p. 157).

Bielanski (1975), in his review of the evaluation of stallion semen, says that in general there have been no significant changes in the methods of semen evaluation over the past 15 years which enable us to evaluate potential male fertility any more accurately than was possible before 1960. He quotes from Anderson (1952): 'considerable success has been achieved in the field of examinations of semen and its relationship to fertility, but no single test, nor combination of tests, seems to be fully reliable so far. It is indeed not to be expected that any single test will suffice, for spermatozoa, in reaching their goal and achieving their object of fertilization, have several functions to perform'. Kenney et al. (1971) agree with observations of MacLeod and McGee (1950) that infertility or subfertility can exist in the presence of apparently normal numbers, motility and morphology of sperm. It is also true that stallions showing very poor semen quality are capable of producing reasonable conception rates if adequately managed. These factors are a major 'stumbling block' to our ability to predict stallion fertility accurately. Kenney (1975) concludes with a practical approach to this problem; if a stallion is to be considered sufficiently fertile to accept a book of 40 mares (or the equivalent if artificial insemination is used) he is expected to demonstrate normal libido, mating behaviour and ejaculation. His genital organs should be visibly and palpably normal and should be free from signs of inflammation or evidence to suggest infection or contamination with potentially pathogenic micro-organisms. He should have the potential for ejaculating 400×10^6 sperm in his first ejaculate, between April and July. 50% should exhibit initial progressive motility, 60% should be morphologically normal, and they should not go below 10% motility in six hours in fresh semen at 22°C. Seasonal effects are taken into consideration. If the stallion does not meet these requirements he is re-examined in 60 or more days. Some stallions fail to meet these requirements with repeated examinations over a period of six months, yet may finally pass. If the horse meets all these criteria he is considered a 'satisfactory prospective breeder', but if border-line in two or more criteria he is considered a 'questionable prospective breeder' and re-examination is recommended. If the horse is very unsatisfactory in two or more criteria or has severe permanent short-comings he is considered an 'unsatisfactory prospective breeder'.

There is no doubt that owners are reluctant to have their stallions evaluated for breeding 'soundness' prior to the breeding season (Pickett & Voss 1972) and in some cases this may lead to costly delays in a breeding programme. As long as our accuracy of prediction is poor (Bielanski 1975; Kenney 1975) despite the use of time-consuming and highly involved testing procedures (one month sexual rest followed by two semen collections one hour apart (Pickett & Voss 1972; Kenney 1975) or seven daily ejaculations to calculate the daily sperm output (Sweistra et al. 1975; Sullivan & Pickett 1975) stallion owners may continue to prefer readily available insurance policies. Such collection schedules are usually impractical prior to sale or export. In our opinion, there is still value in the careful collection and examination of a single semen sample, in full knowledge of the associated limitations, in conjunction with the examination of management and history and a full physical examination.

INFERTILITY

There have been few well documented statistical reports of infertility in the stallion. Examinations are seldom performed unless fertility is obviously low, so that stallions with various levels of subfertility tend to go unnoticed. Many stallions cover too few mares for their reproductive capabilities to be determined accurately (Pickett & Voss 1972). Dimmock (1950) surveyed 150 stallions in the Kentucky area, of which 11% had low or decreasing fertility. Problems of infertility were particularly prevalent in those over 10 years old.

Fertility statistics of different stallions are difficult to compare because of the marked influence of managerial influences. Day (1939) found that the fertility rate in heavy horses was 59%, light horses (premium stallions) 52%, Thoroughbreds at stud 68% and wild ponies 95%. An analysis of the records of 1186 Thoroughbred stallions, at stud during 1976 in the United Kingdom and Eire (Weatherbys 1977), is shown in Table 2.4.

TABLE 2.4 Records of 1186 Thoroughbred stallions at stud, UK and Eire, 1976

	Mean	*Range*	*SD*
Fertility percentage*	73	0–100	23 (50–96)
Total coverings	12	1–135	16 (0–28)
Living produce	7	0–78	9 (0–16)
Dead produce	1	0–8	2 (0–3)
Barren	2	0–30	3 (0–5)
'No returns'	2	0–19	3 (0–5)

$$\text{*Fertility percentage} = \frac{\text{living produce + dead produce}}{\text{mares reported conceived or barren}} \times 100.$$

Fashionable and expensive Thoroughbred stallions, well managed, expect to have recorded fertility in excess of 80%. Many less fashionable and less expensive stallions, who may be forced to accept mares of poor fertility potential, may have recorded fertility percentages lower than this without implying stallion abnormality. A relatively short and unphysiological breeding season contributes to the comparatively poor fertility figures for Thoroughbred stallions.

Managerial influences

Modern systems of stud farm management have a profound effect on a stallion's sexual behaviour and sometimes on his reported fertility percentage. It has been suggested (Merkt et al. 1978) that modern stallion managers are less selective in accepting their complement of mares, in terms of breeding potential, and that mare owners are less willing to cull 'bad breeders' than was previously the custom. This is an explanation for the apparent inability of modern equine stud farm medicine to improve overall fertility rates (see Fig. 1.28, p. 55).

In the wild state stallions cover mares many times during an oestrous period. They remain in contact with the mares throughout and are able to tease them and cover them at their own discretion. Under systems of modern stud farm management, mares and stallions are separated except for the act of mating. Teasing is usually performed by another entire horse, kept specifically for that purpose ('teaser').

Stud grooms and managers usually rely upon advice from the attending veterinary surgeon to decide on the optimal time for covering. Valuable stallions are restricted to two or three matings a day and 40–50 mares per breeding season, each seldom being covered more than twice per oestrus. It is thus vital that teasing, veterinary examinations and the management of the covering process are accurate and effective. General management factors such as lack of or excessive discipline, the stallion's relationships with the stallion man, housing and nutrition may all affect the ability of the stallion to perform his natural function.

Underfeeding the stallion during the breeding season will cause physical deterioration which will adversely affect sexual performance. Emaciation causes testicular atrophy and poor semen quality. Van Demark and Mauger (1964) showed that underfeeding dairy bullocks during their growing period had a limiting effect on sperm production at maturity. Overfeeding the stallion during the season will lead to physical deterioration and poor, slow sexual performance. This is probably a physical and psychological phenomenon rather than a direct effect on semen quality. Incorrect feeding may lead to problems such as laminitis which can have a serious effect on the stallion's sexual performance. Vitamin supplements, especially vitamin E, are occasionally fed to stallions to improve sexual performance or correct reduced libido. Although vitamin E is essential for normal reproductive function in the rat, there is no evidence that additional vitamin E is helpful in the stallion. There is no reliable evidence that mineral deficiencies have a specific effect on the reproductive tract of the stallion. A stallion's reproductive performance will not be adversely affected by nutritional deficiencies if a normal balanced ration is fed. Provided food intake is adequate and work and exercise correctly balanced, the benefit of feeding supplements is questionable.

In the arbitrarily arranged breeding season, stallions are required to mate outside the optimal period of the year for libido and at times of the day when their natural inclination may dictate otherwise. In these circumstances the number of services per day may be significant and particular individuals may suffer from overwork if called upon to mate two or three times in 12 hours for seven consecutive days and several consecutive weeks. This may result not only in a loss of libido but also, early in the breeding season, in the depletion of extragonadal sperm reserves and the ejaculation of semen of low sperm density. Cooper and Wert (1975) suggested that such problems might be avoided by artificially increasing daylight length during the winter or early spring to improve semen quality and sexual behaviour (see Chapter 1).

Failure to recognize ejaculation is one of the most serious defects of management in the covering yard and can be a substantial cause of subfertility. Some stallions show obvious signs of tail-flagging; others are very deceptive. The only reliable method of diagnosis is to place a hand lightly on the under-surface of the penis after intromission and feel the ejaculatory pulsations in the urethra (Fig. 2.20).

Abnormal behaviour

Behavioural patterns at mating are formed of a natural sequence of events; man's interference is most unlikely to improve on the process. The most common cause of abnormal sexual behaviour is mis-management (Pickett & Voss 1972). In many instances, if a young stallion develops behavioural abnormalities such as difficulties in intromission or ejaculation, the remedy is to encourage coitus without restraint of mare or stallion.

Pickett and Voss (1972, 1975) and Kenney (1975) all consider that the disciplinary measures presented to race-horses in training may result in a suppression of normal sexual behaviour when a stallion first retires to stud. Maiden stallions vary in the ease with which they learn to cover. The process is an instinctive phenomenon which environmental factors either help or hinder. Some maiden stallions present no problems but others need a great deal of patience and understanding. A quiet, experienced mare well in oestrus and with an unsutured vulva is a good subject for a first mating. A traumatic first experience for a young stallion may cause lasting psychological problems. A young stallion may become confused if too much human guidance is given. Failure at the first attempt should not give rise to anxiety and further attempts are best delayed for several hours. Firmness is essential on the part of the stallion man to protect animals and humans from injury and to ensure good covering yard routine; but too much physical or verbal chastisement will only confuse the stallion and affect sexual performance adversely. The establishment of a good stallion/handler relationship is essential for good breeding routine and adequate sexual performance. For this reason only one man should handle the stallion and he should be patient and understanding, yet capable of intelligent firmness.

Pickett and Voss (1972) found that there were variations in the number of mounts per ejaculation, reaction time and other less definable aspects of sexual behaviour in and out of the natural breeding season (see p. 124). There was a greater tendency for stallions to show aggressive behaviour towards mares out of the breeding season. It is difficult to cure a stallion of an aberrant behavioural pattern once established. Such stallions may become excessively vicious, biting and kicking the mare instead of mounting. These stallions should be kept firmly in check and the mare fitted with a leather collar or hood to protect her from injury.

Systemic illness or pain may result in abnormal sexual behaviour, often manifest as reduced libido or failure of erection, intromission or ejaculation. Any stallion showing abnormal sexual behaviour should receive a thorough physical examination for systemic illness resulting in elevation of body temperature, evidence of pain throughout the musculoskeletal system, e.g. laminitis, muscular damage or lumbar vertebral spondylitis. The genital organs should be examined for signs of injury or infection. Haematological tests and urine analysis should be used to search for evidence of disease.

The mature stallion who loses his libido halfway through the stud season may have problems involving management, general health, injury or inheritance. Failing libido may follow overwork, detrimental handling or adverse changes in the stallion's environment. A particular mare to which a horse takes a dislike or with which he has had a painful experience may reduce his confidence, especially if management persists in attempts to force a successful mating. A stallion that shows little or no sexual interest may be lunged for half an hour before presentation of the mare. This, or a change in surroundings at mating time, may increase libido. The stallion may be used to tease mares in the morning and this may accentuate sexual desire in the covering yard. In most cases, however, it is difficult to evaluate therapy and many techniques may have to be tried before the condition is corrected or corrects itself.

The habit of prolonged delay in mounting or ejaculating, so that a service takes 30–60 minutes, frustrates horse and management. Various procedures can be tried to encourage more speedy performance, from the use of hippomanes to injections of testosterone, from the administration of LH, GnRH or β-carotene to women's perfume applied to the mare's hind-quarters. No remedy appears to have had consistent success. Perhaps the best advice is to limit the stallion to a maximum number of mounts – say three – before returning him to his box. A further attempt is then made an hour later. Stallions who take a long time to cover may have to be restricted to a reduced number of mares during each season. In certain instances turning the stallion loose with a mare in oestrus may help to restore his confidence and reduce the time he takes to mate.

Pickett and Voss (1972, 1975) recognized four main categories of abnormal stallion sexual behaviour:

1. Failure to obtain or maintain erection.
2. Incomplete intromission or lack of pelvic thrusts after intromission.
3. Dismounting at the onset of ejaculation.
4. Failure to ejaculate in spite of a complete prolonged erection and repeated intromissions. Some stallions in this category respond to a few days of sexual rest, although libido remains very high.

These authors found that many of their cases were primarily psychological and responded to a retraining process. This consisted of presenting the stallion to a mare or a series of mares, observing his behaviour and then letting him act independently until a given situation elicited a favourable sexual response. Extreme patience and time were often required but after the stallion had repeatedly ejaculated successfully, he was subjected to gradual discipline. The authors report that all but the most severely maladjusted stallions respond favourably to this process. Each case is different and successful treatment requires close observation. Sometimes such a case may respond to the sight of another stallion covering a mare.

Rasbeck (1975) suggested that ejaculatory disorders may be more prevalent than previously suspected. Clinical signs were normal libido and erection of the penis followed by a number of copulatory movements which terminated in partial or complete failure of ejaculation. In some stallions the condition occurred during the first two or three seasons at stud and in others it developed after several seasons of normal activity. It could be transitory, intermittent or permanent. Some stallions appear distressed and/or exhausted following several unsuccessful attempts at ejaculation. 'Tail-flagging' sometimes gave a false impression that ejaculation had occurred. Post mortem examination of four cases revealed no pathological changes in the reproductive organs or elsewhere. It has been postulated that a functional disturbance of the nervous mechanism controlling ejaculation may be caused by environmental or genetic factors or could be acquired and of psychological or physical origin. Eleven cases of ejaculatory disorders in normal healthy stallions were investigated by Rasbeck (1975) and three of these animals recovered after simple correction of environmental factors, including the number of mares served. Of the eight stallions which did not respond to environmental changes, one recovered after treatment with pilocarpine and one after treatment with ephedrine. This author described the possible causes of failure of the nervous regulation of the reproductive tract and explained the rationale behind his medical treatments.

Kenney and Cooper (1974) have described the use of a phantom mare for semen collection and in overcoming or controlling undesirable stallion breeding behaviour. They first re-train the stallion by teaching him to use an artificial vagina. The mare's hind-quarters are then covered by a canvas shroud, during semen collection, and this is then transferred to a mattress over a teasing rail. The overall height of the phantom described was originally 127 cm but later the phantom was constructed to be adjustable for height. Stallions may become conditioned to using an artificial vagina while mounted on a dummy. An in-oestrus mare is held to one side at first but later this is unnecessary. A phantom may be useful in overcoming abnormal sexual behaviour such as 'mare shyness' after an injury or associated with pain or lameness, delayed ejaculation, inability to ejaculate and excessively vicious behaviour.

Genetic factors

Sterile or subfertile stallions with no history of trauma, infectious disease or managerial problems are often considered to have genetic inadequacies. These may be associated with semen abnormalities or, in rarer cases, chromosomal abnormalities. Hermaphrodites and genetic mosaics have been reported but are usually associated with obvious abnormalities of the genitalia. Penile size is probably determined genetically and in some cases may produce mechanical difficulties at covering. Ideally, horses suffering from heritable conditions should not be used for breeding, as abnormalities may thus be spread among the horse population. Cryptorchidism is a heritable condition and may be associated with degrees of testicular hypoplasia in pony stallions (Bishop et al. 1966). We have seen abnormal bilateral testicular degeneration, probably associated with testicular hypoplasia, in a miniature pony stallion (Fig. 2.24). There may be no diminution of fertility in monorchidism. Increased male sexual behaviour with associated nervousness and irritability is seen in cryptorchid horses (rigs). This is thought to be the result of increased secretion of androgenic hormones by the retained testis. Some authors have suggested that testicular descent may occur up to two years of age and this has led to much confusion. When examining yearlings for sale it is essential that animals with only one palpable testis in the scrotum are classified as cryptochid. In such cases the inguinal canal ventral to the external inguinal ring must be carefully explored to detect those testes that have been pulled up due to the action of the cremaster muscles. There is no evidence that testes can be pulled up through the external inguinal ring and then descend again at will.

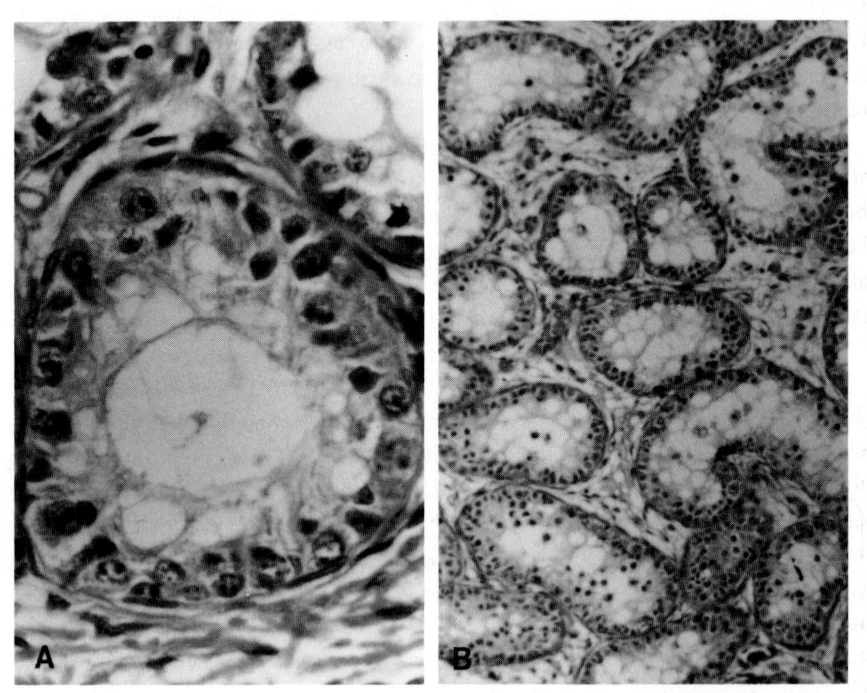

Fig. 2.24. Testicular biopsy showing degeneration, probably associated with testicular hypoplasia in a miniature pony stallion. A, Transverse section of seminiferous tubule showing loss of germinal cells and resulting vacuole formation (c.f. Fig. 2.2). H & E × 400. B, Low-power photomicrograph showing diffuse lesion. H & E × 100.

Umbilical and inguinal hernias may be genetically determined and in many cases are corrected before the horse becomes a stallion. This produces an ethical problem which is difficult to solve. If they are not corrected they may cause unwillingness to cover due to pain or discomfort during attempts to mount.

Hormonal factors

There are no reports in the literature of the correlation of blood hormone levels with fertility problems and, although endocrinological inadequacies are frequently blamed for infertility or subfertility in the stallion, hormonal treatment rarely causes lasting improvement.

Berndstone et al. (1979) advised against the use of exogenous testosterone on the grounds that daily doses of 200 μg/kg reduced testicular weight. After 74–90 days, this produced a depression of sperm output. This dose rate doubled peripheral testosterone levels but reduced peripheral LH levels by one-third. Recovery after treatment was very slow and incomplete after 90 days. LH therapy has been used on maiden stallions, with apparent success, at the start of their first covering season. Some authorities have discouraged its use on the ground that it could, theoretically, produce anaphylaxis as it is not of equine origin. Roser et al. (1979) monitored the development of antibodies to repeated injections of HCG in five cycling mares and found no abnormalities of ovulation or fertility and no evidence of allergic reactions. It will be interesting to see if gonadotrophic releasing factors are successful in the treatment of low libido and deficient spermiogenesis of possible hormonal origin in stallions.

The results of hormonal 'profiles' in 'normal' mares or stallions must be correlated with the target organ effects, if hormone therapy is to be put on a more scientific basis. In the meantime the clinician is advised to administer 3000 units of luteinizing hormone intravenously, one hour before coitus, to stallions of low libido. Cox et al. (1973) have shown that administration increases blood testosterone levels, but its effect on libido must be judged on individual results.

Abnormalities of the penis and prepuce

The penis and prepuce are very vulnerable to traumatic injury. If kicked when erect, the penis may swell rapidly and massively from vascular rupture and haemorrhage. Immediate first aid for such an injury should include removal of the mare, quietening the stallion and the application of cold water either by hose or with wet towels. A similar rupture of a superficial penile blood vessel may occur when covering a tightly sutured mare, without prior episiotomy, or when a mare moves suddenly while the stallion is thrusting. Traumatic damage to the penis may occur after prolonged penile prolapse or priapism following the use of some tranquillizers (Kenney 1975; Pearson & Weaver 1978).

Voss and Pickett (1975) described the diagnosis and treatment of haemospermia, resulting from bacterial or viral urethritis, urethral abnormality or damage to the glans penis by suture material in the mare's vulva. Diagnosis was achieved by demonstration of blood in semen samples and this appeared to result in infertility. Suggested treatment was sexual rest and the use of specific antibacterial medication, if indicated. The results of treatment were varied. Surgical removal of urethral strictures was performed in one case and in another haemospermia was associated with the demonstration of *Strongylus edentatus* larvae in the ejaculate.

Tumours of the penis are uncommon and are usually squamous-cell carcinomas of low malignancy (Roberts 1971). Papillomas, angiomas and melanomas have been recorded in or on the sheath and penis of horses. Carcinomas often ulcerate and usually bleed at the time of service. These lesions must be differentiated from granulomas caused by *Habronema* larvae ('summer sores') in countries where this condition occurs. Sarcoids may involve the prepuce, causing severe discomfort (see p. 456).

The herpesvirus associated with coital exanthema causes painful vesicles on the glans penis (see Fig. 1.54) (Gibbs et al. 1970; Pascoe & Baggust 1975) (see p. 103).

Abnormalities of the scrotum, testis and epididymes

The scrotum is subject to traumatic injury. Oedema of the scrotum may reflect systemic illness, especially hepatic disease and more specifically equine infectious anaemia (see p. 428) (Roberts 1971; Kenney 1975). Such a condition may cause inhibition of spermatogenesis by interfering with heat exchange.

Incompetence of the inguinal rings may result in herniation of peritoneal fat and small intestine into the scrotum. Strangulation of the hernial contents is recognized by acute colic and hard tense painful scrotum. It is most often seen in horses up to three years old. In very early cases, it may be possible to retrieve the herniated tissues by digital manipulation per rectum. In other cases urgent surgical intervention is essential.

Torsion of the testis may occur in degrees varying from those that produce no pain or semen abnormalities at all to those that are associated with vascular obstruction and acute colic. Some cases of testicular torsion appear to be transient (Kenney 1975).

Orchitis may be a complication of injury, for instance a kick, or of infection, for instance with *Str. zooepidemicus, Str. equi, Brucella abortus, Pfeiferella mallei, Salmonella abortus equi* or equid herpesviruses I and II (Roberts 1971). The testes become swollen, hot and painful and epididymitis frequently accompanies the condition. The stallion may refuse to cover, but if he ejaculates the semen may contain large numbers of leucocytes, sometimes appearing as clots. Spermatozoal morphology and motility are abnormal. The most frequently isolated organism is *Str. zooepidemicus* which may be cultured from semen or observed directly on a Gram-stained smear. The prognosis is always guarded and the condition may become chronic, with testicular fibrosis and poor semen quality, which may have a permanent effect on the stallion's fertility. Acute orchitis should be treated with systemic antibiotics. The choice depends on the sensitivity of any organism recovered, otherwise a broad-spectrum antibiotic should be given. Cold-water therapy to the scrotum also gives relief and reduces blood supply and further swelling. It is known that in man an acute orchitis, of infectious or traumatic origin, can sometimes lead to the release of testicular antigens to which the body has not previously been exposed. This may lead to the production of autoantibodies which may lead to degeneration of the other testis. Thus in some human cases a severe acute orchitis of one testis is treated by rapid surgical removal to prevent damage to the other one. It is not known whether this phenomenon occurs in the stallion but the removal of the abnormal testis in severe cases may be contemplated.

Testicular hypoplasia may be associated with cryptorchisism (Bishop et al. 1966).

Testicular degeneration may be associated with thermal factors following the elevation of body temperature by systemic infection, very high ambient temperatures and possibly conformation factors resulting in an incompetant heat-exchange system. Testicular torsion and scrotal hernia may interfere with testicular blood vessels, resulting in congestion, pain and elevation of testicular temperature. Contusion and inflammation of the testes has been reported in racing stallions, particularly Standardbreds. Inflammation of the testicular artery in the horse may be caused by strongyle larvae, the equine arteritis virus and other unknown agents. These may produce areas of testicular degeneration (McEntee 1970) and strongyle larvae may produce testicular adhestions. Varicocele is sometimes seen in association with the spermatic vein in stallions (Roberts 1971). McLeod and McGee (1950) describe degeneration of the testes, based on semen examinations, in ageing stallions. Discrepancies between testicular size, measured by calipers, and daily sperm output may suggest the diagnosis of testicular degeneration (Thompson et al. 1979) (see p. 139). Testicular biopsy may provide interesting data in some cases of testicular degeneration, but this procedure has not been widely used and is not without reported risk (Smith 1974).

Kenney (1975) states that few diseases of the stallion's epididymis are known. Granulomas and *Streptococcus zooepidemicus* abscess have been described.

Testicular and epididymal tumours, dermoid cysts, teratomas, seminomas, adenocarcinomas, interstitial and sertoli cell tumours have all been rarely reported (Roberts 1971). A melanoma of the scrotum has been reported and lipomas are not uncommon on the surface of the testis (McEntee 1970).

Abnormalities of secondary sexual organs

Seminal vesiculitis is uncommon in the stallion but has been reported in association with a *Brucella abortus* infection (Vandeplassche & Devoss 1960). Klug et al. (1979) have described a surgical technique for the removal of these organs which was used in one case of seminal vesiculitis in a stallion. The condition may be diagnosed by rectal palpation. One or both vesicles are enlarged and sensitive. The stallion may refuse to cover, or may try to do so but be unable to ejaculate. If ejaculation does occur, the semen will contain many leucocytes and bacterial culture will reveal pathogenic organisms. The chronic form of the condition is associated with poor prognosis and treatment should consist of early systemic antibiotic therapy usually with complete sexual rest. There may be a case, however, for allowing daily ejaculation during the period of antibiotic therapy, attempting to 'flush out' the genital tract.

Apparent blockage of semen in the efferent ducts, somewhere between the testis and penis, has been encountered (Cooper & Kenney, personal communication). We have seen this condition in a five-year-old Thoroughbred stallion during his second season at stud. During his first season, fertility appeared normal but during the first two months of his second breeding season, no conceptions were produced despite normal libido and apparently normal mating and ejaculation. Following excessive sexual excitement the stallion produced a semen sample which was of the constituency of thick cream. It contained 600 million spermatozoa per ml, the majority of which were dead and tailless. Following the apparent removal of this 'blockage', semen samples contained live, morphologically normal and motile spermatozoa and fertility returned to normal. The exact site of blockage in this case was not determined.

Specific genital infections

Equine coital exanthema

Coital exanthema is a specific venereal infection caused by a herpesvirus distinct from equid herpesviruses I and II (Pascoe & Bagust 1975). The virus affects both stallions and mares (see Fig. 1.53), but the manifestations in the stallion are usually more severe and systemic signs may occur (Gibbs et al. 1970). The infection is brought into the stud farm by a visiting mare, usually a symptomless carrier. She then infects the stallion, who infects other mares, before he shows clinical signs and mating is stopped. Pascoe and Bagust (1975) reported experimental infections in stallions which suggested that the incubation period varied from five to ten days. The time to healing and disappearance of the virus was as long as 40 days but in the field lesions often heal rapidly and stallions can normally recommence their duties in 10–14 days after the first signs. In the stallion, lesions appear in the form of papules, vesicles or pustules on the penis and there may be associated dullness, anorexia and unwillingness to work. Pyrexia may be present and palpation of the genital area is often resented. Treatment is by systemic and local antibiotics (to combat secondary bacterial infection) and sexual rest. All mares covered by the stallion during the previous ten days should be examined, treated if necessary and isolated. Pascoe and Bagust (1975) demonstrated serological responses to this infection, including the production of complement-fixing and serum-neutralizing antibodies which reached a maximum at 14–21 days after infection. CF antibodies declined rapidly and were not detectable by 60 days after infection whereas SN antibodies remain for at least one year. If readily available, these serological tests might be useful, in association with epidemiological data, in the identification of carrier mares.

Dourine

Dourine is a condition caused by *Trypanosoma equiperdum* which occurs in Asia, Africa, South America, southern and eastern Europe and Mexico, but not in the United Kingdom. Clinical signs include fever, inappetence, oedema of the genitalia and discharge from the urethra and vagina. Urticarial plaques occur on the body and progressive muscular paralysis develops. The incubation period is two to 12 weeks and the disease is spread by coitus. Diagnosis is made by recognizing the organism in smears of exudative fluid or inocculation into rabbits; or by a complement fixation test. Treatment of choice is by quinapyramine sulphate (Ristic 1972). This disease is now notifiable in the United Kingdom.

Bacterial infections

Stallions harbour many kinds of potentially pathogenic and non-pathogenic bacteria on their external genitalia, particularly in the prepuce and associated smegma (Hughes et al. 1967; Burns et al. 1975; Kenney et al. 1975). The stallion does not usually suffer clinical signs and the bacteria are more important for their effect on the fertility of his mares. Bacteria isolated may be classified according to their effect on the mare (see p. 170):

1. Those organisms not associated with infection and endometritis in the mare, e.g. diphtheroids, *Neisseria* spp., *Streptococcus faecalis* and *Staphylococcus albus.*

2. Organisms capable of causing infection and endometritis in mares who have depressed local natural defence mechanisms (Hughes & Loy 1969; Peterson et al. 1969; Kenney et al. 1975), e.g. *Streptococcus zooepidemicus* (β-haemolytic streptococci), *Staphylococcus aureus* (coagulase-positive), haemolytic *E. coli, Proteus* species and some *Klebsiella aerogenes* capsule types (e.g. type 7).

3. Organisms capable of causing primary infection and endometritis in mares with normal local defence mechanisms, and outbreaks of venereal disease, e.g. some *Kl. aerogenes* capsule types (e.g. 1 and 5), some strains of *Ps. aeruginosa* and *H. equigenitalis*.

Any of these organisms may be mechanically transmitted directly into the uterus of the mare at coitus (Kenney et al. 1975). It is impossible to sterilize the penis and prepuce before service and coitus results in further bacterial challenge to the endometrium (Hughes & Loy 1969; Peterson et al. 1969; Kenney et al. 1975).

Crouch et al. (1972) found that it was possible to culture *Kl. aerogenes* capsule type 5 from the urethra and accessory glands of a stallion that had been transmitting the disease, although showing no clinical signs himself. Similarly, with contagious equine metritis stallions show no systemic signs during an outbreak in their mares and, unlike the mare, show no serological antibody response.

For the detection of possible venereal-disease-producing bacteria on the genital organs of stallions, swabs should be taken from the urethra, urethral fossa, prepuce and pre-ejaculatory fluid on a number of occasions (David et al. 1977) (see p. 139). Unfortunately, the interpretation of bacteriological findings is not always straightforward. Certain capsular strains of *Kl. aerogenes* have been associated with outbreaks of venereal disease, especially types 1 and 5 (Crouch et al. 1972; Atherton 1975; Merkt et al. 1975*a*; Platt et al. 1976), but there are so many capsular strains about which we have little or no epidemiological knowledge that it is sometimes impossible to rule out the possibility of venereal spread without transmission experiments using maiden mares. This is difficult to organize in practice, but in some cases may be essential before one can advise that an affected stallion is fit to cover his mares. Laboratories have reported finding micro-aerophilic organisms which appear almost indistinguishable from *Haemophilus equigenitalis* and this may prove a further problem for diagnosis in the future.

Treatment for the genital organs of a stallion infected with bacteria which have the potential to produce venereal disease is difficult and fraught with dangers. *H. equigenitalis* has been found to be widely sensitive to antibiotics and penicillin, ampicillin and chlorhexidine have been recommended. *Kl. aerogenes* and *Ps. aeruginosa* are frequently very resistant to antibiotics, as judged by in vitro sensitivity tests. Gentamicin and polymyxin are the two which appear to be most useful. Possibly because of their capsulated form and ability to invade the urinary system, *Klebsiella* and *Pseudomonas* infections often respond to treatment less well than *H. equigenitalis* infections. Systemic treatment with gentamicin at a dose rate of 4.4 mg/kg intravenously, twice daily for up to 34 days, has been used successfully to treat *Ps. aeruginosa* and *Kl. aerogenes* infections in stallions (Hamm 1978). The stallion's penis is a very sensitive organ and severe local reactions may follow local treatment. Removal of the natural smegma and oils by repeated local treatments, which is necessary to remove the offending organism, may result in soreness, cracking of the penile integument and haemorrhage. In an attempt to avoid this, lanolin may be added to the treatment material. Local treatment with antibiotics or antiseptics may remove some of the natural bacterial flora and allow multiplication of the more resistant species, notably *Kl. aerogenes* and *Ps. aeruginosa.* For these reasons, prophylactic treatment of the stallion's penis with antibiotics or disinfectants is contraindicated. Recently we have heard that a 1% water-miscible solution of silver sulphadiazine has been used successfully to treat a stallion with *Pseudomonas* contaminating the external genitalia.

ARTIFICIAL INSEMINATION

Artificial insemination in the horse has been reviewed by Bowen (1969), a practical manual of techniques has been produced by Pickett and Back (1973) and experiences with its use under conditions of Standardbred stud farm management has been described (Cooper & Wert 1975). The technique for unfrozen semen is simple and easy to perform and is now used routinely in the Standardbred and Quarterhorse breeding industries in the United States. The semen is collected by an artificial vagina, with the stallion mounting an in-oestrus mare or phantom (see p. 140). The semen may then be used in one of three ways:

1. The whole ejaculate, without dilution, may be inseminated into a single mare.

2. The semen may be diluted with an extender at room temperature, for insemination into one or more mares. The extended semen may be fractionated depending on mares available and semen quality.

3. The sperm may be 'washed' by repeated centrifugation and dilution with semen extender containing antibiotics as part of a 'minimal contamination technique' (Kenney et al. 1975). Semen samples plus an equal volume of extender are carefully centrifuged at 1500 rpm for three minutes so as to produce a soft pellet. Centrifugation does not appear to damage sperm motility (Pickett et al. 1975*b*). The supernatant is removed and the pellet is resuspended in an appropriate volume of warm extender for the number of mares to be inseminated.

The choice of technique used depends on the stud farm management, the number of mares to be inseminated, semen quality, the presence of potentially pathogenic bacteria in the semen and/or the susceptibility of the mare's uterus to infection. The mares are prepared in a collection area and are inseminated with the semen into the uterus via plastic sterile pipettes.

With good technique, a high fertility percentage can be achieved by the use of an artificial insemination programme (Cooper & Wert 1975). The exact number of normal motile sperm needed per insemination is not known. Success with as few as 100×10^6 normal motile sperm has been reported but in the absence of more accurate data, and to give a practical safety margin, 500×10^6 normal motile sperm is recommended (Pickett & Back 1973). Raw (undiluted) semen is normally inseminated within one hour of collection and so is used within the confines of the stud farm. The semen is maintained at 30–35°C and precautions are taken to prevent 'cold shock'.

For short-term storage (up to three days) of stallions semen, the semen may be diluted immediately with extender, usually in a 2 : 1 proportion (Allen et al. 1976). The extended semen is then cooled slowly to 4°C over one to four hours and held at that temperature until used.

Much more information is now available on the techniques of freezing stallion's semen, which is significantly more fragile than bull semen. This is a highly specialized field. Those who are interested in this subject are referred to Barker and Gandier (1957), Buell (1963), Polge and Minotakis (1964), Rajamannam (1968), Tischner (1979), Krug et al. (1975), Merkt et al. (1975*b*), Nishikawa (1975), and Pace and Sullivan (1975).

Artificial insemination is widely used throughout the world in non-Thoroughbred horses. Thoroughbred registration authorities refuse to accept progeny produced by artificial insemination and thus effectively prevent veterinary surgeons from providing their clients with this potentially valuable service (Rossdale 1978; Rossdale et al. 1979). The advantages and disadvantages of artificial insemination systems have been discussed by Bowen (1969), Pickett and Voss (1973), and Allen et al. (1976). The advantages are as follows:

1. *Disease control.* By providing a system where there need be no direct physical contact between the stallion and mare, the risk of spread of contagious infectious disease, either venereal (equine coital exanthema, *Kl. aerogenes, Ps. aeruginosa* and *Haemophilus equigentalis*) or non-venereal (equine infectious anaemia, strangles, equid herpesvirus I abortion, equine influenza), may be very much reduced or eliminated. Seminal extenders and minimal contamination techniques (Burns et al. 1975; Kenney et al. 1975; Simpson et al. 1975) may be used to treat semen containing potentially pathogenic organisms or to reduce the normal seminal bacterial contaminants, as a prophylatic measure, in mares suffering from an increased susceptibility to uterine infection.

2. *Overcoming physical deformities in mares.* Mares that have tightly stitched vulvas may be inseminated without the need for continually re-opening and re-closing the suture line. Mares with physical conditions or behavioural problems which make natural service difficult or hazardous may also be inseminated.

3. *Overcoming abnormal or unwanted stallion behaviour.* Stallions with abnormal

sexual behaviour may be retrained to an artificial insemination programme; vicious stallions may be taught to use a phantom, thus eliminating the risk of damage to the mare.

4. *Managerial advantages.* The collection and fractionation of semen with an artificial vagina could significantly reduce the covering load of a stallion. This might be a great help in avoiding the deterioration of semen quality during busy periods and in reducing the time spent by stud farm personnel in the covering yard. The insemination of in-oestrus mares on alternate days throughout the oestrous period might reduce the number of repeated rectal examinations performed by the veterinary surgeon.

It is possible to synchronize oestrus (Hyland & Bristol 1978) using prostaglandin and HCG treatment, and then to inseminate, resulting in a reduction in the spread of foaling the following year. Such a system, if widely used, could reduce the length of the breeding season with all the economic advantages that would accrue. Using freezing techniques, costs could be reduced by transporting semen rather than mares from country to country. An artificial insemination system could increase the breeding efficiency of any particular stallion and could, if considered desirable, significantly increase the number of mares he inseminates. Similarly, using freezing techniques, the breeding life of the stallion could be increased.

Registration authorities have traditionally been worried by the risk of exploitation of fashionable sires, reduction of the individual value of bloodstock through oversupply and the increased risk of fraud. There is also a worry that the traditional organization and structure of the breeding industry would change from stud farms to stallion stations. Many of these worries stem from an ignorance of how equine artificial insemination systems are run and the misconception that a system such as used in dairy cows might be directly applicable to horses. There is little similarity between either the needs of the two industries or the necessary technical methods for handling the two types of semen. It is a great mistake to compare these two different systems. We recommend that until such time as the Thoroughbred breeding industry satisfies itself that the widespread use of artificial insemination is in its own best interests and can be adequately controlled, artificial insemination is allowed for disease control only, under direct veterinary supervision. The progeny of such matings could be checked by parentage control which has now reached an advanced stage of development (Towers-Clark 1977). Such a system would not change the structural organization of the Thoroughbred breeding industry, but would reduce the incidence and spread of infectious and venereal diseases and might allow the improvement of fertility rates in 'problem' mares.

Following such limited use of artificial insemination, and further research into the needs of the industry, the wider use of artificial insemination might be allowed. Such a system would need built-in safe-guards such as the limiting of the number of mares to be covered per season by a particular stallion (this may not be possible under restrictive practice legislation in some countries), the registration only of progeny born to matings which had been nominated to the registration authorities, prior to the start of the breeding season, strict veterinary supervision and certification, and the checking of indentities by blood parentage control. It would also be necessary to ensure that artifical insemination was not knowingly used to perpetuate or disseminate genetic abnormalities and that any increased in-breeding would not be detrimental to the breed.

In order to attain the excellent conception rates possible by artificial insemination, and reported by those who are highly experienced in the use of the technique under practical stud farm conditions (Pickett & Voss 1972; Cooper & Wert 1975), there would be a stimulus for stud farm management and veterinary supervision to become highly proficient and efficient in all aspects of fertility control. This can only be to the long-term advantage of the industry.

References and further reading

Allen, W.R., Bowen, J.H., Frank, C.J., Jeffcott, L.B. & Rossdale, P.D. (1976) The current position of A.I. in horse breeding. *Equine vet. J.*, **8**, 72.

Aman, R.P., Thompson, D.L., Squires, E.L. & Pickett, B.W. (1978) Effects of age and frequency of ejaculation on spermatozoa and production and extragonadal spermatozoal reserves in stallions. *J. Reprod. Fert.*, Suppl. **27**, 1

Anderson, J. (1952) The examination of semen and the relationship to fertility. *Proc. 2nd int. Congr. Phys. Path. Anim. Reprod. artific. Insem., Copenhagen*, **3**, 7.

Atherton, J.G. (1975) The identification of equine genital strains of *Klebsiella* and *Enterobacter* species. *Equine vet. J.*, 7, 207.

Barker, C.A.V. & Gandier, J.C.C. (1957) Pregnancy in a mare resulting from frozen epididymal spermatozoa. *Can. J. comp. Med.*, **21**, 47.

Berndstone, W.R., Hoyer, J.H., Squires, E.L. & Pickett, B.W. (1979) Influence of exogenous testosterone on sperm production, seminal quality and libido of stallions. *J. Reprod. Fert.*, Suppl. **27**, 19.

Berndstone, W.E., Pickett, B.W. & Nett, T.H. (1974) Reproductive physiology of the stallion and seasonal changes in the testosterone concentrates of peripheral plasma. *J. Reprod. Fert.*, Suppl. **39**, 115.

Bielanski, W. (1975) The evaluation of stallions semen in aspects of fertility control and its use for artificial insemination. *J. Reprod. Fert.*, Suppl. **23**, 19.

Bishop, M.W.H., David, J.S.E. & Messervy, A. (1966) Cryptorchidism in the stallion. *Proc. R. Soc. Med.*, **59**, 769.

Blom, E. (1946) A comparing chamber for microscopic examination of undiluted bull semen. *Br. vet. J.*, **102**, 252.

Bowen, J.M. (1969) Artificial insemination in the horse. *Equine vet. J.*, **1**, 98.

Buell, R. (1963) A method of freezing stallion semen and tests of its fertility. *Vet. Rec.*, **75**, 900.

Burns, S.J., Simpson, R.B. & Snell, J.R. (1975) Control of microflora in stallion semen with a semen extender. *J. Reprod. Fert.*, Suppl. **23**, 139.

Cooper, W.L. & Wert, N. (1975) Wintertime breeding of mares using artificial light and insemination: six years experience. *Proc. 1st ann. Conv. Am. Ass. equine Practnrs*, 245.

Cox, J.E. & Williams, J.H. (1975) Some aspects of the reproductive endocrinology of the stallion and cryptorchid. *J. Reprod. Fert.*, Suppl. **23**, 75.

Cox, J.E., Williams, J.H., Rowe, P.H. & Smith, J.A. (1973) Testosterone in normal, cryptorchid and castrated male horses. *Equine vet. J.*, **5**, 85.

Crouch, J.R.F., Atherton, J.G. & Platt, H. (1972) Venereal transmission of *Klebsiella aerogenes* in a Thoroughbred stud from a persistently infected stallion. *Vet. Rec.*, **90**, 21.

Day, F.T. (1939) Some observations on the causes of infertility in horse breeding. *Vet. Rec.*, **51**, 581.

David, J.S.E., Frank, G.J. & Powell, D.G. (1977) Contagious metritis 1977. *Vet. Rec.*, **101**, 189.

Dimock, W.W. (1950) Fertility and infertility of stallions. *Bull. Ky agric. Exp. Stn,* 68.

Dott, H.M. (1975) Morphology of stallion spermatozoa. *J. Reprod. Fert.,* Supp.. **23**, 41.

Dott, H.M. & Foster, G.C. (1972) A technique for studying the morphology of mammalian spermatozoa which are eosinophilic in a differential live/dead stain. *J. Reprod. Fert.,* **29**, 443.

Dott, H.M. & Foster, G.C. (1975) Preservation of different staining of spermatozoa by formol citrate. *J. Reprod. Fert.,* **45**, 57.

Elliott, F.E., Sherman, J.K., Elliott, E.J. & Sullivan, J.L. (1973) A photographic method of measuring percentage of progressing motile sperm cells using dark field microscopy. *VIIIth int. Symp. Zootech., Milan,* **160**.

Ganjam, V.K. (1978) Episodic nature of the Δ4 and Δ5 steroidogenic pathways and their relation to adreno-gonadal axis in stallions. *J. Reprod. Fert.,* Suppl. **27**, 67.

Ganjam, V.K. & Kenney, R.M. (1975) Androgens and oestrogens in normal and cryptorchid stallions. *J. Reprod. Fert.,* Suppl. **23**, 67.

Gebauer, M.R., Pickett, B.W. & Swierstra, E.E. (1974*a*) Reproductive physiology of the stallions II daily production and output of sperm. *J. Anim. Sci.,* **39**, 732.

Gebauer, M.R., Pickett, B.W., Voss, J.L. & Swierstra, E.E. (1974*b*) Reproductive physiology of the stallion: daily sperm output and testicular measurements. *J. Am. vet. med. Ass.,* **165**, 711.

Gibbs, E.P.J., Roberts, M.C. & Morris, J.M. (1970) Equine coital exanthem in the United Kingdom. *Equine vet. J.,* **4**, 74.

Hamm, D.H. (1978) Gentamicin therapy of genital tract infections in stallions. *J. equine Med. Surg.,* **2**, 243.

Hughes, J.P., Asbury, A.C., Loy, R.G. & Burd, H.G. (1967) The occurrence of *Pseudomonas* in the genital tract of stallions and its effect on fertility. *Cornell Vet.,* **57**, 53.

Hughes, J.P. & Loy, R.G. (1969) Investigations on the effect of intra-uterine inoculations of *Streptococcus zooepidemicus* in the mare. *Proc. 15th ann. Conv. Am. Ass. equine Practnrs,* 289.

Hyland, J.H. & Bristol, F. (1979) Synchronisation of oestrus and timed insemination of mares. *J. Reprod. Fert.,* Suppl. **27**, 251.

Kenney, R.M. (1975) Clinical fertility evaluation of the stallion. *Proc. 21st ann. Conv. Am. Ass. equine Practnrs,* 336.

Kenney, R.M., Bergmann, R.V., Cooper, W.L. & Morse, G.W. (1975) Minimal contamination techniques for breeding mares: technique and preliminary findings. *Proc. 21st ann. Conv. Am. Ass. equine Practnrs,* 327.

Kenney, R.M. & Cooper, W.L. (1974) Therapeutic use of a phantom mare for semen collection from a stallion. *J. Am. vet. med. Ass.,* **165**, 706.

Kenney, R.M., Kingston, R.S., Rajamannam, A.H. & Ramberg, C.F. (1971) Stallion semen characteristics for predicting fertility. *Proc. 17th ann. Conv. Am. Ass. equine Practnrs,* 53.

Klug, E., Deegen, E., Lieske, R., Freytag, K., Martin, J.C., Gunzel, A.R. & Bader, H. (1979) The effect of vesiculectomy on seminal characteristics in the stallion. *J. Reprod. Fert.,* Suppl. **27**, 61.

Klug, E., Treu, H., Hillman, H. & Heinze, H. (1975) Results of insemination of mares with fresh and frozen semen. *J. Reprod. Fert.,* Suppl. **23**, 107.

Kosiniak, K. (1975) Characteristics of the successive jets of ejaculated semen of stallions. *J. Reprod. Fert.,* Suppl. **23**, 59.

McEntee, K. (1970) The female genital system. In *Pathology of Domestic Animals,* ed. K.V.F. Jubb & P.C. Kennedy, 2nd ed., vol. I. New York and London: Academic Press.

McLeod, J. & McGee, W.R. (1950) The semen of the Thoroughbred. *Cornell Vet.,* **40**, 233.

Mann, T. (1975) Biochemistry of stallion semen. *J. Reprod. Fert.,* Suppl. **23**, 47.

Merkt, H., Jacobs, K.O., Klug, E. & Aukes, E. (1978) An analysis of stallion fertility rates (foals born alive) from the breeding documents of the Langestut Celle over a 158 year period. *J. Reprod. Fert.,* **27**, 73.

Merkt, H., Klug, E., Bohm, K.H. & Weiss, R. (1975*a*) Recent observations concerning *Klebsiella* infections in stallions. *J. Reprod. Fert.,* Suppl. **23**, 143.

Merkt, H., Klug, E., Krause, D. & Bader, H. (1975*b*) Results of long term storage of stallion semen frozen by the pellet method. *J. Reprod. Fert.,* Suppl. **23**, 105.

Nishikawa, Y. (1959) Studies on reproduction in horses: Singularity and artificial organ control. In *Reproductive Phenomena.* Tokyo: Japan Racing Association.

Nishikawa, Y. (1975) Studies on the preservation of raw and frozen horse semen. *J. Reprod. Fert.*, Suppl. **23**, 99.

Pace, M.M. & Sullivan, J.J. (1975) Effect of timing of insemination, numbers of spermatozoa and extender components on the pregnancy rate in mares inseminated with frozen stallion semen. *J. Reprod. Fert.*, Suppl. **23**, 115.

Pascoe, R.R. & Bagust, J.L. (1975) Coital exanthema in stallions. *J. Reprod. Fert.*, Suppl. **23**, 147.

Pearson, H. & Weaver, B.M.Q. (1978) Priapism after sedation, neuroleptanalgesia and anaesthesia in the horse. *Equine vet. J.*, **20**, 85.

Peterson, F.B., McFeely, R.A. & David, J.S.E. (1969) Studies on the pathogenesis of endometritis in the mare. *Proc. 15th ann. Conv. Am. Ass. equine Practnrs,* 279.

Pickett, B.W. (1974) Evaluation of semen. In: *Lameness in Horses*, ed. O.R. Adams, 3rd ed. Philadelphia: Lea & Febiger.

Pickett, B.W. & Back, D.G. (1973) Procedures for preparation, collection evaluation and inseminating of stallion semen. *Bull. Colo. St. Univ. agric. Exp. Stn Anim. Reprod. Lab. gen. Ser.*, 935.

Pickett, B.W. Faulkner, L.C., & Sutherland, T.N. (1970) Effect of month and stallion on seminal characteristics and sexual behaviour. *J. Anim. Sci.*, **31**, 713.

Pickett, B.W., Faulkner, L.C. & Voss, J.L. (1975*a*) Effect of season on some characteristics of stallion semen. *J. Reprod. Fert.*, Suppl. **23**, 25.

Pickett, B.W., Sullivan, J.J., Byers, M.S., Pace, M.M. & Rommenga, E.E. (1975*b*) Effect of centrifugation and seminal plasma on motility and fertility of stallions and bull spermatozoa. *Fert. Steril.*, **26**, 167.

Pickett, B.W. & Voss, J.L. (1972) Reproductive management of stallions. *Proc. 18th ann. Conv. Am. Ass. equine Practnrs,* 501.

Pickett, B.W. & Voss, J.L. (1973) Reproductive management of the stallion. *Bull. Colo. St. Univ. agric. Exp. Stn Anim. Reprod. Lab. gen. Ser,* 934.

Pickett, B.W. & Voss, J.L. (1975) Abnormalities of mating behaviour in domestic stallions. *J. Reprod. Fert.*, Suppl. **23**, 129.

Platt, H., Atherton, J.G. & Ørskov, I. (1976) *Klebsiella* and *Enterobacter* organisms isolated from horses. *J. Hyg., Camb.*, **77**, 401.

Platt, H., Atherton, J.G., Simpson, D.J. Taylor, C.E.D., Rosenthal, R.O., Brown, D.F.J. & Wreghitt, T.G. (1977) Genital infections in mares. *Vet. Rec.*, **101**, 20.

Plewinska-Wierzobska, D. & Bielanski, W. (1970) The methods of evaluation of the speed and sort of movement of spermatozoa. *Medycyna Wet.*, **26**, 237.

Polge, C. & Minotakis, C. (1964) Deep freezing of jackass and stallion semen. *Proc. 5th int. Cong. Anim. Reprod. artif. Insem., Trento, Italy, VII,* 545.

Rajamannam, A.H.J. (1968) Freezing and fertilizing studies with stallion semen. *Proc. 6th int. Congr. Anim. Reprod. AI, Paris, France,* 1601.

Rasbeck, N.O. (1975) Ejaculatory disorders of the stallion. *J. Reprod. Fert.*, Suppl. **23**, 123.

Ristic, M. (1972) Protozoal disease. In *Equine Medicine and Surgery*, ed. E.J. Cattcott & J.F. Smithcors, 2nd ed., pp. 137–155. Wheaton, I11.: American Veterinary Publications.

Roberts, S.J. (1971) Artificial insemination in the horse. *Veterinary Obstetrics and Genital Diseases* (*Theriogenology*), 2nd ed., pp. 740–743. Ithaca, N.Y.: Roberts (distributed by Edwards Bros Inc., Ann Abor, Michigan).

Rossdale, P.D. (1978) Artificial insemination to help control CEM. *Vet. Rec.*, **102**, 291.

Rossdale, P.D., Hunt, M.D.N., Peace, C.K., Hopes, R., Ricketts, S.W. & Wingfield Digby, N.J. (1979) The case for AI. *Vet. Rec.*, **104**, 536.

Roser, J.F., Kiefer, B.L., Evans, J.W., Neely, D.P. & Pachecoe, C.A. (1979) The development of antibodies to human chorionic gonadatrophin following its repeated injection in the cyclic mare. *J. Reprod. Fert.*, Suppl. **27**, 173.

Sano, M.E. (1949) Trichrome stain for tissue section culture or smear. *Am. J. clin. Path.*, **19**, 898.

Simpson, R.B., Burns, S.J. & Snell, J.R. (1975) Microflora in stallion semen and their control with a semen extender. *Proc. 21st ann. Conv. Am. Ass. equine Practnrs,* 255.

Smith, J.A., (1974) Biopsy and the testicular artery of the horse. *Equine vet. J.*, **6**, 81.

Squires, E.L., Pickett, B.W. & Amann, R.P. (1979) Effect of successive ejaculation on stallion seminal characteristics. *J. Reprod. Fert.*, Suppl. **27**, 7.

Sullivan, J.J. & Pickett, B.W. (1975) Influence of ejaculation frequency of stallions on characteristics of semen and output of spermatozoa. *J. Reprod. Fert.*, Suppl. **23**, 29.

Sweistra, E.E., Pickett, B.W. & Gebauer, M.R. (1975) Spermatogenesis and duration of transit of spermatozoa through the excurrent ducts of stallions. *J. Reprod. Fert.*, Suppl. **23**, 53.

Swerczek, T.W. (1975) Immature germ cells in the semen of thoroughbreds. *J. Reprod. Fert.*, Suppl. **23**, 135.

Taylor, C.E.D., Rosenthal, R.G. & Brown, D.F.J. (1978) The causative organisms of contagious equine metritis 1977; Proposal for a new species to be known as *Haemophilus equigenitalis. Equine vet. J.*, **10**, 136.

Thompson, D.L., jun., Pickett, B.W., Squires, E.L. & Amman, R.P. (1979) Testicular measurements and reproductive characteristics in stallions. *J. Reprod. Fert.*, Suppl. **27**, *13*.

Tischner, M. (1979) Evaluation of deep frozen semen in stallions. *J. Reprod. Fert.*, Suppl. **27**, 53.

Tischner, M., Kosiniak, K. & Bielanski, W. (1974) Analysis of the pattern of ejaculation in stallions. *J. Reprod. Fert.*, **41**, 329.

Towers-Clark, P. (1977) The success of Weatherbys' blood typing scheme. *Stud and Stable*, June 1977.

Vandeplassche, M. & Devoss, A. (1960) Excretion of *Brucella abortus* in the semen of a stallion. *Vlaams Diergeneesk. Tijschr.*, **29**, 199.

Van Demark, N.I. & Mauger, R.E. (1964) Effect of energy intake on reproductive performance of dairy bulls. I. Growth: reproductive organs and puberty. *J. Dairy Sci.*, **47**, 798.

Voss, J.L. & Pickett, B.W. (1975) Diagnosis and treatment of haemospermia in the stallion. *J. Reprod. Fert.*, Suppl. **23**, 151.

Voss, J.L., Pickett, B.W. & Cheadler, R.K. (1976) The effect of haemospermia on fertility in horses. *Proc. VIIIth int. Congr. Anim. Reprod. AI, Krnbow*, **4**, 1093.

Weatherbys (1977) *The Statistical Record*, 1st Suppl. **38** of the General Stud Boo. Wellingborough: Weatherbys and *Stud and Stable*.

Wierzbowski, S. (1966) The scheme of sexual behaviour in bulls, rams and stallions. *Wld Rev. Anim. Prod.*, **2**, 2.

Gestation 3

Gestation begins when the ovum is fertilized and ends at birth. It is a period of fetal development and growth to a state at which the new individual is sufficiently mature to survive in the extrauterine environment, a period of particular biological interest. It includes the unique event of fertilization by which the genetic material of the parents is brought together in the zygote, the single cell destined to contribute to a cell life which continues until death. The development of the zygote into a full-term fetus is of supreme concern to embryologists; the structure and function of the placenta to anatomists and physiologists; the mechanisms that control and end gestation to endocrinologists; and the peculiarity of the immune status in which the maternal tissues accept a foreign organism to immunologists.

The clinician must recognize the practical implications of these disciplines, especially the areas in which failure or dysfunction presents problems of abortion, neonatal illness and errors in fetal development. Yet the fetus is remote, hidden from direct view and usual methods of clinical investigation. Diagnosis depends solely on the effects that fetal pathology has on the mare, until the fetus is expelled by adoption or birth. We will describe the gestational points of particular interest to clinicians. These include the salient features of fetal development and endocrinology, an account of management and husbandry of the pregnant mare, pregnancy diagnosis, the fetal environment and abortion.

EMBRYOLOGY

Embryology is the study of the development of the individual from the single-celled zygote. Three types of activity – growth, cell division and differentiation – are involved. Growth and cell division are readily understood since they form part of extrauterine life, but differentiation is largely an activity of fetal existence. The basis of differentiation is the forming of certain sets of cells into germ-layers – endoderm, mesoderm and ectoderm – each of which is responsible for definite sets of organs. Successive stages of subdivision complete the process of differentiation. For example, ectoderm is divided into epidermis, sense organs and nervous system; these subsequently become definite divisions with special histological characteristics of cellular shape and size.

This is not the place for a detailed description of embryological development and we shall concentrate on those features which are peculiar to Equidae or have particular relevance to recognizable clinical events such as abortion. For a description of early embryonic development in the horse see Van Niekerk and Allen (1975) and Flood and Marrable (1975).

Tubular transport

Fertilization occurs in the proximal end of the fallopian tube and the zygote descends into the uterus; unfertilized ova remain in the tube degenerating over seven to eight months (Van Niekerk & Gerneke 1966). It seems that developing embryos influence their own transport to the uterus, because they can overtake old, unfertilized, eggs en route (Betteridge & Mitchell 1975; Onuma & Ohnami 1975). It is not known how horse embryos exert this influence but it has been suggested that they may produce humoral substances that overcome resistance at the isthmo-ampullary junction where retention most often occurs (Flood et al. 1979). The results of experiments conducted by Betteridge et al. (1979) suggest that development beyond at least the two- to four-cell stage is necessary for normal transport and that a unilateral interaction with a corpus luteum is not necessary for the transport of the embryo to the uterus.

The ovum loses its corona radiata cells before ovulation and becomes surrounded by a sticky gelatinous mass at ovulation. It remains 'fertilizable' up to four hours after ovulation (Nelsen 1953). A newly ovulated ovum possesses one polar body and sperm entry appears to stimulate the second meiotic division (Van Niekerk & Gerneke 1966). Clinical experience suggests that conception can occur up to 36 hours after ovulation as determined by rectal palpation, although such cases are comparatively rare and may follow a second and undetected ovulation. Hamilton and Day (1945) recovered a 15-cell stage morula from the fallopian tube of a pony mare 98 hours after ovulation.

But Van Niekerk and Gerneke (1966) concluded that 9% of unfertilized ova undergo further genetic division and suggest that early cleavage states illustrated by Hamilton and Day fit the description of degenerating and parthenogenetically dividing ova.

The fertilized ovum arrives in the uterus about five days after ovulation and by Day 14 has formed a globular-shaped blastocyst 1.3 cm in diameter (Ewart 1915). By 21 days it is pear-shaped, measures 6 × 7 cm and contains the embryo at the broad rounded end. Vitelline vessels, a sinus terminalis, minute circular projections (trophoblastic discs) and semi-opaque depressions are present in the surface of the blastocyst at this age (Fig. 3.1). The outer surface of the blastocyst is the trophoblast consisting of columnar epithelial cells which probably 'absorb' uterine secretions and so provide the fetus with nourishment through the yolk sac ectoderm and vitelline veins. The trophoblastic discs may help to fix the blastocyst in position but they disappear by the end of four weeks and a close attachment to

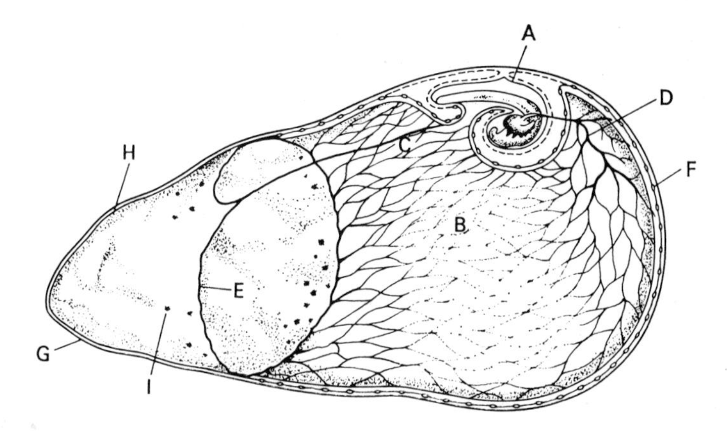

Fig. 3.1. Semi-diagrammatic drawing of a 21-day blastocyst. The embryo can be seen (top right) surrounded by the amnion (A) and connected to the yolk sac (B). Other structures are left and right vitelline arteries and vein (C, D), sinus terminalis (E), mesoderm (F), trophoblast (G), endoderm (H) and trophoblastic discs (I).

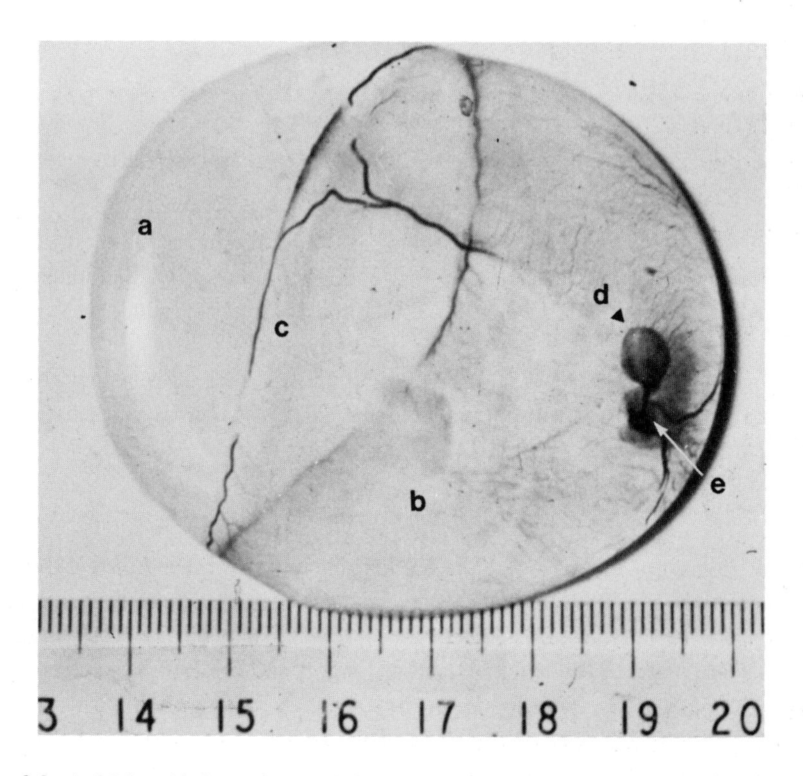

Fig. 3.2. A 25-day-old fetus showing bilaminar (a) and trilaminar (b) omphalopleurs, sinus terminalis (c), developing allantois (d) and embryo (e). (*By kind permission of R. V. Short*)

the uterine mucosa does not develop until after eight weeks. The yolk sac is small and functions only in the first 20 days of fetal growth. By about Day 21 the allantois begins to form and the sinus terminalis, which marks the division between bilaminar and trilaminar omphalopleur, is equatorial in position (Fig. 3.2). Also the long axis of the blastocyst is parallel to that of the uterine horn (Short 1969). The sinus terminalis moves down the blastocyst and at the same time the allantois grows to surround the fetus. By Day 40 it has converted the yolk sac to a true chorio-allantoic placenta. The front of the chorio-allantois forms a band which advances across the surface of the blastocyst and produces a specialized girdle of

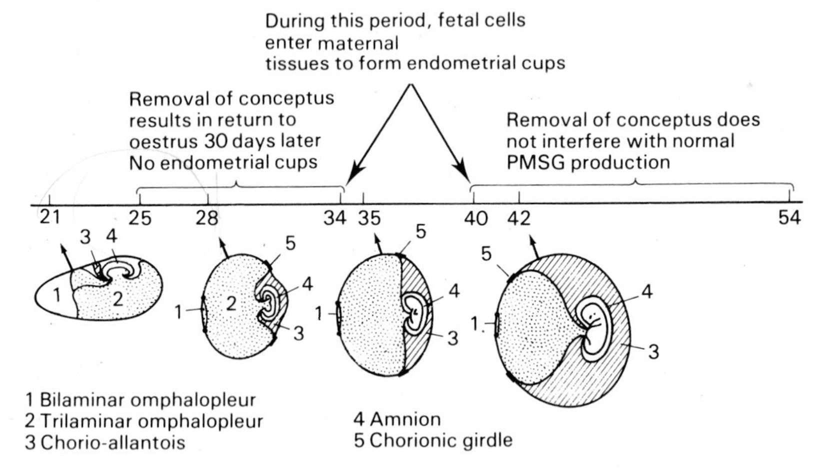

Fig. 3.3. Development of the fetal membranes and endometrial cups between Days 21 and 54. (*After Allen 1970 and Allen & Moor 1972*)

cells on the outer surface of the placenta (Fig. 3.3). Close to Day 37 these separate and rapidly invade the adjacent maternal endometrium to form the endometrial cups (Allen & Moor 1972). We shall see later that these cells produce the hormone PMSG.

Douglas and Ginther (1975) examined morphological changes in the fetus and placenta of pony mares with known breeding dates. A summary of their findings is presented in Table 3.1.

Fetal growth

By Day 30 most of the organs are present in rudimentary form and the eyes, mouth and limb buds are visible. By Day 40 eyelids and auditory pinnae have appeared. By Day 60 the lips, nostrils and feet are developing and by Day 90 hooves and mammae are present. The external genitalia, ergots and orbital areas are visible by Day 120 and fine hair starts to appear, by Day 180, on lips, orbital arch, nose and eyelids. Hair covering spreads to include mane, tail, back and distal parts of extremities by Day 240. By Day 270 short, fine hairs cover the entire body. By Day 320 the coat is complete and the testes have descended through the inguinal ring.

TABLE 3.1 Time of appearance of prenatal characteristics in relation to crown–rump length of the fetus of the pony

Days after end of oestrus	*No. of mares*	*Characteristic*	*Crown–rump length* (mm)
10	3	Yolk-sac placenta	–
14	4	Primitive streak formation	–
18	4	Somites	–
24	3	Heart beat	5–6
		Visible fore-limb bud	5–6
		Visible hind-limb bud	5–6
		Embryo C-shaped	5–6
30	2	Chorio-allantoic placenta	9–10
40	2	Differentiated nostrils and eyes	22–25
		External genitalia	22–25
		Endometrial cups	22–25
		Placental attachment (macroscopic)	22–25
50	3	Differentiated appendages	35–51
50–60		Exocoelom of pregnant horn filled with chorio-allantois	35–75
60	3	'L'-shaped fetus	58–75
		Eyelids close	58–75
60–80		Exocoelom of non-pregnant horn filled with chorio-allantois	58–136
80	3	Endometrial cups in early desquamation	120–136
100	3	Endometrial cups completely desquamated	170–181
100		Amniotic nodules	170–181
160	2	Hair around eyes and muzzle	310–319
220	1	Hair at tip of tail and mane	505

After Douglas and Ginther (1975).

Body weight increases 100-fold from 0.2 g at Day 30 to 20 g at Day 60; 50-fold between Days 60 and 120 (20 to 2000 g); five-fold between Days 120 and 180 (1 to 5 kg); three-fold between Day 180 and Day 240 (5 to 15 kg); two and a half times between Day 240 and Day 300 (15 to 37 kg); and about one and a half times to full term at 340 Days (37 to 54 kg). The weight of the fetus varies according to breed and normality of placental function. Published data at different gestational ages are summarized in Fig. 3.9.

Crown-to-rump (C/R) length increases from 1 cm at Day 30 to about 7 cm at Day 60, 20 cm at Day 120, 60 cm at Day 180, 80 cm at Day 240, 120 cm at Day 300 and 150 cm at Day 340. The limits of variation which are affected by breed and placental efficiency are shown in Fig. 3.10.

Fetal gonads

The fetal gonads reach a maximal weight between Days 180 and 200. Douglas and Ginther (1975) found no significant differences between the weights of fetal ovaries and fetal testes throughout the period of hypertrophy. They reported that the gonads, at 80 days gestation, weighed 1.4 g, at 140–160 days 18.7 g, at 180–200 days 48 g and at full term 31.4 g. The increase in size of the gonads results from hypertrophy and hyperplasia of the interstitial cells (Cole et al. 1933).

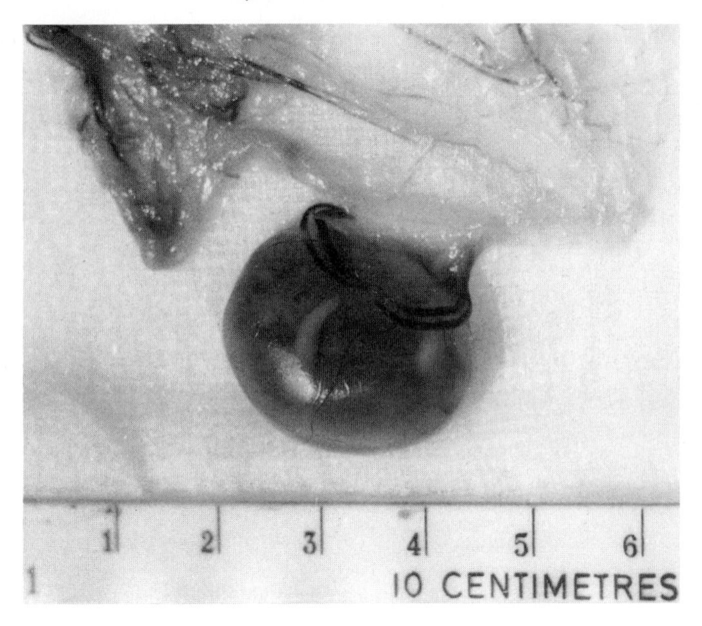

Fig. 3.4. A 37-day fetus enclosed in amnion (crown-to-rump length 2 cm).

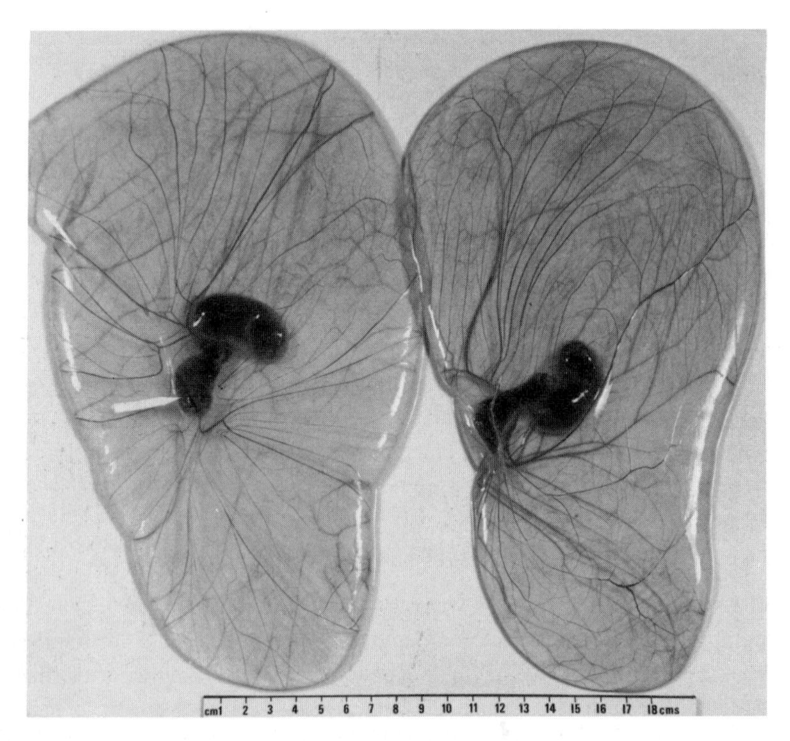

Fig. 3.5. The uterus opened to show embryos, one vestigial yolk sac (arrowed) and placentae (57 days). (*By kind permission of W.R. Allen*)

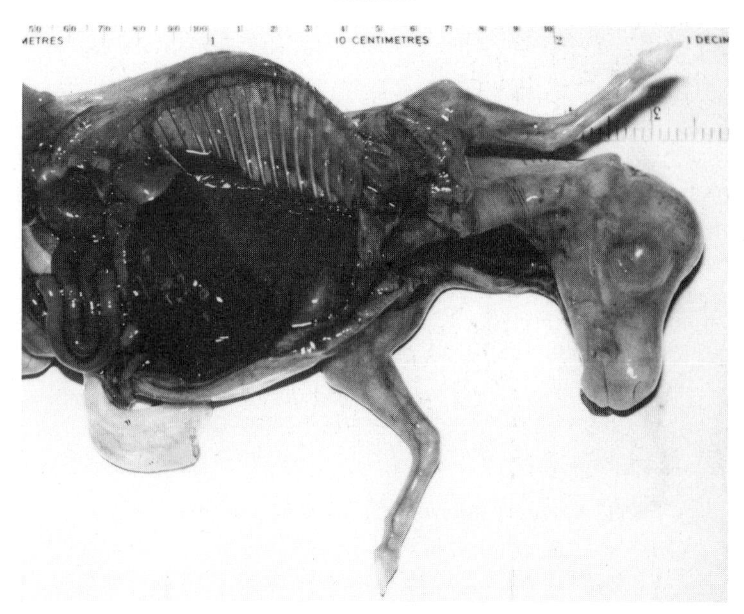

Fig. 3.6. A 97-day fetus opened to show the thoracic and abdominal contents. Note that the gonad (top left) is relatively large at this age. Crown-to-rump length 20 cm.

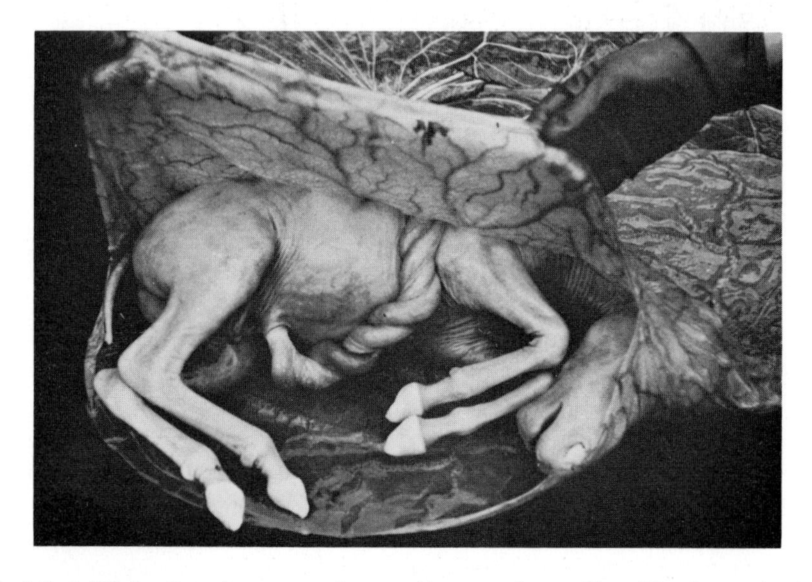

Fig. 3.7. A 203-day fetus from a mare destroyed because of an accident. The placenta has been removed and the amnion laid open. Note the twists in the umbilical cord. Crown-to-rump length 60 cm.

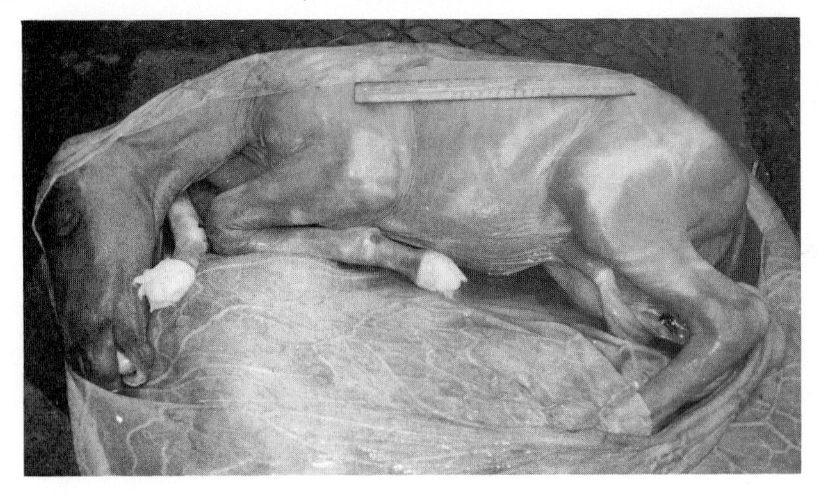

Fig. 3.8. A 250-day fetus. Crown-to-rump length 80 cm.

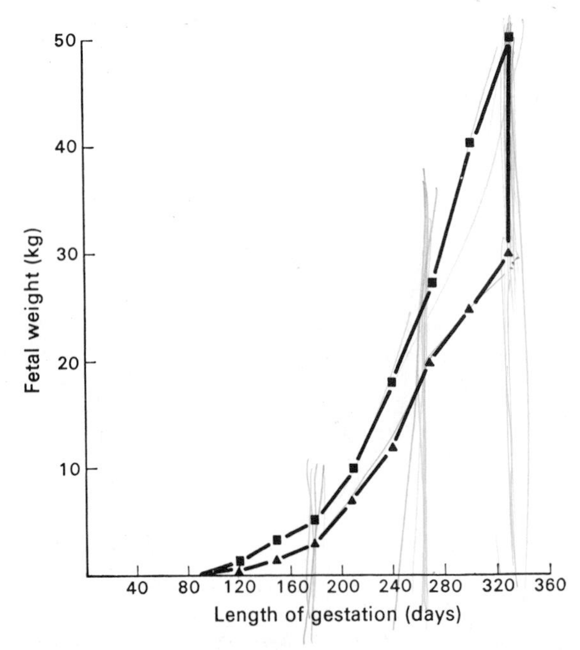

Fig. 3.9. The expected fetal weight at various gestational ages. (*After Roberts 1971*)

The development of the equine ovary and ovulation fossa has been reported by Walt et al. (1979). At 40–45 days of gestation the fetal ovaries are enclosed in the cortical layer surrounded by a surface germinal epithelium. At all times of development this epithelium lines only cortical tissue. Sexual differentiation appears to occur between Days 39 and 45. Migrational contraction of the cortical layer from the hilar region initiated by Day 60 continues through gestation with the cortical movement occurring more rapidly at the anterior portion of the ovary. The equine ovary is peculiar in that the surface germinal epithelium is restricted to a portion of the ovary and ovulation is possible only through an ovulation fossa. From 120 to 180 days of gestation ovarian size averages 35 × 20 × 19 mm. The enlargement of the ovary is caused by hyperplasia at the fetal medullary interstitial cells with the

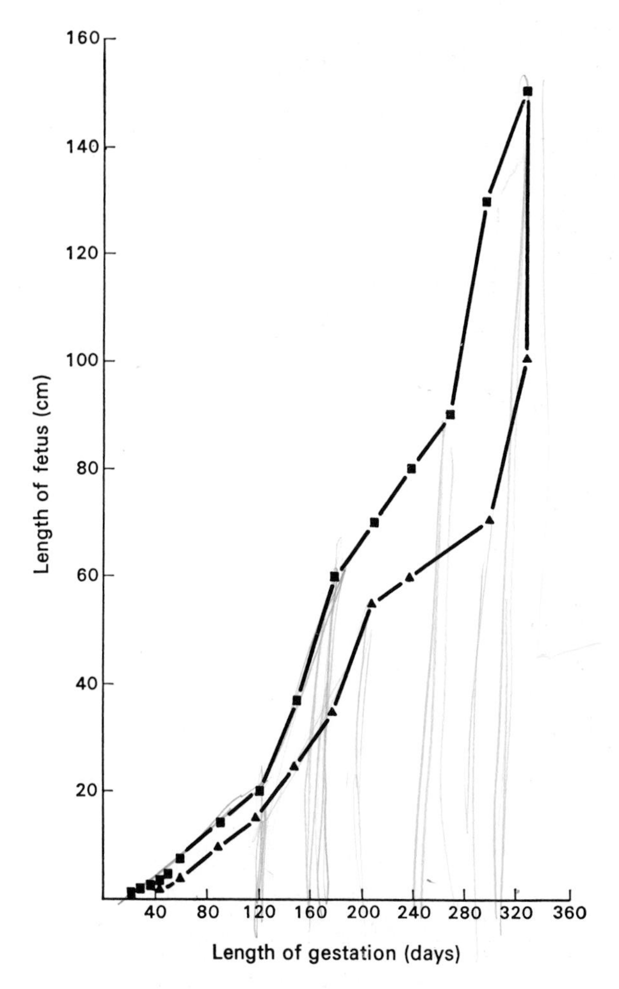

Fig. 3.10. The expected crown-to-rump length at various gestational ages. (*After Roberts 1971*)

result that the cortex covers only approximately one-half of the gonad. The average size of the ovaries at 180–270 days gestation is 44 × 28 × 26 mm and the cortex covers only one-third of the ovarian surface. Between 270 days gestation and birth ovarian size is 45 × 30 × 23 mm and the borders of the cortex are delineated on the posterior pole by the utero-ovarian ligament and on the anterior pole by the fimbria. Follicular development is present during this period although ovulation does not appear to occur.

The reader is referred to the following for further information on the development of the fetal horse ovary: Deanesly (1975), Hay and Allen (1975), Gonzalez-Angulo et al. (1975) and Walt et al. (1979).

Placenta

The equine placenta is diffuse (i.e. it covers the entire uterine surface) and is epitheliochorial, i.e. six cell layers separate maternal from fetal capillaries (Grosser 1927).

The surface of the placenta is smooth in early pregnancy but by Day 70 it becomes velvety due to the development of minute villi. The microhistology and vascular supply has been described by Tsutsumi (1962) and Steven (1968). Small

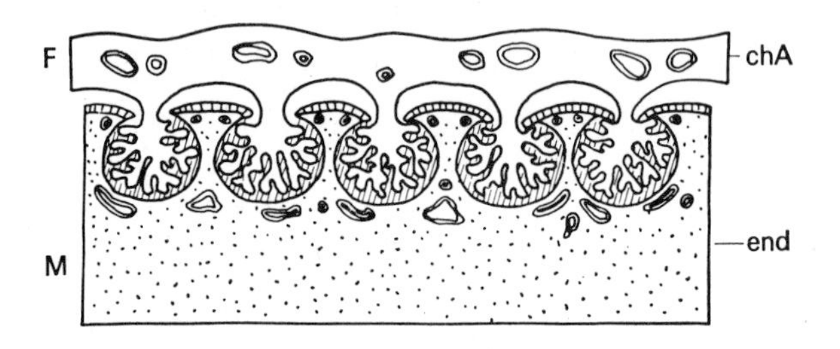

Fig. 3.11. The macroscopic structure of the mare's placenta, illustrating microcotyledonary structures. chA, chorio-allantois; end, endometrium; F, fetal; M, maternal. (*After Steven 1968*)

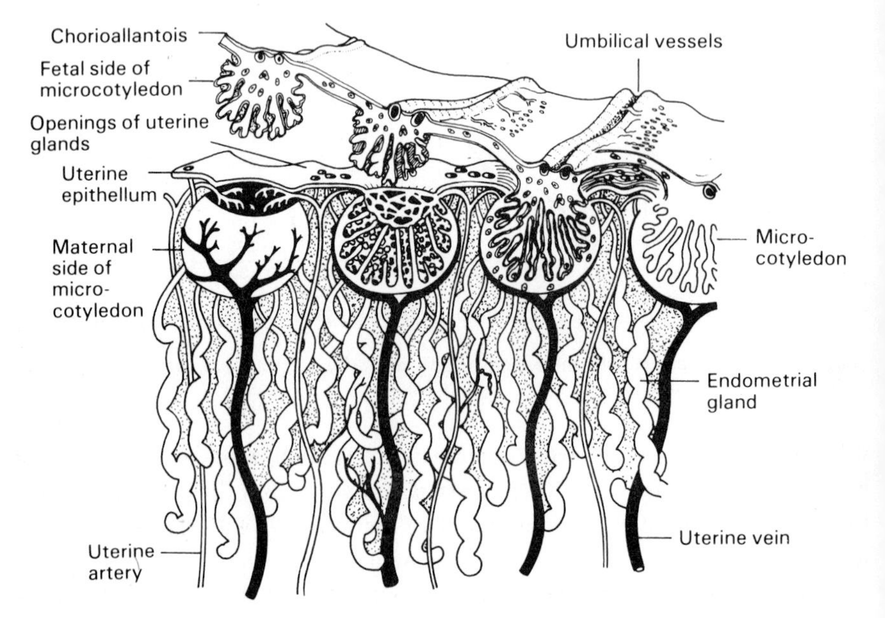

Fig. 3.12. The mature equine placenta, showing the nature of the cotyledons. (*After Steven and Samuel 1975*)

tufts of chorionic villi project into the corresponding invagination of the endometrium to form small globular structures of microcotyledons (Figs 3.11, 3.12). Uterine arteries enter the endometrium and pass to the deep surface of the endometrial epithelium where they divide into branches which give rise to dense capillary networks in the wall of the maternal crypts (Fig. 3.13). This network drains to a single vein which passes to the subendometrial plexus. The placental

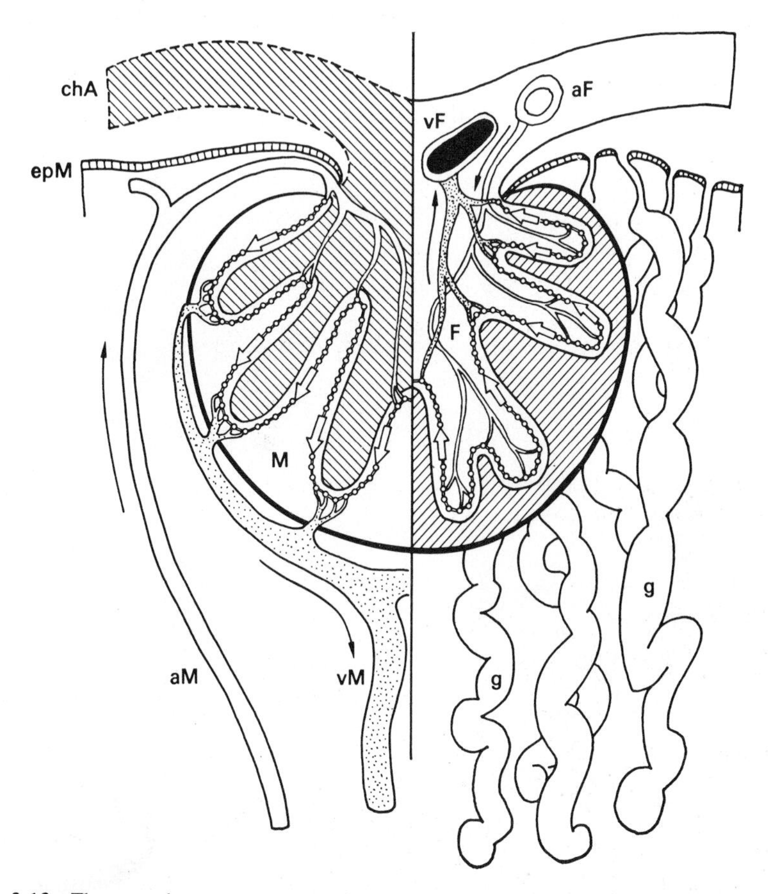

Fig. 3.13. The vascular arrangements of an equine placental microcotyledon. Small open arrows show the postulated direction of flow in fetal and maternal capillaries. aM, maternal artery; vM, maternal vein; chA, chorio-allantois; epM, uterine epithelium; g, endometrial glands; aF, fetal artery; vF, fetal vein; F, fetal; M, maternal. (*After Tsutsumi 1962*)

villi are supplied by branches of the umbilical arteries and veins. According to Tsutsumi the veins do not extend as far as the arteries and capillary flow is from the tip to the base of the villus and therefore in the opposite direction to that of the maternal capillary flow.

The microcotyledons are fully formed by Day 150. The maternal epithelium is greatly reduced in height between Days 60 and 150 but no change occurs on the fetal side of the placenta. Between Days 100 and 250 gestation there is a progressive indentation of the epithelium by fetal capillaries which reduces the effective thickness of the placental barrier (Silver et al. 1973). The anatomy of the placental barrier has been described by Steven and Samuel (1975) who have pointed to the similarity of the uteroplacental junction and the air–blood barrier of the mammalian lung. In both tissues, capillary blood is contained by a thin non-fenestrated endothelium, an intermediate layer is formed by fusion of the basement membranes of endothelium and epithelium and an attenuated epithelium forms the outermost boundary. In the lung this boundary is in contact with air and in the placenta it is in intimate apposition to the endometrial epithelium. The thickness between the maternal and fetal capillaries, in the last two months of gestation, is 2.4–3 μm,

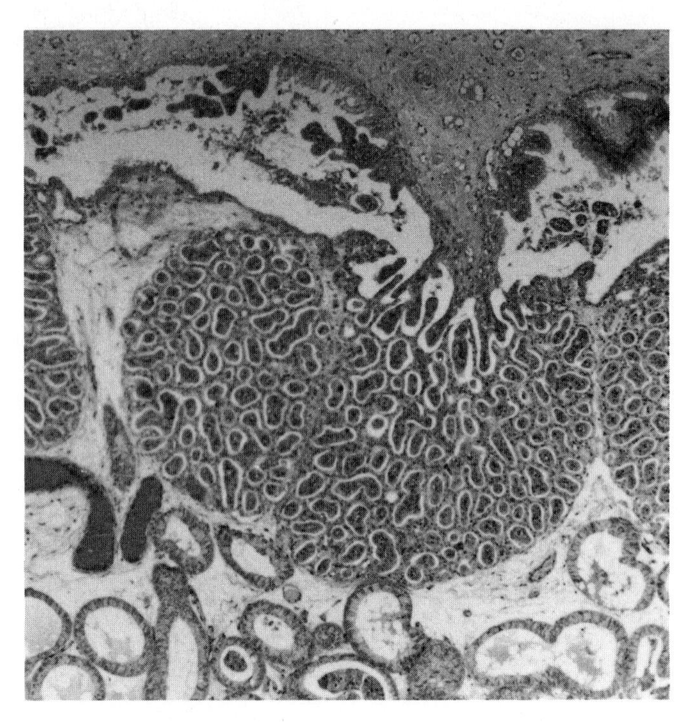

Fig. 3.14. Microcotyledon at full term with chorio-allantois above and endometrium below. H & E × 30.

thus the diffusion pathway over the fetal side of the placenta appears to be greater in the mare than in domestic ruminants. However, the total diffusion distance from maternal to fetal capillaries is less than that of the cow or sheep (Silver et al. 1973). The rate of diffusion does not appear to be a limiting factor in the transport of oxygen across the placenta, but the amount of oxygen transferred to the fetus may be influenced by the metabolically active tissues within the diffusion pathway. A full-term microcotyledon is shown in Fig. 3.14.

At full term the placenta weighs about 4 kg (range 1.5–8 kg); its surface area approximates 14 000 cm^2 (range 4500–18 500 cm^2) and it is 1 mm thick (range

0.45–2.7 mm). The foal's birth-weight is directly proportional to placental surface area, but no correlation exists with weight or thickness of the membrane (Rossdale 1966).

There are three types of twin placentation (Jeffcott & Whitwell 1973) (Fig. 3.15).

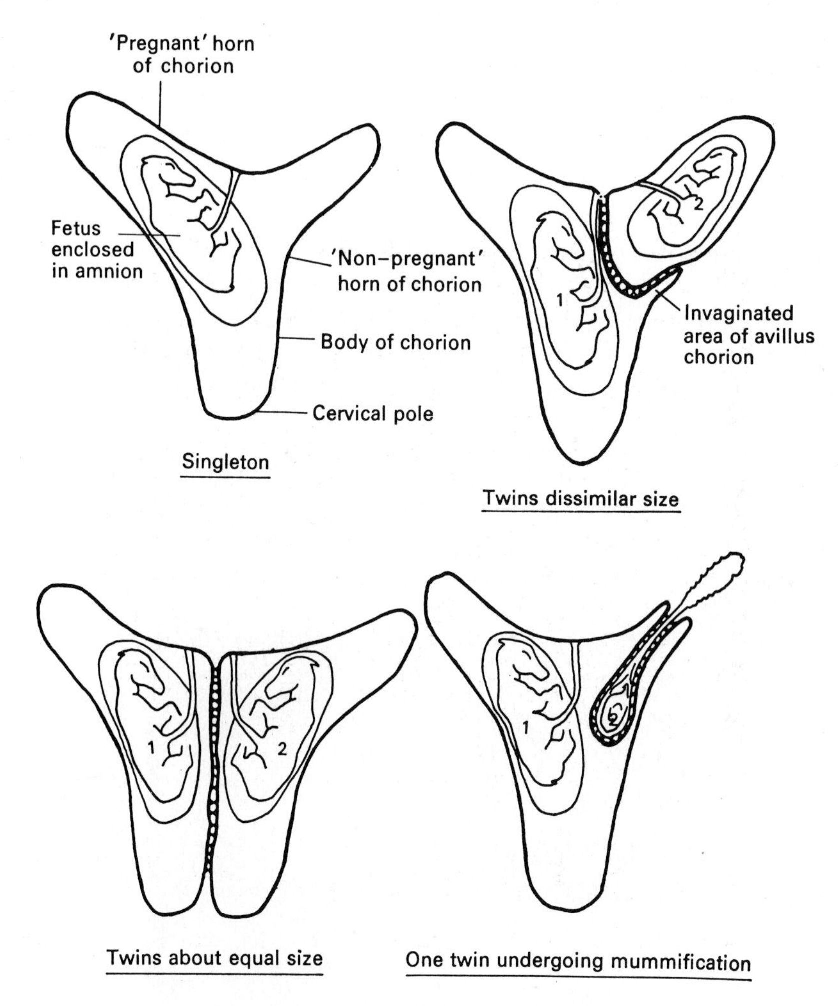

Fig. 3.15. Various types of twin placentation. (*After Jeffcott & Whitwell 1973*)

1. One twin occupies the uterine body and one horn and possesses 68% of the functional surface area. Where the two chorions abut there is usually a degree of invagination of the smaller into the other.

2. The chorion of one twin almost totally excludes the other, occupying the uterine body, one horn and most of the other.

3. Equal division of surface area with no invagination of one chorion by the other.

Jeffcott and Whitwell found mean functional surface areas between twins of 12640 : 5476 cm^2 in type 1; 12204 : 2216 cm^2 in type 2; and 10711 : 9069 cm^2 in type 3. In each category, mean avillous areas where chorions abutted were 1610 to 5068 cm^2. These areas showed considerable inflammatory reaction and small anastamoses of blood vessels, although no evidence of useful sharing was found.

Allantoic fluid

Allantoic fluid is formed from the chorio-allantoic membrane and it receives urinary fluid through the urachus. During gestation there is a steady increase in total nitrogen and in sodium, potassium, calcium, magnesium and phosphate ions. The volume increases from about 110 ml to 1300 ml between Days 45 and 60, to 3000 ml by Day 128, and to 8500 ml by Day 310, although individuals and breeds vary. The allantoic fluid changes from a clear yellow in the first trimester to a turbid brown or yellowish-brown by mid-term. The fluid contains desquamated epithelium, small chorio-allantoic peduncles and a single hippomane.

Hippomane

The hippomane is a soft, flat, roughly oval-shaped structure found in allantoic fluid. It is brown or cream in colour, about 14 × 1.5 cm and contains high concentrations of nitrogen, hexosamine, calcium, phosphorus, sodium, potassium and magnesium.

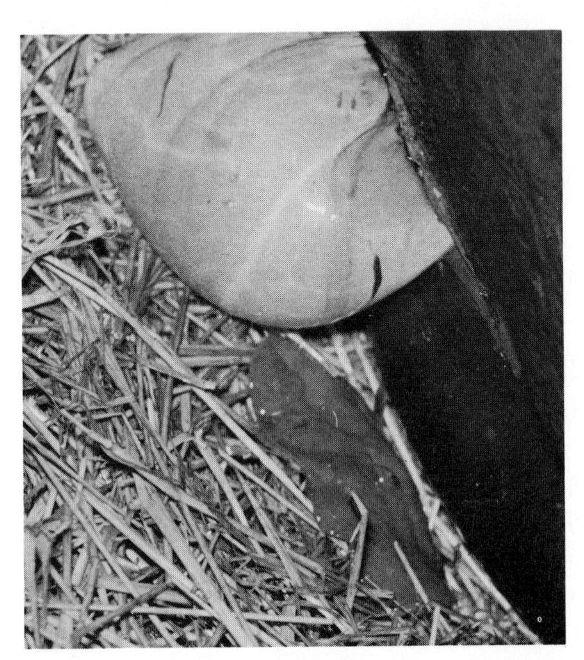

Fig. 3.16. The hippomane, seen here on the straw bedding, may be passed during second-stage birth.

TABLE 3.2 The composition of hippomane compared with that of the allantoic fluid in which it was found

	160 days		*182 days*		*203 days*		*310 days*		*340 days: Parturition*	
	Hippomanes	Allantoic fluid	Hippomanes	Allantoic fluid	Hippomanes	Allantoic fluid	Hippomanes	Allantoic fluid	Hippomanes	Allantoic fluid
Weight (g)	5.67	–	7.41	–	11.04	–	25.2	–	56.3	–
Water (g)	792	–	796	–	786	–	748	–	821	–
Total nitrogen (g)	21.6	2.50	24.1	2.75	22.1	3.79	–	4.61	18.5	3.42
Hexosamine (g)	4.94	0.54	4.45	1.15	6.18	1.10	5.16	1.50	4.60	2.09
Na (mmol)	29.8	36.2	26.2	23.0	9.0	10.5	33.3	62.8	106	96
K (mmol)	0.5	5.0	31.0	42.0	24.0	30.5	94.4	1.1	13.5	11.4
P (mmol)	56.4	3.0	121	7.7	56.4	3.5	363	31.0	274	64.9
Ca (mmol)	411	15	287	21.2	420	23.8	630	85.8	285	15.9
Mg (mmol)	28.5	12.4	38.0	29.2	69.0	21.4	9.16	34.8	76.0	3.88
Na/K (mmol/mmol)	59.5	7.3	0.85	0.55	0.38	0.34	0.35	57.0	7.85	8.43
Ca/P (mmol/mmol)	7.3	4.8	2.5	2.7	7.5	6.8	17.8	2.7	1.05	0.25

After Dickerson et al. (1967).
Values are expressed per kg of hippomane and per litre of allantoic fluid.

The composition of a hippomane compared with allantoic fluid is shown in Table 3.2. The hippomane occurs singly in the allantoic fluid and is passed during or after second-stage delivery (Fig. 3.16). Its development has been described by King (1967) and Dickerson et al. (1967). It is first found in the allantoic fluid at about Day 85 and is flat, white, oval or rectangular, little more than 1 cm long and with a matt surface and elastic consistency. There is no evidence to implicate the chorio-allantoic pouches, yolk sac or amnion in the formation of the true hippomane. The only contribution from the fetal membranes is desquamated epithelium which provides a nucleus of tissue debris for the subsequent formation of a soft allantoic calculus. King suggests that the hippomane's specific gravity, being higher than that of allantoic fluid, has an important bearing on its singularity and shape. He reviewed the literature and is of the opinion that confusion has surrounded the word 'hippomane' because of its loose application to almost any object that occurs in the extraembryonic sac of mammals: in his view the use of the term should be confined to Equidae since the translation of this Greek word is 'horse madness'.

Amnion

The amnion develops about Day 17 and is complete by Day 21. It is closely allied to the embryo up to Day 56 and becomes separated as the quantity of amniotic fluid increases. From Day 70 'amniotic pustules' appear on the inner surface of the amnion. These are local accumulations of ectoderm in which glycogen is stored (Amoroso 1952). At full term the amnion weighs 2.4 kg (range 0.5–4 kg) and consists of a fine transparent membrane interlaced by a network of blood vessels.

Amniotic fluid

The electrolyte and salt content of amniotic fluids shows very little change during gestation but there appear to be substantial changes in hormone levels and surfactant content. Its circulation and source have not been established but its composition is approximately that of a serum ultrafiltrate (Table 3.3). The amnion and kidneys may contribute to it and exchange of fluids and solutes occurs in the respiratory tract, and absorption is through the intestinal tract.

TABLE 3.3 The composition of amniotic fluid

	59 days	*95 days*	*120 days*	*160 days*	*182 days*	*203 days*	*310 days*
Total N (g)	0.68	0.38	0.62	0.70	0.50	0.61	0.56
Hexosamine (mg)	0.12	0.075	0.075	0.115	0.073	0.125	0.058
Na (mmol)	131	94	115	130	123	127	96
K (mmol)	6.0	4.9	5.6	4.5	4.0	6.1	3.1
Ca (mmol)	1.1	1.9	2.8	2.05	2.5	2.5	2.8
Mg (mmol)	–	0.9	1.4	0.8	0.8	0.5	0.6
P (mmol)	0.6	1.3	2.0	1.5	0.5	0.5	0.6

After Dickerson et al. (1967).
Values expressed per litre of amniotic fluid.

Amniotic fluid is opalescent, straw-coloured, slightly mucoid and sweet-smelling with a mean pH of 6.928 (range 6.75–7.05) and mean $P\text{CO}_2$ of 56.18 mmHg (range 31–84 mmHg) at birth (Rossdale 1968). The fluid normally contains desquamated skin cells and 10–1000 leucocytes/mm^3. Volume increases from about 400 ml in the first trimester to 3.5 litres at full term (Dickerson et al. 1967).

Umbilical cord

The umbilical cord develops from an expansion of the two fetal sacs surrounding the remnants of the yoke sac and the vitelline duct. It attaches to the original implantation site on the dorsal wall of the uterus. The cord contains two arteries, a vein and a urachus. It is divided equally into allantoic and amniotic portions. In a series of 143 normal Thoroughbred foals the mean umbilical cord length was 55 cm (95% of values were 36–83 cm) (Whitwell & Jeffcott 1975). Amniotic pustules may be present on the cord surface and plaques or minute nodules of hyperplastic epithelium may be present on the surface of the amniotic portion of the cord. Within the allantoic portion is a narrow, smooth-walled cavity, the infundibulum, a remnant of the extraembryonic coelom in which the vestigial yoke sac is found. The remnant grows in size from a small fusiform body up to 20 cm or more in diameter. The largest specimen may hang down in to the allantoic cavity and plaques of bone are often present in the wall of these structures and may be erroneously referred to as amorphus globosus. Whitwell (1975) suggested that increased cord length was associated with untoward consequences for the fetus by (*a*) strangulation causing death of the fetus between Days 212 and 287 or (*b*) excessive torsion resulting in urachal obstruction and vascular accretion. She described mild urachal obstruction causing multiple urachal dilatations in two case cases of cord length 98 and 110 cm. Larger urachal dilatations and bladder distensions were described and it was suggested that high urachal obstruction could predispose to congenital or intrapartum rupture of the bladder. Excessive twisting of the umbilical cord may lead to the obstruction of the blood vessels followed by fetal death. Organ autolysis may be found in these cases when an interval occurs between death and subsequent expulsion of the fetus.

UTERINE CHANGES

During gestation the uterus grows to accommodate the developing fetus. The mechanisms which allow for the enormous increase in size are unknown but are probably hormonal. Throughout most of pregnancy the connective tissue resists stretch to an extent that permits slow distension of the body of the uterus, where the proportion of connective tissue is low, but maintains closure of the cervix, where the proportion is high. This property of uterine connective tissue is derived from tightly packed bundles of collagen fibres lying in the relatively sparse proteoglycan matrix (Liggins 1979). Changes in the matrix of the cervix render it capable

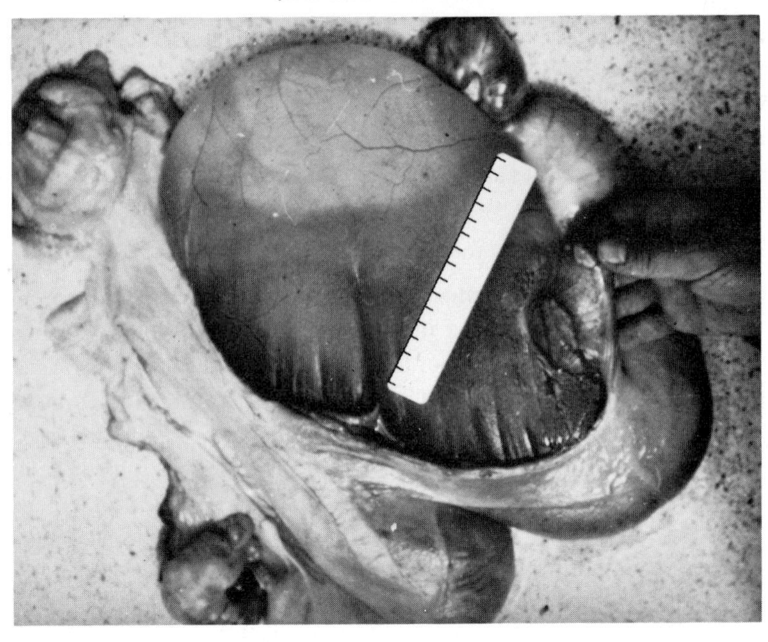

Fig. 3.17. An 80-day fetus and its membranes exposed after part of the uterine walls had been removed. An endometrial cup is held in the hand.

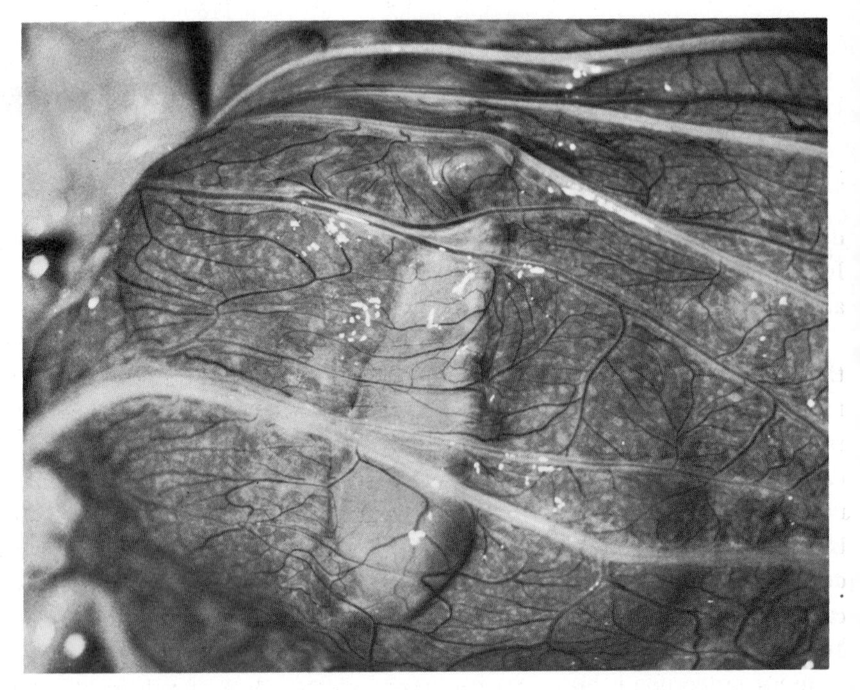

Fig. 3.18. An endometrial cup measuring 3 × 1 cm in the wall of a uterus from which a 97-day fetus had been removed.

of dilating under endocrine control to allow passage of the fetus at full term (Danforth et al. 1974).

Another aspect not yet fully explained is the uterine tolerance to the presence of fetal tissue, tissue which is essentially foreign to the maternal immunological system. The lack of reaction to the placenta contrasts with the response to fetal cells which invade the endometrium at the 'cups' and which are eventually rejected by the maternal tissues.

Endometrial cups (Schauder 1912; Cole & Goss 1943; Amoroso 1951) are structures which begin to form on about Day 36 as discrete circumscribed, well-defined ulcers in the endometrium (Figs 3.17, 3.18). These are specialized areas which develop at predetermined sites around the base of the pregnant horn (Clegg et al. 1954; Amoroso 1955) and which first become apparent macroscopically about Day 40. They occur opposite a well-defined thickening of the chorion and are composed of small round cells and a densely packed mass of large epithelioid decidual-like cells which are of fetal origin (Allen & Moor 1972).

Firm attachment between the cells of the chorionic girdle and the adjacent endometrium occurs on Day 36 (Moor et al. 1975). Girdle cells then rapidly invade and phagocytose the endometrial epithelium. They migrate into the endometrial glands and the uterine stroma where they differentiate into large sessile endometrial cup cells and secrete gonadotrophin (PMSG) until about Day 90.

Allen (1970) has suggested that at this time a maternal immunological response (associated with densely accumulated lymphocyte and plasma cells in the cups) rejects the 'foreign' fetal tissue. The circle formed by the cups at the base of the pregnant horn regresses during the rest of pregnancy and the cups are not visible in the barren uterus; scarring may remain on the placenta for some months after the cups have ceased to function.

If abortion occurs once the cups have become established, i.e. after about 42 days gestation, the secretion of PMSG continues in the absence of the conceptus. In these circumstances PMSG may remain detectable in the blood up to 130 days after conception (Mitchell 1971; Mitchell & Allen 1975).

Hershman and Douglas (1979) performed experiments to determine the critical time at which the equine blastocyst must be present within the uterus of the mare to prevent regression of the corpus luteum. A non-surgical blastocyst collection technique was developed and results demonstrated that the cyclic life-span of the corpus luteum is not affected by the presence of the blastocyst within the mare's uterus until after Day 14 from ovulation. Luteal function was prolonged when blastocysts were removed on Day 15 or later. However, this change in CL status does not appear to be the result of a corresponding change in prostaglandin-binding capacity of the corpus luteum because this has been found to be high between Days 16 and 18 of pregnancy (Vernon et al. 1979).

Bain (1967*a*) found intense ovarian activity between Days 25 and 150 on routine rectal examination including an increase in ovarian size and the presence of numerous follicles in one or both ovaries. Cole et al. (1931) used experimental methods to divide pregnancy into four periods:

1. Days 1–40. The ovaries have a CL and follicles of variable size.

2. Days 40–150. There is progressive activity including formation of follicles and ovulation.

3. Day 150 to an undetermined date. There is a decrease in lutein tissue and absence of follicles.

4. The period towards the end of pregnancy. No CL is present. These changes are part of the endocrinological mechanisms which maintain pregnancy.

More recent work (Squires & Ginther 1975) suggests that the primary CL of pregnancy may remain functional until at least Day 160 of gestation. However, it seems that primary and secondary CLs and the placenta or uterus contribute to the total progesterone pool in mares during pregnancy. Eleven of the 20 mares ovariectomized between Days 50 and 70 failed to produce abortion in the study reported by Holtan et al. (1979). These results suggest that the ovaries may not be essential to continuing pregnancy from a much earlier time than was hitherto assumed.

ENDOCRINOLOGY

The endocrinology of pregnancy is summarized in Fig. 3.19.

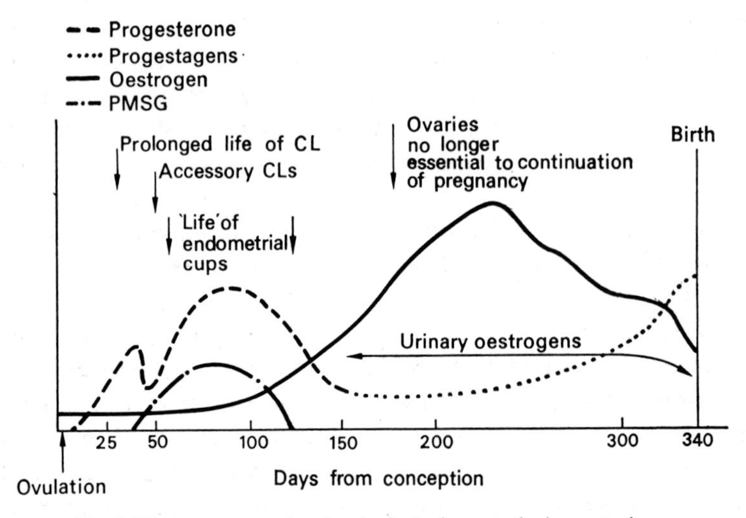

Fig. 3.19. A summary of endocrinological events during gestation.

Conception to Day 150

Gestation is associated with a sequence of endocrinological activity in which the maternal ovaries and fetal organs, including the placenta, play a major role. The mechanism by which the maternal tissues recognize a fertilized ovum is unknown, but there is evidence that the presence of a blastocyst after Day 15 is associated with the prolongation of the functional life of the corpus luteum (Hershman &

Douglas 1979). As we have seen, the zygote arrives in the uterus about five days after conception and by Day 15 the corpus luteum of dioestrus is maintained and continues to function for a further 160 days (Squires & Ginther 1975). The mechanism which determines prolonged functional life is unknown, but presumably it involves prostaglandin, either by reducing secretion or by blocking its luteolytic effect. Doubt has been thrown on the latter hypothesis by Vernon et al. (1979), who found high PGF-binding capacity in the corpus luteum between Days 16 and 18 of pregnancy. Ginther and First (1971) have shown that the uterine effect on the corpus luteum does not involve a local or unilateral utero-ovarian mechanism.

The ovaries become increasingly active after Days 20–30 (Van Niekerk 1965*a*; Bain 1967*a*). Follicular development and ovulation provide a second crop of corpora lutea which function until about Days 120–150.

Blood plasma levels of progesterone reach peak levels of 12–20 ng/ml between Days 16 and 25 and, after falling, rise to a new peak at about Day 45, again falling to minimal levels by Day 150. As already indicated progesterone appears to be produced by non-ovarian sources and the possibility that the placenta contributes to the progestagen pool at a much earlier age than was hitherto suspected is gaining increasing credibility. Steroidogenesis in the equine blastocyst has been reported by several workers from as early as ten days after conception (Flood et al. 1979). Nett and Pickett (1979) noticed a positive correlation between maternal serum concentrations of LH and progesterone between Days 5 and 28 of gestation.

Blood levels of PMSG first appear at about Day 40, reaching a maximum between Days 50 and 70 and falling to low levels by Day 130. There are reports of PMSG being present in peripheral maternal blood to well past Day 130. For example, Spincemaille et al. (1975) detected PMSG in peripheral maternal blood up to 265 days in the progeny of matings between twin brothers and sisters. This finding confirms the immunological concept of fetal cell rejection within the cups put forward by Allen and Moor (1972), because it indicates a degree of immunological tolerance between tissues of similar genotypes.

Allen (1969*b*) surveyed PMSG concentrations in Welsh Mountain pony and Thoroughbred mares. In both groups the hormone was first detected in blood serum between Days 35 and 41. The highest concentrations recorded in both groups were 100 to 112 IU PMSG/ml, but one individual produced only 11 IU/ml. Highest concentrations were found in primparous ponies. Surgical removal of the complete conceptus from mares between Days 40 and 54 did not interfere with the subsequent production of PMSG. The explanation for this phenomenon is that the hormone is secreted by fetal cells that cross to the endometrial cups (see p. 183) at about Day 37 (Allen & Moor 1972). Blood levels of PMSG decline in successive pregnancies (Day & Rowlands 1947) and the genotype of the fetus affects the concentration. Clegg et al. (1962) have shown that a mare carrying a mule fetus produces less than if she were carrying a horse fetus. The role of PMSG is unknown but in certain circumstances it seems to have a strong antagonizing effect on exogenous prostaglandins and may prevent effective luteolysis of the CL between Days

40 and 90 (Allen & Rossdale 1973). Squires and Ginther (1975) concluded that PMSG does not stimulate follicular development but prolongs the life-span of the primary CL and induces ovulation or luteinization of secondary follicles and Allen, W.R. (1975) suggests that PMSG is synergistic with pituitary gonadotrophins which are the primary stimulus on the ovary. It is possible that PMSG plays some part in suppressing the immune response of the endometrium to the presence of the conceptus although this hypothesis remains, as yet, untested.

Perhaps the most challenging endocrinological finding reported in recent years has come from Lincoln College in New Zealand where a radio-immunoassay developed for equine FSH and LH revealed a mid-dioestrous surge of FSH which appeared to be important for further development of follicles destined to ovulate 10–13 days later (Evans & Irvine 1975). These mid-cycle surges of FSH continued to occur during the 30-day period studied in early pregnancy and again in the period two to three weeks before parturition. It seems probable that this cyclic pattern represents an inherent pituitary rhythm that is influenced but not abolished by intrinsic physiological variations and external environmental factors.

Day 150 to full term

Although earlier work suggested that ovariectomy could be performed only at the end of the sixth month of pregnancy without abortion (Hart & Cole 1934) more recent work discussed above suggests that the continuance of pregnancy is independent of the ovaries from a much earlier time in gestation (Holtan et al. 1979).

Progestagen levels fluctuate between 8 and 25 ng/ml until about Day 20 when they decline slowly to basal levels of about 1–3 ng/ml by Days 150–200. They remain low until 10–20 days before term when they again increase, rising to a peak at parturition, after which they drop rapidly to less than 1 ng/ml within the few hours following delivery (Allen & Hadley 1974; Barnes et al. 1975). The variable rise in levels prior to term is due mainly to an increase in 5α-pregnane metabolites of progesterone (Holtan et al. 1975). Three major metabolites have recently been identified, one secreted mainly by the fetus, one by maternal tissues and the third, a combined placental and maternal source (Moss et al. 1979). Progesterone is present in high concentration in umbilical cord blood (Short 1959) and Barnes et al. (1975), using long-term catheterized pony mares, found that fetal oestrogen and progestagen concentrations in late gestation were much higher than maternal values. These workers reported a large venous arterial difference in progestagens and total oestrogens throughout late gestation, thus suggesting a metabolic cycle in the fetus. In one pony mare and fetus, fetal plasma prostagen fell 24–36 hours before parturition when maternal peripheral progestagen concentrations remained high.

The oestrogen pattern during early pregnancy has been reported by Terqui and Palmer (1979). They found that plasma total (conjugated plus unconjugated) oestrogens were similar to those during dioestrus from Day 0 to 35 gestation but an increase occurred between Days 35 and 40 followed by a plateau of 3 ng/ml between Days 40 and 60. The first increase in total oestrogen level was thought to be produced by the ovaries because values were suppressed after ovariectomy. The increase was considered to be due indirectly to PMSG causing follicular growth. After Day 60, a second increase was detected which was not suppressed by ovariectomy and it was, therefore, thought to be of fetoplacental origin. By Day 85 oestrogen concentrations exceeded those detected in non-pregnant mares, thus

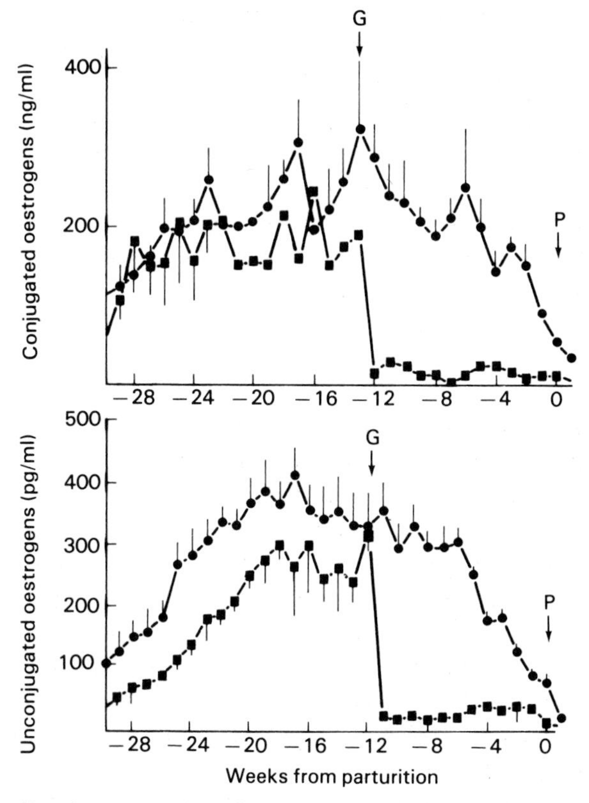

Fig. 3.20. Mean (± SE) concentration of conjugated and unconjugated oestrogens in the peripheral plasma of mares carrying normal and sham-operated (●) (n = 5 in (a), 10 in (b)) and gonadectomized (■) (n = 4 in (a) and (b)) fetuses during the second half of pregnancy. G = gonadectomy; P = parturition. (*After Pashen & Allen 1979b*)

providing a means of pregnancy diagnosis. This rise in oestrogens occurs at a time when the fetal gonads are undergoing hypertrophy and hyperplasia and an association between the two phenomena has often been suggested (Cole et al. 1933). The gonads have organelles associated with steroid biosynthesis (Hay & Allen 1975) and venous drainage of the gonads contains higher levels of the oestrogen precursor dehydroepiandrosterone sulphate (DHAS) than does the gonadal artery, suggesting production by the gonads (Raeside et al. 1979). Fetal gonadectomy results in an immediate drop in oestrogen levels (Pashen & Allen 1979*a*). In this study, surgical removal of the gonads from four fetuses between 197 and 250 days of gestation resulted in an immediate drop, from near-peak concentrations, to basal levels of both conjugated and unconjugated oestrogens in maternal plasma within 48 hours of operation. Having fallen in this manner, the concentrations remained very low throughout the rest of pregnancy (Fig. 3.20), the subsequent birth of the foals occurring spontaneously in all the mares between Days 306 and 327 gestation. Thus, the placenta relies on the fetal gonads for precursors in the formation of oestrogens, whereas maternal precursors are necessary for progesterone synthesis. In normal mares blood plasma oestrogen levels increase rapidly after Day 80 and reach maximal levels at Day 210 after which they decrease to parturition (Nett et al. 1973) (Fig. 3.21).

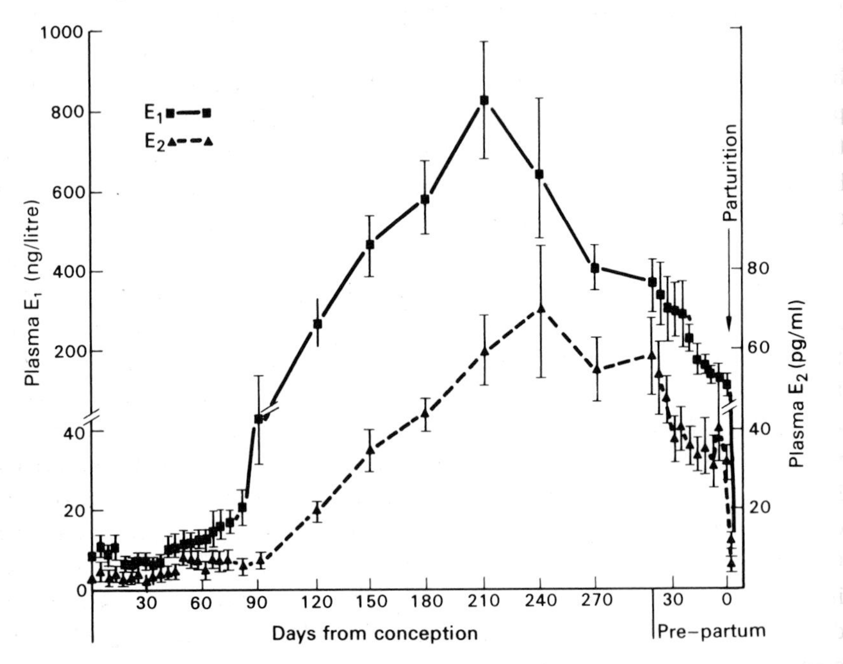

Fig. 3.21. The concentration of plasma oestrogens in mares from conception to parturition (mean ± SE, $n = 4$). E_1, oestrone, equilenin, E_2, oestradiol. (*After Nett et al.* 1973)

Maternal plasma levels of primary prostaglandins show little change during pregnancy (Silver et al. 1979) and although they increase gradually towards term, significant increments are observed only at parturition and following surgery for the insertion of catheters or during starvation (Barnes et al. 1978). In the fetus, levels of both $PGF_2\alpha$ and PGE_2 in the plasma and allantoic fluid increased during the last weeks of gestation, but the prostaglandin metabolite (PGFM) concentration remained almost unchanged (Silver et al. 1979). For further discussion on the role of prostaglandins see Chapter 4.

Maintenance of pregnancy

The maintenance of pregnancy is an important clinical subject, particularly in the inverse relationship that it has to gestational failures. We shall see, when discussing abortion, that a substantial proportion of fetal deaths appear to be the result of some dysfunction in physiological mechanisms. The diagnosis of some of these idiopathic abortions may rest on as-yet-unidentified processes concerned with the maintenance of pregnancy. Unfortunately, in our present state of knowledge, we can but scratch the surface in terms of available techniques and data necessary for interpreting the underlying mechanisms of the maintenance of pregnancy and the corresponding requirements for the diagnosis of non-infectious abortion. The problems of interpreting simple parameters, such as levels of plasma hormones, is illustrated by Irvine (1979) in discussing the kinetics of gonadotrophins in the mare. He draws attention to the fact that the rates at which hormones are secreted, act on target organs and are metabolized are difficult to determine from measuring blood levels alone. In the case of FSH and LH, sialic acid plays a significant role in preventing hormone degradation by non-target tissues, increasing the half-life and thus the biological potency of the hormones. This, and other similar factors, cannot be measured simply by radio-immunoassay of plasma hormone levels and thus the diagnostic relevance of the results of these assays is correspondingly limited.

The traditional view of progesterone as the hormone of pregnancy has been modified to meet the now well-established concept that synergistic and antagonistic interactions occur with oestrogens and other hormones at differing concentractions. The action of hormones on the target organs is also modified and controlled by local conditions. For example, oestrogens have a 'priming' effect on uterine luminal and glandular epithelium, enhancing the action of progesterone. The way the endometrium prepares to receive the fertilized ovum and then maintains it has not been fully established, but it is unlikely to differ in principle from other mammals. In the mare the origin of progesterone in early pregnancy is the CL of dioestrus and subsequently the accessory corpora lutea. But as already indicated, from Day 50 of gestation the ovaries and therefore the CL become decreasingly important as contributors to the pool of progesterone available for continuing pregnancy. Another question which arises is whether the prolonged luteal life-span of the dioestrous CL is based on a decrease in uterine secretion of prostaglandin or a blocking of its effect on the target organ. Recent work (Vernon et al. 1979) suggests that luteal maintenance during pregnancy is not associated with a reduction of PGF-binding capabilities. Therefore, the suppression of uterine secretion is the more likely mechanism protecting the CL in early pregnancy. Preliminary work with prostaglandin analogues (Allen & Rossdale 1973) suggests that PMSG may protect accessory CLs from luteolytic action; but PMSG is secreted only after 40 days and is not therefore responsible for protecting the dioestrous corpus luteum. In other species prolactin plays an important part in maintaining ovarian secretion of progesterone and thereby ensuring the maintenance of gestation (Heap 1972). Reported levels of prolactin in mares were extremely variable and showed no clear fluctuating patterns during pregnancy (Nett et al. 1975).

A knowledge of endocrinological changes in gestation has an important bearing on clinical measures to prevent abortion but views differ on the efficacy of progesterone therapy and other measures.

Objective reports include those of Gunzel and Merkt (1979), in which 383 mares showing clinical evidence of suspected early fetal resorption, between Days 20 and 60 of gestation, were studied in two groups. 217 mares were treated with a single injection of 200 mg CAP (a synthetic progestagen) and the remaining 166 mares were used as untreated controls. The results indicated that treatment had neither a beneficial nor a detrimental effect on the continuation of pregnancy. In another study plasma progestagen concentration dropped to less than 2 ng/ml after ovariectomy, whether or not pregnancy was maintained, in pony mares from which the ovaries were removed at different stages of pregnancy (Holtan et al. 1979). Mares ovariectomized on Day 25 and injected with 100 mg of progesterone daily for 10 or 20 days remained pregnant during treatment but lost the uterine tone and the fetal sac within four to six days after the end of treatment. Levels of plasma progesterone concentrations resulting from the administration of exogenous progesterone to ovariectomized mares have been reported by Hawkins et al. (1979). In this study progesterone concentrations were not maintained at levels greater than 1 ng/ml for 24 hours when 50 mg/day of progesterone in oil was administered but they remained at levels greater than 1 ng/ml during the last four days of a course of seven daily injections of 100 mg/day and at greater than 1.5 ng/ml throughout the injection sequence of 200 mg/day. Repositol progesterone administered at a dose rate of 500 mg peaked in six hours but returned to near 1 ng/ml in two days. At 1000 mg and 2000 mg, plasma progesterone was maintained at approximately 2 and 4 ng/ml respectively for seven days after injection on Day 1 and was 1.5 and 3.5 ng/ml respectively 11 days after injection on Day 7, indicating a cumulative effect on plasma progesterone following repeated dosages. These figures suggest that claims by clinicians for the efficacy of exogenous progesterone in preventing abortion are open to some doubt on the grounds that the dose administered is usually too small to provide any significant increment in progesterone levels in the plasma or at the uteroplacental junction. For example, progesterone implants inserted through a trocar and cannula often contain only 100 mg progesterone and are claimed to last 250 days. In the authors' experience, plasma progestagen levels in mares aborting between Days 20 and 90 of gestation usually fall after, rather than before, the event. Further, where low levels of plasma progestagen (less than 2 ng/ml) are recorded, individuals will often continue their pregnancy without therapy. In conclusion therefore, the value of progesterone therapy has not been proved by objective studies but, in the absence of any evidence that it is harmful, its use as a placebo cannot be opposed.

Mitchell and Allen (1975) found that plasma progestagen levels showed marked variations in yearling mares that became pregnant and aborted spontaneously between Days 30 and 160. However, the loss of the conceptus was always associated with the drop in progestagen levels and, in some, may have been the result of levels inadequate to maintain pregnancy.

The use of human chorionic gonadotrophin (HCG) has been advocated for use in early pregnancy as a means of promoting luteal activity. However, Allen, W.E. (1975) found in Welsh pony mares that a series of three intravenous injections of 2000 IU HCG on alternate days caused fetal loss when administered before Day 39 but not when administered between Days 40 and 97. The use of HCG in pregnant mares must therefore be contraindicated.

The use of diethylstilboestrol (DES) has been advocated as an anti-abortion therapy on the grounds that it extended the normal life-span of the accessory corpora lutea and its use has been correlated with a decrease in the rate of spontaneous abortion between Days 150 and 200 of pregnancy (Nishikawa 1959). However, Nett and Pickett (1979) concluded that injections of DES did not influence serum concentrations of LH, PMSG or progesterone, affect the length of gestation or influence the maintenance of pregnancy in the mare.

The administration of meclofenamic acid, a prostaglandin synthetase inhibitor, by mouth has been shown to prevent an increase in PGFM associated with fasting and intrauterine surgery (Silver et al. 1979) although its administration in the final stages of gestation does not appear to prevent parturition (Pashen & Allen 1979*b*).

FETAL ENVIRONMENT AND METABOLISM

The environment of the fetus is limited by its dependence on placental function. Environmental control is vested in an interaction between maternal and fetal metabolism. Extreme alterations in physiological status may interfere with normal growth and development, a subject we shall return to later (see Chapter 5).

Information about equine fetal metabolism is limited and that available has come mainly from studies in Cambridge in which chronic catherization and acute preparations have been used.

It appears that the equine placenta may be more efficient than that of the ruminant. There is a relatively small differential between blood gas tensions and pH

TABLE 3.4 Resting P_{O_2}, P_{CO_2} and pH (mean ± SE) in the fetal and maternal blood of seven mares anaesthetized with chloralose or halothane

Blood sample from	P_{O_2} (mmHg)	P_{CO_2} (mmHg)	pH
Maternal artery	92.7 ± 4.3	35.1 ± 1.9	7.40 ± 0.01
Maternal uterine vein	52.1 ± 1.4	40.5 ± 2.1	7.38 ± 0.01
Fetal umbilical vein	48.8 ± 1.4	41.4 ± 2.1	7.35 ± 0.01
Fetal umbilical artery	32.8 ± 1.3	49.6 ± 2.9	7.30 ± 0.01

After Comline and Silver (1970).
Figures were calculated from one or two observations from 11 or 12 animals.

in the blood of the umbilical and maternal uterine veins (Comline & Silver 1970) (Table 3.4); the PO_2 difference in anaesthetized mares was 4 mmHg, compared with 17 mmHg in the ewe and PCO_2 1 mmHg compared with 4 mmHg. When equine maternal PO_2 was raised above 100 mmHg, uterine venous and umbilical venous PO_2 increased and the gradient between the two was reversed (Fig. 3.22).

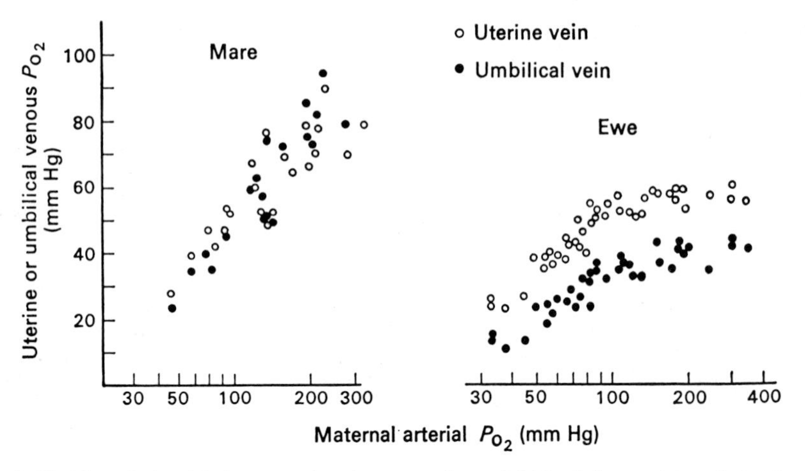

Fig. 3.22. The relationship between Po_2 in maternal arterial blood (log scale) and that in the uterine vein and umbilical vein in seven ewes and seven mares. (*After Silver et al. 1973*)

The effect of variations in umbilical or uterine blood flow on placental blood gas levels has not been examined systematically, but there is a drastic fall in umbilical blood flow with an increased umbilical arteriovenous difference in oxygen tensions when the fetus is removed from the uterus (Silver & Comline 1972). Great variations in flow may occur in the ewe under stress and blood flow may fall during uterine contraction (Greiss 1965). The effect of alterations in the mare's position has not so far been studied.

Silver et al. (1973) reported fetal plasma glucose levels up to 60% of maternal values (Fig. 3.23) and an immediate rise in umbilical plasma glucose when uterine venous levels were increased by glucose infusion into the aorta (Fig. 3.24). Free fatty acid blood levels were also directly related to maternal levels and fetal lactate levels followed those in maternal blood more closely than in ruminants.

The content and output of adrenaline and noradrenaline from the equine fetal adrenal medulla has been investigated by Comline and Silver (1971). Under normal conditions only small amounts were secreted but during anoxia the adrenal discharge was considerable and was independant of nervous mechanism; and both catecholamines were secreted although noradrenaline was predominant. Equine fetal plasma cortisol levels are similar to those of the lamb (about 4 μg/dl) but do not rise before birth (Comline et al. 1973).

Maternal malnutrition may cause retarded fetal growth especially when it occurs during the last third of pregnancy. But a specific relationship between nutritional and maternal environmental factors and equine fetal metabolism has yet to be

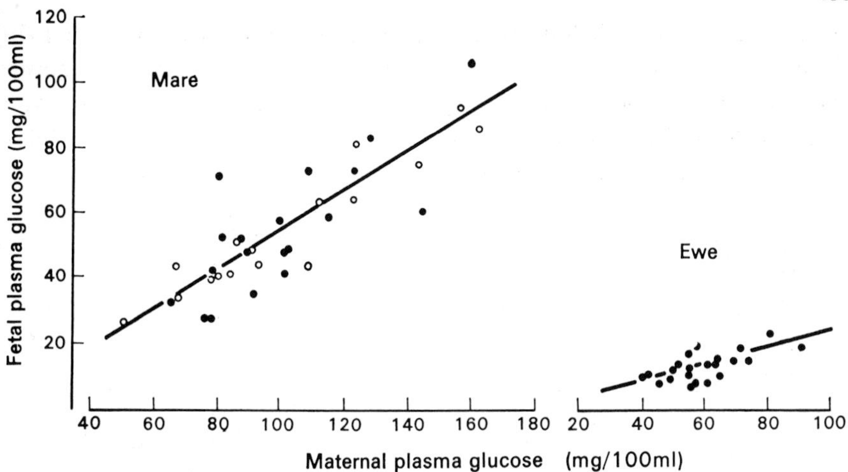

Fig. 3.23. The relationship between maternal and fetal plasma glucose levels in the mare and the ewe. ● Values from chronic preparations. ○ Values from acute preparations (chloralose anaesthesia) with the fetus undisturbed in utero. Two or three values are included per experiment. Regression lines were indicated by the method of least squares. Ewe = 0.26∿ − 2.0; mare = 0.60 ∿ 65.6 Conversion factor: mg/100 ml × 0.0555 = mmol/litre. (*After Silver et al. 1973*)

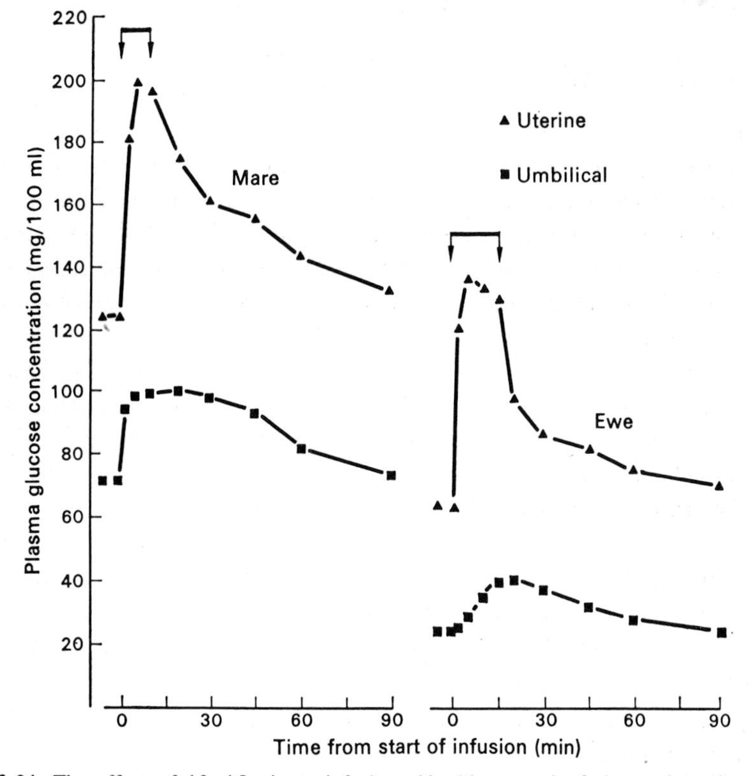

Fig. 3.24. The effect of 10–15-minute infusions (double arrows) of glucose into the uterine circulation (via the lower aorta) on uterine and umbilical venous plasma glucose levels. The mare was anaesthetized (chloralose) and the ewe was conscious with indwelling catheters. Conversion factor: mg/100 ml × 0.0555 = mmol/litre. (*After Silver et al. 1973*)

established. Until more information is available the clinical significance of endocrinological and metabolic changes on the maternal or fetal side will remain obscure.

Fetal stress

The term 'fetal stress' describes major changes in the fetal environment which interfere with normal growth, development and metabolism. The term is one of definition and, although all-embracing, its concept has merit in relation to abortion and neonatal illness.

The clinician must diagnose fetal stress in retrospect by examining the fetus and its membranes after abortion or premature or full-term delivery. Definitive pathology is often present; placentitis, amnionitis and meconium-stained amnionic fluid are easily recognizable.

Stress may be caused by bacteria, viruses or fungi affecting the placenta and/or the fetal body (see Abortion, p. 195 and Chapter 5). The most important non-infectious cause of fetal stress is hypoxia, the effects of which are placentitis, amnionitis and meconium in the amniotic fluid. Damage to fetal organs may follow fetal hypoxia and acidaemia.

The exact relationship of the various aetiological factors has not been established in any species and information in the horse is particularly sparse. It is possible to deduce from the pathology of aborted and dysmature foals that placentitis is the most common single entity in fetal stress. It may be acute, as evidenced by fetal death and abortion or still-birth, or it may be chronic, causing fetal emaciation and subsequent abortion or delivery of an individual which suffers maladjustment.

Because of the diffuse nature of the placenta, comparatively large areas may be partially or completely destroyed and the fetus still survive. Presumably there is a critical level of placental function below which the fetus is at risk. To what extent there can be compensation, e.g. by restricted fetal growth or redirected placental circulation to functional areas, is a matter of speculation. Examples of undersized healthy foals associated with grossly reduced placental area are twins (see p. 177) and singletons accompanied by mycotic placentitis. In some cases involving Thoroughbreds we have found 50% of the placenta to be abnormal and the foal weight to be less than 30 kg (normal 50 kg).

In the absence of experimental or clinical evidence we can only list the possible causes of fetal stress:

1. Alterations in perfusion/perfusion ratios between uterine and placental blood flow, so that the gaseous exchange is subnormal. For example, if uterine flow were directed mainly to the uterine horns and placental flow mainly to that part in apposition to the uterine body, the ratio would be extremely wide and little exchange would be possible.
2. Hypoperfusion of uterine or placental capillary beds causing adverse changes in perfusion/perfusion ratio.

3. Maternal malnutrition in quantitative or qualitative terms.
4. Placentitis from infection or hypoxia.
5. Developmental abnormalities of fetal membranes and especially those which interfere with blood flow through the umbilical vessels.
6. Fetal malposition or posture causing interference with the umbilical cord.
7. Errors in placental implantation and attachment.
8. Local immunological reactions between the uterine mucosa and the placenta.
9. Uterine torsion.
10. Maternal diseases, including infective and metabolic conditions.

Clinical recognition of the particular factor involved in any given case is usually possible only in retrospect and the cause of many abortions remains undiagnosed.

Fetal heart rate

In human medicine fetal heart rate has been used to indicate fetal stress (Larks 1961). In the horse the fetal heart rate has been determined by electrocardiography (Holmes & Darke 1968; Colles et al. 1978) and by ultrasonic detection (Fraser et al. 1973). The rate tends to fall with advancing pregnancy from 180/minute at three months to 100/minute near term. Colles et al. (1978) recorded 595 fetal electrocardiograph traces from 33 mares, employing a bipolar lead system and portable electrocardiogram and using hand-held steel electrodes. They found that clipping the hair was generally unnecessary using hand-held electrodes. They found that the maternal heart rate gradually increased from 150 days gestation to term, while the mean fetal heart rate fell. Before parturition the fetal heart rate was usually faster than the maternal, but this could be temporarily reversed in nervous mares. Fetal tachycardia was defined as a heart rate, for more than five consecutive heart beats, of more than 2 SD above the mean rate of a defined stage of gestation. A persistent tachycardia was recorded in one fetus out of three of aborting Thoroughbreds within five days of abortion. In an aborting pony mare, fetal heart rates reached 166 and 188/minute on Day 245 of gestation some 70 hours before expulsion of the fetus. The amplitude of the fetal electrocardiograph was found to vary considerably and rapidly with the mean amplitude increasing from 150 days to term. Clinical use of this technique is limited, although it may act as a means of pregnancy diagnosis after 150 days. Colles et al. (1978) claim that it may be used to diagnose twins and to provide a permanent record of the presence of a fetus. However, they qualify their opinion by pointing out that the demonstration of a live fetus does not rule out the possibility of a dead twin or of a second fetus with a very small vector deflection.

ABORTION

Abortion is defined as the expulsion of the fetus before Day 300 of gestation, when, due to absolute immaturity, the fetus has little chance of survival, even with intensive care. *Prematurity* is defined as birth between Days 300 and 320.

These are arbitrary divisions, however, and processes which cause fetal stress and abortion in some cases may, in others, be responsible for premature birth, conditions of maladjustment, neonatal septicaemia and anatomical abnormalities.

Abortions are sometimes classified as early or late, depending on whether they are before or after about Day 150. The division has no aetiological or pathological significance and it has been applied in practice mainly because early abortion is not always seen; a mare can be diagnosed as pregnant at, say, Day 40 and found barren some months later. Fetal death, resorption and 'slipping' are synonyms for abortion. Fetal resorption is usually diagnosed where serial palpations reveal the presence of a fetal sac which is small for its age and is reducing in size and softening. Whether complete resorption ever occurs is not known. In most cases, undetected abortion of the dead fetus and membranes probably occurs at some stage.

The reader is referred to the section on maintenance of pregnancy (see p. 188), a process regarded as the obverse of abortion.

Aetiology

Abortion may be due to infective or non-infective causes, although in some cases the division cannot be clear because infection may contribute to the death of a fetus damaged by physiological disturbances; conversely, such disturbances may predispose to infection.

Infective causes. In decreasing order of incidence, these are:

1. Bacterial. *Str. zooepidemicus, E. coli, Klebsiella aerogenes, Staph. aureus* and *Salmonella abortivoequina.*
2. Fungal. Mycotic abortion may be caused by members of *Mucor, Aspergillus* or *Allescheria* families.
3. Viral. Equid herpesvirus I (rhinopneumonitis) and arteritis virus.

Non-infective abortion. Known non-infective causes of abortion are:

1. Twins.
2. Developmental abnormalities of the allantoic or amniotic part of the umbilical cord causing constricted vessels.
3. Nutritional deficiencies (Van Niekerk 1965*b*).

Other possible causes of non-infective abortion are:

4. Endocrinological dysfunction.
5. Twisting of the umbilical cord.
6. Immunological incompatibility.
7. Chromosomal abnormalities.
8. Maternal and/or fetal circulatory disturbances caused by changes in maternal posture, fright or trauma.
9. Overdose of therapeutic drugs or administration of abortifacients.
10. Disturbance of physiological mechanisms including placental function and metabolic stability, as discussed under fetal stress.

Mitchell and Allen (1975) observed a high incidence of early pregnancy loss in yearlings mated between June and August and ascribed this to immaturity, inadequate nutrition and physical stress. They report no significant histological, bacteriological or virological findings in 21 fetuses aborted before Day 160 and conclude that repeated rectal examinations alone were not the cause of the high rate of abortion, a conclusion reached by other experienced clinicians and research workers.

Endometrial incompetence due to chronic degeneration and, in particular, endometrial fibrosis has been suggested as a cause of early embryonic loss (Kenney 1978).

A higher incidence of fetal loss (Finn & Porter 1975; Ricketts 1978) seems to occur in mares that conceive during the foaling heat (Merkt 1966) although no specific cause has, as yet, been detected for this higher rate (Gygax et al. 1979).

Incidence

The incidence of abortion varies with breed, locality and management, and survey results are affected by different methods of collecting and assessing data. Stud book returns are often inaccurate because research into details may not be precise and because breeders' documentation tends to be biased.

Surveys compiled from data collected in the field indicate the abortion rate in groups of mares, but results vary according to the definition of conception, i.e. the time at which pregnancy tests are performed. A summary of published data is set out in Table 3.5. There are few statistical analyses of the gestational age at which abortions occur. Bain (1969) surveyed 1260 Thoroughbred mares during 2562 pregnancies over six years, with a total incidence of 19%, and found no difference in incidence between mares with foals at foot or dry mares. This is at

TABLE 3.5 Incidence of abortion

Country	*Incidence*	*Source*	*Comments*
Italy	13.8%	Matassino (1962)	
South Africa	14%	Du Plessis (1964) Van Niekerk (1965*a, b*)	 Between Days 25 and 31 in mares on low protein grazing
Australia	19%	Bain (1969)	Survey of 1260 TB mares during 2562 pregnancies, 1957–62. Pregnancy diagnosis 20–40 days after service
Great Britain	3.8%	Mahaffey (1968)	Analysis of data from General Stud Book, 1930–52. Includes only abortions in later pregnancy
Great Britain	4.2%	–	Unpublished. Analysis of General Stud Book 1977–9. Includes abortions and mares who 'slipped', expressed as a percentage of total mares covered

variance with the findings of Jennings (1950) and Merkt (1966) who reported a higher incidence in mares with foal at foot and attributed this to embryonic loss after service at the foal heat.

In Bain's series, abortion was not highly repeatable and of mares which had aborted once only 12.5% did so again the following season. However, 19% of the mares that aborted once aborted again during the remaining five years of the survey. The abortion rate was lowest in the three- to six-year age group. Of mares which had aborted and were retained for breeding, 23% failed to produce a live foal during the following three years and the main reason for this was their inability to become pregnant. Poor breeding performance after abortion was also found to increase with age.

Pathogenesis

Abortion represents a rejection of the fetus and its membranes by the uterus. There are two principle pathways:

1. Fetal death caused by viral or bacterial infection which crosses the placental barrier or which interferes with normal placental exchange. Non-infective disturbances may cause cardiac and circulatory failure resulting in fetal death. It is interesting to speculate whether the trigger mechanism of abortion is identical to that of normal birth.

2. Fetal death is not always the precipitating factor in abortion, as some fetuses are delivered with their heart beating and others establish a respiratory rhythm for minutes or even hours. The precipitating factors in these cases probably arise from the maternal side of the placenta, the uteroplacental unit, the fetal endocrinological status or a combination of these.

Examination of the aborted fetus and a uterine biopsy suggest that placental pathology is often a primary factor in abortion. An eroded placental surface and reduced functional area caused by infective or non-infective agents may precipitate abortion or affect the fetus itself. Twins are an example where reduced placental function (in this case due to competition between the placentae, see p. 177) results in one fetal death and eventually to abortion of both fetuses.

Clinical signs

The signs of abortion are similar to those of normal birth, although there is a wide range of premonitory signs. Mammary development, formation of wax on the teat ends and ejection of milk may be apparent weeks before abortion, especially if due to twins. In other cases there is no mammary development and the abortion is spontaneous, as in those caused by equid herpesvirus I infection. There is some evidence that mammary development is associated with placentitis or retention of a dead fetus for some days or weeks before abortion, whereas unheralded abortion is more likely to be caused by sudden fetal death.

First-stage labour may be short and second-stage labour uncomplicated, due to the relatively small fetal size, and in most cases the fetus can be delivered even in abnormal posture, presentation and position without causing dystocia. The chief exception is twins which enter the pelvic inlet together.

Placentitis may cause a prolonged third stage, requiring therapeutic removal of the fetal membranes, but in many abortions the membranes are delivered with the fetus. The behaviour of the mare during abortion is similar to that during normal third-stage birth. After delivery she usually shows maternal signs, although, in the absence of mammary development, she soon loses interest once the aborted conceptus has been taken from her. A more common consequence is uterine infection and nervous symptoms may occur after abortion caused by viral infection (Petzoldt et al. 1972).

Diagnosis and pathology

The diagnosis of abortion depends on a pathological examination of the fetus and its membranes.

Bacterial abortion

Bacterial infection usually causes typical pathological signs of septicaemia in the aborted fetus, i.e. congested mucous membranes and serosal surfaces, pleural pericardial and peritoneal exudates. The muscles are dark red/purple and the myocardium contains splashing along the coronary grooves. Leucocytic infiltrations of parenchymatous organs may be found on microscopic examination but the fetal tissues' response to infection is often limited. Post-mortem changes may obscure the true pathological picture, depending on the interval between fetal death and abortion. A fetus retained in the uterus at 38°C produces considerable autolysis in 24–48 hours. The liver and kidneys are friable and cellular lysis breaks up the normal structure.

Dimock et al. (1947) isolated streptococci in 17% of 1074 fetuses examined. The organism was isolated in many instances from all internal organs but in others from only one or two organs. They believed that if streptococci were isolated only from the stomach and lungs it indicated amniotic infection and that infection of the maternal surface of the chorion was significant. They pointed out that the fetal tissues may not react to bacterial organisms and that the histopathology of abortion may therefore be confined to the placenta.

The affected placenta is thickened and the maternal surface necrotic, with areas covered by a greyish exudate. The non-pregnant horn may be like parchment and adhere to the uterus.

Salmonella abortivoequina infection was once prevalent as a cause of abortion and joint-ill in foals but it is now a rare condition which appears to have completely disappeared from the UK. Mahaffey (personal communcation, 1970) did not find a case during 13 years at the Animal Health Trust's Equine Research Station in Newmarket, nor was the organism found in cervical swabs sent to the station.

Pregnant mares usually abort between the fourth and eighth months and show varying degrees of illness such as fever, colic, diarrhoea and uterine discharge.

The placenta of the aborted fetus is oedematous and haemorrhagic with necrotic areas on the surface; the pleura and peritoneal cavities contain excessive haemorrhagic fluid. But the condition must be diagnosed by bacteriological methods and the causal organism can be cultivated on ordinary laboratory media from fetal organs and membranes. It can also be obtained by culturing cervical swabs as the organism is present in the cervical discharge for several days after abortion. Diagnosis may be confirmed by serological means seven to 14 days after abortion when raised blood titres are present (Bryans et al. 1961).

Mycotic abortion

The pathology is often confined to the placenta but may also occur in the amnion and in a small number of cases within the fetus (Mahaffey & Adam 1964; Mahaffey & Rossdale 1965). There is a substantial thickening of large areas of the placenta and the maternal surface is covered by a brown sticky exudate. Fungal hyphae may be identified on histological examination which also shows widespread necrosis of the chorionic villi. A considerable inflammatory reaction occurs in the subepithelial tissue and giant cells may be present. Amniotic lesions consist of irregular necrotic plaques and the amnion may adhere to the fetal skin. Greyish-white nodules up to 3 mm in diameter may be distributed throughout the lungs, which on histological examination are seen to contain mycelia and giant cells.

The fetus is usually small for its gestational age and its weight may be only a fifth of normal. The body is emaciated but usually free from jaundice and lesions do not occur in the liver.

Viral abortion

Dimock et al. (1947) described its pathology:

> No one assemblage of pathological changes within the fetuses or foals, or the fetal membranes, was present in all cases. Typical specimens were aborted fetuses having the following pathological anatomy. Externally the appearance of ascites, with different degrees of jaundice. Congestion of the liver with pressure on the diaphragm from serous fluid within the thoracic cavity produced an aspect of ascites though no appreciable accumulation of fluid was present in the peritoneal cavity. The organs within the abdominal cavity, the joint cavities, and foot pads appeared icteric. The liver showed the most striking changes and thus the most dependable diagnostic, macroscopic lesion. Beneath the capsule of the liver were a few to many pinhead-sized whitish to yellowish areas of necrosis. In some instances these were scattered over the whole surface of the liver; in others they were more or less limited to individual areas and lobes. These degenerated foci ranged from the border of visibility to 2 mm in diameter. Upon the gross section, similar macroscopic spots became visible in dispersed locations within the parenchyma of the organ. The spleen was hyperaemic with many petechial hemorrhages on its surface. The colic lymph glands were enlarged, congested, and often hemorrhagic.
>
> An abundance of serous fluid often was found in the thoracic cavity. The lungs were edematous and congested with numerous petechial hemorrhages on the surface. In many cases these hemorrhages were classed as ecchymoses. Microscopically, edema was confined to the subcapsular and interstitial tissues of the lungs. In some cases there was more than a normal amount of pericardial fluid. Beneath the epicardium were found numerous petechiae or ecchymoses which for the most part were confined to the ventricles. They followed

the coronary groove and the left longitudinal groove of the heart. The thymus was edematous, hyperemic and sometimes hemorrhagic.

The most pronounced changes observed in the fetal membranes, which usually were expelled completely with the fetus, were in the amnion. In many cases the amnion was edematous in various areas, if not throughout, and was often straw-colored.

The most significant microscopic lesions of this disease, so far observed, were confined to the liver and lungs. In several instances macroscopic examination did not reveal any lesions within these organs though histopathological changes were sufficiently characteristic to justify a diagnosis of virus infection.

Sections of the liver often showed marked hyperemia, in some cases accompanied by hemorrhage. Small degenerated intralobular areas were apparent in the mounted hepatic tissue, varying in location from the border of the central vein to the periphery of the lobule. Some were so small as to be barely visible at 75 diameters magnification, while others occupied a whole lobule. They were numerous or few, diffuse or discrete, depending upon the specimens examined. The typical lesion in which the inclusion bodies were found was an area of focal necrosis with varying degrees of karyorrhexis and pyknosis [Fig. 3.25].

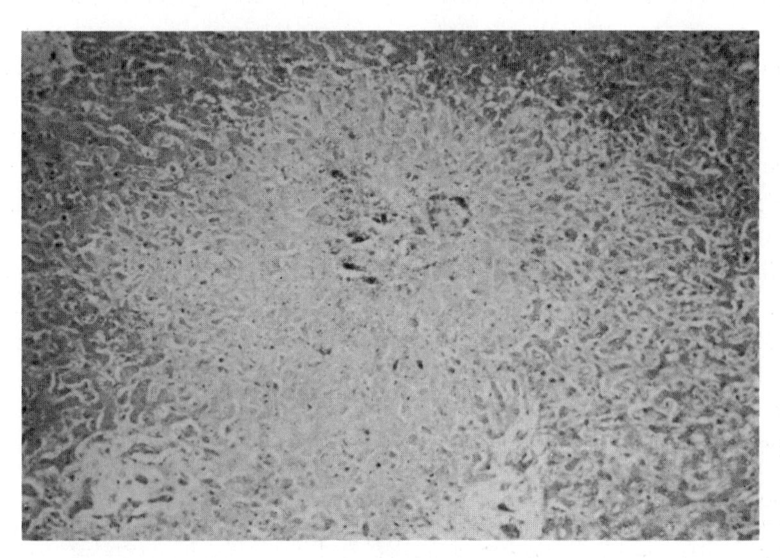

Fig. 3.25. Histological section of equine fetal liver from equid hypesvirus I abortion showing areas of focal necrosis. See also Fig. 3.26. H & E × 120.

Degeneration and destruction of the parenchyma of the liver was shown by accumulation of cellular debris. These lesions were very characteristic, and intra-nuclear inclusions were found in hepatic cells lying in the periphery of the necrotic areas and in adjacent cells. In some cases, similar inclusion bodies were found in the nuclei of epithelial cells lining interlobular bile ducts. The number of inclusions in this location varied from one to many in a cross-section of the duct. Characteristic inclusion bodies were found in the nuclei of endothelial cells lining blood vessels of the liver, in the nuclei of smooth muscle cells and fibroblasts, and in the tunica media and tunica adventitia of the same vessel. Fibroblasts of the connective tissue capsule of the liver also contained typical intranuclear inclusion bodies.

The lungs showed varying degrees of hyperemia and hemorrhage. Cells of the epithelium lining the bronchi, bronchioles, and alveoli often contained intranuclear inclusions. The number of inclusion bodies and their location differed among the specimens examined. When found they were usually in a few areas within a section, although in some instances they were numerous both in the nuclei of epithelium lining the terminal air passages, and in the cells of the alveolar walls. The most striking examples of inclusion bodies within the air passages were in the epithelium of the bronchi. In a few cases the majority of the nuclei within these cells contained large, well-defined bodies. The most common location within the lung tissue, however, was in the epithelium of the bronchioles.

Since this description was written the inclusion bodies have been designated as Cowdry type-A (Fig. 3.26) and Pauli and Alroy (1972) have described lesions in the coronary arteries of aborted fetuses. Techniques of tissue culture have enabled the causal agent to be isolated and studied (Randall et al. 1953; McCollum et al. 1962; Mayr et al. 1965). The virus responsible has been classified as equid rhinopneumonitis (Doll et al. 1959*a, b*) and more recently as equid herpesvirus I (Plummer et al. 1969) and II (see Chapter 6).

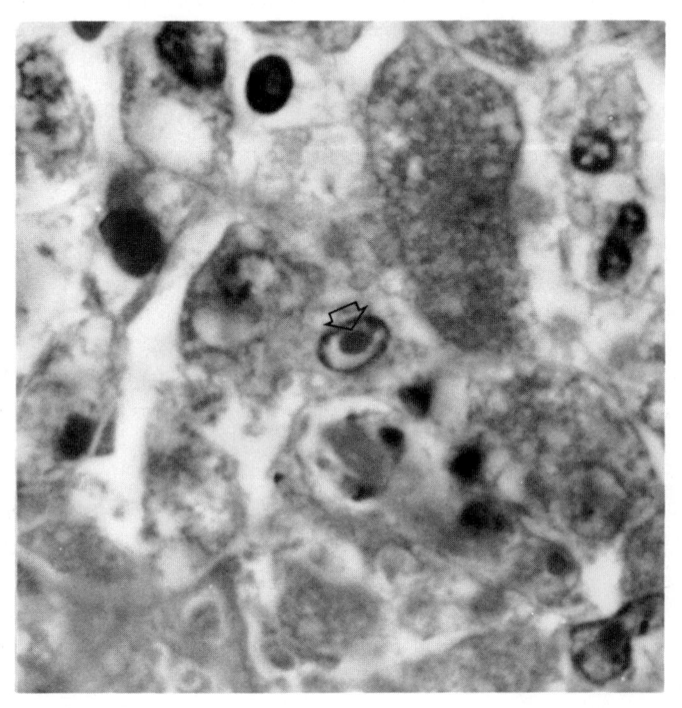

Fig. 3.26. Histological section of liver from an aborted fetus suffering from equid hepesvirus I showing an eosinophilic intranuclear inclusion body (arrowed). H & E × 250.

A comparison of diagnostic methods (Trapp et al. 1972) revealed that those relying on histopathological changes were marginally better than where isolation of the virus was the only method used: agreement between both methods was 88.8%. A cytological method for rapid diagnosis has been described by Correa (1970). Smears (1 × 1 × 0.5 cm) were made from cut areas of liver and, after drying in air, fixed in methanol for five minutes, and stained by various methods, of which Pappenheim's panoptic gave best results. Cytological methods proved better than histological sections for the demonstration of intranuclear inclusion bodies.

Complement-fixing antibodies occur in the sera of infected horses but do not provide a reliable method of diagnosis because they persist for only a few months.

Further, they are present after respiratory infections and their presence has no specific correlation with abortion or risk of abortion.

Gestational age as a guide to diagnosis

Abortion from equid herpesvirus I infection has its greatest incidence in gestational months eight and nine but may be responsible for abortion from six months onwards and for stillbirth or neonatal illness at full term (see p. 308).

Mycotic and twin abortions occur from the sixth month onwards. Bacterial infection is responsible for abortion at any stage of pregnancy although streptococci are more often found in fetuses aborted before, and *E. coli* after, Day 150.

Non-infective abortions may occur at any stage of pregnancy. Protein starvation is known to cause abortion between Days 25 and 31 (Van Niekerk 1965*b*).

Treatment and control

A dual approach to treatment is required. One approach concerns the individual and is aimed at restoring her genital health in preparation for subsequent pregnancies and other the other is concerned with epidemiology and the possible spread of infection to other individuals.

Epidemiology

Apart from the now rare condition of *Salmonella abortivoequina* infection, the only known causes of epidemic abortion are equid herpesvirus I and arteritis virus infection.

Equid herpesvirus I causes mainly upper respiratory tract infections and pneumonitis. Infection is followed by a short-lived immunity and mares can become reinfected each year. From serological surveys it appears that most of the horse population in Britain has experienced infection. Recent evidence sugests that a number of differing subtypes may exist, some of which may be more likely to cause abortion than others. The virus can be isolated in tissue culture from young horses in the early stages of respiratory infection and in large quantities from aborted fetuses. Sporadic abortions occur in Britain but these rarely lead directly or indirectly to epidemics (Mahaffey 1968). Since 1960 two serious epidemics have occurred in England and at least one in Ireland (Condon, personal communication, 1973). The Irish outbreak was associated with paralytic symptoms, a known complication of equid herpesvirus I infection. More recently paralytic signs were observed among mares on a stud farm in Newmarket, associated with at least nine fatalities (Greenwood 1979) (see Chapter 7).

Epidemics tend to occur where mares have had little or no repeated contact with the virus and are subsequently exposed when their immunity is low. Contact with foals and yearlings affected with the respiratory form may therefore have considerable epidemiological significance. In the USA planned-infection campaigns were employed, using attenuated hampster-adapted live virus sprayed into the nostrils of all horses twice yearly (Byrne et al. 1958; Doll & Bryans 1963*a, b*). An inactivated equid herpesvirus vaccine (Pneumabort-K) has been employed in the USA and it is claimed that its use has reduced abortions from EHV-I infection and also the fatality of mares from paralytic disease. The vaccine contains EHV-I chemically inactivated with formaldehyde and combined with a specially prepared oil adjuvant. It is recommended by the manufacturers that a 2 ml dose is given intramuscularly during the fifth, sixth and ninth month of pregnancy in each succeeding year. The efficacy of the vaccine has been reported by Moore and Koonse (1978). A culture-attentuated strain of EHV-I (Rhinomune) has also been employed in vaccination programmes in Canada and the USA. Authorities differ in their opinion on the efficacy and safety of these measures and at present it is illegal to import any of these vaccines into the UK. Eaglesome et al. (1979) investigated the incidence of abortions, still-births and neonatal death on three farms where pregnant mares were vaccinated with a live virus vaccine (Rhinomune). They concluded that, despite vaccination, infection with EHV-I was responsible for most of the fetal and foal mortality observed. These investigators suggested that in practice prophylactic measures should concentrate on management practices designed to minimize the risk of exposure to field virus and to avoid stress on mares at risk.

Because of the large amount of virus in aborted fetuses, it is important to isolate mares that have aborted, pending confirmation of the diagnosis. The aborted fetus and its membranes should be put into a plastic bag and taken direct to an appropriate laboratory for examination. The mare should be confined to the box in which she has aborted and attendants should wear protective clothing and wash their hands and boots in disinfectant before contacting other pregnant mares; preferably, the mare's attendant should not be in charge of other pregnant animals. The mare's hind-quarters and tail should be washed with a weak solution of cetrimide and bedding should be burnt for at least one week after the abortion. If an abortion has occurred in a paddock this should be cleared of grazing horses for at least two weeks and preferably stocked with non-pregnant mares for at least a further two weeks. The area where the fetus has laid should be disinfected and all remnants of the fetal membranes collected and disposed of. Bridles and other equipment should not be applied to an infected mare and then to a pregnant mare without being disinfected. A mare may be considered non-infectious four weeks after aborting.

A complicating factor in epidemiology is the variable interval, in many cases, between infection and abortion. Although spread of infection from an aborted fetus to late-term pregnant mares may start an epidemic of abortions within days of one another, in other cases respiratory spread may occur weeks or months before an individual aborts. In the latter case a mare may become infected and act as a carrier, bringing the infection to susceptible animals at a later date.

Arteritis virus is not known to occur in England and is uncommon in the USA. It has been reported in Switzerland It is unrelated to equid herpesvirus I but it causes a severe respiratory and constitutional illness in horses of all ages. Affected mares suffer a high incidence of abortion and unlike equid herpesvirus I abortion, where the mare shows no visible illness while aborting, arteritis virus is associated with keratitis, nasal occular discharge and swollen extremities.

Measures to be taken in a non-contagious situation

Bacterial, myctoic and non-infective abortions have little or no epidemiological significance. However, each case should be isolated in a manner described for viral abortion until a positive diagnosis has been made in the laboratory.

Infective abortions should be treated for endometritis. Intrauterine infusion of an appropriate antibiotic or antifungal agent should be administered daily for about three days after abortion and repeated between the ninth and twelfth days. Oestrogens and oxytocin may be used to assist uterine involution (see p. 267). Continuing treatment depends on the degree of endometritis and the response to therapy.

Non-infective abortions may require similar treatment for secondary infection although most cases clear up without treatment.

Preventive measures

The most usual prophylactic measure is to give progesterone (see also p.189). Claims have been made for 400 mg subcutaneous implants at Day 120 but this routine has been criticized because the dose is too small to have a likely effect; weekly or monthly injection of hydroxyprogesterone caproate (1 g) in oily solution is suggested as an alternative. Chorionic gonadotrophin 3000 IU intravenously at weekly intervals has been advocated as a rational measure in the first 120 days gestation to stimulate fresh corpora lutea. This may be contraindicated prior to Day 40 (Allen, W.E. 1975) (see p. 191).

Whatever claims are made for success in individual cases there are no reports of controlled trials; nor is there evidence to support the proposition that abortion is due to insufficiency of endogenous progesterone. Until more is known of the factors which cause non-infective abortion, prophylactic measures will remain in the realms of subjective clinical experience.

Mares suffering from infective endometritis before, or at the time of, conception and those with a history of abortion due to bacterial infection may be treated weekly or monthly with parenteral antibiotics. It is difficult to substantiate the efficacy of such measures; in the absence of controls, abortion is more significant than the apparent success of pregnancy continuing to full term.

Endometrial biopsy may reveal the presence of diffuse stromal fibrosis and severe chronic degenerative endometritis. For treatment see p. 88.

In our opinion many cases of non-epidemic abortion or resorption are caused by either fetal abnormalities or endometrial incompetence from progressive 'wear-and-tear' damage (see p. 105). In the case of fetal abnormalities, attempts to delay or prevent fetal loss are contraindicated. The earlier the mare aborts the better it may be for her future breeding career. If the problem is one of endometrial incompetence, an accurate diagnosis and prognosis is essential before attempts at treatment (see p. 108). The effectiveness of treatment should be assessed by repeat biopsy before prophylactic breeding methods are used to try to prevent recurrence. Some cases of endometrial incompetence may be untreatable.

MANAGEMENT OF THE IN-FOAL MARE

Little is known of the relationship between environmental factors and fetal well-being and this prevents us from presenting other than a subjective account of proper management of the mare during pregnancy. Before discussing the subject it is helpful to summarize problems which may be encountered in practice.

Can fetal growth, development (mal-development) and death be affected by (*a*) maternal nutrition; (*b*) changes and traumatic events in the maternal environment, such as injury, frenzied galloping, transport by air, sea or land; (*c*) veterinary measures such as surgery involving local or general anaesthesia, rectal palpation, application of restraint (e.g. twitch) or therapeutic or prophylactic drugs; (*d*) movement of the mare from one environment (stud farm) to another; or (*e*) maternal infectious disease or conditions of colic?

A certain amount is known about the relationship between environmental factors and fetal health (or ill heatlh) but most of the evidence is subjective. We have already referred to Van Niekerk's observations that protein deprivation between Days 25 and 31 may cause abortion; low planes of nutrition and imbalanced diets are associated with prolonged gestation, developmental abnormalities and low birth weight. Comline et al. (1975) and Silver et al. (1979) found that starving pregnant mares prior to surgical procedures caused elevation of serum bilirubin and plasma PGFM. Environmental disturbances such as low-flying aircraft and sale rings have been blamed for abortion. Mahaffey (1968) quotes a case in which a government paid compensation for an abortion after a mare was frightened by low-flying aircraft.

Rectal examinations to diagnose pregnancy have been incriminated as a cause of abortion, partly due to the 'natural' loss of fetuses from Days 40 to 120. These early abortions occur in cases where no rectal examination has been performed and their relatively small incidence (5–12%) does not suggest a close relationship in view of the extensive use of rectal palpation as a routine measure. In our experience, deliberate manipulation of one member of a twin pregnancy from Days 40 to 50 often fails to dislodge either fetus. Allen (1974) and Voss and Pickett (1975) palpated mares daily on Days 19 to 120 and from Days 0 to 50 and found no evidence of fetal loss (see also p. 211). If owners still have strong doubts practioners are advised to use alternative methods of pregnancy diagnosis.

PREGNANCY DIAGNOSIS

Pregnancy diagnosis is required:

1. To confirm the sexual status of the mare during the stud season so that by early diagnosis of the non-pregnant state measures may be taken to return the mare

to oestrus for another chance to conceive. These examinations are usually performed from Days 19 to 90.

2. For purposes of sale or insurance. These examinations are usually required in the last two-thirds of gestation.

3. To meet special requirements, such as no-foal-no-fee arrangements. October 1 is the customary date on which the buyer of a nomination on this basis becomes liable in the northern hemisphere.

Methods of detection

1. Manual. By rectal palpation, applicable to all stages of gestation.
2. Blood test, applicable from Day 45 to Day 90.
3. Urinary test, applicable from Day 150 to full term.
4. Ultrasonic detection, applicable from Day 80 to full term.

Manual examination

The general procedure is as for all rectal examinations (see p. 00) (Bain 1967*b*). The uterus is palpated using the left or right arm. Prior to about Day 60 of gestation the operator should pick up the left or right ovary and pass the hand along the anterior border of the uterine horns, to the opposite ovary. The uterus, at this stage, lies immediately anterior to the pelvic brim and the fetus is contained in one or other of the two horns at the junction with the body. The fetal sac may be felt as a discrete fluid swelling immediately to the left or right of the midline. The size of the fetal sac at various stages is shown in Table 3.6 and Figs 3.27 and 3.28.

TABLE 3.6 Pregnancy diagnosis based on palpation of the fetal sac in the first trimester

Length of gestation (days)	*Diameter of sac* (cm, approx)	*Comments*
19	3	Turgid horns. Fetal sac may be felt as small bulge on anteroventral aspect of pregnant horn
40	8–12	Turgid horns. Fetal sac felt as distinct enlargement
60	20–25	Fetal sac now occupies horn and part of uterine body. Turgid part of horns less readily palpated. Sac losing tenseness
100	30–40	Fetal sac occupies body and both horns. Fetus itself can be palpated

From about Day 18 the uterine walls are thickened and turgid and the horns are felt as firm, clearly delineated, tubular projections on either side of the fetal sac, and readily distinguishable from the flaccid, saccular oestrous state (Solomon 1971). In some cases, however, uterine tone is between these two extremes and the uterus may have a doughy feel. The fetal sac may also vary in size, some feeling small and others large for gestational date. Sometimes the uterine wall is distended with fluid and it is difficult to distinguish the swelling from a fetal sac. Even experienced practitioners may, in a small number of cases, be unable to determine whether a particular mare is pregnant before 50 days.

The problem of fetal death has already been discussed and the earlier pregnancy diagnosis is attempted, the more difficult it is to distinguish between a continuing pregnancy in which the fetal sac is smaller than usual and one in which it is small because the fetus is dead or dying.

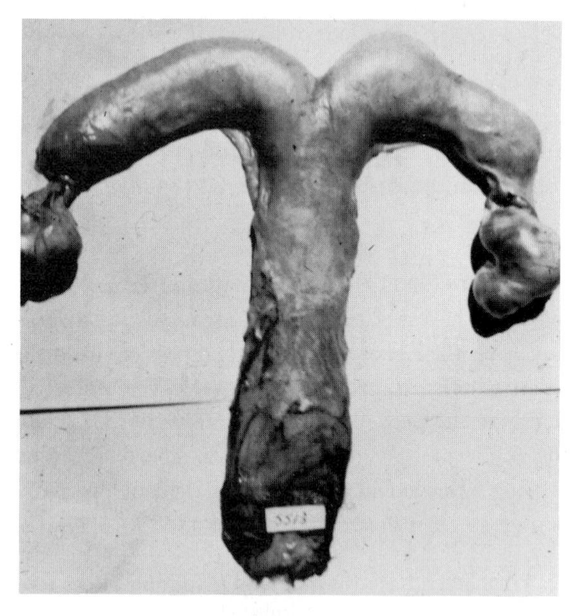

Fig. 3.27. A 21-day pregnant uterus with a fetal sac in the right horn. Note the turgid appearance of the uterine horns and the small swelling at the junction of the horns and the body. This swelling may sometimes be felt per rectum at this stage on the anteroventral aspect. (*By kind permission of C.H. Van Niekerk*)

Diagnosis at 18 days after ovulation is subjective and the clinician should adopt a suitable set of criteria by which results may be recorded and interpreted. The following system is suggested:

- Category A Turgid uterine wall with maximum tone and fetal sac definitely palpated in left or right horn – positive.
- Category B Maximum tone but no fetal sac detected – probably positive.
- Category C Uterine tone between B and D firm or dough-like – probably negative.
- Category D Flaccid uterine wall with minimum tone – negative.

Definite diagnoses may be given only for categories A and D.

Early diagnosis may be hampered by the mare straining on the operator's arm or because the uterus lies posterior to the pubic brim where it is difficult to palpate. In these cases a speculum should be inserted into the vagina so that this part becomes ballooned with air. This helps to push the uterus in an anterior direction and the operator can pass the hand to the anterior edge of the uterine horns.

Up to Day 60 it may be helpful to locate the non-pregnant horn and its corresponding ovary before passing the hand over the fetal sac in the pregnant horn. It is then important to locate the corresponding ovary and to pass the hand from one

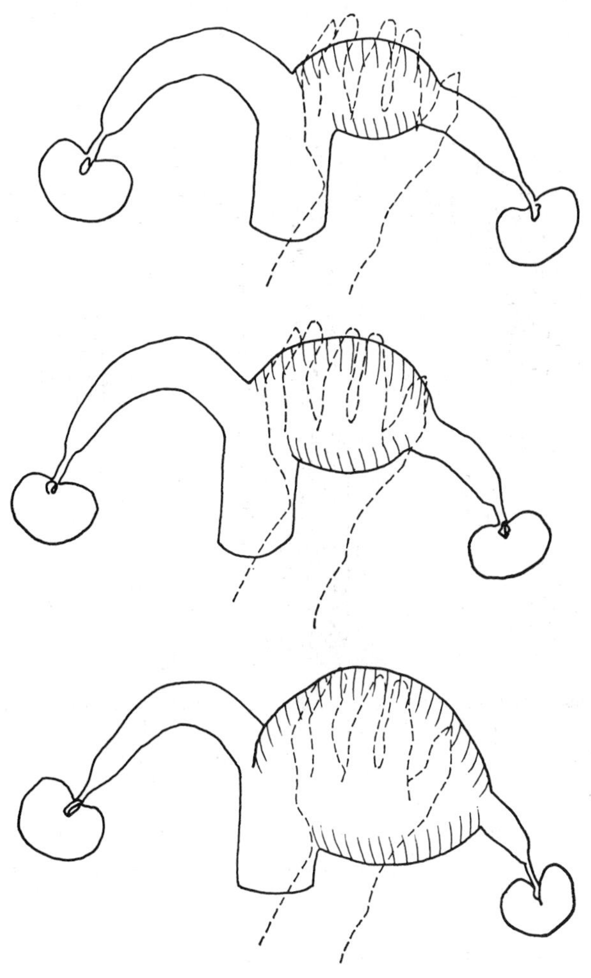

Fig. 3.28. The size and position of the fetal sac relative to the human hand during pregnancy diagnosis at 33, 42 and 60 days.

ovary to the other. This manoeuvre helps to differentiate the pregnant uterus from a coil of small intestine which may sometimes give the impression of turgidity similar to the gravid uterus.

Examination of the cervix may aid diagnosis, although the state of this organ varies considerably in pregnancy. In most cases of pregnancy the cervix is tightly closed, white to pink in colour and covered by sticky mucus. In some instances it may be moist and occasionally it is red and relaxed. Conversely, many non-pregnant mares may have the closed white apperance of pregnancy. However, taken in conjunction with the results of rectal examination, the state of the cervix sometimes helps to confirm the non-pregnant state. It is of little help in confirming pregnancy.

Blood plasma progesterone levels are helpful only in cases where blood levels are zero or below 4 ng/ml. These results suggest the non-pregnant state but higher levels are diagnostic of only a functional corpus luteum, which may be present in the non-pregnant, dioestrous state.

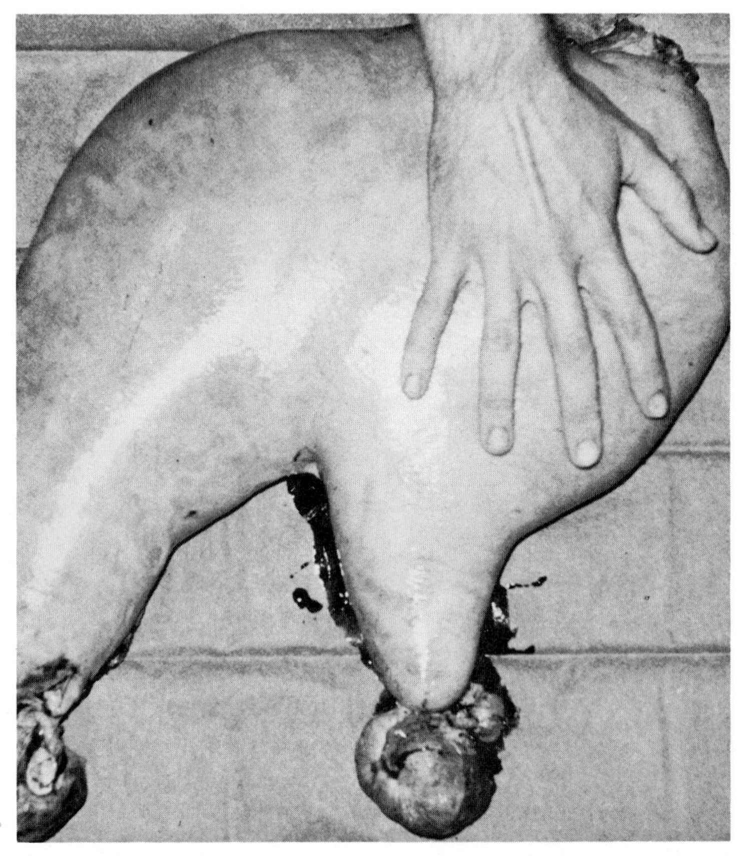

Fig. 3.29. A 97-day pregnant uterus illustrating the size in relation to the human hand. At this stage of gestation the margins of the uterus can be palpated only with difficulty.

From about Day 60 the fetal sac starts to extend into the uterine body. Its size and decreasing tone make it difficult for the operator to feel the anterior margin of the uterus, as the organ is carried forward and downwards by the weight of the fetus and fetal fluids. Inexperienced operators may find the examination around Day 60 to be the most difficult. At this time the fetus is moving into the uterine body and is not yet big enough to be easily palpated; nor is tension in the fetal fluid sufficient to make the uterus feel taut. The operator should feel for the distended uterine surface, passing the hand gently from one side to the other (Fig. 3.29). Up to about Day 140 the uterine horns and ovaries may still be palpated, although in many cases only with difficulty. The ovaries are drawn towards the midline as pregnancy proceeds and it is necessary to feel farther into the abdominal cavity and direct the arm obliquely downward from the pelvis. The fetus may sometimes be felt through the uterine wall as a firm object, like a piece of wood floating in water. In many cases it is surprisingly difficult to palpate the fetus, although with patience and by passing the hand to the lateral surface of the uterine swelling contact can usually be made. Pyometritis and the urinary bladder must be distinguished from a pregnant uterus. The bladder is circumscribed and lies immediately below the pubic brim. Pyometritis is comparatively rare and can be differentiated only by palpating the fetal body or appendages.

From Day 200 to full term the fetus becomes more readily palpable, although from 200 to 260 days it may still be situated low in the abdomen, and the uterus is felt as a large fluid-filled mass under what seems to be considerable tension. At some stage between Days 200 and 260 the tension is reduced and the fetus passes upwards towards the pelvic inlet where it can be readily palpated on rectal examination.

The uterine contents of mares in foal for the first time are usually nearer the pelvic inlet than those that have carried in previous years.

The subject of possible harmful effects of manual examinations is often raised by laymen and discussed at veterinary gatherings. There is no objective evidence to determine conclusively whether or not the examinations may cause abortion at any particular stage of pregnancy. Allen (1974) palpated Welsh pony mares for examination purposes daily from Days 19 to 120 of pregnancy and concluded that 'there was no evidence that vigorous palpation of a healthy conceptus is a cause of fetal death'. Voss and Pickett (1975) vigorously palpated mares daily for the first 50 days of pregnancy and found no evidence that it caused fetal loss. Clinical experience in vigorous squeezing, at about Day 40 of pregnancy, in an attempt to eliminate one of two members of twins, demonstrates clearly the difficulty in causing abortion, because in many cases such action fails to dislodge either of the fetuses. On the other hand, measurement of myometrial electrical activity shows that this is increased by palpation of the genital tract per rectum and by vaginoscopic examination. Further, Osborne (1975) is of the opinion that stress plays a significant part in some causes of abortion. We are inclined to the view that pregnancy diagnosis and other stressful influences may cause abortion in a very small number of cases, but the individuals involved are probably predisposed to the event and might be expected to abort for one reason or another.

Blood tests

The basis of the blood test is the presence of gonadotrophin (PMSG) in the serum between Days 40 and 100. Hart and Cole (1932) first described a technique of injecting mare's serum into immature mice or rats. 0.5 ml of serum is injected subcutaneously into each of two 17–21-day-old female mice. At 48 hours the mice are killed by chloroform and the uterus and ovaries examined. A positive result is a congested, enlarged uterus. The ovaries are enlarged and contain follicles. One or two mice may be used as a control. The test is sensitive to 1 IU of PMSG/ml.

Immunological methods of PMSG detection have been described by Wide and Wide (1963) and Allen (1969*a, b*). Serum is incubated for several hours with anti-PMSG obtained from rabbits by hyperimmunization. The mixture is then added to an indicator system consisting of sheep erythrocytes sensitized by PMSG (Wide & Gemzell 1960). The reactions are illustrated in Fig. 3.30. The biological and

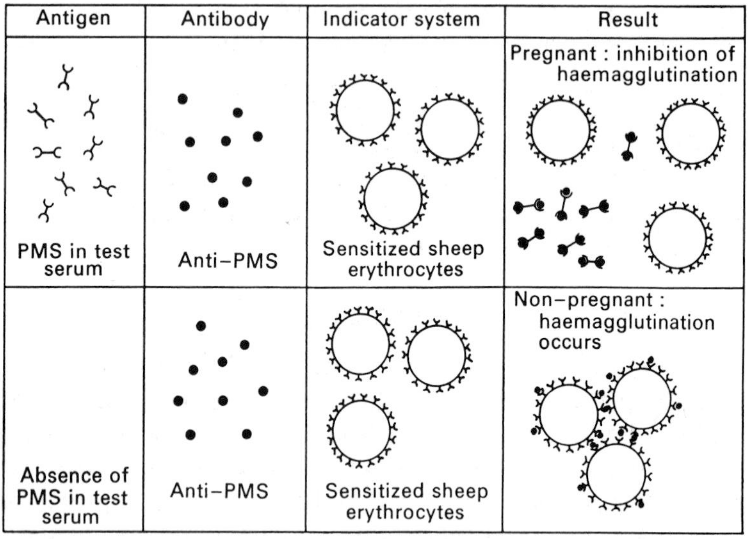

Antigen	Antibody	Indicator system	Result
PMS in test serum	Anti–PMS	Sensitized sheep erythrocytes	Pregnant : inhibition of haemagglutination
Absence of PMS in test serum	Anti–PMS	Sensitized sheep erythrocytes	Non–pregnant : haemagglutination occurs

Fig. 3.30. The haemagglutination test. (*After Jeffcott et al. 1969*)

immunological tests for PMSG are accurate to 90% (Cox & Galina 1970; Henriksen & Jorgensen 1972). False positives are more frequent than false negatives, due in part to the continuation of PMSG secretion by the endometrial cups after the fetus has died or been removed (Allen & Moor 1972). We have encountered a small number of mares who have produced false negative reactions to this method, in successive pregnancies. A quantitative method may be preferable for such cases (Allen 1969*a*). Walker (1977) describes a quantative 'bioassay' involving the injection of measured quantities of test serum into immature female mice. 24 hours later the mice are sacrificed and the utero-ovarian weight is expressed as a percentage of body weight, 24 hours previously. Marked endometrial stromal oedema occurs in the mice injected with pregnant mare serum and this results in an increase in utero-ovarian weight. Walker claims that the biological assay is slightly more sensitive than the haemagglutination inhibition test method.

Shaw and Morton (1980) have described the detection of an immunosuppressive early pregnancy factor (EPF) in the blood of several species from as early as six hours after mating. They suggest that this may in the future form the basis of a highly accurate method for early pregnancy diagnosis in the mare.

Urine tests

Tests for urinary oestrogens are chemical (Cuboni 1934; Mayer 1955; Lunaas 1962) and biological (Miller 1934). Cox (1971) considered that Cuboni's test was the method of choice and was reliable after Day 150. In this method 3 ml of concentrated hydrochloric acid are added to 15 ml of urine and heated over a boiling water bath for ten minutes. After cooling, the hydrolysed urine is extracted with 18 ml of benzene. The benzene is transferred to a test-tube and 10 ml of concentrated sulphuric acid are poured down the side of the tube to lie under the benzene. The tube is stoppered, inverted gently once and heated at 80°C for five minutes. Results are read in reflected daylight and under an ultra-violet Wood's lamp. A green fluorescence is positive.

Ultrasonic detection

Fraser et al. (1973) have described a technique of ultrasonic pregnancy diagnosis by transducer probe placed in the rectum. A fetal pulse was detected as early as Day 42 and was consistently found from Day 120 to full term.

GESTATIONAL LENGTH

On Thoroughbred stud farms it is usual to calculate the expected date of parturition as 11 calendar months from the last service, i.e. a gestational length of 333–336 days. Statistical surveys based on the interval between service and birth indicate mean gestational lengths in Thoroughbreds of 338–340 days (Uppenborn 1933; Bilek 1936; Jennings 1941; Rossdale 1967), with a range of 310–374 days. In other breeds means of 322–345 days have been reported (Kenneth & Ritchie 1953). Ropiha et al. (1969) calculated gestational length as the interval between ovulation and birth and found a mean of 345.3 days for births in October (southern hemisphere season) and 337.9 days in December. They found no significant difference attributable to the sire of the foal, sire of the dam, age of the sire or dam, or year; but sex of the foal, month of conception and the dam had significant effects on duration of pregnancy.

The fetus determines the duration of its own intrauterine life and its phenotype has an important bearing as evidenced by crosses of stallion and mare (340 days), stallion and jennet (350 days), jack and mare (355 days), jack and jennet (365 days). Howell and Rollins (1951) found a heritability of 36% and that environmental influences, especially nutrition, affect gestational length.

The physiological mechanisms which end gestation are discussed in the following chapter and the clinical implications of gestational length *vis à vis* prematurity in Chapter 5.

PRENATAL MAMMARY DEVELOPMENT

The mare has two mammary glands, each a short flattened cone consisting of a glandular body and a teat with two small openings.

Two main phases of mammary development occur during pregnancy, i.e. growth and secretion. Special milk secretions known as colostrum are found in the last four weeks of pregnancy and stored in the glands until birth. Sometimes this secretion is lost prematurely and the mare 'runs milk' hours, days or even weeks before parturition.

The precise hormones necessary to initiate and maintain lactation are unknown. Anterior pituitary hormones such as prolactin, growth hormone and adrenocorticotrophin have roles in both mammary growth and milk secretion in other species (Cowie 1972), but no account has thrown light on the process in the mare.

Mammary growth begins about a month before parturition but the major increment in size occurs in the last two weeks, at a time when progesterone levels are rising and oestrogen levels falling. The effect of these hormones on mammary development has been reviewed by Folley (1952) but no information is available on the horse. Mammary development and milk secretion sometimes occur in barren and maiden mares during spring and autumn flushes of grass growth, but the significance of this phenomenon and its possible relationship to endogenous or exogenous oestrogen is a matter for speculation. Changes in mammary secretions during late pregnancy in the mare have been described by Peaker et al. (1979) (see p. 227).

References and further reading

Allen, W.E. (1974) Palpable development of the conceptus and fetus in Welsh pony mares. *Equine vet. J.*, **6**, 69.

Allen, W.E. (1975) Pregnancy failure induced by human chorionic gonadotrophin in pony mares. *Vet. Rec.*, **96**, 88.

Allen, W.E. & Hadley, J.C. (1974) Blood progesterone concentrations in pregnant and non-pregnant mares. *Equine vet. J.*, **6**, 87.

Allen, W.R. (1969*a*) A quantitative immunological assay for pregnant mare serum gonadotrophin. *J. Endocr.*, **43**, 581.

Allen, W.R. (1969*b*) The immunological measurement of pregnant mare serum gonadotrophin. *J. Endocr.*, **43**, 593.

Allen, W.R. (1970) Endocrinology of early pregnancy in the mare. *Equine vet. J.*, **2**, 64.

Allen, W.R. (1975) Ovarian changes during early pregnancy in pony mares in relation to PMSG production. *J. Reprod. Fert.*, Suppl. **23**, 425.

Allen, W.R. & Moor, R.M. (1972) The origin of the equine endometrial cups. I. Production of PMSG by fetal trophoblast cells. *J. Reprod. Fert.*, **29**, 313.

Allen, W.R. & Rossdale, P.D. (1973) Preliminary studies upon the use of prostaglandins for inducing and synchronizing oestrus in Thoroughbred mares. *Equine vet. J.*, **5**, 137.

Amoroso, E.C. (1951) The decidual reaction in the mare's placenta. *J. Physiol., Lond.*, **113**, 3.

Amoroso, E.C. (1952) Placentation. In *Marshall's Physiology of Reproduction,* ed. A.S. Parkes, vol. 2, p. 127. London: Longmans Green.

Amoroso, E.C. (1955) Endocrinology of pregnancy. *Br. med. Bull.*, **11**, 117.

Bain, A.M. (1963) Common bacterial infections of fetuses and foals and association of the infection with the dam. *Aust. vet. J.*, **29**, 413.

Bain, A.M. (1967*a*) The ovaries of the mare during early pregnancy. *Vet. Rec.*, **80**, 229.

Bain, A.M. (1967*b*) The manual diagnosis of pregnancy in the Thoroughbred mare. *N.Z. vet. J.*, **15**, 227.

Bain, A.M. (1969) Fetal losses during pregnancy in the Thoroughbred mare: a record of 2562 pregnancies. *N.Z. vet. J.*, **17**, 155.

Barnes, R.J., Comline, R.S., Jeffcott, L.B., Mitchell, M.D., Rossdale, P.D. & Silver, M. (1978) Fetal and maternal concentrations of 13,14-dihydro-15-oxo-prostaglandin F in the mare during late pregnancy and at parturition. *J. Endocr.*, 78, 201.

Barnes, R.J., Nathanielsz, P.W., Rossdale, P.D., Comline, R.S. & Silver, M. (1975) Plasma progestagens and oestrogens in fetus and mother in late pregnancy. *J. Reprod. Fert.,* Suppl. **23**, 617.

Betteridge, K.J., Eaglesome, M.D. & Flood, P.F. (1979) Embryo transport through the mare's oviduct depends upon cleavage and is independent of the ipsilateral corpus luteum. *J. Reprod. Fert.,* Suppl. **27**, 387.

Betteridge, K.J. & Mitchell, D. (1975) A surgical technique applied to the study of tubal eggs in the mare. *J. Reprod. Fert.,* Suppl. **23**, 519.

Bilek, F. (1936) *Neue Forschungen in Tierzucht und Abstammungslehre,* 17. Bern: Duerst.

Bryans, J.T., Fallow, E.H. & Shephard, B.P. (1961) Equine salmonellosis. *Cornell Vet.,* **51**, 468.

Byrne, R.J., Quan, A.L. & Kaschula, V.R. (1958) Responses of horses to a neurotropic strain of influenza virus. *Am. J. vet. Res.,* **19**, 655.

Clegg, M.T., Boda, J.M. & Cole, H.H. (1954) The endometrial cups and allantochorionic pouches in the mare with emphasis on the source of equine gonadotrphin. *Endocrinology,* **54**, 448.

Clegg, M.T., Cole, H.H., Howard, C.B. & Pigon, H. (1962) The influence of fetal genotype on equine gonadotrophin secretion. *J. Endocr.,* **25**, 245.

Cole, H.H. & Goss, H. (1943) Source of equine gonadotrophins. In *Essays in Biology in Honor of Herbert M. Evans,* p. 107. Berkeley, Calif.: University of California Press.

Cole, H.H., Hart, G.H., Lyons, W.R. & Catchpole, H.R. (1933) The development and hormonal content of fetal horse gonads. *Anat. Rec.,* **56**, 275.

Cole, H.H., Howell, C.E. & Hart, G.H. (1931) The changes occurring in the ovary of the mare during pregnancy. *Anat. Rec.,* **49**, 199.

Colles, C.M., Parkes, R.D. & May, C.J. (1978) Fetal electrocardiogarphy in the mare. *Equine vet. J.,* **10**, 32.

Comline, R.S., Hall, L.W., Lavelle, R. & Silver, M. (1975) The use of intravascular catheters for long-term studies on the mare and foetus. *J. Reprod. Fert.,* Suppl. **23**, 583.

Comline, R.S. & Silver, M. (1970) pO_2, pCO_2 and pH levels in the umbilical and uterine blood of the mare and ewe. *J. Physiol., Lond.,* **209**, 587.

Comline, R.S. & Silver, M. (1971) Catecholamine secretion by the adrenal medulla of the fetal and newborn foal. *J. Physiol., Lond.,* **216**, 659.

Comline, R.S., Silver, M., Nathanielsz, P.W. & Hall, L.W. (1973) Parturition in the larger herbivores. In *Fetal and Neonatal Physiology,* ed. R.S. Comline, K.W. Cross, G.S. Dawes & P.W. Nathanielsz. Cambridge: Cambridge University Press.

Correa, W.M. (1970) A rapid method for the diagnosis of equine virus abortion. *Can. J. comp. Med.,* **34**, 164.

Cowie, A.T. (1972) Lactation and its hormonal control. In *Reproduction in Mammals. 3. Hormones in Reproduction,* ed. C.R. Austin & R.V. Short, p. 106. Cambridge: Cambridge University Press.

Cox, J.E. (1971) Urine tests for pregnancy in the mare. *Vet. Rec.,* **89**, 606.

Cox, J.E. & Galina, C.S. (1970) A comparison of the chemical tests for oestrogens used in equine pregnancy diagnosis. *Vet. Rec.,* **86**, 97.

Cuboni, E. (1934) Uber einer einfache und schnelle chemische-hormonald Schwanger schaftsekretion. *Klin. Wschr.,* **13**, 302.

Danforth, D.M. Veis, A., Breen, M., Weinstein, H.G., Buckingham, J.C. & Manalo, P. (1974) The effect of pregnancy and labour on the human cervix – changes in collagen glycoproteins and glycosaminoglycans. *Am. J. Obstet. Gynec.,* **121**, 641.

Day, F.T. & Rowlands, I.W. (1947) Serum gonadotrophin in Welsh and Shetland ponies. *J. Endocr.,* **5**, 1.

Deanesly, R. (1975) Germ cell development and the meiotic prophase in the fetal horse ovary. *J. Reprod. Fert.,* Suppl. **23**, 547.

Dickerson, J.W.T., Southgare, D.A.T. & King, J.M. (1967) The origin and development of the hippomanes in the horse and zebra. 2. The chemical composition of the fetal fluids and hippomanes. *J. Anat.,* **101**, 285.

Dimock, W.W., Edwards, P.R. & Bruner, D.W. (1947) Infections of fetuses and foals. *Bull. Ky agric. Exp. Stn,* 509.

Doll, E.R. & Bryans, J.T. (1963*a*) A planned infection program for immunising mares against viral rhinopneumonitis. *Cornell Vet.,* **53**, 249.

Doll, E.R. & Bryans, J.T. (1963*b*) Epizootiology of equine viral rhinopneumonitis. *J. Am. vet. med. Ass.,* **142**, 31.

Doll, E.R., Crow, M.E., McCollum, W.H. & Bryans, J.T. (1959*a*) In vitro serum neutralisation of hamster-propagated equine rhinopneumonitis virus. *Cornell Vet.*, **49**, 28.

Doll, E.R., McCollum, W.H., Bryans, J.T. & Crowe, M.E. (1959*b*) Effect of physical and chemical environment on the viability of equine rhinopneumonitis virus propagated in hamsters. *Cornell Vet.*, **49**, 75.

Douglas, R.H. & Ginther, O.J. (1975) Development of the equine fetus and placenta. *J. Reprod. Fert.*, Suppl. **23**, 503.

Du Plessis, J.L. (1964) Some observations and data in Thoroughbred breeding. *J.S. Afr. vet. med. Ass.*, **35**, 215.

Eaglesome, M.D., Mitchell, D. & Henry, J.N.R. (1979) Control and prevention of equine herpesvirus I abortion. *J. Reprod. Fert.*, Suppl. **27**, 607.

Evans, M. J. & Irvine, C.H.G. (1975) Serum concentrations of FSH, LH and progesterone during the oestrous cycle and early pregnancy in the mare. *J. Reprod. Fert.*, Suppl. **23**, 193.

Ewart, J.C. (1915) Studies on the development of the horse. I. The development during the third week. *Trans. R. Soc. Edin.*, **51**, 287.

Finn, C.A. & Porter, D.G. (1975) The uterus. In *Handbook of Reproductive Biology*, vol. 1. London: Elek Science.

Flood, P.F., Betteridge, K.J. & Irvine, D.S. (1979) Oestrogens and androgens in blastocoelic fluid and cultures of cells from equine conceptuses of 10–22 days gestation. *J. Reprod. Fert.*, Suppl. **27**, 413.

Flood, P.F. & Marrable, A.W. (1975) A histochemical study of steroid metabolism in the equine fetus and placenta. *J. Reprod. Fert.*, Suppl. **23**, 495.

Folley, S.J. (1952) Lactation. In *Marshall's Physiology of Reproduction*, ed. A.S. Parkes, vol. 2, p. 525. London: Longmans Green.

Fraser, A.F., Keith, N.W. & Hastie, H. (1973) Summarised observations on the ultrasonic detection of pregnancy and foetal life in the mare. *Vet. Rec.*, **92**, 20.

Ginther, O.J. & First, N.L. (1971) Maintenance of the corpus luteum in hysterectomized mares. *Am. J. vet. Res.*, **32**, 1687.

Gonzalez-Angulo, A., Hernandez-Jauregui, P. & Martinez-Zedilo, G. (1975) Fine structure of the gonads of the horse and its functional implications. *J. Reprod. Fert.*, Suppl. **23**, 563.

Greenwood, R.E.S. (1979) Equine rhinopneumonitis outbreak at Newmarket. *Vet. Rec.*, **104**, 534.

Greiss, F.C. (1965) Effect of labor on uterine blood flow. Observations on gravid ewes. *Am. J. Obstet. Gynec.*, **93**, 917.

Grosser, O. (1927) *Frühentwicklung, Einhautbildung und Placentation.* Munich: Bergmann.

Gunzel, A. & Merkt, H. (1979) Oestrus and fertility following progestagen treatment of mares showing clinical evidence of early pregnancy failure. *J. Reprod. Fert.*, Suppl. **27**, 453.

Gygax, A.P., Ganjam, V.K. & Kenney, R.M. (1979) Clinical, microbiological and histological changes associated with uterine involution in the mare. *J. Reprod. Fert.*, Suppl. **27**, 571.

Hamilton, W.J. & Day, F.T. (1945) Cleavage stages of the ova of the horse, with notes on ovulation. *J. Anat.*, **79**, 127.

Hart, G.H. & Cole, H.H. (1932) A practical method for the diagnosis of pregnancy in the mare. *J. Am. vet. med. Ass.*, **80**, 604.

Hart, G.H. & Cole, H.H. (1934) The source of oestrin in the pregnant mare. *Am. J. Physiol.*, **109**, 320.

Hawkins, D.L., Neely, D.P. & Stabenfeldt, G.H. (1979) Plasma progesterone concentrations derived from the administration of exogenous progesterone to ovariectomised mares. *J. Reprod. Fert.*, Suppl. **27**, 211.

Hay, M.F. & Allen, W.R. (1975) An ultrastructural and histochemical study of the interstitial cells in the gonads of the fetal horse. *J. Reprod. Fert.*, Suppl. **23**, 557.

Heap, R.B. (1972) Role of hormones in pregnancy. In *Reproduction in Mammals. 3. Hormones in Reproduction*, ed. C.R. Austin & R.V. Short, p. 73. Cambridge: Cambridge University Press.

Henriksen, S.A. & Jorgensen, J.B. (1972) Pregnancy diagnosis in mares, II. Comparison between an immunological and a biological method. *Nord. VetMed.*, **24**, 17.

Hershman, L. & Douglas, R.H. (1979) The critical period for maternal recognition of pregnancy in mares. *J. Reprod. Fert.*, Suppl. **27**, 395.

Holmes, J.R. & Darke, P.G.G. (1968) Fetal electrocardiography in the mare. *Vet. Rec.*, **82**, 651.

Holtan, D.W., Nett, T.M. & Estergreen, V.L. (1975) Plasma progestagens in pregnant mares. *J. Reprod. Fert.*, Suppl. **23**, 419.

Holtan, D.W., Squires, E.L., Lapin, D.R. & Ginther, O.J. (1979) Effect of ovariectomy on pregnancy in mares. *J. Reprod. Fert.*, Suppl. **27**, 457.
Howell, C.E. & Rollins, W.C. (1951) Environmental sources of variation in the gestation length of the horse. *J. Anim. Sci.*, **10**, 789.
Irvine, C.H.G. (1979) Kinetics of gonadotrophins in the mare. *J. Reprod. Fert.*, Suppl. **27**, 131.
Jeffcott, L.B., Atherton, J.G. & Mingay, J. (1969) Equine pregnancy diagnosis. A comparison of two methods for the detection of gonadotrophin in serum. *Vet. Rec.*, **84**, 80.
Jeffcott, L.B. & Whitwell, K.E. (1973) Twinning as a cause of fetal and neonatal loss in the Thoroughbred mare. *J. comp. Path.*, **83**, 91.
Jennings, W.E. (1941) Equine abortion and diseases of foals. *Vet. Med.*, **36**, 452.
Jennings, W.E. (1950) Twelve years of horse breeding in the army. *J. Am. vet. med. Ass.*, **116**, 11.
Kenney, R.M. (1978) Cyclic and pathologic changes of the mare endometrium as detected by biopsy, with a note on early embryonic death. *J. Am. vet. med. Ass.*, **172**, 241.
Kenneth, J.H. & Ritchie, G.R. (1953) *Gestation Periods,* 3rd ed. Slough: Commonwealth Agricultural Bureaux.
King, J.M. (1967) The origin and development of the hippomanes in the horse and zebra. I. The location, morphology and histology of the hippomanes. *J. Anat.*, **101**, 277.
Larks, S.D. (1961) *Foetal Electrocardiography.* Springfield, Ill.: Charles C. Thomas.
Liggins, G.C. (1979) Initiation of parturition. *Br. med. Bull.*, **35**, 145.
Lunaas, T. (1962) A rapid method for the quantitative estimation of urinary oestrogens in the pregnant mare. *Acta chem. scand.*, **16**, 2064.
McCollum, W.H., Doll, E.R., Wilson, J.C. & Johnson, C.B. (1962) Isolation and propagation of equine rhinopneumonitis virus in primary monoler kidney cultures of domestic animals. *Cornell Vet.*, **52**, 164.
Mahaffey, L.W. (1968) Abortion in mares. *Vet. Rec.*, **82**, 681.
Mahaffey, L.W. & Adam, N.M. (1964) Abortions associated with mycotic lesions of the placenta in mares. *J. Am. vet. med. Ass.*, **144**, 24.
Mahaffey, L.W. & Rossdale, P.D. (1965) An abortion due to *Allescheria boydii* and general observations concerning mycotic abortions of mares. *Vet. Rec.*, **77**, 541.
Matassino, D. (1962) A study of the vital statistics of Hafling mares in Southern Italy. I. Services, conception, non-pregnancies, abortions, parturitions and average age at different parturitions. *Annali Fac. Sci. Agric. Univ. Napoli,* **28**, 249 (*Anim. Breed. Abstr.*, **31**, 1788).
Mayer, D.T. (1944) A comparative study of two biologic and two chemical techniques of pregnancy diagnosis in the mare. *Am. J. vet. Res.*, **5**, 209.
Mayr, A., Bohm, H.O., Brill, J. & Wayciechowska, S. (1965) Charakteristung einer Staten-abortvirus aus Polen und Vergleichung mit bekannten Rhinopneumonitis Virusstannen der Pferdes. *Arch. ges. Virusforsch.*, **17**, 216.
Merkt, H. (1966) Foal heat and embryonic resorption. *Zuchthygiene,* **1**, 102 (*Anim. Breed. Abstr.*, **35**, 1035).
Miller, W.C. (1934) Biological methods of diagnosing equine pregnancy. I. The mouse test. *Proc. R. Soc. Lond.*, **116**, 237.
Mitchell, D. (1971) Early fetal death and a serum gonadotrophin test for pregnancy in the mare. *Can. vet. J.*, **12**, 41.
Mitchell, D. & Allen, W.R. (1975) Observations on reproductive performance in the yearling mare. *J. Reprod. Fert.*, Suppl. **23**, 531.
Moor, R.M., Allen, W.R. & Hamilton, D.W. (1975) Origin and histogenesis of equine endometrial cups. *J. Reprod. Fert.*, Suppl. **23**, 391.
Moore, B.O. & Koonse, H.J. (1978) Inactivated equine herpesvirus I vaccine – Pneumabort K. *Proc. 24th ann. Conv. Am. Ass. equine Practnrs,* 75.
Moss, G.E., Estergreen, V.L., Becker, S.R. & Grant, B.D. (1979) The source of the 5α-pregnanes that occur during gestation in mares. *J. Reprod. Fert.*, Suppl. **27**, 511.
Nelsen, O.E. (1953) *Comparative Embryology of the Vertebrates.* New York: Blakiston.
Nett, T.M., Holtan, D.W. & Estergreen, V.L. (1973) Plasma estrogens in pregnant mares. *J. Anim. Sci.*, **37**, 962.
Nett, T.M., Holtan, D.W. & Estergreen, V.L. (1975) Oestrogens, LH, PMSG and prolactin in serum of pregnant mares. *J. Reprod. Fert.*, Suppl. **23**, 457.
Nett, T.M. & Pickett, B.W. (1979) Effect of diethylstilboestrol on the relationship between LH, PMSG and progesterone during pregnancy in the mare. *J. Reprod. Fert.*, Suppl. **27**, 465.
Nishikawa, Y. (1959) *Studies on Reproduction in Horses.* Tokyo: Japan Racing Association.

Onuma, H. & Ohnami, Y. (1975) Retention of tubal eggs in mares. *J. Reprod. Fert.*, Suppl. **23**, 507.

Osborne, V.E. (1975) Factors influencing foaling percentages in Australian mares. *J. Reprod. Fert.*, Suppl. **23**, 477.

Pashen, R.L. & Allen, W.R. (1979*a*) Endocrine changes after foetal gonadectomy and during normal and induced parturition in the mare. *Anim. Reprod. Sci.*, **2**, 271.

Pashen, R.L. & Allen, W.R. (1979*b*) The role of the fetal gonads and placenta in steroid production, maintenance of pregnancy and parturition in the mare. *J. Reprod. Fert.*, Suppl. **27**, 499.

Pauli, B. & Alroy, J. (1972) Lesions in the coronary arteries of equine fetuses and unweaned foals a few days old. *Schweiz. Arch. Tierheilk.*, **114**, 83.

Peaker, M., Rossdale, P.D., Forsyth, I.A. & Falk, M. (1979) Changes in mammary development and the composition of secretion during late pregnancy in the mare. *J. Reprod. Fert.*, Suppl. **27**, 555.

Petzoldt, K., Luttmann, U., Pohlenz, J. & Teichert, U. (1972) Virological studies on the central nervous system of equine fetuses and the lesions in mares with central nervous symptoms after abortion caused by equine herpesvirus I. *Schweiz. Arch. Tierheilk.*, **114**, 129.

Plummer, G., Bowling, C.P. & Goodheart, C.R. (1969) Comparison of 4 horse herpesviruses. *J. Virol.*, **4**, 738.

Raeside, J.I., Liptrap, R.M., McDonnell, W.N. & Milne, F.J. (1979) A precursor role for DHA in a feto-placental unit for oestrogen formation in the mare. *J. Reprod. Fert.*, Suppl. **27**, 493.

Randall, C.C. Ryden, S.W., Doll, E.R. & Schenell, F.S. (1953) Cultivation of equine abortion virus in fetal horse tissue in vitro. *Am. J. Path.*, **29**, 139.

Ricketts, S.W. (1978) Histological and histopathological studies of the endometrium of the mare. Fellowship thesis, Royal College of Veterinary Surgeons.

Roberts, S.J. (1971) *Veterinary Obstetrics and Genital Disease.* Ann Arbor, Mich.: Edwards.

Ropiha, R.T., Matthews, R.G., Butterfield, R.M., Moss, F.P. & McFadden, W.J. (1969) The duration of pregnancy in Thoroughbred mares. *Vet. Rec.*, **84**, 552.

Rossdale, P.D. (1966) A Clinical and Laboratory Assessment of the Health Status of the Newborn Thoroughbred Foal. Fellowship Thesis, Royal College of Veterinary Surgeons.

Rossdale, P.D. (1967) Clinical studies on the newborn Thoroughbred foal, I. Perinatal behaviour. *Br. vet. J.*, **123**, 470.

Rossdale, P.D. (1968) pH and pCO_2 of equine amniotic fluid at the time of birth. *Biol. Neonat.*, **12**, 378.

Schauder, W. (1912) Untersuchungen uber die Eihaute und Embryotrophe des Pferde. *Arch. Anat. Physiol.*, **259**, 259.

Shaw, F.D. & Morton, H. (1980) The immunological approach to pregnancy diagnosis: a review. *Vet. Rec.*, **106**, 268.

Short, R.V. (1959) Progesterone in blood, IV. Progesterone in the blood of mares. *J. Endocr.*, **19**, 207.

Short, R.V. (1969) Implantation and maternal recognition of pregnancy. In *Ciba Foundation Symposium on Foetal Autonomy*, ed. G.E.W. Wolstenholme & Maeve O'Connor, pp. 2–31. London: Churchill.

Silver, M., Barnes, R.J., Comline, R.S., Fowden, A.L., Clover, L. & Mitchell, M.D. (1979) Prostaglandins in maternal and fetal plasma and in allantoic fluid during the second half of gestation in the mare. *J. Reprod. Fert.*, Suppl. **27**, 531.

Silver, M. & Comline, R.S. (1972) Some observations on the umbilical circulation of the foal compared with the ruminant. In *Placental Gas Exchange*, ed. L.D. Longo & H. Bartells, p. 113. WIHB-316. Washington, DC: DHEW.

Silver, M., Steven, D.H. & Comline, R.S. (1973) Placental exchange and morphology in ruminants and mares. In *Foetal and Neonatal Physiology*, ed. R.S. Comline, K.W. Cross, G.S. Dawes & P.W. Nathanielsz, p. 245. Cambridge: Cambridge University Press.

Solomon, W.J. (1971) Rectal examination of the cervix and its significance in early pregnancy evaluation of the mare. *Proc. 17th ann. Conv. Am. Ass. equine Practnrs*, 73.

Spincemaille, J., Bouters, R., Vandeplassche, M. & Bonte, P. (1975) Some aspects of endometrial cup formation and PMSG production. *J. Reprod. Fert.*, Suppl. **23**, 415.

Squires, E.L. & Ginther, O.J. (1975) Follicular and luteal development in pregnant mares. *J. Reprod. Fert.*, Suppl. **23**, 429.

Steven, D.H. (1968) Structural differences between exchange units in the sheep and horse placenta. *J. Physiol., Lond.*, **196**, 24.

Steven, D.H. & Samuel, C.A. (1975) Anatomy of the placental barrier in the mare. *J. Reprod. Fert.*, Suppl. **23**, 579.

Terqui, M. & Palmer, E. (1979) Oestrogen pattern during early pregnancy in the mare. *J. Reprod. Fert.*, Suppl. **27**, 441.

Trapp, A.L., Roberts, A.W. & Carter, G.R. (1972) Comparison of methods for diagnosing equine rhinopneumonitis virus abortion. *Vet. Med.*, **67**, 895.

Tsutsumi, Y. (1962) The vascular pattern of the placenta in farm animals. *J. Fac. Agric. Hokkaido (imp.) Univ.*, **52**, 372.

Uppenborn, W. (1933) Untersuchungen uber die Trachtigkeitsdauer der Suten mit einem Anhang: Untersuchungen uber Zwillingsbeburten beim Pferd. *Z. Zuchthyg., B,* **28**, 1.

Van Niekerk, C.H. (1965*a*) I. Early clinical diagnosis of pregnancy in mares. *J.S. Afr. vet. med. Ass.*, **36**, 53.

Van Niekerk, C.H. (1965*b*) II. Early embryonic resorption in mares. A preliminary report. *J.S. Afr. vet. med. Ass.*, **36**, 61.

Van Niekerk, C.H. & Allen, W.E. (1975) Early embryonic development in the horse. *J. Reprod. Fert.*, Suppl. **23**, 495.

Van Niekerk, C.H. & Gerneke, W.H. (1966) Persistence and pathogenetic cleavage of tubal ova in the mare. *Onderstepoort J. vet. Res.*, **31**, 195.

Vernon, M.W., Strauss, S., Simonelli, M., Zavy, M.T. & Sharp, D.C. (1979) Specific $PGF_2\alpha$ binding by the corpus luteum of the pregnant and non-pregnant mare. *J. Reprod. Fert.*, Suppl. **27**, 421.

Voss, J.L. & Pickett, B.W. (1975) The effect of rectal palpation on the fertility of cyclic mares. *J. Reprod. Fert.*, Suppl. **23**, 285.

Walker, D. (1977) Laboratory methods of equine pregnancy diagnosis. *Vet. Rec.*, **100**, 396.

Walt, M.L., Stabenfeldt, G.H., Hughes, J.P., Neely, D.P. & Bradbury, R. (1979) Development of the equine ovary and ovulation forssa. *J. Reprod. Fert.*, Suppl. **27**, 471.

Whitwell, K.E. (1975) Morphology and pathology of the equine umbilical cord. *J. Reprod. Fert.*, Suppl. **23**, 599.

Whitwell, K.E. & Jeffcott, L.B. (1975) Morphological studies on the foetal membranes of the normal singleton foal at term. *Res. vet. Sci.*, **19**, 44.

Wide, L. & Gemzell, C.A. (1960) An immunological pregnancy test. *Acta endocr.*, **35**, 261.

Wide, M. & Wide, L. (1963) Diagnosis of pregnancy in mares by an immunological method. *Nature, Lond.*, **198**, 1017

Birth 4

Birth is the process of expelling the fetus and its membranes from the uterus. It marks the end of gestation and the beginning of independent existence. In the horse it is an event of remarkable rapidity, lasting on average about 45 minutes. For descriptive purposes it is convenient to divide birth into three stages: the first leading up to rupture of the chorio-allantoic membrane, the second delivery of the foal through the birth canal and the third when the after-birth is expelled from the uterus.

Most studies of equine birth have been made on mares confined to yards or loose boxes and under supervision (Fleming 1878; Wright 1943; Rossdale 1967; Jeffcott 1972). Studies of feral breeds (Tyler 1972) suggest that parturient mares often move away from the herd and seek a sheltered area, but that the birth does not differ much in varying circumstances.

Birth concerns two individuals and although we have chosen to describe the event as it affects each in turn, the distinction is academic in physiological terms. For example, birth is initiated by a complex interaction of maternal and fetal function; maternal behaviour appears to be altered by the disposition of the fetus; dystocia may be caused by maternal or fetal factors and affect the mare or foal.

Birth presents peculiar problems to the clinician and those responsible for managing the event. In the majority of cases it is normal, but because of its rapidity and the fetus's delicate physiological balance during passage through the birth canal, accurate diagnosis of abnormality is essential. Any corrective measure must be applied immediately if it is to succeed. Our description is aimed therefore at a better understanding of the process from the practical viewpoint.

INITIATION AND ENDOCRINOLOGY OF BIRTH

Clinical and experimental investigations throw light upon, but do not explain, the timing of metabolic interactions leading to the onset of parturition in mammals. Nor is it possible, except in general terms, to relate information obtained from one species to another. That the fetus determines the length of gestation in the horse has been discussed in the previous chapter, but maternal influence is indicated by the majority of equine births being in the period of least daylight (Zwolinski & Siudinski 1965; Rossdale & Short 1967) (Fig. 4.1). The mare's ability to control the time of birth is mediated, presumably, through her pituitary gland.

The genetic influence is indicated by the gestational length of hybrid pregnancies in reciprocal inter-species matings. The horse has an average gestation of 340 days, the donkey 380 days. In cross-matings the gestational length tends to follow the normal gestation of the paternal species. For example, mule foals (donkey stallion

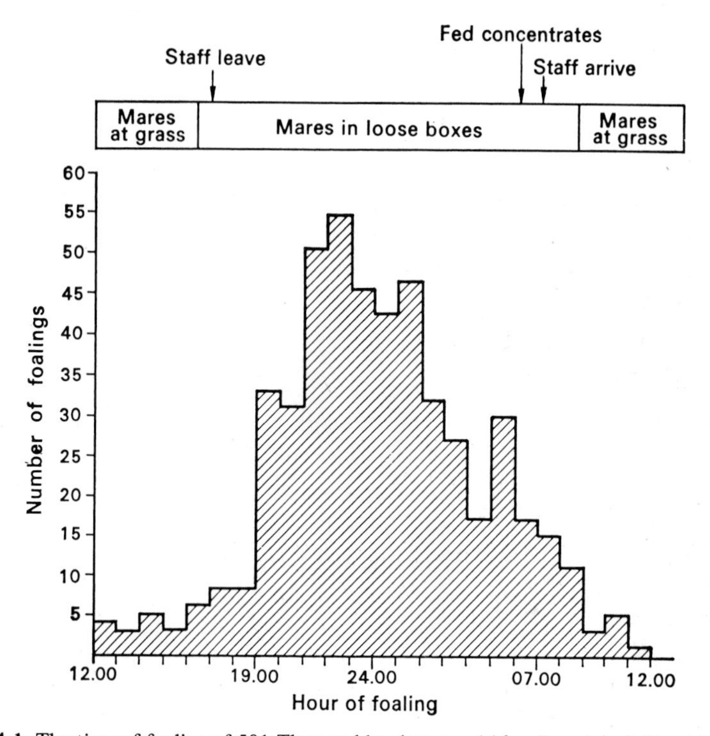

Fig. 4.1. The time of foaling of 501 Thoroughbred mares. (*After Rossdale & Short 1967*).

cross mare) may be carried up to 380 days, whereas hinny foals (horse stallion cross donkey) tend to have a gestational length of 340 days (Asdell 1946; Howell & Rollins 1951).

The basis of birth is myometrial activity. This is inhibited by progesterone and increased by oestrogens, prostaglandins and oxytocin. A uterine contraction requires the more-or-less simultaneous activity of all smooth muscle cells in the uterus. To understand the mechanism involved we must examine not only how a single smooth muscle cell is activated but also how the activity is spread from one group of cells to another. The reader is referred to Liggins (1979) for a review of the physiology of excitation and propagation of uterine muscle activity and various pathways by which the uterus is affected by hormonal and biochemical influences. He concludes that the conceptus probably dominates the mechanisms stimulating the onset of parturition in most mammalian species. In some, control is mediated by fetal adrenal glands; in others, extrafetal tissues, perhaps the chorion, seem more important. In human pregnancy, the fetal adrenal makes a minor contribution to the timing mechanism and parturition is probably initiated by the release of prostaglandin F_2 from the uterine epithelium. In general, synthesis and release of PGF_2 is stimulated by an increase in the oestrogen/progesterone ratio. In humans and some other species in which the ratio is unaltered in the circulation it is necessary to postulate changes at a cellular level.

In sheep, parturition is initiated by a system involving the fetal pituitary and adrenal glands (Liggins 1969; Thorburn et al. 1977). A complex hormonal interaction occurs; an increase in fetal corticosteroids induces placental enzyme systems which permit the conversion of progesterone to oestrogen. This changed metabolism of progesterone is in part responsible for the surge in oestrogens and drop in progesterone seen in the 48 hours prior to birth in this species (Flint et al. 1979). These hormonal changes are then responsible for increased uterine prostaglandin production, a change needed to alter the uterus from 'inert' to reactive in which forceful contractions will bring about birth of the fetus. Similar mechanisms exist to initiate parturition in the goat, cow and pig. In all these species parturition is preceeded by a fall in maternal progesterone levels, which is triggered by a rise in the level of cortisol in the fetal circulation.

Comparatively less is known about the initiation of parturition in equidae and whether the mechanisms controlling foaling are similar to those of birth in the sheep or goat, with the fetal stimuli dominating timing, or are more similar to the human, where a built-in, genetically controlled, maturation signal starts in the fetal membranes (Liggins et al. 1977). Investigations have been frustrated by problems in techniques which have been found useful in other species. Fetal surgery and the insertion of catheters into fetal preparations in the mare, which have been used to identify the changing hormonal patterns associated with parturition in other species, have failed to a large extent when applied to the mare (Comline et al. 1975).

It has been suggested (Pashen & Allen 1979*a*) that interactions between placental and fetal size and uterine capacity influence gestation length in the mare, although this does not appear to be the case in other species (Davies & Ryan 1972). However, although non-hormonal factors may influence gestation length in the horse, the endocrine pathways must be the final arbiter of when foaling occurs. Present-day knowledge of the hormonal profile of pregnancy and parturition has been reviewed by Pashen and Allen (1979*a*).

Maternal unconjugated oestrogens decrease from peak plasma levels (700 pg/ml oestrone and 200 pg/ml oestradiol-17β) to basal levels at birth of 150 pg/ml and 40 pg/ml respectively (Fig. 3.2) (Nett et al. 1973; Barnes et al. 1975). The oestrogens are composed of the phenolic oestrogens, oestrone and oestradiol-17β, and the ring-B unsaturated oestrogens, equilin and equilenin (Gaudrey & Glen 1959; Pashen & Allen 1979*a*). As the source of these oestrogens is the fetoplacental unit (Pashen & Allen 1979*b*) levels reach base-line values within a few hours after birth of the foal and expulsion of the placenta. For further discussion of the endocrine patterns of gestation see pp. 184–8.

Plasma progestagen levels (Fig. 4.2) rise to peak levels about ten days pre-partum and remain high (10–15 ng/ml) until second-stage delivery has started (Barnes et al. 1975). This rise in levels prior to term is mainly due to an increase in 5α-pregnane metabolites rather than progesterone itself (Atkins et al. 1974; Holtan et al. 1975; Lovell et al. 1975). Recent work (Moss et al. 1979) suggests that the metabolites represent an alteration in placental, endometrial and fetal metabolism of steroids during the final stages of pregnancy. A similar change in progesterone metabolism occurs in the peripartum rhesus monkey (Scholl et al. 1979). It is suggested that as these 5α-pregnanes occupy progesterone bonding sites, their increase at the expense of progesterone would cause an effective progesterone withdrawal from the myometrium.

The stable prostaglandin F metabolite 13,14 dihydro-15-oxoprostaglandin $F_2\alpha$ (PGFM) shows a dramatic rise in the peripheral plasma of the mare at term (Barnes et al. 1978) (Fig. 4.3). This rise occurs during second-stage labour and it appears in oxytocin- and fluprostenol-induced foalings at full term. PGFM was also found to rise in fetal plasma during the last two hours before delivery in chronic catheterized preparations (Barnes et al. 1978).

Silver et al. (1979) measured the concentrations of primary prostaglandins $PFG_2\alpha$ and PGE_2 and the metabolite PGFM in maternal and fetal plasma and in allantoic fluid in chronically catheterized mares and fetuses. A gradual rise in all three PGs occurred with increasing gestational age. PGE_2 and $PGF_2\alpha$ levels were highest in the allantoic fluid and lowest in the maternal plasma, whereas PGFM concentrations were greatest in maternal plasma. Significant venous–arterial plasma differences in PGFM concentration were detected across the uterine circulation between 180 and 280 days of gestation, suggesting that uterine tissues are the main site of PGF metabolism at this time. Increases in PGE_2 and $PGF_2\alpha$ in the fetal fluids preceded premature delivery of the foal, while PG changes in maternal plasma were minimal before delivery. Pashen and Allen (1979*a*) reported higher levels of $PGF_2\alpha$ and PGE_2 than of PGFM in amniotic fluid in a limited series of observations. The increase in PGE levels in the fetal circulation is probably important in fetal vascular mechanics, especially in the maintenance of a patent ductus arteriosus (Coceani et al. 1976) during late pregnancy.

A close link is known to exist between the actions of oxytocin and of prostaglandin $F_2\alpha$. The fact that oxytocin levels remain constant throughout late pregnancy, and only rise during second-stage labour (Allen et al. 1973) when prostaglandin levels are also rising (Barnes et al. 1978; Pashen & Allen 1980). supports this argument. It is therefore likely that the major hormonal stimuli to the strong uterine contractions of second stage labour are oxytocin and prostaglandin $F_2\alpha$.

Maternal plasma cortisol levels remain relatively constant throughout gestation. The only significant rise occurs during foaling, presumably reflecting the stress of

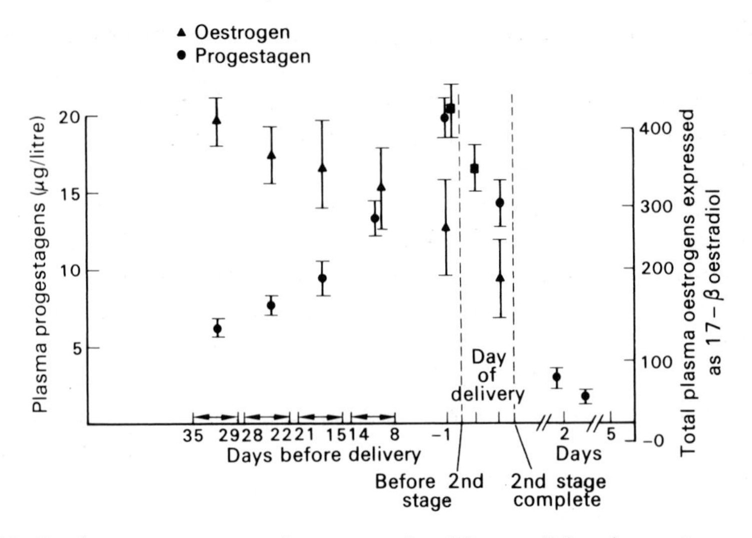

Fig. 4.2. Total oestrogen concentration, expressed as 17β-oestradiol, and progestagen concentration in peripheral plasma of seven pregnant mares (mean ± SE). Progestagen concentrations in four of the mares on the day before labour and the day of foaling (before the second stage) are also shown (mean ± SE). Samples taken on the day of foaling were divided into those before the second stage and those taken within 15 minutes of delivery. (*After Barnes et al. 1975*)

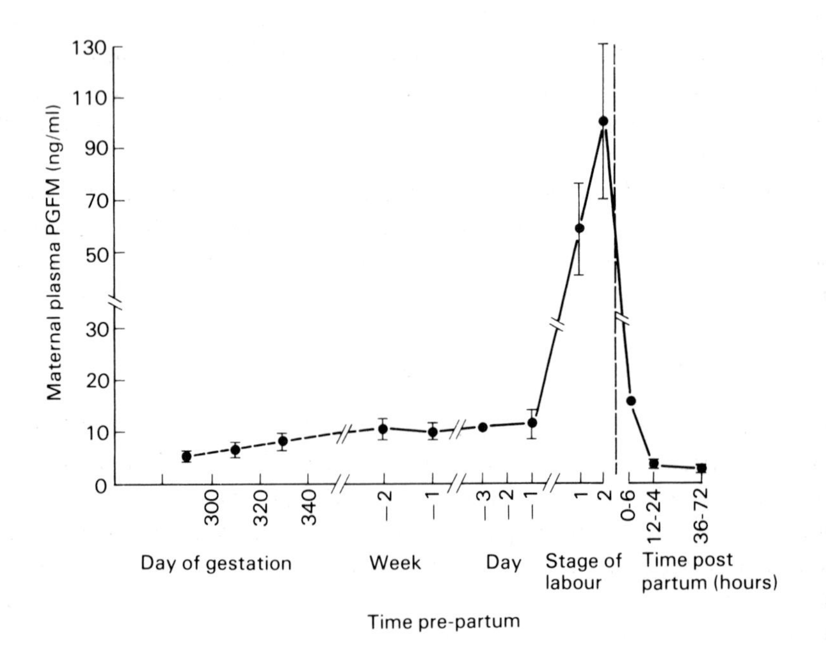

Fig. 4.3. The concentrations of 13-14-dihydro-15-oxo-prostaglandin F (PGFM) (means ± SE) in the plasma of four Thoroughbred mares before, during and after the delivery of live healthy foals. Arrow and vertical broken line indicate time of delivery. (*After Barnes et al. 1978*)

labour. The pronounced rise in fetal plasma cortisol levels which occurs in other species has not been noted in the horse (Rossdale et al. 1973; Nathanielsz et al. 1975). Failure to detect such a rise may be due to inability to obtain fetal blood samples from stable chronically catheterized fetal preparations over the last days of gestation. A less pronounced rise has, however, been noted in amniotic fluid cortisol levels (from 3 ng/ml at 200–250 days to 13 ng/ml at parturition) during this period (Pashen & Allen 1979*a*). The source of this cortisol is likely to be the fetus or the fetal membranes, as it appears there is little transplacental transfer of cortisol in the mare (Nathanielsz et al. 1975). The increase seems to be gradual and therefore unlike the surge of cortisol which acts as a trigger to parturition in the sheep and goat (Flint et al. 1979). Cortisol is known to be important in the activation and maturation of organ enzyme systems (Liggins et al. 1979). The rise in amniotic fluid levels and the marked rise in the foal following delivery could be related to such phenomena. The main organs of adaption for extrauterine life are those of the respiratory and alimentary tracts.

In summary, the initial stimulus to parturition in the mare remains unknown. There is no evidence concerning the factors influencing cervical dilatation and changes in cervical collagen at the time of foaling. In the ewe, high levels of PGE have been reported as occurring in the cervical vein compared to those found in the cervical artery during parturition (Ellwood et al. 1979). Changes in maternal and fetal hormone levels probably play a major role but the relatively high levels of progestagens and low levels of oestrogens are in contrast to the findings in other species such as sheep and cattle. Technical problems of chronic catheterization in mares have, so far, restricted the amount of information available on fetal hormonal changes, but what evidence exists does suggest that equine birth is initiated on the fetal, rather than on the maternal, side of the placenta.

From a practical viewpoint a knowledge of the endocrinology of foaling is relevant only in so far as it may be used to diagnose abnormal birth, throw light on prematurity or, most importantly, provide a safe and effective means of inducing foaling.

INDUCTION

Experiences of induced foaling extend over many years (Britton 1963). The use of oxytocin alone or in combination with oestrogen has been reported by Britten (1972), Purvis (1972), Klug and von Lepel (1974), Hillman (1975) and Rossdale and Jeffcott (1975). More recently fluprostenol, a synthetic prostaglandin analogue (Rossdale et al. 1976) and a natural prostaglandin $F_2\alpha$ in combination with flumethasone and oestrogen (Van Niekerk & Morgenthal 1976) have been successfully used to induce foaling at full term.

The administration of corticosteroids, which is successful at inducing birth in ruminants (Drost & Holm 1968; Adams & Wagner 1970), does not appear to be as successful when administered to mares. The reason for this is apparent when the difference between the endocrinology of parturition in the horse and that of ruminants is taken into account (see p. 192). In ruminants, increased corticosteroid levels alter placental enzyme systems and thus steroid and prostaglandin biosynthesis. These changes do not appear to occur in equidae.

Methods for inducing foaling have been reviewed by Jeffcott and Rossdale (1977). More recently endocrine changes occurring in the mare have been studied by Barnes et al. (1978) and Hillman and Ganjam (1979) using oxytocin and by Rossdale et al. (1979) using fluprostenol.

Indications for induced foaling

The indications for induced foaling may be managerial, clinical or for the purposes of teaching and research.

There are economic advantages in causing mares to foal at specified hours during daylight or early evening and in this way the cost of having attendants watch mares all night (sitting up) may be reduced or entirely eliminated. Planned birth may also help to reduce the risks associated with foaling in circumstances where management has reduced resources of man-power and experience as, for example, where an owner has only one or two mares. In these circumstances it is often not possible to arrange a system of 'sitting up' and veterinarians or schooled personnel may not be easily available for urgent assistance. Similar economic considerations apply at the end of a breeding season, even on large stud farms. The breeding season now extends, in the UK, to 15 July, but only a small number of mares are likely to foal in June. The stud farm management may often find itself facing the prospect of having attendants 'sit up' nightly for several nights just for one or two mares at the tail-end of the season. It may be highly beneficial to employ induced foaling in these circumstances.

Suggested indications for induction have included uterine atony, prolonged gestation, loss of colostrum, preparturient colic, pelvic or other injury of the mare, ventral rupture and arthritic or other painful skeletal disease which may become more severe as pregnancy nears full term. The objective of elective induction is to alleviate the maternal condition and allow delivery to occur when veterinary assistance is immediately available.

An induced foaling enables veterinary and agricultural students to observe and assist at foalings with a minimum of explanatory time and teaching resources. These occasions may supplement teaching of or be used concurrently in research on such aspects as the efficacy of various inducing agents, parturient and neonatal physiology and maternal/fetal risks at parturition.

Safety

We feel that no method can give complete safety in our present state of knowledge. To put this in another perspective, there is no evidence to suggest that induced foaling can be more natural and therefore more normal than natural delivery. The risks are largely to the fetus rather than to the mare herself, although either may be damaged depending on the degree to which the event differs from normal parturition. The mare is at risk from over-forceful efforts, possibly related to the nature or dose rate of the inducing drug. Contraction of the uterus and complications in the delivery may also injure the fetus physically as it passes it through the birth canal and also because of premature and abnormal placental separation before delivery is complete. Perhaps the biggest risk to the fetus, however, is that it will be expelled from the uterine environment before it is sufficiently mature to survive the extra-uterine environment.

The assessment of fetal maturity is essential before induction is contemplated for clinical or managerial purposes. 'Full term' implies a gestational length sufficient for the fetus to have achieved the maturity necessary for successful adaptation. The criteria by which fetal maturity can be assessed are somewhat limited in our present state of knowledge. The clinician, before deciding to induce foaling, should consider the length of gestation, the state of mammary development and secretion, cervical relaxation, fetal position, posture and heart rate and maternal endocrinology.

Mammary development

Although the actual size of the udder may be affected by variables such as parity, breed and nutritional status, a substantial increase in size should occur before foaling is induced. A scale based on subjective observations ranging from 0 to +++ is suggested (Table 4.1). The presence of oedema of the udder and ventral body wall are additional indications of full term. However, the most important indication is the presence of colostrum in the mammae. Typically, mammary secretions pass from straw or amber colour to cloudy straw in the weeks preceding parturition

TABLE 4.1 Assessment of changes in mammary size during late pregnancy

Time before parturition (days)	*Arbitrary scale*					*Median value*
	+	+/++	++	++/+++	+++	
8	1 (8)	4 (33)	6 (50)	1 (8)	0 (0)	++
7	2 (18)	2 (18)	6 (55)	1 (9)	0 (0)	++
6	3 (21)	3 (21)	6 (43)	2 (14)	0 (0)	++
5	1 (11)	0 (0)	5 (56)	3 (33)	0 (0)	++
4	1 (8)	1 (8)	7 (54)	3 (23)	1 (8)	++
3	1 (5)	1 (5)	9 (47)	6 (32)	2 (10)	++
2	0 (0)	1 (5)	9 (45)	5 (25)	5 (25)	++/+++
1	0 (0)	0 (0)	3 (13)	6 (26)	14 (61)	+++
0	0 (0)	0 (0)	2 (10)	1 (5)	18 (85)	+++

After Peaker et al. (1979).

Values shown are the number of mares, with the percentage of the total number examined on that day in parentheses.

Mammary glands were examined visually and by palpation and judged as +, ++ or +++ on an arbitrary scale ascending in magnitude; in cases of uncertainty, two intermediate categories were used.

and then to yellow or yellowish white and viscous, close to the natural termination of pregnancy. In most mares, a bead of colostrum dries at the teat end as wax one to four days before foaling. Some individuals, however, may run milk and lose variable quantities of milk-like secretion. In general, induction should not be practiced unless a readily available supply of colostrum or milk-like secretion is present in the mammae.

Preparturient mammary secretions have been studied by Forsyth et al. (1975) and Peaker et al. (1979). The main changes observed were:

1. The presence of milky-white secretion, the incidence of which increased from 9% on Day 4 to 77% on the day of foaling. This suggests that true milk secretion starts during the last few days of pregnancy in most mares.

2. Of any of the constituents measured prior to foaling in normal mares at full term total calcium concentration showed the most consistent increase close to foaling. An arbitrary limit of 10 mmol/litre appears to provide a simple test that foaling is imminent.

3. In the study by Peaker et al. (1979), performed in the last three weeks of pregnancy, the concentrations of sodium (118–24 mmol/litre) and chloride (91–33 mmol/litre) decreased, while those of potassium (13–36 mmol/litre), lactose (26–107 mmol/litre), citrate (0.58–3.68 g/litre), dialysable inorganic phosphate (P_{id}) (0.007–0.12 g/litre), total magnesium (3–13 mmol/litre) and total protein (20–170 g/litre) increased, 'but not in a fashion that absolute or changing values could be used to predict the imminence of parturition in any particular individual'.

It must be emphasized that the values quoted may provide a useful guide to the imminence of parturition but do not necessarily relate to the maturity of the fetus. It is reasonable to suppose that if changes have occurred in the composition of the secretions to levels quoted, especially where calcium has risen above 10 mmol/litre, the fetus will be relatively mature; the converse cannot be claimed in cases where the parameters are significantly different from those quoted because it is possible that the fetus may reach sufficient maturity for survival at some time before actual parturition occurs.

Relaxation of the cervix and pelvic ligaments

The cervix has been described as becoming softer and relaxed shortly before full term. Hillman (1975) advocates that a two-finger-sized dilatation should be present before foaling is induced. In our limited experience of natural birth we have found that the cervix may be widely dilated before the fetus moves into the birth canal. However, we have successfully induced several mares in which the cervix remained firmly closed and covered in tacky mucus until the end of first-stage labour.

In the mare the relaxation of the pelvic ligaments (i.e. sacroiliac and sacrosciatic) is a much less obvious sign of impending parturition than it is in the cow. There is a degree of hollowing and softening of the quarters in some mares and this may be accompanied by relaxation and lengthening of the vulva.

In conclusion, the decision to induce must be taken in the absence of any absolute knowledge of fetal maturity. The three criteria considered to be essential for full-term induction are a gestational length greater than 320 days, substantial mammary development and the presence of colostrum in the mammae with wax on the teats. Daily examinations are recommended because a changing situation is considered more significant than one that is static.

Methods

The clinician must make a subjective decision on the method of induction in the absence of definitive studies. The techniques in current use are summarized in Table 4.2. This information is intended to provide a guide for any practitioner

TABLE 4.2 Summary of current methods for the induction of parturition in mares

Induction agent	*Method of administration*		*Reference*
	Dose	*Route*	
Oxytocin	0.04–0.26 IU kg	i.m. or i.v.	Britton (1972); Purvis (1972); Klug and von Lepel (1974); Hillman (1975); Rossdale and Jeffcott (1975)
Oxytocin + stilboestrol	0.04–0.26 IU kg + 12–30 mg	i.m.	Britton (1972); Purvis (1972); Hillman (1975)
Dexamethasone	100 mg for 3–4 days	i.m.	Rossdale and Jeffcott (1975)
Prostaglandin (fluprostenol)	250–1000 μg	i.m.	Rossdale et al. (1976, 1979)
Prostaglandin $F_2\alpha$ + stilboestrol + flumethasone	10 mg + 10 mg + 7.5 mg 30 mg 10 mg	i.m.	Van Niekerk and Morganthal (1976)

After Jeffcott and Rossdale (1977).

who wishes to induce foaling but is not familiar with the methods available. In our experience, 250 μg of fluprostenol, administered intramuscularly, is sufficient to cause parturition within two hours in a mare that it at full term. If the mare is not at full term, fluprostenol appears to have little, if any, action although if a second or third dose is administered it may be possible to induce foaling after several hours. The results of inducing foaling using intramuscular fluprostenol in 17 mares are shown in Table 4.3 (Rossdale et al. 1979). Problems were encountered in foaling and in the foal following birth. It should be pointed out that this study was for experimental purposes and the mares were induced so that the fetus could be catheterized during delivery. It was not a clinical study and therefore the results

TABLE 4.3 Results of induction using intramuscular fluprostenol in 20 mares

No.	*Age* (years) *and type**		*Gestation length* (days)	*Dose rate* (μg)	*Delivery time* (min)	*Time for foal to stand* (min)	*Placenta expelled* (min)	*Remarks*
1	4	Pony	332	250	95	84	48	Foal normal after birth
2	7	Pony	325	250	105	55	50	Foal normal after birth
3	14	Pony	322	250	42	27	51	Foal normal after birth
4	24	TB	341	500	56	52	27	Foal normal after birth
5	3	Pony	334	350	100	27	37	Foal normal after birth
6	7	Pony	318	250	163	22	8	Foal normal after birth
7	6	TB	339	500	92	140	29	Foal weak initially: ? fractured ribs; at one month developed joint-ill
8	4	Pony	325	500	72†	40	55	Foal normal
9	10	TB	367	500	63†	112	27	Foal weak initially but improved by 24 hours
10	4	TB	328	1000	205†	–	25	Difficult delivery and foal suffered fractured ribs; foal very weak and destroyed at 48 hours
11	7	Pony	330	250	110	–	–	Foal weak initially but gradually improved over the first week of life
12	5	Pony	334	250	140†	–	–	Foal died during labour, elective caesarean: cervix failed to dilate, mare not ready for induction
13	4	Pony	342	250	133	33	7	Foal normal. Rapid expulsion of placenta

*TB = Thoroughbred.
† From last injection of fluprostenol.

are not necessarily those which one would expect to obtain in practice if full-term mares were carefully selected for the purpose of induced foalings.

It is our opinion that foaling induced by fluprostenol is more physiological than by any other method, but this applies only to cases that are at full term. If the mare is not at full term there is little doubt that oxytocin is the agent of choice. In most cases reported from the field 60–120 IU have been used intramuscularly or intravenously. Pashen (1980) claims that these high rates are unnecessary to commence the chain of hormonal changes resulting in birth. He has shown that 5 IU of oxytocin intravenously can cause parturition in some instances. However, it should be emphasized that, whatever agent is used and at whatever dosage, it is probably the individual's endocrinological status at the time which determines whether or not foaling takes place, how long it will take and how physiological it will be. There have been far too few critical studies for any dogmatic assertions to be made as to the safety of induction by any methods or for clinicans to be completely confident of the results. This is not to suggest that induction cannot be used safely and effectively, but rather that it must be employed with caution.

Corticosteroids have been used to induce birth but the experiences with low dosage rates (10–40 mg daily) (Campbell 1971; Drost 1972) showed them to be insufficient whereas 100 mg daily could induce premature parturition (Alm et al. 1974) but with serious complications and dystocia in some cases (Rossdale & Jeffcott 1975). From the physiological evidence available to date it would appear that corticosteroids do not directly induce parturition in the horse.

THE FORCES OF DELIVERY

The myometrium is composed of smooth muscle which can contract in rhythmic waves. During the first stage the waves pass down the horns and body towards the cervix, thereby bringing pressure to bear on the uterine contents (Fig. 4.4). These painful contractions are responsible for the signs of the first stage which will be described later. They may be transitory and occur without dilatation of the cervix. In these cases the mare shows signs of the first stage and then 'cools off'.

If birth is to proceed, the cervix dilates and the mounting pressure in the uterus causes the placenta to bulge into the cervical aperture. The membrane is usually particularly thin at this point (the 'cervical star') and ruptures to allow escape of allantoic fluid (Fig. 4.5). This event marks the onset of the second stage, i.e. delivery. In this stage the presure transmitted to the uterine contents by contractions of the myometrium is powerfully supplemented by pressure from the abdominal musculature. The stimulus which initiates these muscular contractions is unknown but they become apparent shortly after escape of allantoic fluid and continue until the fetus has been expelled from the birth canal. Rossdale et al. (1979) made observations on the maternal endocrinology of mares in which the fetus and fetal membranes were manipulated during delivery. Closely timed samples taken during vaginal and cervical manipulations produced no rise in peripheral PGFM levels

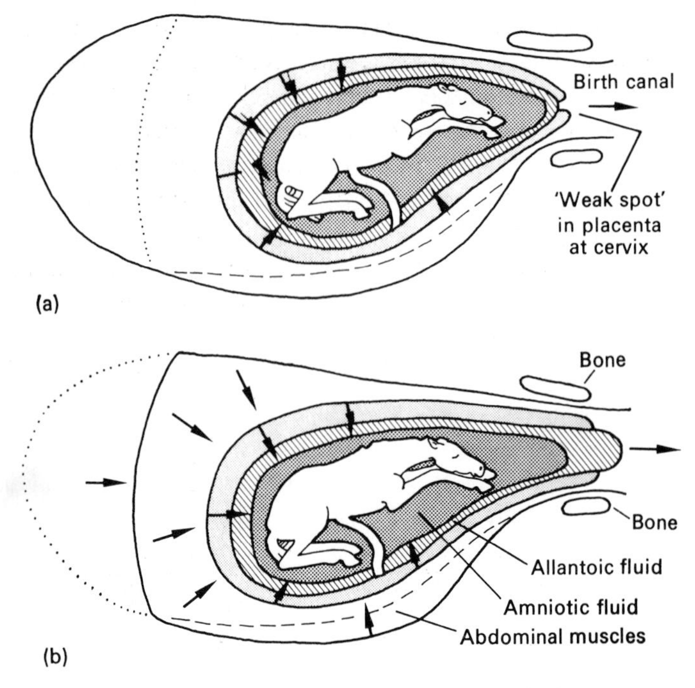

Fig. 4.4. The forces involved in expelling the fetus during birth. (*a*) First-stage contractions of the uterus. (*b*) Second-stage straining and uterine contractions.

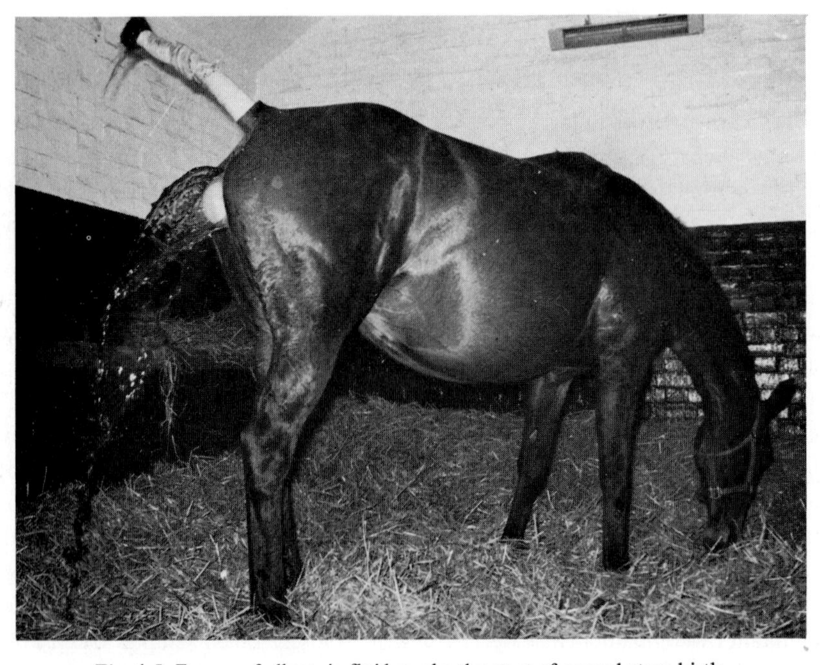

Fig. 4.5. Escape of allantoic fluid marks the start of second-stage birth.

(Fig. 4.6), nor did rupture of the chorio-allantoic membrane. However, in one mare traction was applied to the foal's fore-legs and during this procedure a peak of PGFM levels appeared which was accompanied by straining from the mare. It appears, therefore, and this is substantiated by our experience in the field, that movement of the fetus through the birth canal, as produced by traction, is more effective at stimulating contractions than is the actual presence of the fetus itself in the birth canal. The contractions are further stimulated by endogenous prostaglandin and oxytocin release due to the movement and stretching of the cervix and vagina by the fetus, and so the contractions become self-promoting.

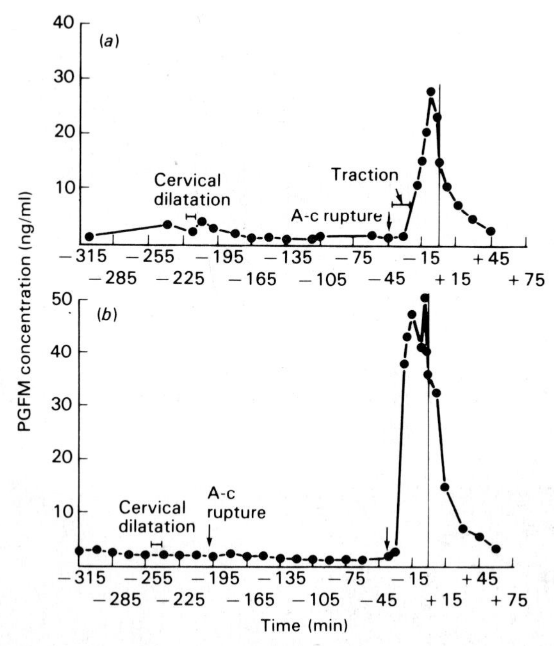

Fig. 4.6. Plasma PGFM concentrations in mares after cervical manipulation and rupture of the allantochorionic membrane (A-c) followed by (*a*) traction on the foal or (*b*) an intravenous injection of 10 IU oxytocin (O). Complete delivery is denoted by the vertical line at zero time. (*After Rossdale et al.* 1979)

The basis of voluntary straining is as follows: the mare breathes in and holds the rib cage and diaphragm at the position of maximum inspiration; the abdominal muscles are then caused to contract the abdominal contents and pressure is transmitted to the uterine contents. Most mares strain only when recumbent, a position which increases intra-abdominal pressure. The combined forces of the uterine and abdominal muscles 'push' the fetus through the birth canal, which is lubricated by the allantoic and amniotic fluids.

ANATOMY OF BIRTH

Birth canal

The canal includes the cervix, vagina and vulva, each of which can expand sufficiently to accommodate the fetus. During the first stage the cervix dilates, the vulva relaxes and the vaginal secretions become moist. The mechanism of cervical dilatation is not fully understood. The connective tissue of the pregnant uterus serves to support the smooth muscle but also acts as a means of retaining the conceptus within the uterus until term. The proportion of collagenous tissue increases from the body of the uterus to the cervix. The integrity of the cervix depends largely on the collagen it contains. Cervical compliance is, to a large extent, related to the changes that occur in the collagen at the time of parturition. It is possible that prostaglandins play an important role in cervical dilatation. In the ewe PGE has been shown to be involved in cervical dilatation (Ellwood et al. 1979).

Gross studies of the cervix during delivery are difficult since once the vaginal seal has been breached by a speculum for visual examination or by the arm for manual manipulation, subsequent observations may be influenced by the initial and succeeding interference. However, it seems that the equine cervix normally

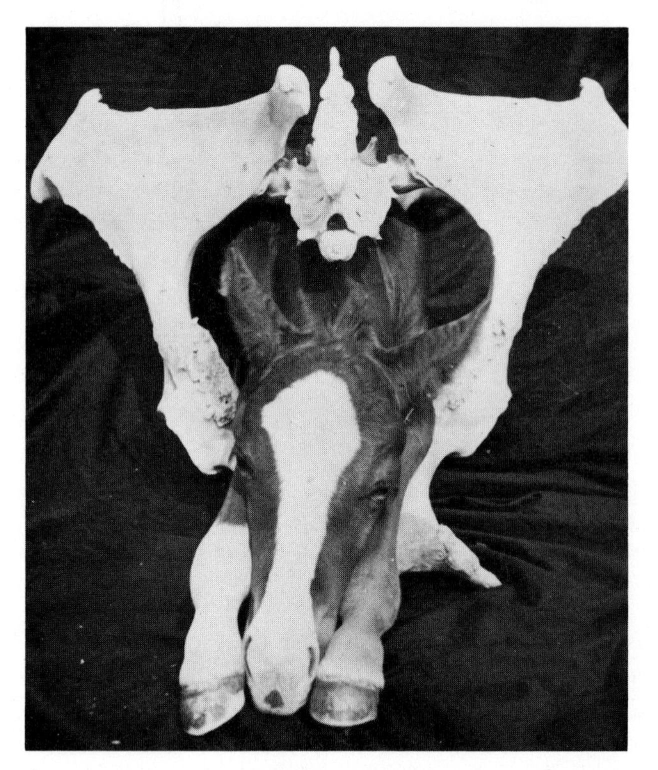

Fig. 4.7. The pelvic outlet.

dilates as the foal's fore-parts press against it during the latter part of the first stage. At this time the vaginal mucosa is covered by a sticky secretion but the cervical plug of mucus present during gestation becomes detached. The fetal forelimbs and muzzle appear to punch against the cervix until eventually they pass through, carrying the placenta with them. The placenta then ruptures and the mucus in the vagina is lubricated by the escaping allantoic fluid. It has been suggested that the fetus makes vigorous movements directed at the cervix because of the impediment to movement presented by the structure as the fetal reflexes become activated (see below). In some cases the placenta, bulging with the pressure of the allantoic fluid, passes through the cervix and appears at the vulval lips before rupturing. This is regarded as abnormal and due to excessive thickness of the placental cervical pole (see Fig. 4.28).

The bones of the pelvis, which surround the soft structures of the canal, form a bony hoop through which the fetus must pass. The pelvic girdle is composed of the os coxae, one on either side, which join ventrally at the symphysis pelvis and articulate dorsally with the sacrum. The os coxae consists of three flat bones – the ilium, ischium and pubis – which join at the acetabulum, the cavity that receives the head of the femur. From an obstetric viewpoint the shape and size of the pelvic outlet is important. The aperture, roughly conical, is formed by the sacrum and first three coccygeal vertebrae above, the ilium, ischium and pubis laterally and below. The opening on the abdominal end (inlet) is somewhat larger than that at the posterior end (outlet) (Fig. 4.7). In a Thoroughbred mare the average diameter of the inlet is about 24 cm and of the outlet above 20 cm. The largest diameter is slightly oblique to the midline. The conformation of the ventral surface of the sacrum and first three coccygeal vertebrae is such as to direct the fetus downwards as it passes through the birth canal. We must now consider the disposition of the fetus in this unyielding bony circumference.

Position, presentation and posture of the fetus

Presentation refers to the region of the fetal body presented to the pelvic inlet, e.g. anterior or posterior. *Position* means the relationship of the fetal vertebral column relative to the dorsal surface of the uterus or maternal vertebral column, e.g. dorsal or ventral. *Posture* denotes the disposition of the head, neck and extremities in relation to the fetal body, e.g. flexed or extended.

Late gestation

In about the sixth month the fetus assumes anterior presentation, ventral position and flexed posture of the head, fore-limbs and hind-limbs (Vandeplassche 1957; Roberts 1971; Arthur 1975). The factors concerned in the alignment of the fetus are poorly understood and the relative roles played by gravity, intrinisic neuro-muscular mechanism of fetal muscular tone and extrinsic pressures exerted on the uterine contents are largely unknown. The specific nature of the control, however, is illustrated by the high incidence of anterior presentation; less than 1 in 500 presentations are posterior. Fraser et al. (1975) studied fetal kinesis using a Doppler ultrasound technique. They showed that considerable reflex activity involving the fetal head, neck and fore-limbs occurred before foaling. A radiographic study (Jeffcott & Rossdale 1979) confirmed these findings and showed that the fetus tends to extend its head and distal fore-limbs in what appears to be a purposeful

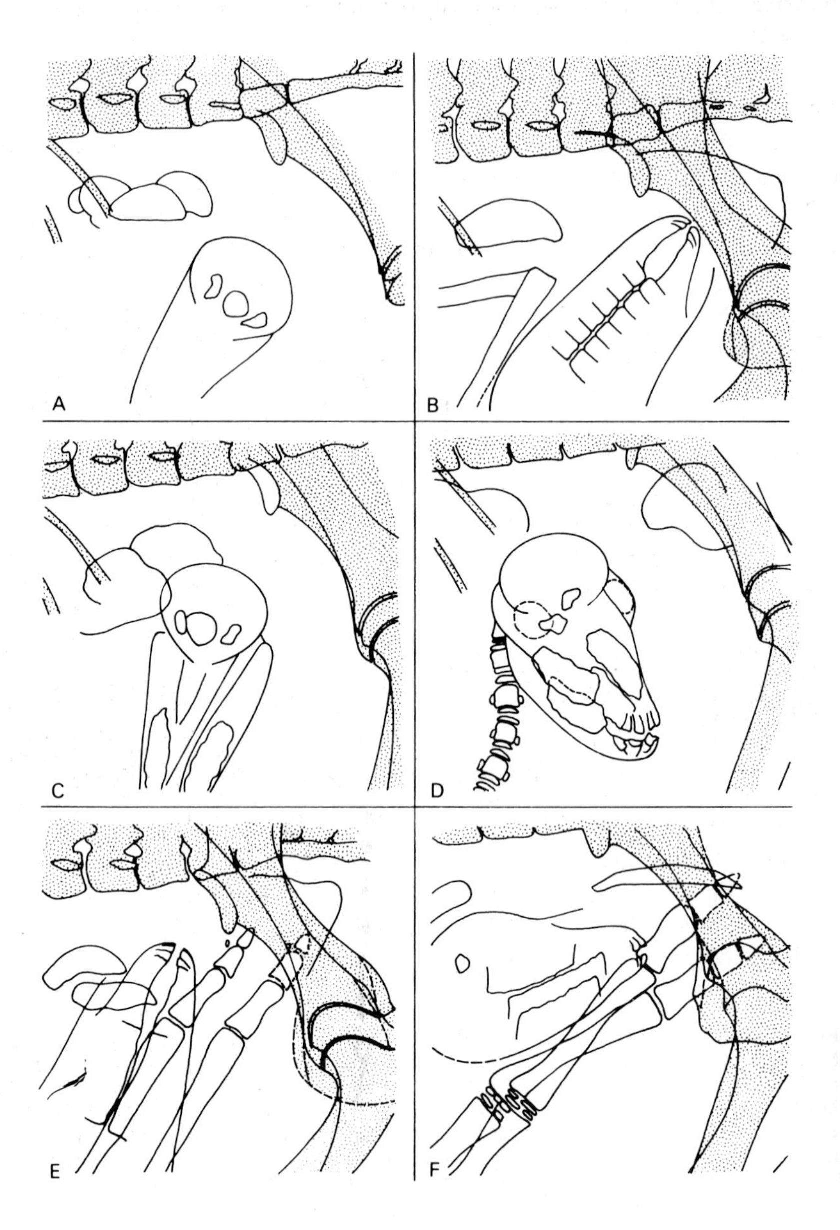

Fig. 4.8. Sequence of fetal movements in a mare during natural parturition (335 days gestation). Maternal bones are stippled. A, Fetus lying on its side with head and poll flexed and fore-limbs flexed out of view. B, Radiograph taken 180 minutes before delivery of the foal, the fetal head is extended and the distal fore-limbs partly extended. C, 100 minutes before delivery, the fetal head is again in flexion and the fore-limbs are flexed out of view. D, 85 minutes before delivery, the fetal head is raised towards the pelvic inlet and partly rotated while the fore-limbs, in flexion, are out of view. E, 35 minutes before delivery and fetal head and fore-limbs are in extension but still in the ventral position. F, 10 minutes before delivery the fetal head and extended fore-limbs have rotated into the dorsal position and engaged in the birth canal for normal delivery. (*From Jeffcott & Rossdale 1979*)

movement during first stage, followed by rotation into the dorsal position (Figs 4.8, 4.9).

First-stage labour

The change to extended posture by the head and fore-limbs followed by the rotation of the fetal body may be assisted by myometrial contractions, the influence of the mare getting up and down, changing from recumbency on one side to the other and rolling, as well as by the escape of the allantoic fluid at the onset

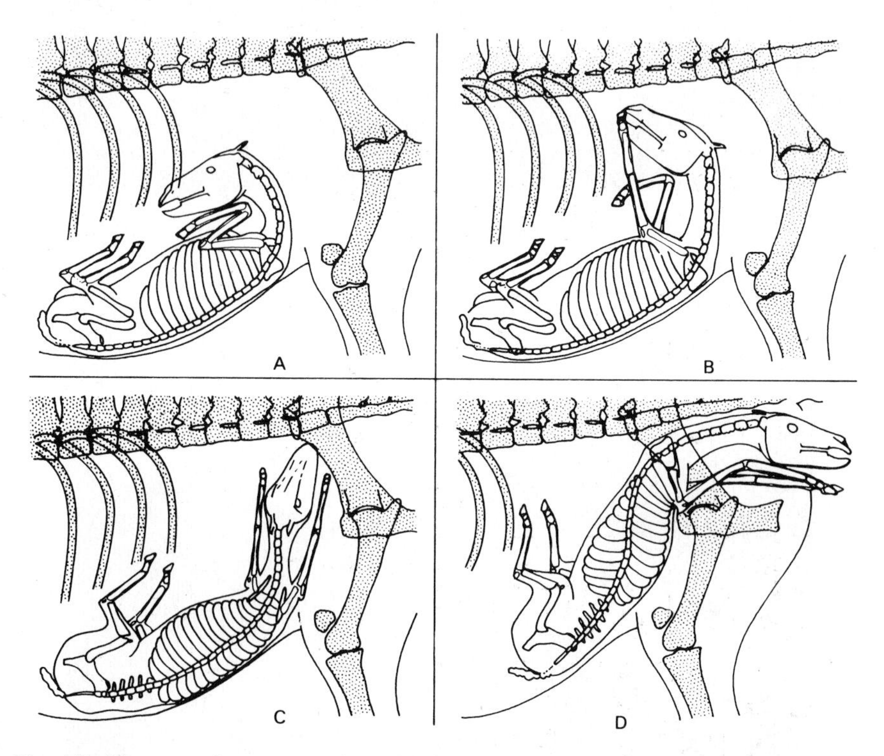

Fig. 4.9. Diagrammatic representation of fetal movements during parturition in the mare. Maternal bones are stippled. A, Near-term fetus is lying in ventral or ventrolateral position with head and fore-limbs flexed. B, Before first-stage labour fetal movements are chiefly confined to head, upper neck and distal fore-limbs. C, During first-stage labour the head and fore-limbs extend and rotate into dorsal position for delivery. D, At second-stage labour the fetus engages in the birth canal although the distal vertebral column and hind-limbs are still in ventral position. (*From Jeffcott & Rossdale 1979*)

of second stage. Radiographic studies suggest that part of the fetal movement is due to its own reflex activity and part due to outside influences exerted by the mare and by gravity. The sequence of turning is usually complete by the time that the fetus enters the birth canal.

During the first stage and the early part of the second stage pressure caused by myometrial contractions and the escape of the allantoic fluid brings the fetus from ventral to dorsal position and its head and limb posture to extension. The fetus

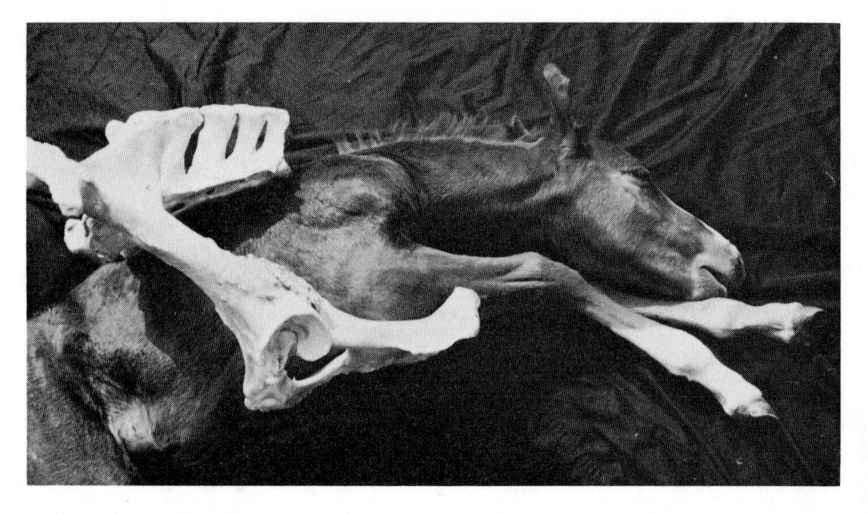

Fig. 4.10. The fetal disposition during passage through the maternal pelvis.

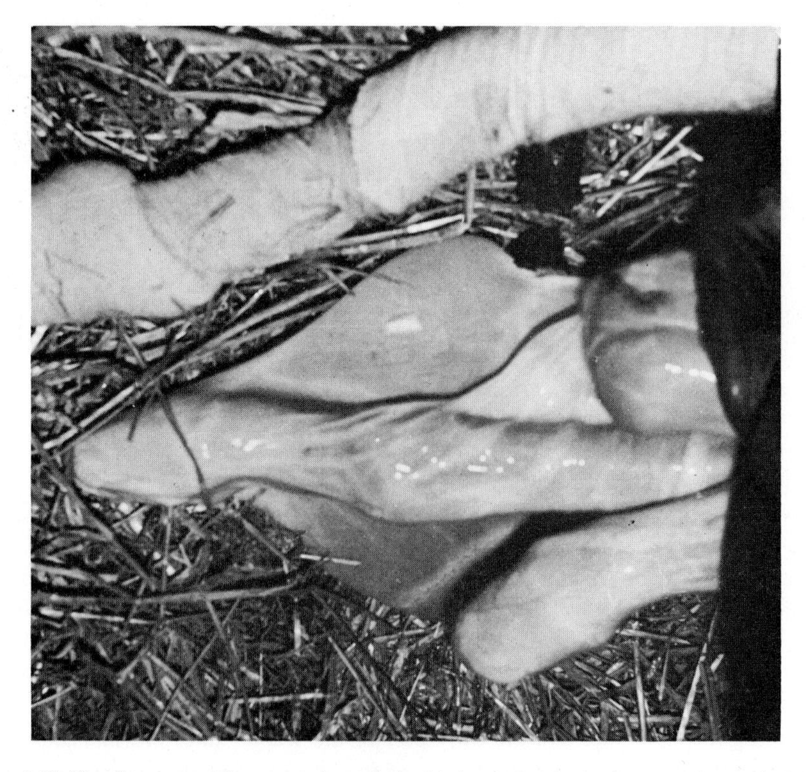

Fig. 4.11. The fetus normally passes through the birth canal with one fore-leg advanced slightly more than the other.

normally enters the maternal pelvis in anterior presentation, dorsal position and extended posture; no other disposition can be regarded as normal (Fig. 4.10).

Second-stage labour

There is little change in fetal position during expulsion through the birth canal. The dorsoventral axis of the thorax deviates slightly from the midline, thus bringing the greatest dimension of the fetal chest to lie in the longest axis of the pelvic canal. One fore-leg is usually slightly in advance of the other, so that the foot of one leg is level with the fetlock joint of the other (Fig. 4.11). This discrepancy may sometimes be increased as the olecranon becomes temporarily lodged against the maternal pelvis (Fig. 4.12). The alignment of the fore-limbs appears to minimize

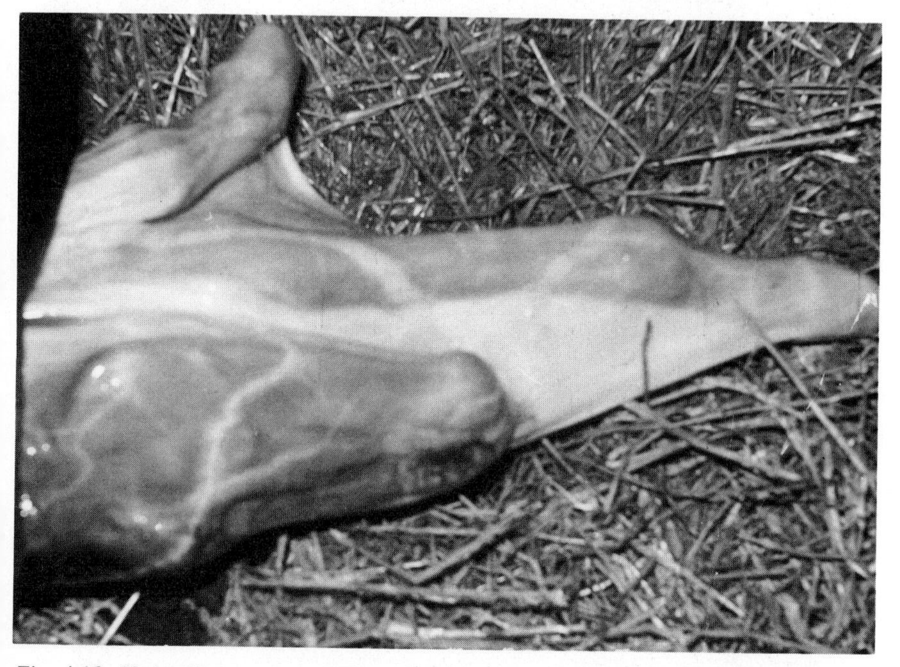

Fig. 4.12. If the discrepancy between the fore-legs is too great, the retarded leg should be eased gently forward.

the total cross-section of the thorax and may have important implications in avoiding thoracic trauma. The head rests above or between the knees, although in some cases it may hang below. Delivery is completed with the foal in the same posture and position. Final delivery places the fore-legs and head in the region of the mare's hocks and its hind-legs remain in the vagina (Fig. 4.13).

MATERNAL BEHAVIOUR

First-stage labour

Signs of the first stage (Figs 4.14, 4.15) occur in increasingly frequent waves but the intensity of pain, or its appreciation, seems to vary considerably. Some mares

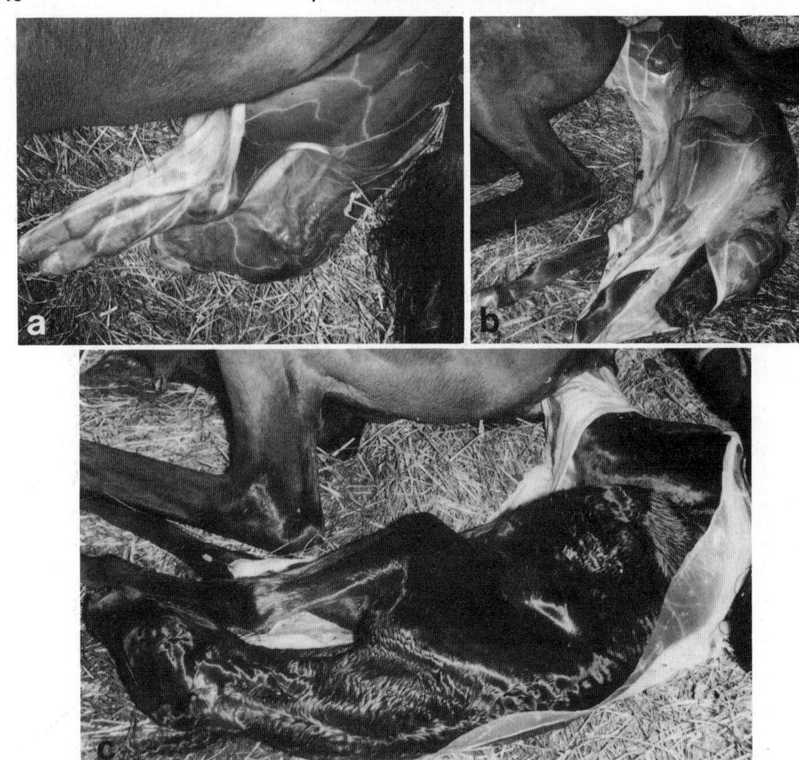

Fig. 4.13. Delivery is complete and the fetus is left with its foreparts close to the mare's hocks. The amnion may be torn during delivery or broken by the foal (*b*) as it makes its first respiratory movements. In (*c*) an attendant has opened the amnion.

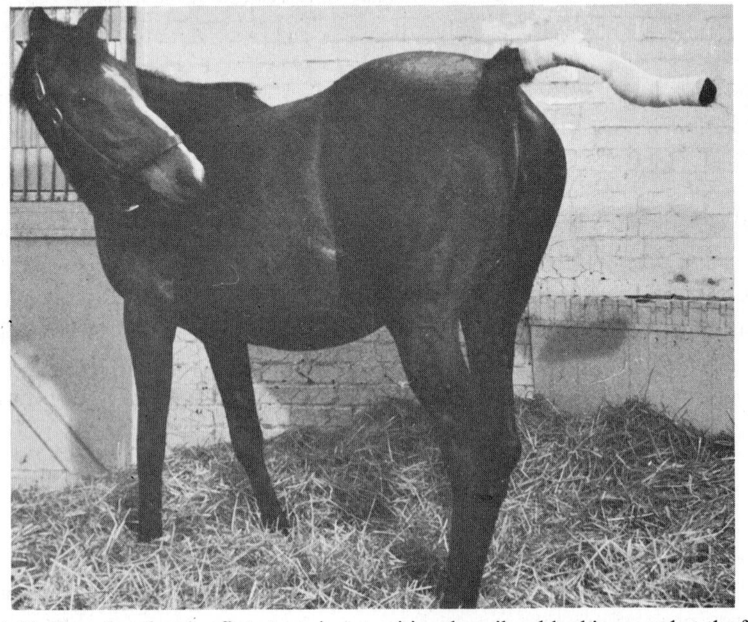

Fig. 4.14. The mare showing first-stage signs – raising the tail and looking round at the flanks.

show only minimal premonitory signs and others marked distress for several hours. Signs, some or all of which may be present, are: increased skin temperature, patchy or profuse sweating, uneasiness, pawing the ground, looking round at the flanks, pacing uneasily around the box with an anxious facial expression, cringing at the hind-quarters and clamping the tail on the perineum. Occasionally a mare may rub her hind-quarters against a wall. Curling of the upper lip in the *Flehmen* posture is common. Milk may drip or spurt from the teats and considerable amounts of

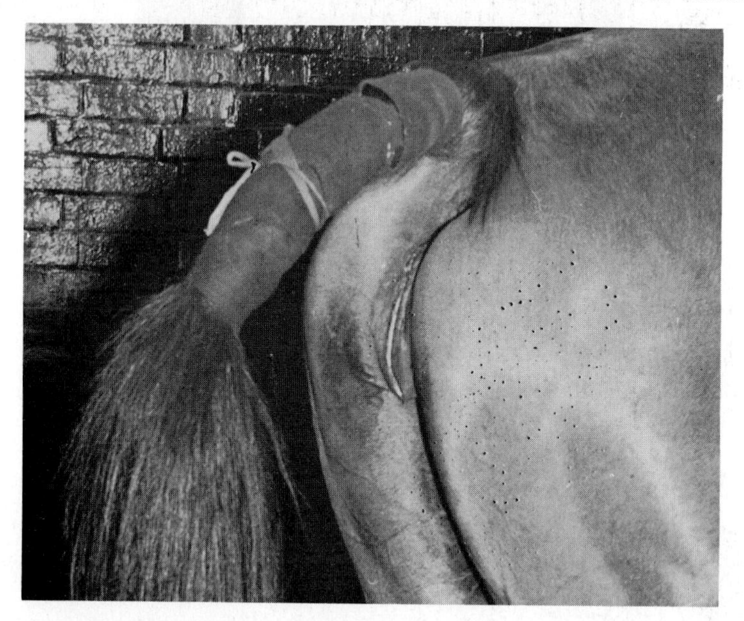

Fig. 4.15. A first-stage sign – lengthening of the vulva.

colostrum are sometimes lost. During intervals between painful bouts the mare may eat or rest quietly. The signs of first-stage labour are associated with peak levels of prostaglandin and oxytocin in the blood stream of the mare.

Sometimes first-stage signs may appear but are not followed by second-stage labour. The event is 'postponed' for a matter of hours or days and then preceded by fresh signs of first stage. Repetitive 'false alarms' or premature first stage, during which the mare 'warms up' and 'cools off', are common in Thoroughbred mares. The extent to which factors in the environment may be responsible is unknown but it is a well known subjective contention that mares may hold up parturition when attendants are present. Prolonged first stage may be associated with an abnormally thickened placenta which fails to rupture as the cervix dilates.

Second-stage labour

Rupture of the placenta, which marks the onset of the second stage, may occur when the mare is standing or as she becomes recumbent. At first a small trickle of yellow-brown fluid passes (Fig. 4.16) between the vulval lips, or in some cases it is

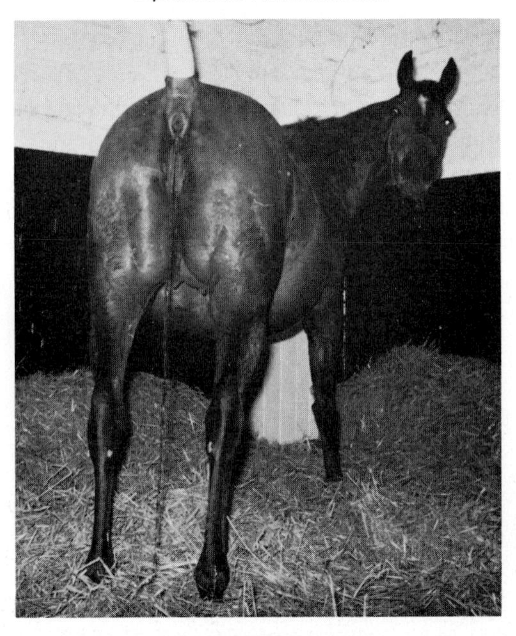

Fig. 4.16. The start of the second stage is marked by rupture of the placental membrane and escape of allantoic fluid.

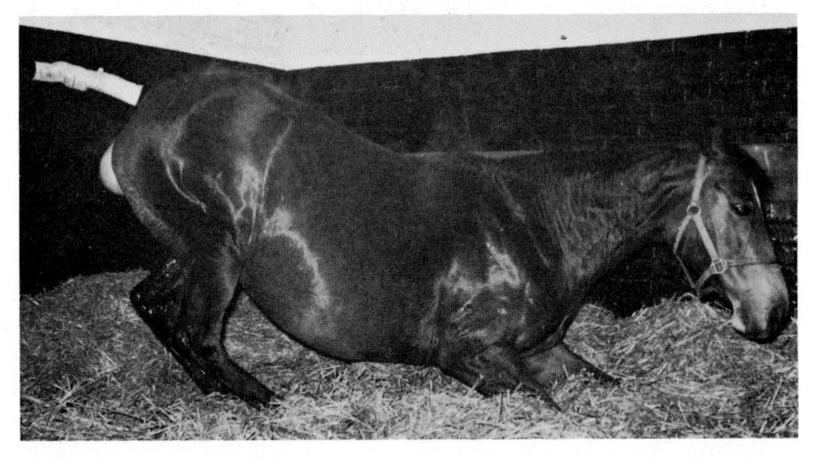

Fig. 4.17. The amnion normally shows at the vulva within about five minutes of the start of the second stage. At about this time the mare lies down. Steam can be seen rising from the mare's coat.

a copious stream. The amount of fluid voided at any one moment during the second stage depends on total quantity of fluid and the strength of uterine contractions. Although 'breaking water', as the event is described by studmen, is usually recognized easily, some mares may start the second stage with so little fluid escaping that the onset is missed.

Within about five minutes of placental rupture the amnion should appear between the vulval lips (Fig. 4.17). Visible straining begins soon after the start of second stage and usually after the mare has become recumbent. Some mares make expulsive efforts in the standing position but this may be the result of disturbed environment, as is inevitable in the presence of attendants. About 95% of mares make their final expulsive efforts while recumbent and spend the majority of the second stage lying down, although they may change their position many times in the process of delivery. Mares that stay on their feet for most of second stage or during final delivery may do so in succeeding parturitions.

Expulsive efforts appear more successful when the mare is lying stretched out (Fig. 4.18). During parturition in a confined space, mares frequently lie with their withers and quarters pressed against a partition wall as if this helps their expulsive efforts.

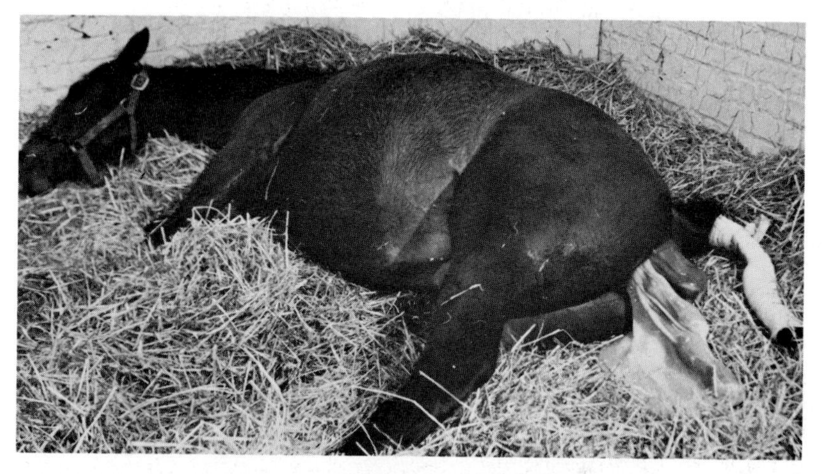

Fig. 4.18. During the second stage expulsive efforts are most effective when the mare is recumbent. A mare often seems to prefer to lie with her withers and back pressed against a wall.

Most mares return to the standing position at least once before final delivery is accomplished (Fig. 4.19). Clinical impression suggests that the fetus may be wrongly aligned if the mare repeatedly alters her posture from standing to recumbency or from left to right recumbency. Some individuals may roll or remain in a semi-recumbent posture with hind-quarters raised for several seconds.

A notable feature of the mare's behaviour during the second stage is the licking of allantoic fluid that has fallen on the straw bedding, her own skin or the clothes of attendants (Fig. 4.20). The extent to which the taste or smell of allantoic fluid influences subsequent maternal behaviour is unknown, but its presence on the ground may help to define the territory on which birth is to proceed. As the second stage continues mares will often turn their heads towards their hind-quarters, nicker or whinny.

Once the fetal head is delivered past the level of the vulva the mare, unless disturbed, will remain recumbent until expulsion is complete. After the fetal hips have passed from the vagina, straining ceases abruptly and the mare remains lying

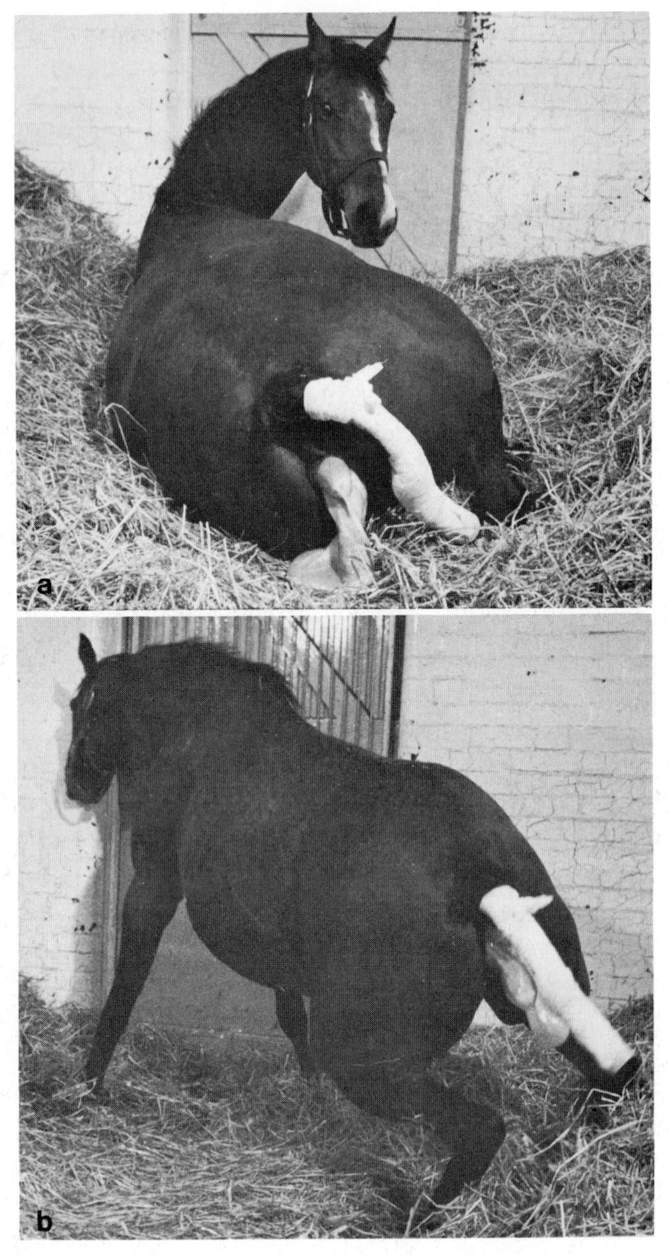

Fig. 4.19. Straining while on the brisket (*a*) and rolling and changing position (*b*) are features of second-stage behaviour.

stretched out or in a position of sternal recumbency for up to 40 minutes (Fig. 4.21). In some cases the mare may get to her feet immediately the foal is delivered but this is abnormal and is usually caused by environmental factors. On Thoroughbred stud farms the presence of men in the foaling box, or an episiotomy performed

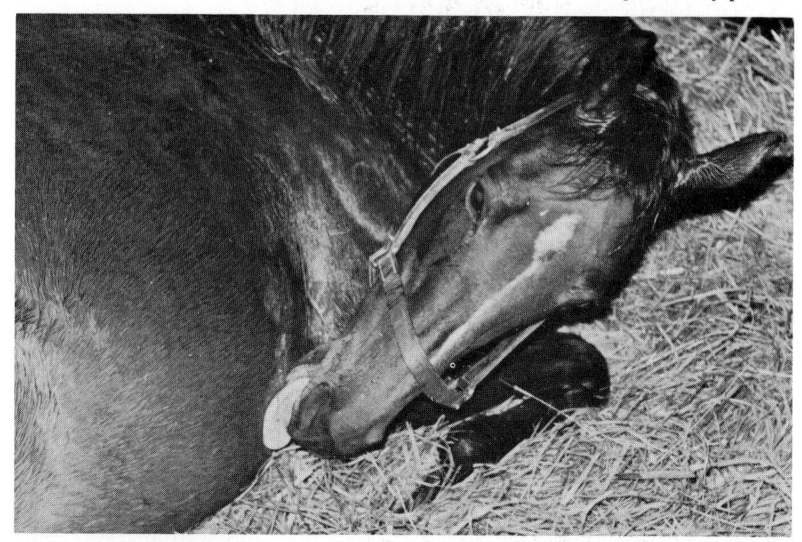

Fig. 4.20. Licking behaviour starts in the first stage and is well established by the middle of the second stage.

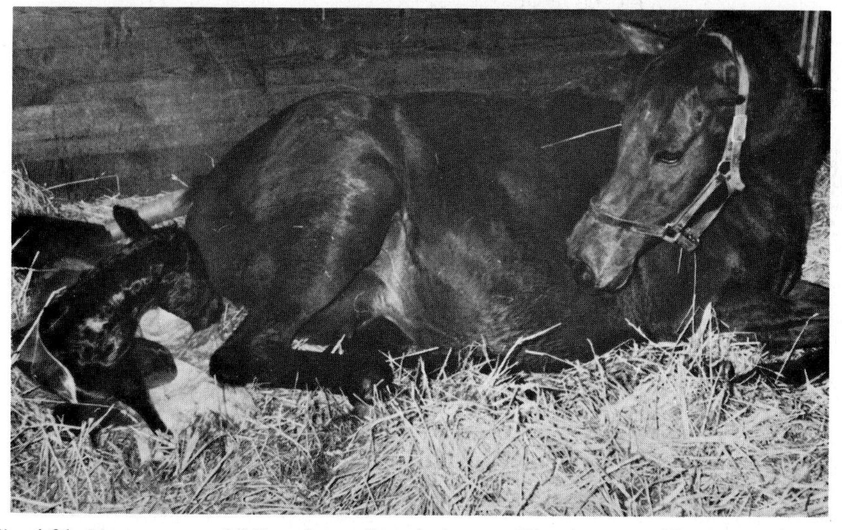

Fig. 4.21. Most mares exhibit a phase of marked tranquillity for up to 40 minutes after the fetus has been delivered. During this phase they remain recumbent.

during the second stage, disturbs normal behaviour patterns. In most cases, however, mares appear to be affected by a strong 'tranquillizing' influence during the post-delivery phase. Most mares are reluctant to get to their feet and pay intermittent attention to their foal, turning their head, nickering and licking the nearest

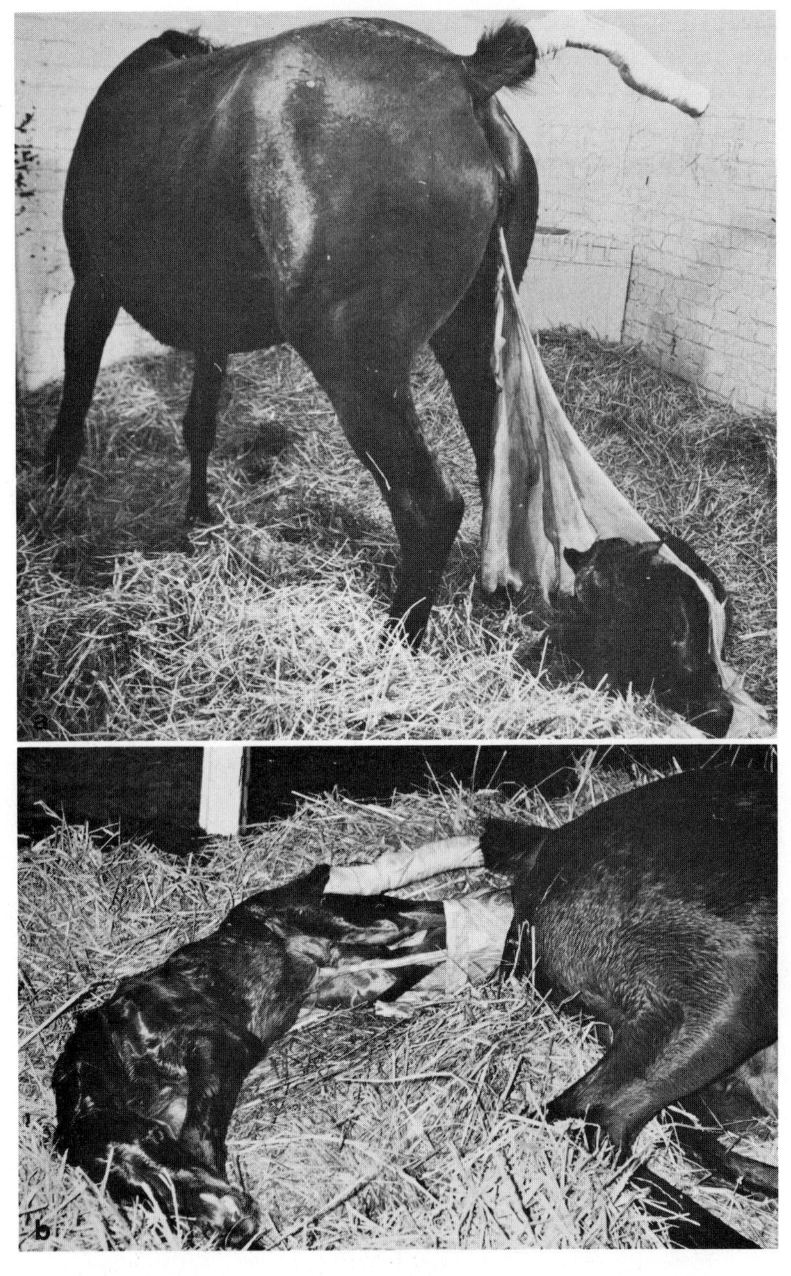

Fig. 4.22. The umbilical cord is normally ruptured by tension, either because the mare gets to her feet or because the foal moves away in trying to stand.

part, which is generally the foal's muzzle or head. They may eat straw, hay or grass within their reach. A few individuals show great excitement, rising to their feet, snorting and whinnying, pawing the ground and perhaps the foal, as if it were a strange object. This type of behaviour is not confined to mares foaling for the first time, but is sometimes noted in a mare at successive parturitions. The second stage lasts five to 60 minutes (average 20 minutes). In general, mares foaling for the first time take longer than at subsequent births and individuals that have a prolonged first stage often have a short second stage.

Third-stage labour

The umbilical cord remains intact after delivery of the foal. It is normally ruptured either by the mare rising to her feet or by the foal struggling to stand for the first time (Fig. 4.22). The first causes a sudden and the second a gradual build-up of

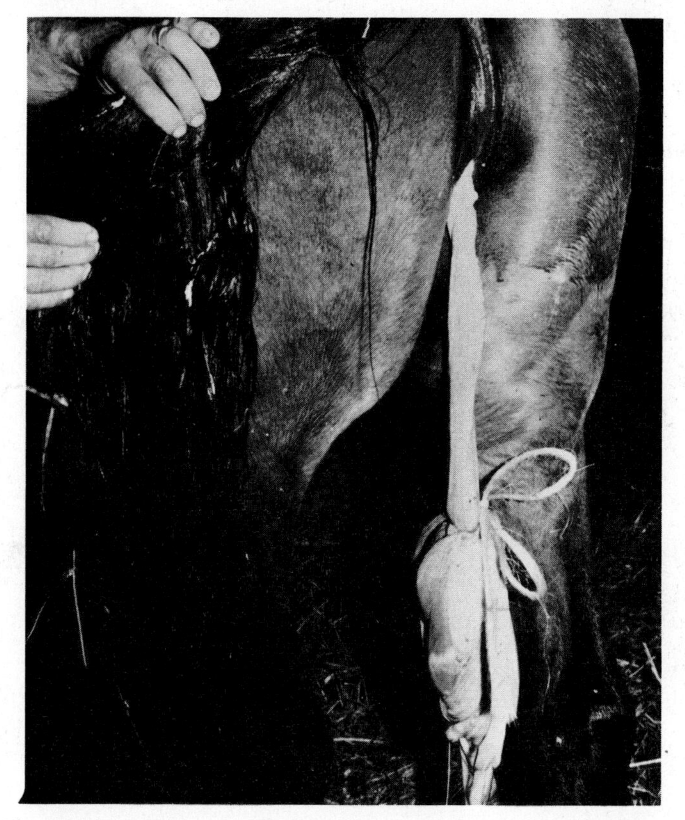

Fig. 4.23. The amnion is usually tied to the cord after the foal has been born.

tension, ending in separation at a predetermined point of relative weakness in the cord structure about 3 cm from the abdomen. During much of the time the cord remains intact its blood vessels are patent. After rupture of the cord attendants usually tie the amnion to the cord with string (Fig. 4.23). This is thought to help

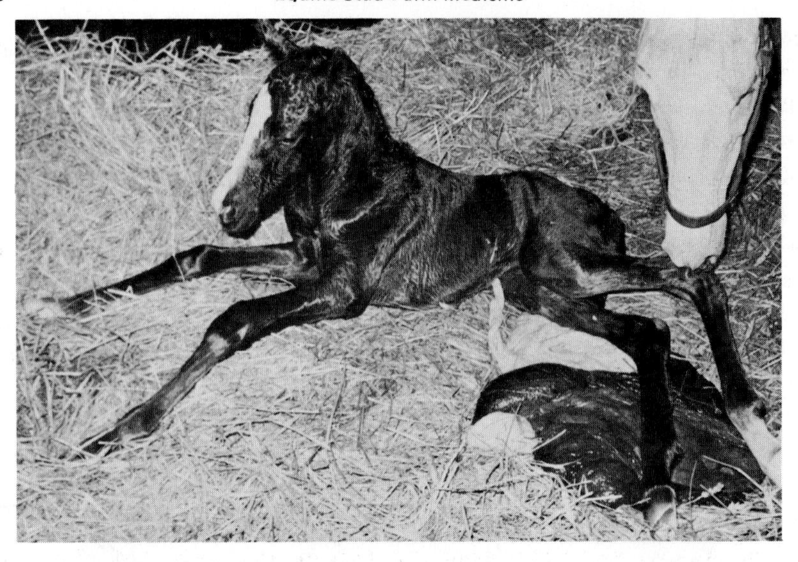

Fig. 4.24. The placenta is expelled before the cord has been broken.

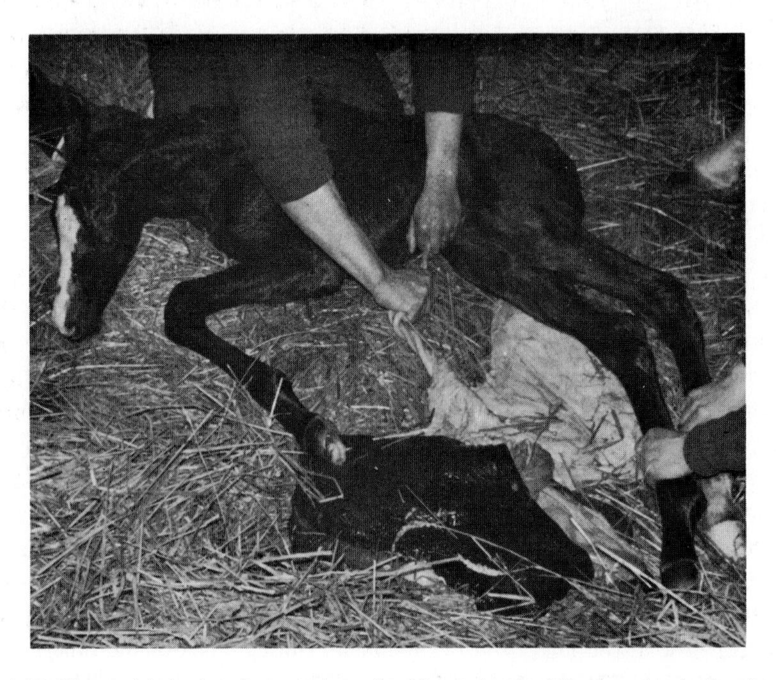

Fig. 4.25. The cord is broken by a strong pull with one hand while the other is placed on the foal's abdomen.

expulsion by providing weight and it prevents the mare from tearing or kicking at the amnion.

The placenta is expelled with the chorio-allantoic surface outermost in most cases and in some instances with the chorionic surface exposed. The duration of third stage is 60 minutes on average following the foal's final delivery. Occasionally the placenta is expelled before the cord breaks (Fig. 4.24). In this event the cord should be severed manually (Fig. 4.25). During the third stage mares may show signs of pain – rolling, sweating, pawing the ground, unease and retracting the upper lip. Mares do not normally attempt to eat parts of the afterbirth, although some will lick the amnion and placenta, especially if their foal fails to make active movements or is removed from the loose box.

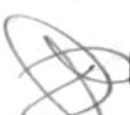

Retention of the afterbirth

There are no criteria by which to define retention of the afterbirth as pathological. The usual practice is to allow about ten hours to elapse after parturition before action is taken.

Vandeplassche et al. (1971) found that retention of the fetal membranes nearly always occurs in the non-gravid horn and that it is a localized phenomenon. They noted that the thickness of the chorio-allantois and the length of villi and degree of attachment to the endometrium decrease from the non-gravid to gravid horn and to the body of the uterus. The microcotyledons of the placenta are firmly attached by the fifth month of gestation and from this stage onwards the fetal membranes may become retained if the mare aborts. Retention is particularly common after dystocia and caesarean section. Vandeplassche et al. (1971) believe that the causes may be hormonal imbalance and abnormal myometrial activity.

The following treatments are recommended separately or in conjunction.

Manual removal, with the operator wearing a glove and applying the usual aseptic precautions. The tip of the retained horn is frequently difficult to remove. Great care should be taken as prolonged or repeated attempts may cause undue trauma to the endometrium. The optimum procedure is to remove as much of the placenta as can be *easily* detached and to return three or four days later, when the retained portion can usually be freed. A pessary containing antibiotics may be inserted into the uterus on the first occasion and parenteral antibiotics administered daily.

Vandeplassche et al. (1971) recommend 30–60 IU oxytocin intravenously in 1–2 litres of normal saline over a period of 30–60 minutes, followed by manual removal if the membranes are not spontaneously expelled. We have found this method to be very useful in most cases and preferable to immediate manual removal which invariably leaves many microvilli behind (Vandeplassche 1980) and results in delayed uterine involution.

Burns et al. (1977) have described an alternative method for removal of retained placenta in mares. Following tranquillization and thorough perineal cleansing, a gloved hand is introduced into the vagina and the chorio-allantois is grasped and gently pulled outside the vulva. The torn ends of the cervical star are gathered together and a stomach tube is placed through the opening into the collapsed chorio-allantoic space. 9–12 litres of dilute povidone iodine solution (15 ml per litre of water) at 37°C are pumped into the cavity. The tube is withdrawn and the chorio-allantoic opening is held closed or tied with a strip of gauze. The mare then attempts to expel the fluid within 5–10 minutes in most cases. Initial efforts may be stimulated by injecting 40 IU of oxytocin intravenously or intramuscularly. As the mare tries to eject the fluid, she will cause sufficient cervical stimulation to maintain a natural oxytocin release. This manifests by the dripping of milk from the teats and increased uterine activity. Each expulsive effort ejects some fluid and placenta. The exposed membrane is held and the fluid squeezed back into the retained portion of the placenta. The mare often displays mild abdominal discomfort at this stage. It may be necessary to allow 15–20 minutes for complete release of the placenta which, if intact, should contain all the fluid, which should not leak. Histological examinations of the placenta removed by this method have shown that the microvilli are intact.

It is difficult to define the effects of placental retention because they are relative to the length and time which the membranes remain in situ. There also appear to be breed differences. Acute metritis and laminitis, the sequelae most often described, do not seem as frequent in Thoroughbreds as in heavy breeds. This may reflect the more intensive managerial and veterinary care which Thoroughbreds usually receive or it might be due to a basic difference in susceptibility.

Environmental factors influencing parturition

In the northern hemisphere Thoroughbred mares are usually confined to boxes and compelled to foal with man in close attendance. In the southern hemisphere mares frequently foal in special paddocks, often flood-lit so that attendants can supervise the event and interfere if necessary. New Forest ponies foal in the open and away from humans and although less is known of their habits it appears that behavioural patterns of the parturient mare are remarkably stereotyped. The hour at which they foal, the position adopted during delivery and the duration of the first, second and third stages fall within a relatively narrow range.

However, there are some aspects in which management clearly alters the natural event. For example Messervy (quoted in Rossdale and Short 1967) noted that when students observed ponies during the night at the Veterinary Field Station at Bristol they tended to foal during the day. But it is during second- and third-stage labour that attendants 'interfere' most. Manipulation and traction of the fore-legs both realign them and shorten the duration of second stage. The degree to which this reduces or increases the hazards of birth must remain a matter of speculation in each particular case. Thoracic trauma and fractured ribs are sometimes found at post-mortem, but it is not usually clear if this is caused by pressure of the elbows, disproportion of the chest relative to the pelvis or the angle at which the thorax passes through the pelvic girdle.

Mares which need an episiotomy and those which are nervous may spend the majority of the second stage standing or may deliver in the standing position. If delivering in recumbency they often get to their feet immediately afterwards, especially if an attendant is present.

The extent to which tying the amnion to the cord hastens the end of the third stage is not known. In Australia one of us (P.D.R.) has been told of mares galloping in fright from the afterbirth trailing behind them. Mares foaling in loose boxes cannot react in this way but some mares may kick violently at the amnion if it is not tied up.

EFFECT OF PARTURITION ON THE FETUS

Extrinsic factors may produce untoward effects in the fetus, which are discussed more fully in the next chapter. Here they are summarized as follows:

1. Trauma due to the natural forces of expulsion and/or the unnatural forces of traction.

2. Asphyxia, i.e. increased blood $P\text{CO}_2$, decreased $P\text{O}_2$ and pH due to (*a*) pressure on the umbilical cord as this is dragged through the birth canal, (*b*) lowering of placental efficiency during uterine contractions, (*c*) uneven distribution of uterine and placental blood flows or (*d*) placental separation from the endometrium.

3. Squeezing of the fetal thorax as it passes through the maternal pelvis. This may compress the lungs and cause evacuation of bronchiolar fluid in preparation for the first breath. Compression of the fore-parts may increase cerebral pressure. The effect of delivery on the fetal circulation is illustrated by pressures of 60–100 mmHg recorded in the jugular veins of foals during second stage (Rossdale, 1973, unpublished).

MANAGEMENT OF THE FOALING MARE

Preparatory period

About six weeks before full term the mare should be taken to premises where she is to foal. This allows her to become accustomed to the particular management and husbandry and ensures that her colostrum will contain antibodies specific to these premises. Tetanus toxoid and influenza vaccine should be given within four weeks of full term. As far as practical the mare should have a regular routine of moving in and out of the paddocks and of feeding. Exercise, laxative diets and free access to water at all times are important. Mammary development should be noted and when this increases the mare should be moved to a foaling box where she can be watched easily during the night.

The foaling unit

The foaling unit box should be at least 3 × 3 m and have good ventilation and as far as possible be free from draughts. The bedding should be of the best straw and every effort should be made to minimize the amount of dust in the atmosphere, particularly during foaling. A Perspex window through which attendants may see all parts of the loose box should be placed in one wall. The box should contain a door to give access from a covered area, and preferably from an adjoining passage or room.

Means of heating the box will be required in certain abnormal conditions which will be described in the next chapter. On some stud farms a special 'incubator' box is set aside for sick foals. The majority of body heat is lost through radiation and adequate insulation of walls and ceiling is therefore required. The best source of heat is radiant lamps or filaments.

Accessory requirements

At every foaling those responsible should have to hand:

1. A pair of surgical scissors with an 8–10 cm straight blade for episiotomy (see below).
2. An oxygen cylinder and flowmeter connected to a rubber tube several meters long; a 50 or 100 ml syringe and large-bore needle and a 500 ml bottle of 5% sodium bicarbonate solution for resuscitation (see p. 331).
3. A suitable antiseptic powder or navel dressing and some sterile tape.
4. A chamois leather or towel to dry the foal if it should show signs of maladjustment (see p. 316).

Management of the first stage

There are no special measures which should be adopted during the first stage. Note should be made of colostrum lost to the milk ejection reflex often present at this time. Preparations may be made for an episiotomy, although this is better performed in the second stage.

Management of the second stage

An episiotomy should, if necessary, be performed shortly after rupture of the chorio-allantois. This can usually be performed without local anaesthesia but if the mare is standing it may be advisable to have a fore-limb raised. A cut should be made in the midline to the upper commissure of the vulval labiae (Fig. 4.26).

About five minutes after the start of the second stage an attendant should insert his arm into the vagina and identify the foal's fore-limbs and muzzle (Fig. 4.27). The amnion should not be broken during this procedure. The colour and thickness of the amniotic membrane should be noted for evidence of amnionitis and meconium staining. If the fetal presentation and position are normal the attendant should leave the box and allow the mare to proceed to completion of second stage.

The second stage should be observed closely but interference is not necessary except in the following circumstances:

1. If there is evidence of meconium staining. In this case it may be advisable, once the head has appeared, to speed delivery by pulling gently on the fore-limbs. The amnion should be removed from the foal's nostrils as the chest is delivered.

2. If the chorio-allantois is abnormally thick (Fig. 4.28) it may be forced through the vagina and appear as a red membrane at the vulva lips. If this occurs it should be ruptured immediately with a hand or a pair of scissors.

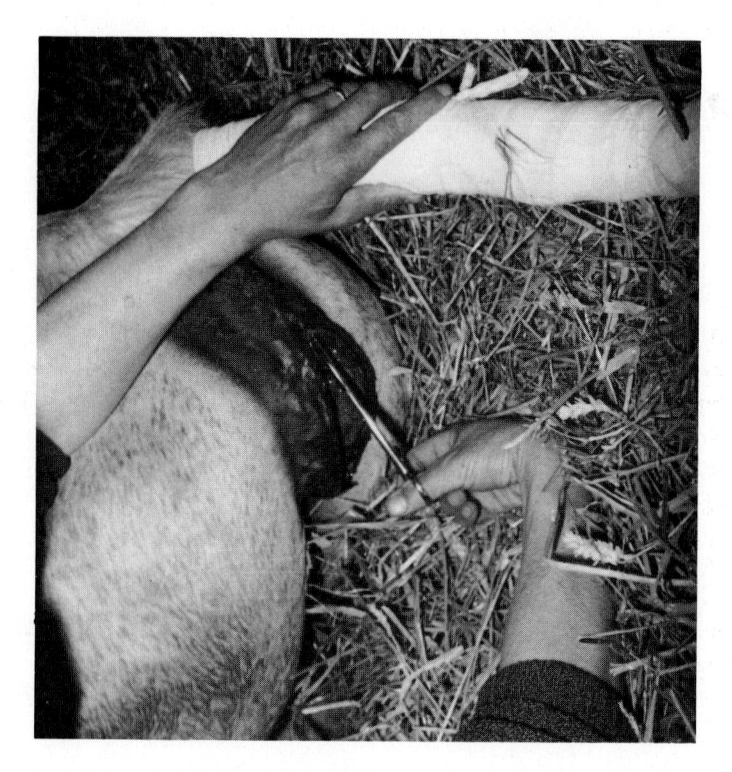

Fig. 4.26. Mares which have had a Caslick operation should have an episiotomy. The vulva should be cut in the midline as soon as the second stage has started.

3. If a fore-leg is driven into the roof of the vagina. If this is not promptly corrected, the foot may penetrate the rectum.

4. If one fore-limb becomes retarded due to the elbow becoming lodged against the pelvis. In this case gentle traction to restore its level with that of the opposite fore-limb may be helpful.

5. If the mare gives the impression that she needs help because delivery does not proceed smoothly despite vigorous straining. Other mares may refrain from straining for long periods. In both cases gentle traction on the fore-limbs is indicated (Fig. 4.29).

6. If an unhealthy foal is suspected. In this case the amnion may be broken and the foal's head lifted out of the amniotic fluid (Fig. 4.30).

7. If an abnormally thick cord does not break naturally. It can be broken by placing one hand on the foal's belly and pulling sharply on the cord with the other (Fig. 4.25). If bleeding from the umbilical stump occurs it can usually be stopped by pinching the vessels between the finger and thumb for a moment or two. Only in

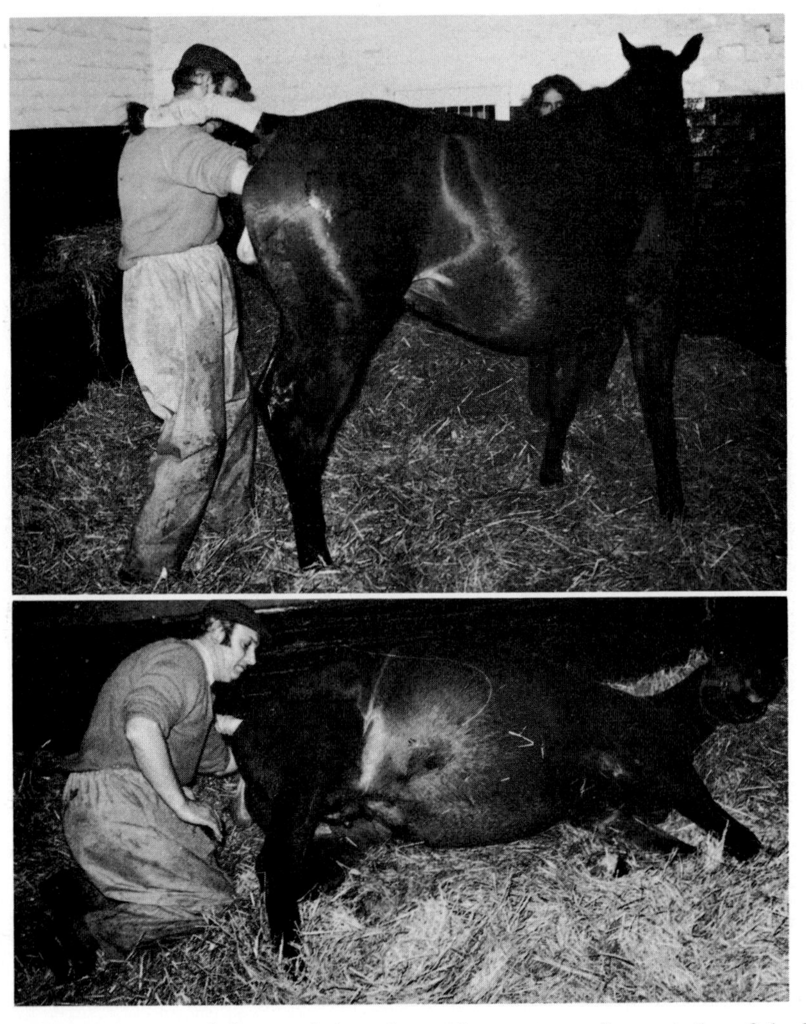

Fig. 4.27. At the start of the second stage the position, posture and presentation of the foal should be checked. This may be done with the mare standing or recumbent. The foal's muzzle and fore-legs are normally easy to identify.

exceptional cases is it necessary to tie a ligature around the stump. Stud grooms were once taught to cut and tie the umbilical cord immediately after delivery, but this deprives the foal of a substantial quantity of placental blood, and the habit is condemned.

Procedure to be followed immediately delivery is completed

1. In normal severance the stump of the umbilical cord is small and should be dressed with antibacterial powder or antiseptic lotion.
2. A hand should be placed gently on the foal's thorax and the heart beat counted over 15–30 seconds (Fig. 4.31). The heart rate provides an index of pathological asphyxia (see p. 290).
3. The amnion can be tied to the cord with string so that it forms a compact mass.

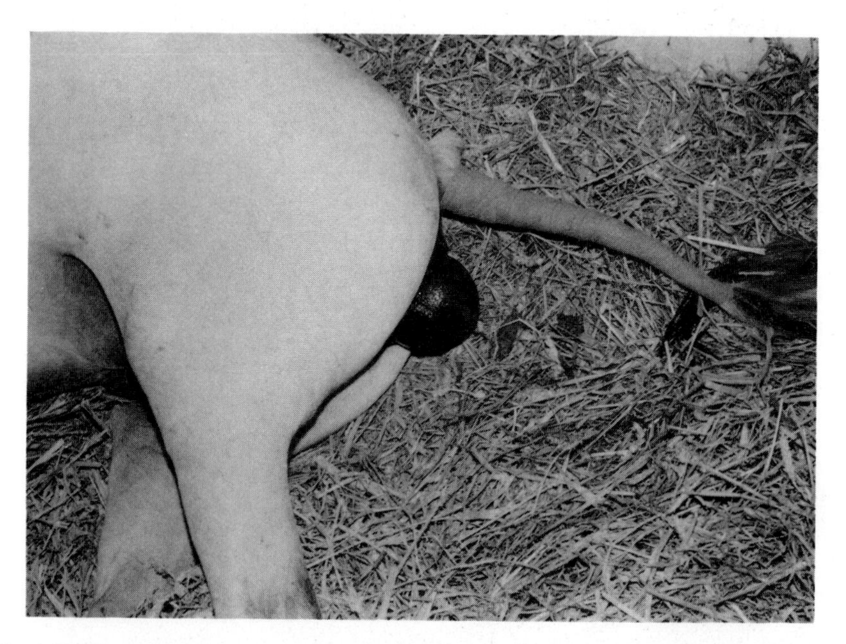

Fig. 4.28. The chorio-allantois may be abnormally thick and appears as a red membrane at the vulva lips. It should be ruptured without delay with the fingers or, carefully, with a pair of scissors.

4. If an episiotomy has been performed the vulva may be resutured within about half an hour of birth without anaesthesia when the mare is recumbent (Fig. 4.32). Suitable alignment is best obtained by suturing from the lower aspect of the episiotomy wound.
5. As far as possible the mare should be left undisturbed and encouraged to remain recumbent. Completion of the third stage before the mare gets up reduces the risk of air being sucked into the genital tract. Temporary use of Michel's clips to hold together the upper commissures of the vulva immediately post-partum may prevent much of the air being aspirated and reduce post-parturient endometritis. The clips are removed after 24–48 hours.
6. The afterbirth should be removed from the loose box and the placental horns checked to ensure that no part remains in the uterus. The surface of the

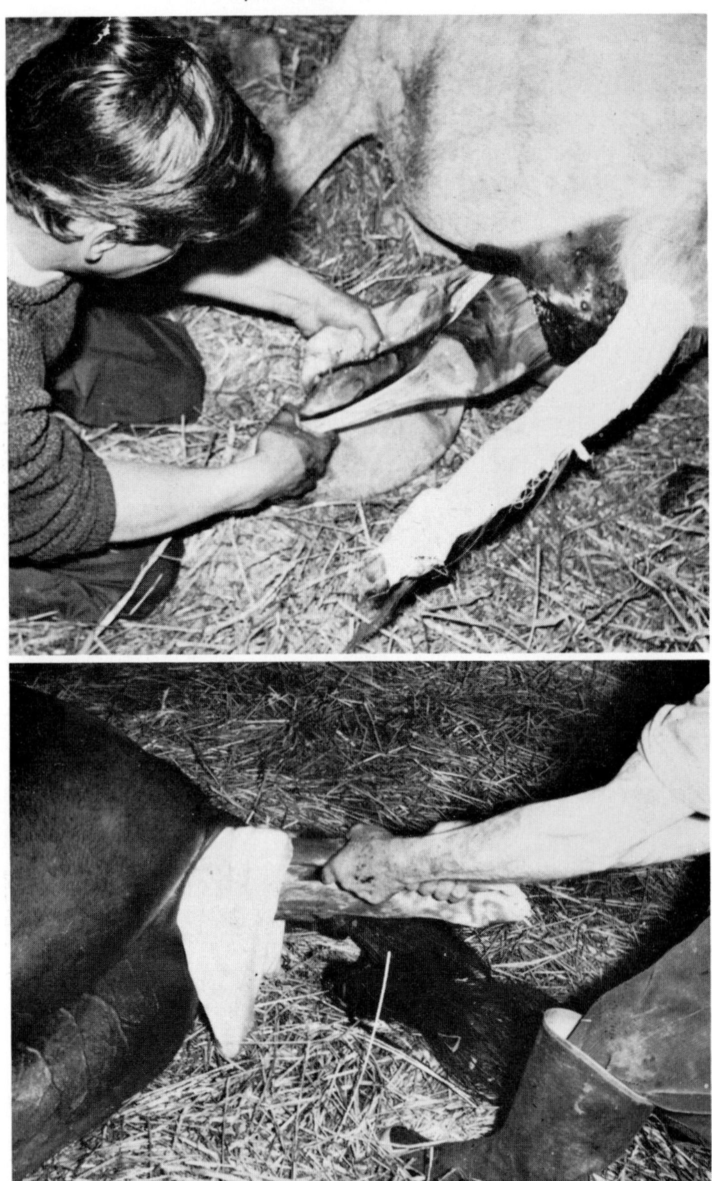

Fig. 4.29. Gentle but firm traction can be applied to the fore-legs during the second stage to hasten the delivery if the fetus is thought to be at risk because of stress or if one fore-leg is abnormally impeded. For full details see text.

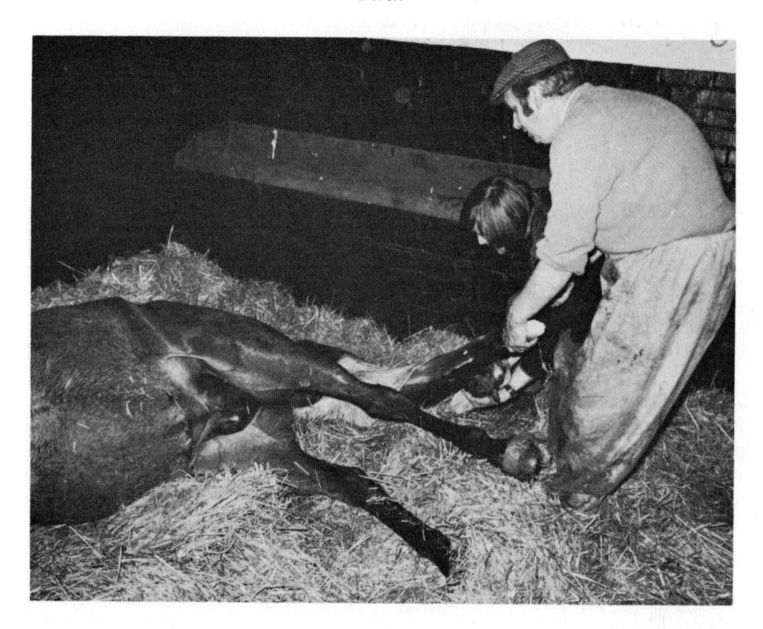

Fig. 4.30. In the final stages of delivery the foal's hips may be eased out of the birth canal and its head guided to a safe position out of the amnion fluid. This is necessary only if the foal is weak or if delivery, as here, is in an awkward situation close to the stable wall.

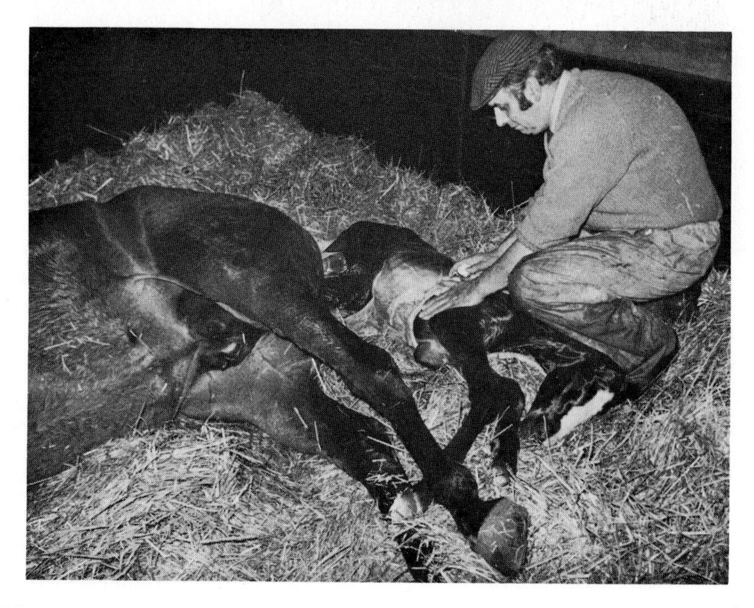

Fig. 4.31. The foal's heart rate should be measured by placing a hand gently on the thorax immediately after delivery.

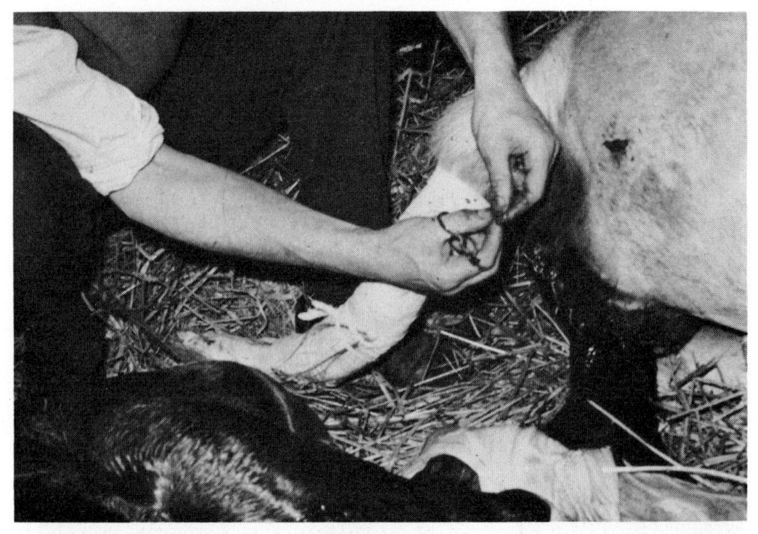

Fig. 4.32. Episiotomy wounds can be repaired once the foal has been born. A local anaesthetic is not normally required within half an hour of delivery. The wound should be sutured from the lowest aspect upwards to obtain correct alignment.

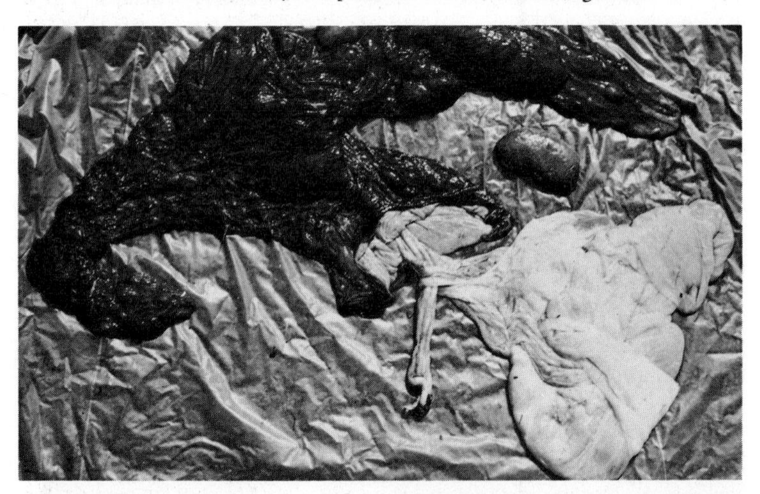

Fig. 4.33. The afterbirth should be examined for evidence of pathological lesions and to see that no part of the horns has been retained. The membranes illustrated here, together with the hippomane, were normal. The chorio-allantois is the darker structure and the amnion the lighter coloured material.

placenta and the amnion should also be examined for evidence of pathological lesions (Fig. 4.33).

The bond between mare and foal strengthens with contact. Human intervention may disturb the delicate relationship during the first two hours, a time when maternal and care-seeking behaviour develops. Maiden mares, or those which make it difficult for their foal to suck from the mammae, may be tranquillized. A twitch should not be applied to the mare for at least 24 hours after foaling because of the possibility that this may provoke internal haemorrhage.

The habit of dragging the foal to the mare's head is unnecessary, although probably not harmful. It is rare for a mare to stand on her foal and accidents that occur are often the result of humans startling the mare and causing her to tread with less than her natural care. Some mares may paw with their fore-leg at the foal,

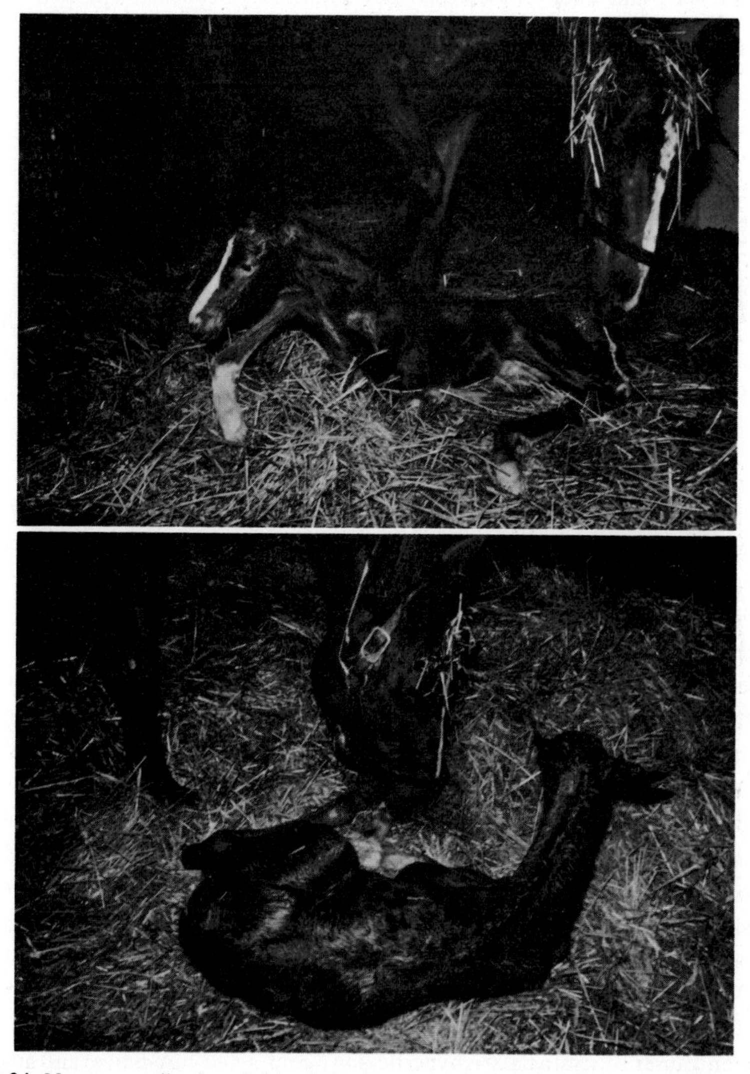

Fig. 4.34. Mares normally show licking behaviour towards their foals, but some may also bite or paw them.

lick it vigorously and occasionally bite it (Fig. 4.34). It is not usually necessary to interfere but a tranquillizing drug or applying a leather bib may occasionally be advisable. Mares with a previous history of aggressive behaviour towards their new-born foals, or who show early signs of such behaviour, should be constantly supervised for the first three or four days post-partum.

Foals that appear weak and take longer than normal to get to their feet or which have difficulty finding the mare's udder may be fed colostrum from a bottle and artificial teat or through a stomach tube to ensure they receive colostrum before they are three hours old.

Warm soap and water or medicinal paraffin used as an enema, with a soft rubber tube, helps the passage of meconium. This is not recommended before the foal has sucked for the first time and care should be taken to avoid rough handling or undue disturbance during this delicate period of adjustment.

DYSTOCIA AND ABNORMAL CONDITIONS OF BIRTH

Dystocia means literally bad birth. It is usually caused by malalignment of the fetal body or appendages. This requires obstetrical correction before delivery can be completed. Dystocia can also be caused by maternal factors, such as uterine inertia or disproportion between fetal size and the maternal birth canal. Certain conditions, such as haemorrhage from the uterine artery or rupture of the caecum, may be associated with birth although they may not directly affect its completion.

Dystocia

Any deviation from normal presentation, posture or position may cause part of the fetus to become impacted against the maternal pelvis. The incidence of dystocia amongst Thoroughbred births is about 4%, although no accurate figures are available from surveys involving large numbers of mares. Benesch and Wright (1950) defined dystocia as some obstacle to parturition whereby the young cannot be delivered by maternal effort alone. Fleming (1878) distinguished maternal dystocia due to abnormal conditions of the birth canal and fetal dystocia due to unnatural conditions of the fetus. Arthur (1965) refers to fetal dystocia arising from failure of gestational orientation or failure of reflex disposition during early labour. Gestational defects comprise posterior or transverse presentation, lateral deviations of the head or neck and hyperflexion of the fore-legs. Dystocia due to failure of reflex disposition of the fetus may be caused by a relatively atonic uterus or an unresponsive fetus. It includes lateral and ventral position, lateral and downward deviation of the head and flexion of one or both fore-limbs. Vandeplassche et al. (1972) and Vandeplassche (1980) state that torsion of the uterus is responsible for 5–10% of all serious cases. But this condition is relatively uncommon among Thoroughbreds, where the most common causes of dystocia are hyperflexion (contracted fore-limbs) and ankylosis of the carpal or metacarpophalangeal joints. The causes of dystocia are summarized in Table 4.4.

Management

The immediate requirement is for early accurate diagnosis that birth is abnormal, followed by an assessment of the cause. Appropriate corrective measures must then be applied. It is essential to recognize normal birth to be able to judge abnormality. The main criteria of abnormality are:

1. The appearance of the chorio-allantois at the vulval lips at the start of the second stage.
2. Failure of the amnion to appear soon after the start of the second stage.
3. The absence of the fetal head and/or fore-limbs in the pelvic inlet at the beginning of the second stage.
4. Absence of straining for prolonged periods during the second stage.
5. Repeated shifting of position and rolling.
6. Straining without progressive delivery.
7. Obstructed fetal hips once the thorax has passed through the maternal pelvis.

Corrective procedures

Diagnosis and correction of abnormal fetal posture and position are best made with the mare standing, except after the fetal chest has passed through the pelvis. In the standing position, gravity causes the fetus to sink back into the uterus, away from the pelvic brim, and the force of the mare's straining is diminished. However, in malaligned fetal posture it may be necessary to abolish or reduce straining by having an attendant pull the mare's tongue forward, out of her mouth, epidural anaesthesia or the administration of muscle relaxants such as proquamezine fumarate. Epidural injections should be made in the first intercoccygeal space. The depression between the first and second coccygeal spines can usually be felt with the finger when the tail is raised, about 2.5 cm in front of the start of the tail hairs. Hall (1971) describes the location of the site as follows: a line drawn over the back joining the two hip joints, crossing the midline at the level of the sacrococcygeal joint. Immediately behind this may be felt the superior spine of the first coccygeal bone and the space immediately posterior to it is the site for the introduction of the needle. The site should be prepared and an insensitive skin weal produced. The depth of the neural canal from the surface is about 8 cm. The operator stands on the left side of the animal adjacent to the hind-limb. The point of the needle is inserted in the centre of the depression between the first and second coccygeal spines and pressed downwards at right angles to the general contour of the croup until the floor of the neural canal is struck. Sometimes it is possible to detect a popping sensation as the interarcual ligament is penetrated. The best evidence that the canal has been entered is the almost complete absence of resistance to the injection of the solution. In our experience about 8–10 ml of 2% procaine hydrochloride solution is sufficient and, indeed, it may be inadvisable to administer any greater quantity because of the risk of causing posterior paralysis.

To correct postural abnormalities, the fetus should, as far as possible, be pushed in an anterior direction to allow room for manipulation. It is sometimes helpful to apply a cord of soft, strong material to the extremities. The cord should have a loop at one end through which to pass the other end to snare the pastern, upper or lower jaws. The appendage may then be pulled towards the pelvic inlet while the operator places a hand on the fetal body and pushes it forward. If the head is presented and the limbs are in carpal flexion then the operator's hand should be placed on the head. If the fetus is presented anteriorly but is malpositioned,

TABLE 4.4 Causes of dystocia

Cause	*Origin*	*Diagnosis*	*Correction*
Malposture or congenital deformity	*a*. Carpal flexion of one or both forelegs	Absence of foot or feet in vagina. Presence of flexed carpi at pelvic inlet	Push back body and carpus, grasp foot and extend carpus
	b. Nape posture	Poll at or below pelvic inlet	Push back limbs and poll, grasp jaw, pulling upwards. Rope looped round lower jaw may be helpful
	c. Neck in lateral flexion	Absence of head at pelvic inlet	Push back limbs and body, grasp muzzle or jaw and pull towards pelvic inlet
	d. Elbow joint(s) extended, leg(s) backwards	Absence of limb in posterior part of uterus	Locate shoulder joint and follow upper part of limb in anterior direction. Push back fetus in posterior direction until limb in carpal flexion
	e. Tarsal flexion and metatarsophalangeal extension	Delivery impeded as thorax is emerging from vagina. Even strong traction fails to cause progress. Tip of toe(s) may be felt with difficulty on pubic brim	Rotate thorax and trunk in attempt to dislodge hind-limbs. Cross fore-legs and grasp withers and elbows to rotate. Measures must be firm, even vigorous
	f. Hyperflexion of fore-legs and ankylosis of carpal and/or metacarphophalangeal joints	As for *a*. Inability to extend fetlock joint	Mild cases, as for *a*. For severely affected individuals embryotomy or caesarean section

	g. Hyperflexion of hind-legs and ankylosis of tarsal and metatarsophalangeal joints	As for *a*	Mild cases as for *a*. For severely affected individuals embryotomy or caesarean section
	h. Wry neck	As for *c*	Caesarean section
	i. Grossly distended bladder	Obstructed delivery when chest is emerging from vagina. Must be differentiated from *e*	Open abdomen with guarded knife and release fluid
Malposition	*j*. Ventral oblique	Sole of fore-feet directed dorsally relative to maternal spine. True ventral position probably rare	Insert arm into uterus and assess optimum side to rotate. Grasp side of neck or head and apply force to rotate in appropriate direction
	k. Dorsal oblique, causing impacted shoulders and, in late second stage, fetal hips against maternal pelvis	Absence of progress in delivery despite straining efforts and traction applied to fore-legs	Rotate body as for *e* and *j*
Malpresentation	*l*. Posterior presentation	Absence of head at pelvic inlet. Hindl-legs identified by feeling hocks	Strong traction to effect speedy delivery. Foal will require resuscitation
Maternal dystocia	*m*. Uterine inertia and/or absence of voluntary straining	Prolonged second stage, undue delay with absence of straining	Assist by gentle but firm pull on fore-legs
	n. Uterine torsion	Signs of colic. Rectal palpation of uterine ligaments	Laparotomy in standing position. Pass hand into abdominal capacity through high flank incision

correction should be attempted by crossing the fore-legs and turning them in a clockwise or anticlockwise direction. The direction depends on the diagnosis of the position of the fetal vertebral column, e.g. if it is at four o'clock the rotation should be anticlockwise but if at eight o'clock it should be clockwise. The diagnosis is made by inserting the arm to establish the position of the withers and neck. These parts may be grasped to assist the movement.

Delivery may be obstructed by the fetal hips or by the hind-feet becoming lodged on the pubic brim. This malposture or malposition should be suspected if delivery is halted as the abdomen is emerging from the vagina and if strong traction at this time does not immediately complete delivery. There are severe risks to fetal survival in this situation because the umbilical cord becomes compressed and the fetus asphyxiated. Corrective measures should be swift. The arm should be 'forced' along the foal's abdomen and the maternal pubic brim located. If one or both fetal hind-feet are palpated an attempt should be made to push them forward. If the operator cannot do this, the foal should be rotated by crossing the fore-legs and grasping the withers and mane. Rotation should be first in one, then in the opposite direction.

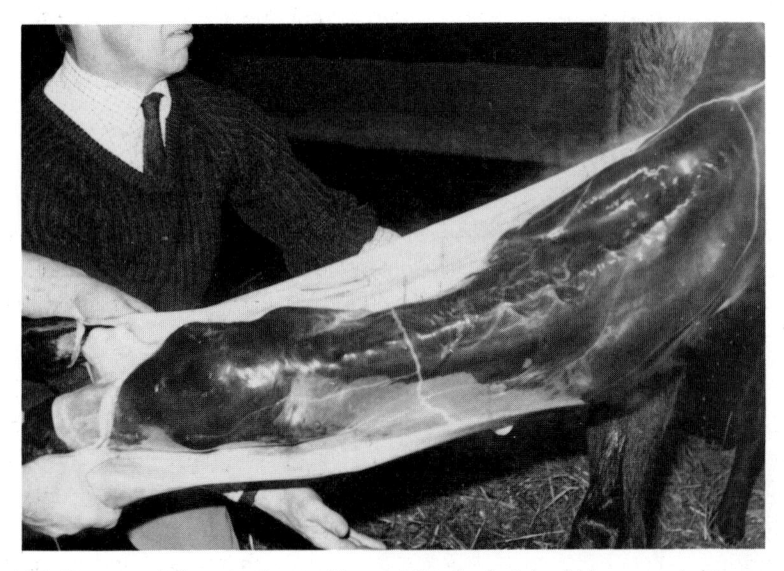

Fig. 4.35. If a mare delivers in the standing position the foal should be supported to prevent it falling.

Posterior presentation is rare; Merkt (1973, personal communication) surveyed 457 foalings and found two cases. It is identified by the presence of the hocks and tail at the pelvic inlet. The fetus should be delivered rapidly by strong traction on the hind-limbs because of the risk of compression of the cord as the thorax is delivered. Delivery is usually unimpeded although some rotation may be required to deliver the fetal hips. If delivered in posterior presentation, the fetus will almost certainly need resuscitating (see p. 331).

It may be necessary to correct minor postural deviations of the fore-legs and head as the chest passes through the maternal pelvis. The fore-limbs may become displaced so that they lie above the head. This posture does not usually impede delivery. It is common, during the first half of the second stage, for one fore-leg to become retarded so that the hoof comes to lie at the level of the knee of the opposite limb. Gentle manipulation of the retarded fore-limb should correct this, but if it cannot be done easily the mare should be made to get up. If she changes her position correction may follow easily.

Once the fetus is in the correct position and extended posture, delivery may be spontaneous. Assistance can be given by pulling on the fore-limbs and, as far as possible, the direction should be in the same plane as that of normal delivery, i.e. horizontally until the chest is engaged in the birth canal and then downwards in an arc directed towards the hocks.

About 5% of mares adopt the standing position for final delivery. Every effort should be made to encourage them to lie down; attendants should withdraw from the box, the lights should be extinguished or dimmed and noise reduced to a minimum. If, despite these measures, the mare is determined to deliver standing, some assistance should be given by pulling gently on the fore-limbs and supporting the foal to prevent it falling heavily on the ground (Fig. 4.35). If possible the cord should be allowed to remain intact until respiration has started.

Abnormal conditions associated with birth

Haemorrhage

Chronic or acute (usually fatal) maternal haemorrhage may occur in the first week after birth, most commonly within 24 hours of parturition. It may be internal, from the middle uterine artery or the utero-ovarian artery, or external, from the lining of the uterus or the wall of the vagina.

Internal haemorrhage from the utero-ovarian, middle uterine or external iliac arteries (Rooney 1964) is probably caused by a combination of factors. The blood vessels in the broad ligament are enlarged at full term and are under considerable tension during birth, the arterial walls may be affected by degenerative processes and it has been suggested that low blood copper levels are associated with fatal haemorrhage (Stowe 1968). Incidence increases with age and the mares most commonly affected are those over eight years. Acute pain, causing the mare to roll violently and sweat profusely, is characteristic. The signs may be masked by, and difficult to distinguish from, second- and third-stage labour. Diagnosis is confirmed by the persistence and intensity of signs. Uneasiness, rapid pulse and sweating after the placenta has been expelled suggest a haemorrhage. If it is severe the mucous membranes become pale and jaundice develops 24–48 hours later. At this time an oedematous swelling often appears in the perineal region on the side the haemorrhage has occurred. The packed cell volume may initially be raised or normal but fall to less than 0.3 litre/litre after 12 hours. On rectal palpation a large, firm swelling may be felt to one side of the midline extending from below the ovary towards the cervix. It is unwise to palpate the area immediately after birth in case this exacerbates the condition and at least two days should elapse before a rectal examination is performed.

The course of the condition depends on the quantity of blood escaping from the ruptured vessel. If the haemorrhage is contained within the peritoneal layers of the broad ligament the case does not usually end fatally. But sufficient blood may be lost to cause shock and profound anaemia (packed cell volume falling to less than 0.2 litre/litre). For several days after the haemorrhage has ceased the mare may be weak and, on suddenly raising the head, suffer from cerebral anaemia and fainting.

The condition is fatal if blood escapes into the peritoneal cavity. If standing, the mare staggers and falls to the ground, her membranes become blanched, the upper lip may be retracted and the body muscles affected by spasms. Death usually supervenes within minutes. Fatal haemorrhage may occur during delivery and the foal should, if possible, be extracted per vaginam and the cord severed. If the foal has not been partially delivered a rapid incision should be made through the flank and uterus and the foal removed by this route.

The treatment of chronic internal haemorrhage is aimed at reducing blood loss, combating shock, controlling pain and restoring circulating blood volume. Small doses of tranquillizing drugs help to reduce excitability that may precipitate further haemorrhages. Most tranquillizing drugs tend to reduce blood pressure and this is helpful, except where large volumes of blood have been lost or in shock. Pain-relieving drugs such as pethidine or hyoscine butylbromide should be administered intramuscularly. Intravenous or intramuscular oxytocin aids uterine involution. Corticosteroids help to combat shock. Intravenous administration of whole blood or dextran is the therapy of choice but, because of the large quantities necessary, this may be impractical. The total blood circulating volume of the mare is about 50 litres. Where only a small amount is lost, transfusion is unnecessary. If a larger amount is lost 15–20 litres of blood must be readily to hand.

The swelling caused by the haemorrhage and associated oedema may partially obstruct the pelvic cavity and make defaecation difficult. The intestinal contents may become dry due to loss of body fluid and it is therefore advisable to give a mixture of salt, water and liquid paraffin by stomach tube on the second and third days after haemorrhage.

The course of the case can be judged on packed cell volume, heart and respiratory rates, degree of jaundice and absence of painful signs. Exercise should be restricted until the packed cell volume is above 0.25 litre/litre.

External haemorrhage may occur from the vaginal wall due to haemorrhage from the posterior uterine artery or because of a haematoma. It is quite common to find a haematoma at the entrance to the vagina, due to bruising during second-stage labour. It may be seen and palpated as a red soft swelling of 3–4 cm in diameter, or may be an extensive area extending towards the cervix and bulging from between the vulval labiae. Occasionally the mucosal surface is lacerated and considerable, even fatal, loss of blood occurs, especially if a substantial branch of the posterior uterine artery is involved.

Contained haematomas should be treated by parenteral antibiotics and small doses of corticosteroids may control inflammation and reduce swelling. If the surface is broken the haemorrhage may be stopped by temporarily holding a cotton wool pad on the area, packing the 'wound' with sterile swabs (held in position by sutures) and ligating obvious bleeding points with catgut sutures. Bleeding is usually arrested without difficulty but in rare cases of rupture of a major vessel it may be necessary to explore the area surgically and to tie off the offending vessel. In some cases the point of haemorrhage may be too far forward to reach and bleeding continues until the mare dies.

Haemorrhage from the endometrium is not often severe. The placenta is non-deciduate, i.e. it does not erode the uterine surface, and therefore its separation does not normally cause bleeding. In some cases unusually large quantities of blood and blood-stained fluid are expelled from the uterus during the first two or three days after foaling. This may be associated with delay in uterine involution and the collecting of placental blood and fluid. True uterine bleeding occurs after manipulation and embryotomy of the fetus or manual removal of the placenta. It is not usually serious unless the uterus has been torn or infective metritis supervenes.

Hypocalcaemia

Hypocalcaemia is generally not recognized as occurring in mares after foaling. However, after the administration of calcium borogluconate many clinicians have recognized an improvement in the condition of mares that appear to have become involuntarily recumbent for long periods following parturition, especially those associated with dystocia or caesarean section.

Delayed uterine involution

The time the uterus takes to return to the non-pregnant size varies considerably. Within a few hours of expelling the placenta the uterus has normally contracted to about a quarter of its fully expanded state. By the seventh day post-partum the organ can be felt per rectum as a turgid mass about two or three times the size of that of a barren mare. In most cases the uterus of a foaling mare is relatively enlarged until 30–60 days post-partum and in some individuals considerably longer. The definition of delayed involution therefore rests on subjective observation. Histological confirmation can be obtained by endometrial biopsy. A voluminous uterus with little tone and a dilated cervix at the foal heat may be abnormal and certainly is if found after 30 days post-partum. Delayed involution may be associated with a depressed position of the cervix so that, on vaginal examination, the cervix is viewed at an angle below the horizontal. This condition is often accompanied by pooling of urine and fluid on the vaginal floor. Delayed uterine involution follows retained placenta, abortion, dystocia and placentitis. Signs include uterine discharge and in some cases, especially in the first two to three days post-partum, dullness, inappetence and mild pain.

The treatment of delayed uterine involution is the intravenous administration of 60 IU of oxytocin in 500 ml of saline over one hour, repeated daily until normal uterine size and tone are restored. Exercise helps to evacuate the uterine contents.

Antibiotics may be administered prophylactically by the parenteral and intrauterine routes. See also Chapter 1.

Post-parturient metritis

Bacterial or, less commonly, mycotic infection of the uterus may follow delayed involution, haemorrhage, dystocia, retained placenta or uterine prolapse. Dust-contaminated air may enter the uterus after foaling, especially if the mare gets to her feet with the placenta still in situ.

Signs are similar to those of delayed involution but in severe cases may be accompanied by general malaise, laminitis and fever. Less severe cases develop a uterine discharge and show little or no general signs.

Treatment should consist of parenteral and intrauterine administration of antibiotics selected after laboratory examination of the organism present in the uterus. Injections of oxytocin and exercise are recommended.

Uterine prolapse

Uterine prolapse may occur post-partum or, less commmonly, post-abortion; parturition may be normal or abnormal. The incidence is small (Benesch & Wright 1950) and few reports of the condition are available in the literature (Brewer & Kliest 1963). The condition affects primi- and multiparous mares.

Diagnosis is on the presence of the prolapsed organ hanging from the vagina as a soft mass with a red corrugated surface. As soon as the prolapse occurs attendants should attempt to keep the mare standing pending veterinary help. A large warm wet towel or sheet may be wrapped around the organ to protect and support it.

Epidural anaesthesia or a muscle relaxant such as proquamezine fumerate should be administered to reduce straining. It may help to tranquillize the mare with acetylpromazine or a similar drug. Tetanus antitoxin serum and oxytocin 50 IU should be administered intramuscularly; corticosteroids may be used to combat shock and parenteral antibiotics given as a prophylactic measure.

The uterus should be washed with warm, normal saline and massaged gently but firmly towards the pelvic outlet. Initially, replacement is easier with the mare recumbent, but once the majority of the organ has been replaced, gravity may have more effect if the mare is standing. Great care must be taken not to push a finger through the uterus when attempting to replace it. This is especially important if the endometrium is becoming friable.

Once the organ has been replaced, several tape sutures may be inserted in the vulval labiae to prevent another complete prolapse. Further oxytocin and sedatives during the following 24 hours may help to prevent another prolapse.

The prognosis for future breeding is good if the replacement is uncomplicated and the condition does not usually occur at subsequent parturitions. Fatal complications include rupture of the uterus and prolapse of the intestines, haemorrhage from one of the uterine arteries and oedema of the uterus preventing replacement of the organ.

Uterine rupture

Uterine rupture is uncommon but when it occurs early in the second stage it may cause uterine inertia and reduce or abolish voluntary straining. Diagnosis can be made only after birth, if the opening is palpated through the cervix or if the intestines prolapse through the vagina. In the latter event surgical intervention is required and the tear should be repaired under general anaesthesia, through a laparotomy wound. Minor tears should be treated as for delayed involution.

Rupture of the caecum and colon

Rupture of the large intestine during first and second stage is followed by reduced straining efforts and signs of shock (sweating, trembling, depression, rapid heart rate and fever). Voss (1969) suggests that it may be caused by large amounts of feed offered before parturition.

Fracture of the femur or pelvic bones

Accidents may occur if a mare slips or does the splits in getting to her feet while the fetus is half delivered. Such cases invariably have to be slaughtered on humane grounds. The floor of the foaling box should be of a non-slip variety and attendants should not make a mare get to her feet once delivery has progressed beyond the fetal head.

Uterine torsion

Vandeplassche et al. (1972) reported that 5–10% of all serious dystocias in the mare are due to uterine torsion, usually in an anticlockwise direction. Other workers have not found this. Day (1972) encountered only three cases. Uterine torsion should, however, be considered in cases of severe colic during late pregnancy. Diagnosis is made by rectal examination of the uterine ligaments (Vandeplassche et al. 1972). Wheat and Meagher (1972) described five cases in which the direction of torsion was clockwise. In two mares the uterus ruptured, allowing the fetus to escape into the abdominal cavity. Laparotomy is the optimal therapy to save the mare and fetus (Vandeplassche et al. 1961). The operation is performed with the mare standing in stocks; she is under epidural and local infiltration anaesthesia and tranquillization. A high flank incision is made and a hand passed into the abdominal cavity to rotate the uterus. At term, manual reposition through the cervix is recommended. When this is not possible a caesarean operation should be undertaken.

Uterine retroflection

Vandeplassche (1980) described this condition in 18 mares who showed signs of severe colic near term. Rectal palpation revealed a live foal, in the posture of birth, in the pelvic canal. The fetus could be easily pushed cranially into the abdominal cavity but this increased the severity of colic symptoms and the fetus rapidly regained the intrapelvic position. Vandeplassche reports that 200 mg of isoxsuprine lactate, a smooth muscle relaxant, injected intramuscularly at intervals, relieved the colic symptoms and allowed the fetus to return to the cranial inlet of the pelvic canal. Normal parturition then followed.

Perineal lacerations

Lacerations are classified according to their severity. First-degree are superficial and involve the vaginal and vulval mucous membranes; second-degree involve the vaginal wall and vulva; third-degree tears penetrate the rectum causing a fistula; and fourth-degree lacerations form a common opening with the vagina and rectum (cloaca).

Surgical repair of errors in vulval and perineal conformation, perineal lacerations and rectovaginal fistula have been described by Bemis (1930), Caslick (1937), Straub and Fowler (1961) and Aanes (1964).

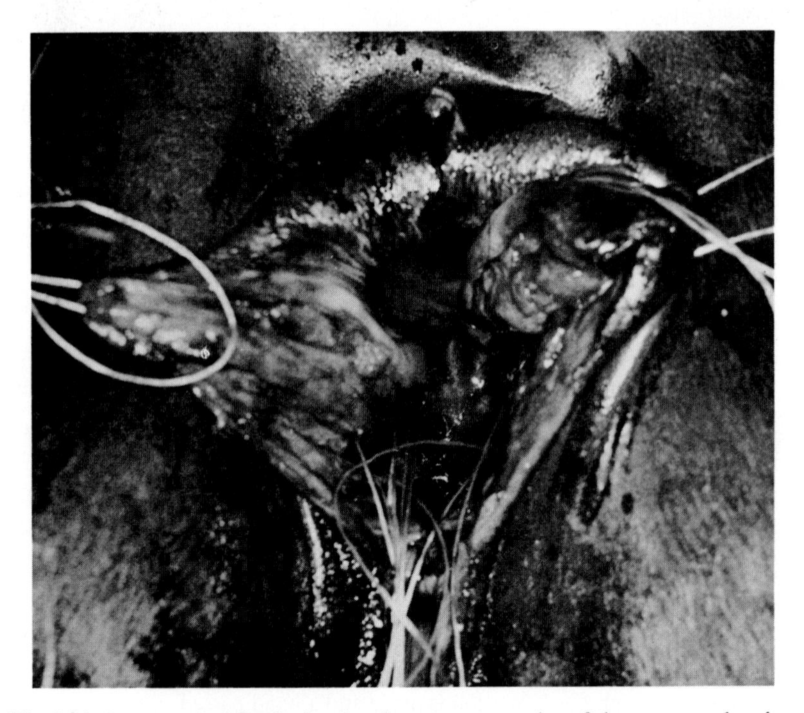

Fig. 4.36. A rectovaginal fistula showing the common opening of the rectum and vagina.

Rectovaginal fistulas may be caused by the foal's foot being driven through the vaginal roof in the early part of second stage. If not corrected immediately the head may follow and a common opening between the rectum and vagina result (Fig. 4.36). Repair is often difficult because of faecal matter penetrating the rectal fascia and establishing a fistula to the vagina.

Aanes (1964) described a two-phase operation for third-degree perineal lacerations (rectovaginal fistula). A shelf of tissue is constructed between the rectum and vagina and the perineal area between anal sphincter and dorsal commissure of the vulva is allowed to remain open. A second operation is performed on the perineal area when the shelf has healed. Modified operations include inserting a sheet of inert water-repellent material beneath the rectal mucosa which is left unsutured. The sheet is removed after a week (Fig. 4.37) (Peace 1973, personal communication).

Geering (1979) has suggested the use of a temporary colostomy to allow the immediate repair of rectovaginal fistulas, without postoperative faecal contamination of the surgical site in order to minimize faecal contamination of the uterus before operation.

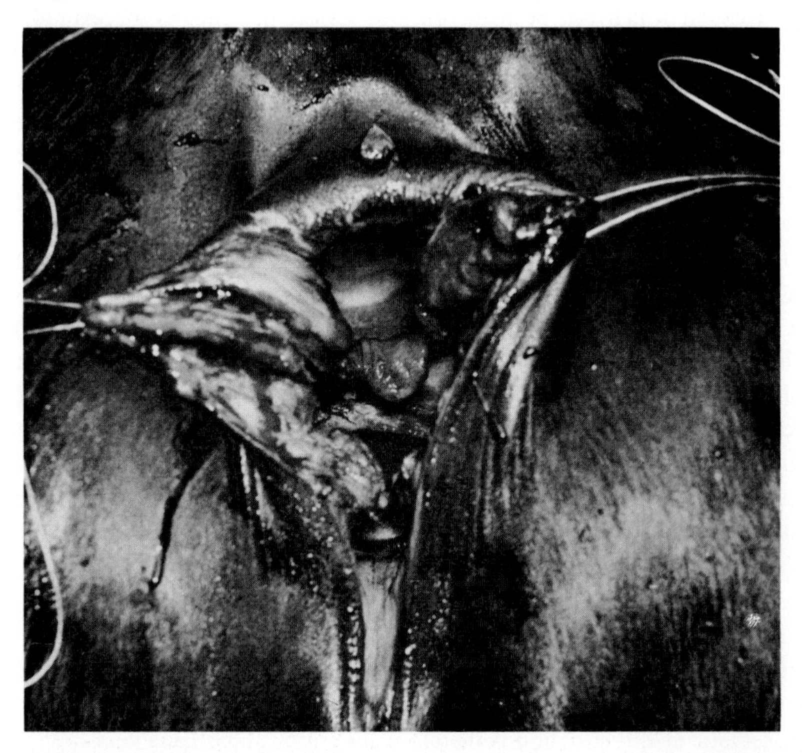

Fig. 4.37. The repair of a rectovaginal fistula, showing the sutures to take the sailcloth which will be stitched in position below the rectum and removed at the end of one week. For details see text.

CAESAREAN SECTION VERSUS EMBRYOTOMY

If a realignment of the fetal parts is impossible the clinician is faced with the decision of whether to perform an embryotomy or a caesarean section. Much will depend on the experience of the operator and the facilities available.

Embryotomy in the hands of a skilled person provides a relatively simple opportunity to dismember the fetus and deliver it part by part. The disadvantage is that, even with the greatest care, the mare's cervix and uterus may be damaged by the wire used for cutting or by bony projections from the dismembered fetus. Injuries to the genital tract may cause permanent infertility. Embryotomy is considered only if a fetus is dead or so severely deformed as to be not worth saving.

In considering caesarean section, the clinician may wish to try first an intermediate course, namely to anaesthetize the mare and restrain her on the operating table and to attempt to manipulate the fetus for delivery per vaginam. This manoeuvre is sometimes successful, especially if the surface of the operating table can be tilted so that the fetus may be fixed whilst the mare is rotated. Another manoeuvre which may be helpful is to tilt the table so that the fetus is drawn away from the pelvis for the purpose of re-alignment. However, the decision as to how delivery should be accomplished – embryotomy, traction, or caesarean section – is a judgement which can be made only by experience and its success judged in retrospect. If the operator decides not to perform a caesarean section and the fetus becomes lodged in the birth canal, the decision not to operate will have serious consequences. On the other hand, the performance of a caesarean section when the fetus could be delivered under general anaesthesia through the birth canal obviously subjects the mare to different but none-the-less serious risks.

Caesarean section poses less risk to future fertility. It is relatively safe and simple with modern anaesthetics and antibiotics. It has the advantage that the fetus can be delivered alive, although the chances of survival are small if a mare has been in the second stage for long. The disadvantage of caesarean section is that it requires a surgical team and a dust-free area in which to perform the operation (although many successful caesareans have been carried out by practitioners working with unskilled assistants and in far from ideal conditions). The procedure is not without surgical risks to the mare. Vandeplassche et al. (1972) recorded maternal mortality of 12 of 63 caesarean sections. Death was due to postoperative haemorrhage, peritonitis, shock, sacroiliac fracture or infection. Maternal mortality after embryotomy was 13 of 127.

Caesarean section has been reviewed by Roberts (1971). Indications are malposture and malposition causing dystocia which cannot be corrected by manipulation. It is unusual for an elective caesarean section to be performed and death of the fetus has usually occurred before a decision to operate is reached. The type of anaesthetic in this situation is therefore not critical. Fluothane inhalation anaesthesia, following induction by intravenous thiopentone and premedication, is preferred. If the fetus is alive care should be taken to ensure adequate maternal ventilation from the moment anaesthesia is induced since long periods of maternal apnoea may cause fetal hypoxia. An alternative method of anaesthesia is the use of epidural combined with low level narcosis by chloral hydrate and glyceryl guaiacolate (Vandeplassche et al. 1972).

A variety of incision sites has been used successfully in the mare. The most popular is that used by Vandeplassche and known as the 'Marsenac approach'. This extends 25–40 cm from the middle of the last rib on the left flank caudally and ventrally towards the stifle. Other incision sites include the upper left flank, left paramedian or midline. Operations in the right flank area are complicated by the caecum. Roberts (1971) considers that incision of the uterus should be on its greatest curvature, over a fetal prominence.

If the placenta comes away easily it should be removed, otherwise it should be left in situ to be expelled per vaginam. Diffuse bleeding may occur from the uterine submucosa and Vandeplassche recommends that a continuous suture of catgut should be placed around the uterine incision and through the endometrium, submucosa and serosa, taking care not to include the placenta. This suture is then inverted into the uterine cavity by a double row of Lembert sutures. The peritoneum, muscle and fascial layers of the abdominal wall should be sutured separately with strong chromic catgut and the skin incision closed with non-absorbent nylon sutures.

Aftercare should include tetanus antitoxin, oxytocin and broad-spectrum antibiotics.

A method for elective caesarean section in the mare, used for the production of gnotobiotic foals, has been described by Edwards et al. (1974). Their timing was based on the average gestation period for the stud farm during the previous years. In order to minimize the depressant effect on the foal, anaesthesia was with methohexitone sodium at a dose rate of 1 g/200 kg body weight. Anaesthesia was maintained with halothane and oxygen via an endotracheal tube and the plane of anaesthesia was maintained as low as possible throughout the operation. A flank approach was made because of better attachment and access to the surgical isolator. A cranioventral abdominal incision was made low in the left flank, 12 cm behind and parallel with the last rib. On entering the abdominal cavity, the part of the uterus adjacent to the foal's hocks was located and brought to the incision. It was then carefully incised along its greatest curvature, avoiding large vessels where possible, and the foal was delivered in posterior presentation. The foal was resuscitated as necessary and the umbilical cord was left intact until the arterial pulse was no longer palpable and, whenever possible, until the foal was breathing spontaneously. Before closing the uterus, the chorio-allantois was separated for 5 cm from the margin of the uterine incision and a continuous haemostatic suture of No. 1 plain catgut placed around the entire margin. This technique is indicated because the equine endometrium is only loosely attached to the myometrium and the large plexus of intervening veins makes venous bleeding a serious problem. The technique consists of a simple over-and-over pattern penetrating the three layers of the uterus. Closure of the uterine incision was accomplished with a single Cushing suture using No. 3 chromic catgut. The flank incision was closed in three layers. The peritoneum and aponeurosis of the transversalis muscle was closed with a continuous horizontal mattress suture using No. 3 chromic catgut and the oblique muscles and abdominal tunic with simple interrupted sutures of the same material. The skin and subcutaneous muscles were closed using vertical mattress sutures of braided nylon. Fourteen elective caesarean sections were performed by this method on 12 mares at a mean gestational age of 323 days: 11 foals were reared successfully and 13 mares made uneventful recoveries. The remaining mare suffered uterine prolapse and dehiscence of the abdominal incision, 72 hours postoperatively, during violent abdominal straining. The main complication seen was retention of the placenta which was retained for a mean of 29 hours. Severe metritis and laminitis did not develop in these mares. Uterine prolapse occurred on three occasions and in these cases retention of the placenta was involved. Postoperative skin wound infection occurred in three cases but this was simply treated by removal of the skin sutures and the provision of adequate drainage. The authors conclude that their technique was designed for use with elective surgery to produce a live fetus into a specialized surgical isolator. In field cases, where caesarean section is indicated, the foal is often already dead and then the choice of anaesthetic is not critical. They also suggest that a ventral midline approach may be preferable because of easy entry to the abdominal cavity, ready access to the uterus and less postoperative swelling.

References and further reading

Aanes, W.A. (1964) Surgical repair of third-degree perineal laceration and rectovaginal fistula in the mare. *J. Am. vet. med. Ass.*, **144**, 485.

Adams, W.M. & Wagner, W.C. (1970) Role of corticosteroids in parturition. *Biol. Reprod.*, **3**, 223.

Allen, W.E., Chard, T. & Forsling, M.E. (1973) Peripheral plasma levels of oxytocin and vasopressin in the mare during parturition. *J. Endocr.*, **57**, 175.

Alm, C.C., Sullivan, J.J. & First, N.L. (1974) Induction of premature parturition by parenteral administration of dexamethasone in the mare. *J. Am. vet. med. Ass.*, **165**, 721.

Arthur, G.H. (1965) A rational veterinary approach to equine parturition. *Proc. 4th ann. Congr. Br. equine vet. Ass.*, 3.

Arthur, G.H. (1975) *Veterinary Reproduction and Obstetrics*, 4th ed. London: Baillière Tindall.

Asdell, S.A. (1946) *Patterns of Mammalian Reproduction.* New York: Comstock.

Atkins, D.T., Sorensen, A.M. & Fleeger, J.L. (1974) 5-Dihydroneprogesterone in the pregnant mare. *J. Anim. Sci.*, **39**, 196A.

Barnes, R.J., Comline, R.S., Jeffcott, L.B., Mitchell, M.D., Rossdale, P.D. & Silver, M. (1978) Foetal and maternal plasma concentrations of 13,14 dihydro-15-oxo prostaglandin F in the mare during late preganncy and at parturition. *J. Endocr.*, **78**, 201.

Barnes, R.J., Nathanielsz, P.W., Rossdale, P.D., Comline, R.S. & Silver, M. (1975) Plasma progestagens and oestrogens in fetus and mother in late pregnancy. *J. Reprod. Fert.*, Suppl. **23**, 617.

Bemis, H.E. (1930) A new operation for rectovaginal fistula. *N. Am. Vet.*, **11**, 37.

Benesch, F. & Wright, J.G. (1950) *Veterinary Obstetrics.* London: Baillière Tindall & Cox.

Brewer, R.L. & Kliest, G.J. (1963) Uterine prolapse in the mare. *J. Am. vet. med. Ass.*, **142**, 1118.

Britton, J.W. (1963) Breeding farm practices. In *Equine Medicine and Surgery,* ed. E.J. Catcott & J.F. Smithcors, p. 649. Wheaton, I11.: American Veterinary Publications.

Britton, J.W. (1972) Discussion of elective induction of labor and parturition in the mare. *Proc. 18th ann. Conv. Am. Ass. equine Practnrs,* 116.

Burns, S.J., Judge, N.G., Martin, J.E. & Adams, L.G. (1977) Management of retained placenta in mares. *Proc. 23rd ann. Conv. Am. Ass. equine Practnrs,* 381.

Campbell, D.L. (1971) Corticosteroids in the first trimester of pregnant mares. *SWest. Vet.*, 103.

Caslick, E.A. (1937) The vulva and vulvo-vaginal orifice and its relation to genital health of the Thoroughbred mare. *Cornell Vet.*, **27**, 178.

Coceani, F., Olley, P.M. & Bodach, E. (1976) Prostaglandins: a possible regulator of muscle tone in the ductus arteriosus. *Adv. Prostaglandin Res.*, **1**, 417.

Comline, R.S., Hall, L.W., Lavelle, R. & Silver, M. (1975) The use of intravascular catheters for long term studies on the mare and foetus. *J. Reprod. Fert.*, Suppl. **23**, 583.

Davies, J. & Ryan K.J. (1972) Comparative endocrinology of gestation. *Vitam. Hormones,* **30**, 223.

Day, F.T. (1972) In discussion of Vandeplassche et al. (1972).

Drost, M. (1972) Failure to induce parturition in pony mares with dexamethasone. *J. Am. vet. med. Ass.*, **160**, 321.

Drost, M. & Holm, L.W. (1968) Prolonged gestation in ewes after foetal adrenalectomy. *J. Endocr.*, **40**, 293.

Edwards, G.B., Allen, W.E. & Newcombe, J.R. (1974) Elective Caesarean section in the mare for the production of gnotobiotic foals. *Equine vet. J.*, **6**, 122.

Ellwood, D.A., Mitchell, M.D., Anderson, A.B.M. & Turnbull, A.C. (1979) Prostaglandins and cervical ripening during parturition in the sheep. *Acta endocr.*, Suppl. **225**, 117.

Fleming, G. (1878) *A Textbook of Veterinary Obstetrics*, p. 209. London: Baillière.

Flint, A.P.F., Ricketts, A.P.F. & Craig, V.A. (1979) The control of placental steroid synthesis at parturition in domestic animals. *Anim. Reprod. Sci.*, **2**, 239.

Forsyth, I.A., Rossdale, P.D. & Thomas, C.R. (1975) Studies on milk composition and lactogenic hormones in the mare. *J. Reprod. Fert.*, Suppl. **23**, 631.

Fraser, A.F., Hastie, H., Callicott, R.B. & Brownlie, S. (1975) An exploratory ultrasonic study on quantitative foetal kinesis in the horse. *Appl. Anim. Ethol.*, **1**, 395.

Gaudry, R. & Glen, W.L. (1959) Sur la fraction steroide de l'urine de la jument gravide. *Étud. belge*, Suppl. **2**, 435.

Geering, R.R. (1979) An alternative approach to treatment of recto-vaginal fistula. *18th ann. Congr. Br. equine vet. Ass., Exeter.*

Hall, L.W. (1971) *Wright's Veterinary Anaesthesia and Analgesia*, 7th ed. London: Baillière Tindall.

Hillman, R.B. (1975) Induction of parturition in mares. *J. Reprod. Fert.*, Suppl. **23**, 641.

Hillman, R.B. & Ganjam, V.K. (1979) Hormonal changes in the mare and foal associated with oxytocin induction of parturition. *J. Reprod. Fert.*, Suppl. **27**, 541.

Holtan, D.W., Nett, T.M. & Estergreen, V.L. (1975) Plasma progestins in pregnant post partum and cycling mares. *J. Anim. Sci.*, **40**, 251.

Howell, L.E. & Rollins, W.C. (1951) Environmental sources of variation in the gestation length of the horse. *J. Anim. Sci.*, **10**, 789.

Jeffcott, L.B. (1972) Observations on parturition in Crossbred pony mares. *Equine vet. J.*, **4**, 209.

Jeffcott, L.B. & Rossdale, P.D. (1977) A critical review of current methods of induction of parturition in the mare. *Equine vet. J.*, **9**, 208.

Jeffcott, L.B. & Rossdale, P.D. (1979) A radiographic study of the foetus in late pregnancy and during foaling. *J. Reprod. Fert.*, Suppl. **27**, 563.

Klug, E. & von Lepel, J.D. (1974) Possibilities of initiating normal birth in the mare with oxytocin. *Dt. tierarztl. Wschr.*, **81**, 349.

Liggins, G.C. (1969) Premature delivery of foetal lambs infused with glucocorticoids. *J. Endocr.*, **45**, 515.

Liggins, G.C. (1979) Initiation of parturition. *Br. med. Bull.*, **35**, 145.

Liggins, G.C., Forster, C.S., Grieves, S.A. & Schwartz, A.L. (1977) Control of parturition in man. *Biol. Reprod.*, **16**, 39.

Liggins, G.C., Ritterman, J.A. & Forster, C.S. (1979) Foetal maturation related to parturition. *Anim. Reprod. Sci.*, **2**, 193.

Lovell, J.D., Stabenfeldt, G.H., Hughes, J.P. & Evans, J.W. (1975) Endocrine patterns of the mare at term. *J. Reprod. Fert.*, Suppl. **23**, 449.

Moss, G.E., Estergreen, V.L., Becker, S.R. & Grant, B.D. (1979) The source of the 5α-pregnanes that occur during gestation in mares. *J. Reprod. Fert.*, Suppl. **27**, 511.

Nathanielsz, P.W., Rossdale, P.D., Silver, M. & Comline, R.S. (1975) Studies on foetal, neonatal and maternal cortisol metabolism in the mare. *J. Reprod. Fert.*, Suppl. **23**, 625.

Nett, T.M., Holtan, D.W. & Estergreen, V.L. (1973) Plasma estrogens in pregnant mares. *J. Anim. Sci.*, **37**, 962.

Pashen, R.L. (1980) Low doses of oxytocin can induce foaling at term. *Equine vet. J.*, **12**, 85.

Pashen, R.L. & Allen, W.R. (1979*a*) Endocrine changes after foetal gonadectomy and during normal and induced parturition in the mare. *Anim. Reprod. Sci.*, **2**, 271.

Pashen, R.L. & Allen, W.R. (1979*b*) The role of the foetal gonads and placenta in steroid production, maintenance of pregnancy and parturition in the mare. *J. Reprod. Fert.*, Suppl. **27**, 499.

Pashen, R.L. & Allen, W.R. (1980) The role of prostaglandins in parturition in the mare. *Acta vet. scand.*, in the press,

Peaker, M., Rossdale, P.D., Forsyth, I.A. & Falk, M. (1979) Changes in mammary development and the composition of secretion during late pregnancy in the mare. *J. Reprod. Fert.*, Suppl. **27**, 555.

Purvis, A.D. (1972) Elective induction of labour and parturition in the mare. *Proc. 18th ann. Conv. Am. Ass. equine Practnrs,* 113.

Roberts, S.J. (1971) *Veterinary Obstetrics and Genital Diseases.* Ann Arbor, Mich.: Edwards.

Rooney, J.R. (1964) Internal haemorrhage related to gestation in the mare. *Cornell Vet.,* **54**, 11.

Rossdale, P.D. (1967) Clinical studies on the newborn Thoroughbred foal. I. Perinatal behaviour. *Br. vet. J.,* **123**, 470.

Rossdale, P.D. & Jeffcott, L.B. (1975) Problems encountered during induced foaling in pony mares. *Vet. Rec.,* **97**, 371.

Rossdale, P.D., Jeffcott, L.B. & Allen, W.R. (1976) Foaling produced by a synthetic prostaglandin analogue (fluoprostenol) to induce foaling. *J. Reprod. Fert.,* Suppl. **27**, 521.

Rossdale, P.D., Pashen, R.L. & Jeffcott, L.B. (1979) The use of synthetic prostaglandin analogue (fluprostenol) to induce foaling. *J. Reprod. Fert.,* Suppl. **27**, 521.

Rossdale, P.D. & Short, R.V. (1967) The time of foaling of Thoroughbred mares. *J. Reprod. Fert.,* **13**, 341.

Rossdale, P.D., Silver, M., Comline, R.S., Hall, L.W. & Nathanielsz, P.W. (1973) Plasma cortisol in the foal during the late foetal and early neonatal period. *Res. vet. Sci.,* **15**, 395.

Scholl, S.A., Robinson, J.A. & Wolf, R.C. (1979) Progesterone and 5α-pregnane-3,20-dione in serum of peripartum rhesus monkeys. *Endocrinology,* **104**, 329.

Silver, M., Barnes, R.J., Comline, R.S., Fowden, A.L., Clover, L. & Mitchell, M.D. (1979) Prostaglandins in maternal and foetal plasma and in allantoic fluid during the second half of gestation in the mare. *J. Reprod. Fert.,* Suppl. **27**, 531.

Stowe, H.D. (1968) Effects of age and impending parturition upon serum copper of Thoroughbred mares. *J. Nutr.,* **95**, 179.

Straub, O.C. & Fowler, M.E. (1961) Repair of perineal lacerations in the mare and cow. *J. Am. vet. med. Ass.,* **138**, 659.

Thorburn, G.D., Challis, J.R.G. & Currie, W.B. (1977) Control of parturition in domestic animals. *Biol. Reprod.,* **16**, 18.

Tyler, S.J. (1972) The behaviour and social organisation of the New Forest ponies. *Anim. Behav. Monogr.,* **5**, 2.

Vandeplassche, M. (1957) The normal and abnormal presentation, position and posture of the foal-fetus during gestation and at parturition. *Meded. VeeartSch. Rijksuniv., Gent,* **1**, 36 (Suppl. *Vlaams Diergeneesk. Tijdschr.,* **7**, 26).

Vandeplassche, M. (1980) Obstetricians' views of the physiology of equine parturition and dystocia. *Equine vet. J.,* **12**, 45.

Vandeplassche, M., Paredis, F. & Bouters, R. (1961) Flanksnede bij de rechtstaande of neerliggende merrie voor het ontdraaien van torsio uteri. *Vlaams Diergeneesk. Tijdschr.,* **30**, 1.

Vandeplassche, M., Spincemaille, J. & Bouters, R. (1971) Aetiology, pathogenesis and treatment of retained placenta in the mare. *Equine vet. J.,* **3**, 144.

Vandeplassche, M., Spincemaille, J., Bouters, R. & Bonte, P. (1972) Some aspects of equine obstetrics. *Equine vet. J.,* **4**, 105.

Van Niekerk, C.H. & Morgenthal, J.C. (1976) Plasma progesterone and oestrogen concentrations during induction of parturition with flumethasone and prostaglandin. *Proc. 8th ann. Congr. Anim. Reprod. artif. Insem.,* **3**, 1114.

Voss, J.L. (1969) Rupture of the caecum and ventral colon of mares during parturition. *J. Am. med. Ass.,* **155**, 745.

Wheat, J.D. & Meagher, D.M. (1972) Uterine torsion and rupture in mares. *J. Am. vet. med. Ass.,* **160**, 881.

Wright, J.G. (1943) Parturition in the mare. *J. comp. Path.,* **53**, 212.

Zwolinski, J. & Siudinski, S. (1965) Dobowy rozklad wyzrebien u klaczy. *Medycyna wet.,* **21**, 614.

The Adaptive Period 5

Successful adaptation to the extrauterine environment is based on certain physiological changes. These may be anatomical (e.g. closure of the ductus arteriosus and foramen ovale (Figs 5.1, 5.2); functional (expansion of the lungs with air); or biochemical (associated with newly acquired characteristics of alimentation and increased metabolism).

Clinicians recognize underlying physiological alterations by corresponding changes in behaviour, breathing movements, heart rate, rectal temperature and laboratory measurements of haematology and blood biochemistry.

The adjustment does not affect each body system to the same extent; for instance, cardiopulmonary adaptation involves the most dramatic change and forms the basis on which further adjustment depends. We cannot be precise about when the adaptive period ends; for some purposes it is at weaning time, for others when the skeleton is fully mature. In the present context adaptation refers to the first four days after birth, by which time the major physiological changes are over and any associated signs of maladjustment have appeared. During this period clinicians are faced with shifting base-lines against which to measure findings. For example, in the first half hour after birth normal respiratory rate is double that at age 12 hours and mean levels of blood pH rise from 7.260 to 7.376. Before discussing the abnormal it is appropriate, therefore, to consider first the clinical status of the normal foal; a summary of the major features of change that can be recognized by the clinician is provided in Fig. 5.3.

THE NORMAL NEWBORN FOAL

The mare's final expulsive effort delivers the foal so that it is lying on its side with the hind-legs to the level of the hocks still in the vagina and the cord intact (Fig. 5.4). Exceptions include delivery in the standing position or if the mare rises to her feet immediately after delivery. Also, the mare's final expulsive effort (perhaps aided by an attendant pulling on the fore-legs of the foal) may completely deliver the hind-legs and rupture the cord.

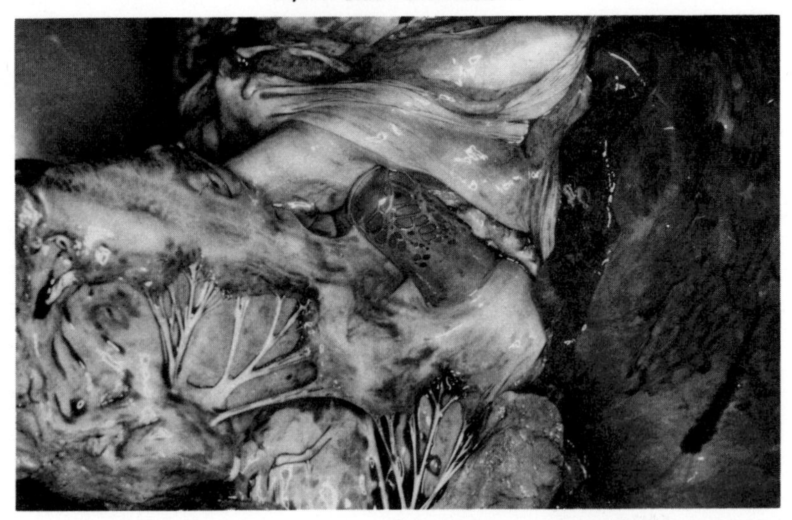

Fig. 5.1. The left ventricle of a newborn foal opened to show the foramen ovale into which a test tube has been inserted through the vena cava. The AV valves can be seen (bottom left) and the left lung with apical lobe removed (right).

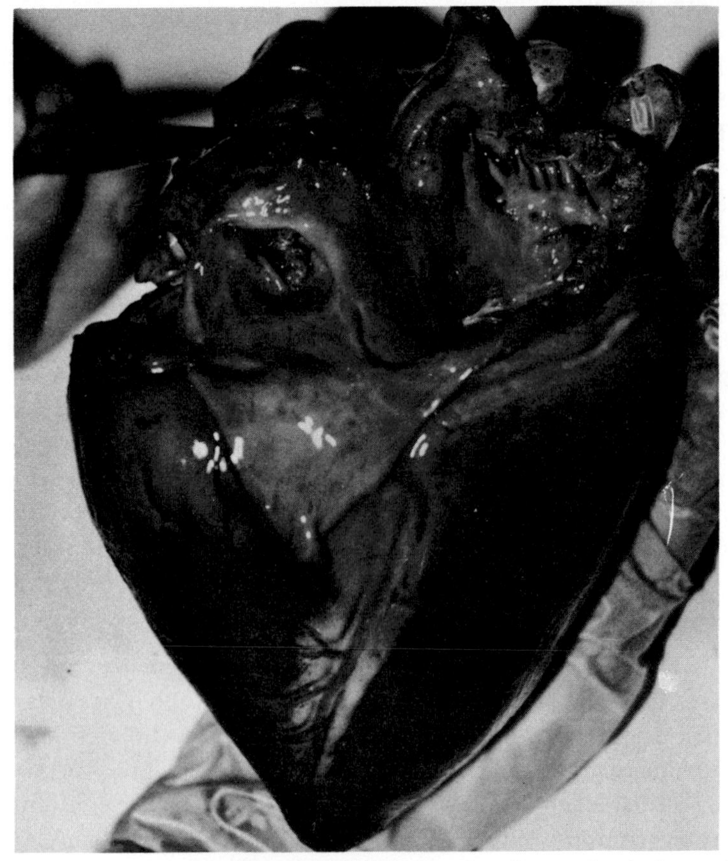

Fig. 5.2. The right atrium of a seven-day-old foal opened to show a cicatrized area of closed foramen ovale (below point of forceps).

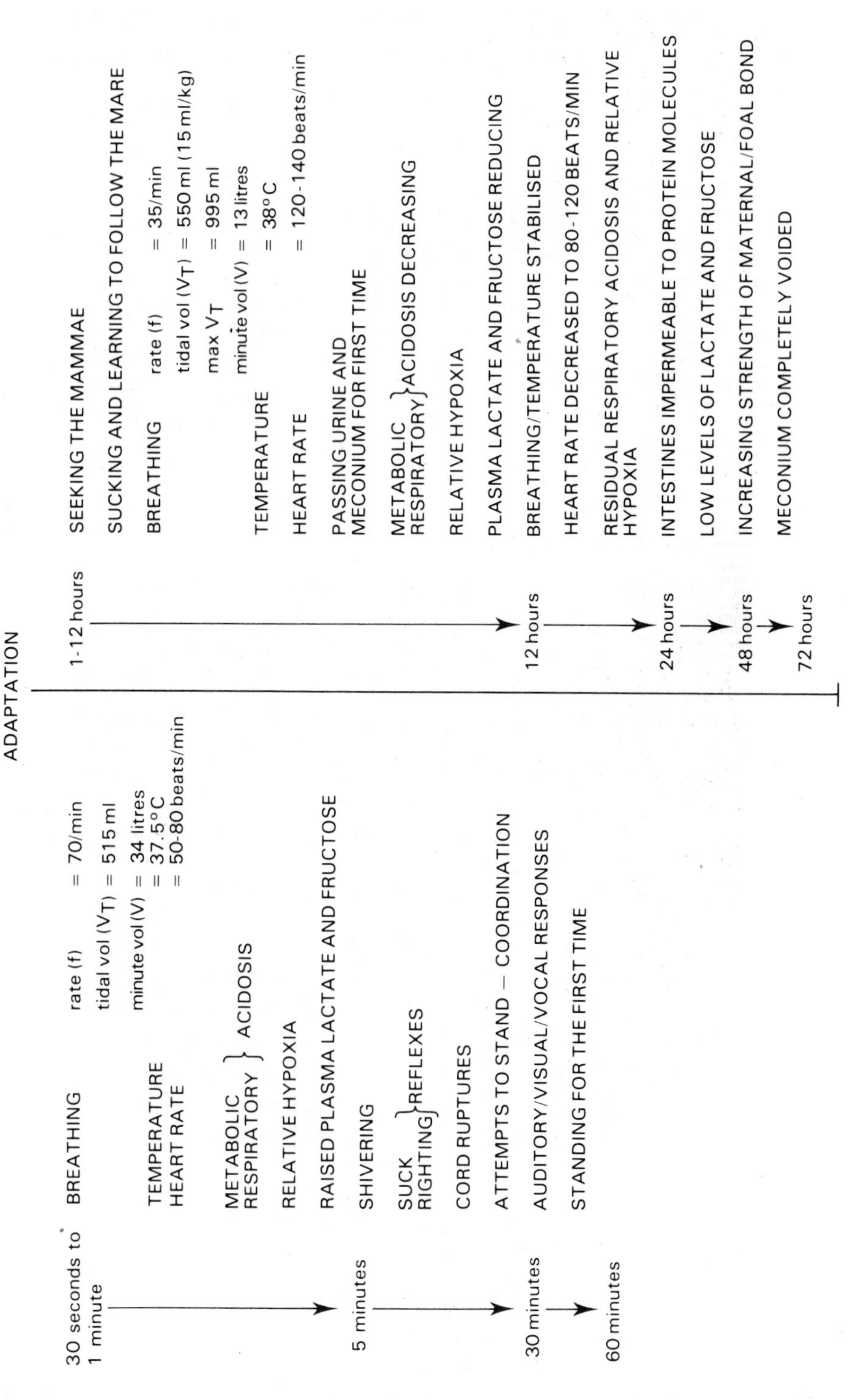

Fig. 5.3. Summary of changes in the early adaptive period (mean values or ranges).

Breathing rhythm

Respiratory movements of the abdomen and chest start within 30 seconds of final delivery and may be preceded by a series of gasps accompanied by arching of the neck. The amnion is normally broken by opposing movements of the fore-legs

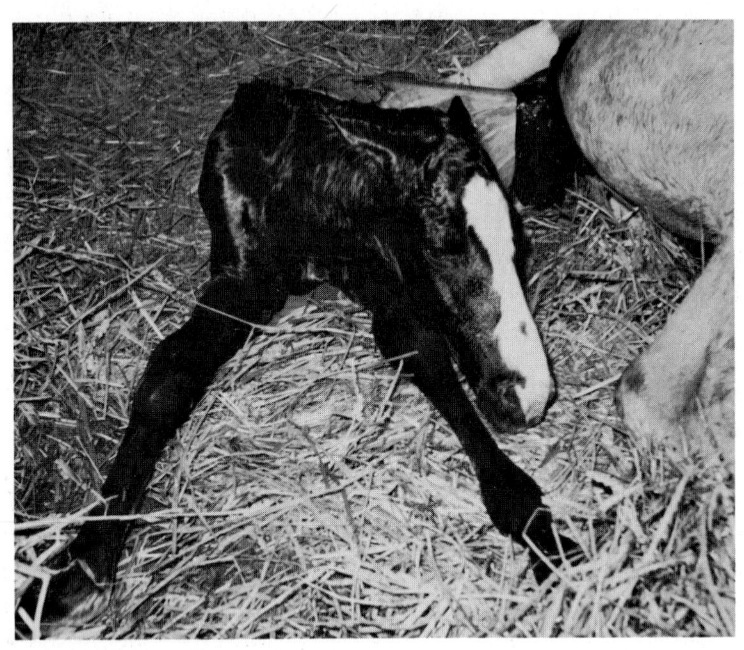

Fig. 5.4. Final delivery normally leaves the foal with its hind-legs in the mare's vagina and the umbilical cord intact.

and head as breathing begins. Once established, the respiratory rhythm sharply raises blood oxygen levels and thereby activates reflex and muscular activity.

Development of reflexes and sensory awareness

Within five minutes of delivery the foal responds to painful stimuli and handling and shows evidence of righting reflexes. These raise the head and neck, extend the front-legs and flex the hind-legs to bring the body into the sternal or dog-sitting position. Sucking movements, blink and pupillary reflexes are apparent and the foal becomes aware of auditory stimuli and may whinny or nicker. The foal often shows rhythmic bobbing movements of the head while making sucking movements with the lips.

Umbilical cord

Mares usually stay recumbent for up to 40 minutes after delivery and the umbilical cord stays intact until ruptured by increasing tension, produced by the foal's attempts to stand or by the mare rising to her feet. If the cord is not artificially severed nor the mare disturbed, the cord will rupture on average about eight minutes after delivery. During this time there is a decreasing blood circulation.

Studies were carried out on 46 Thoroughbred foals in which the cord was severed (*a*) immediately on delivery; (*b*) one to five minutes after delivery, but when one or both of the umbilical arteries were pulsating, and (*c*) one to nine minutes after delivery when no arterial pulses could be detected. These indicated that the foal may be deprived of up to 1 litre of total circulating blood by immediate severance (Fig. 5.5). Rupture of the cord normally occurs about 3 cm from the abdominal wall and if the cord remains intact for several minutes the point of rupture becomes white and constricted (Figs 5.6, 5.7).

Standing for the first time

The foal appears to have an inborn pattern of behavioural responses by which it stands. This is identical to that of the older foal and adult. The fore-legs are extended, the hocks flexed and the foal raises the front part of the spinal axis, followed by the hind part. A foal may make several attempts to stand before it succeeds and some are more clumsy in their efforts than others.

Thoroughbred foals stand on average within 60 minutes of birth, although there is a considerable variation, some doing so by 20 minutes. The distribution of times of first standing in a group of 249 Thoroughbred foals is shown in Fig. 5.8. Crossbred pony foals stand on average by 32 minutes (Jeffcott 1972). Tyler (1972) reported that she saw New Forest ponies which took 33–45 minutes to stand for the first time. Rossdale (1973, unpublished) found no significant relationship between the foal's birth weight and the time taken to stand (15–175 minutes) in 94 Thoroughbred foals weighing between 40 and 63.6 kg. Weight *per se* does not appear to influence standing time.

For clinical purposes, foals which take longer than two hours to stand for the first time should be regarded as potentially abnormal.

Sucking and affinity for mare

Sucking behaviour in the foal is elicited by contact with soft surfaces such as its own or its mother's skin. Soon after the foal stands for the first time it shows directional activity towards the mare's mammary region (Fig. 5.9). The foal is attracted towards dark surfaces and usually starts its search at the mare's brisket, passing eventually along the flanks to the stifle at which it often sucks quite vigorously. Eventually it reaches the udder and finally takes hold of one of the teats. The foal may be confused by handling and the approach of attendants and some make sucking movements in the air or at a wall or manger surface. Many mares help the foal during its care-seeking activity by nudging it and by flexing the opposite hind-leg to the approach side. The mean time at which Thoroughbred foals first suck from the mare is 111 minutes (range 35–420 minutes) (Fig. 5.10), compared with a mean of 65 minutes (range 45–135 minutes) in Crossbred pony foals (Jeffcott 1972).

Once the foal has established an affinity for the mare it follows readily, seeking the udder and sucking with increasing assurance at intervals of 30–60 minutes.

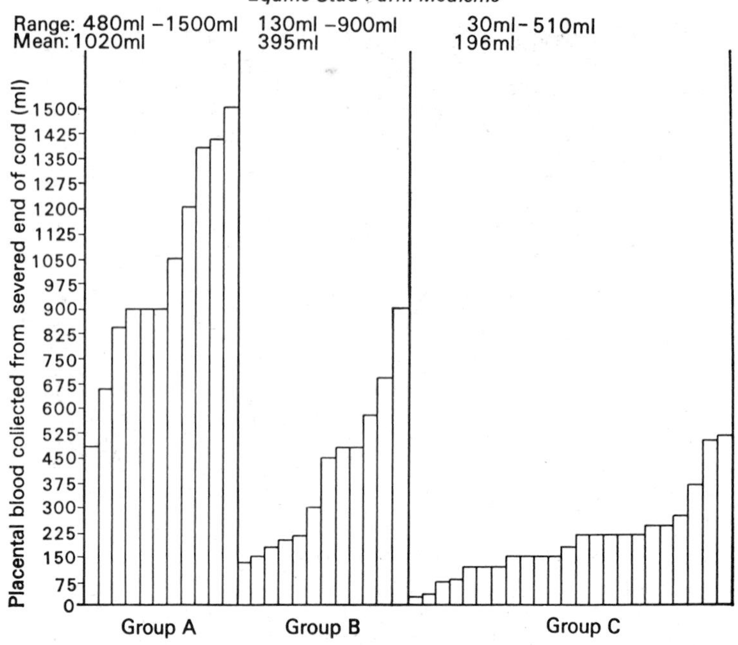

Fig. 5.5. The amount of blood collected from the severed end of the cord of 46 Thoroughbred foals. In Group A (11 cases) the cord was severed immediately on delivery. In Group B (12 cases) the cord was severed while the cord vessels were pulsating (1–5 minutes). In Group C (23 cases) the cord was severed after pulsation had ceased (1–9 minutes). (*After Rossdale 1967a*)

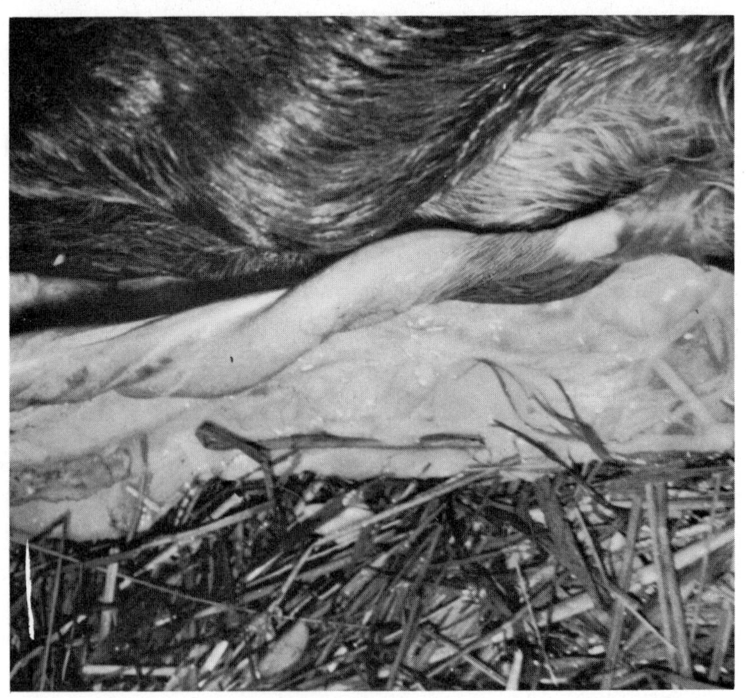

Fig. 5.6. If the umbilical cord is allowed to remain intact for several minutes after delivery, it becomes white at the natural breaking point close to the umbilicus.

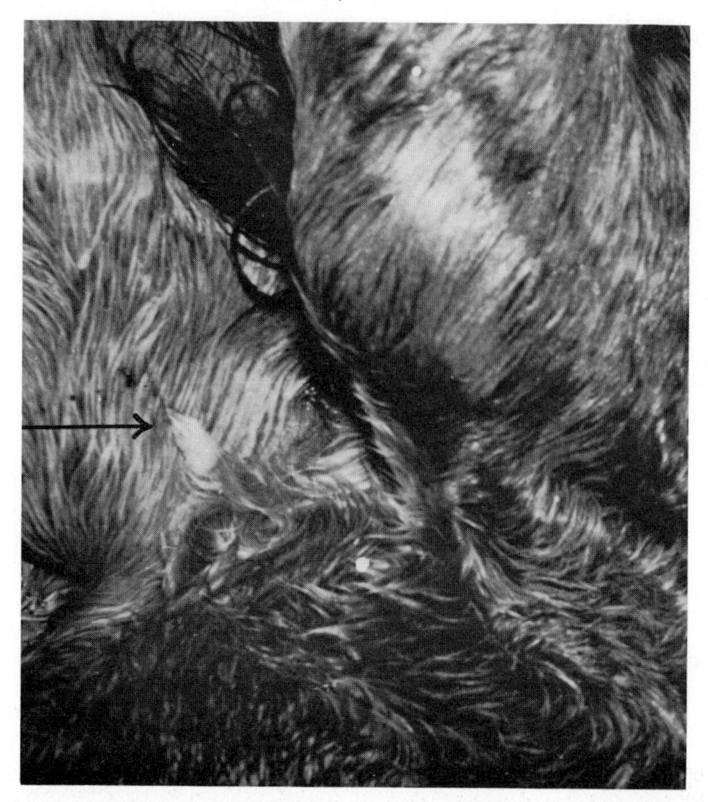

Fig. 5.7. The cord ruptures naturally about 3 cm from the umbilicus to leave a stump (arrowed).

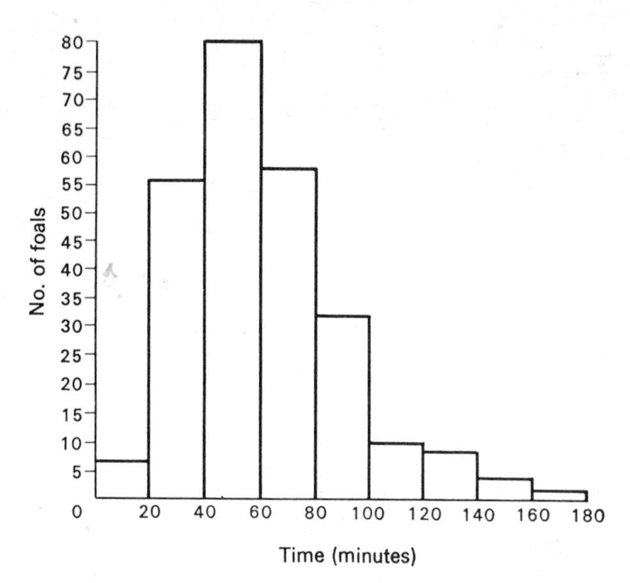

Fig. 5.8. The time taken to stand for the first time, as observed in 249 Thoroughbred foals (*After Rossdale 1967a*)

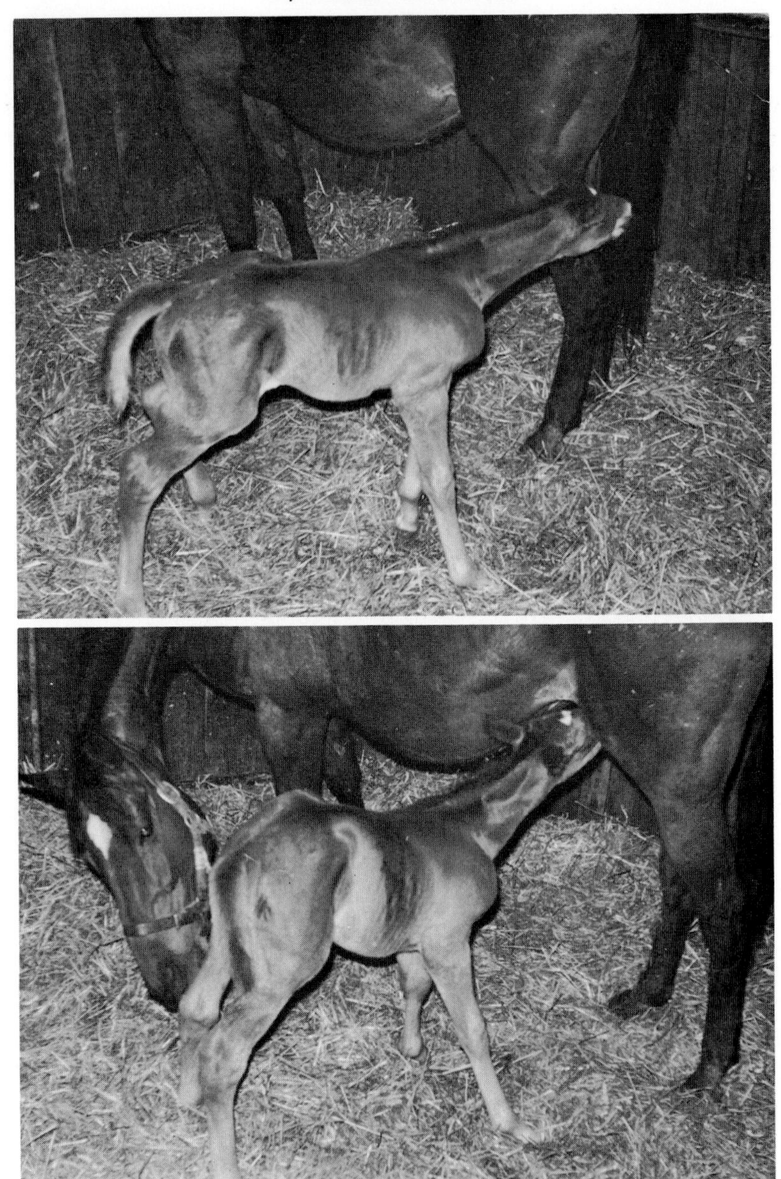

Fig. 5.9. A newborn foal exhibiting sucking activity.

Foals that take longer than three hours to suck must be regarded as potentially abnormal.

After achieving the standing position and the first suck the foal more readily accepts restraint and handling. The manner of getting up and down follows the adult pattern; in lying down the foal lowers its withers first then the hind-quarters. The movement is accomplished in a smooth sequential manner. Periods of rest, play (circling the mare) and sucking form the basis of behavioural patterns and

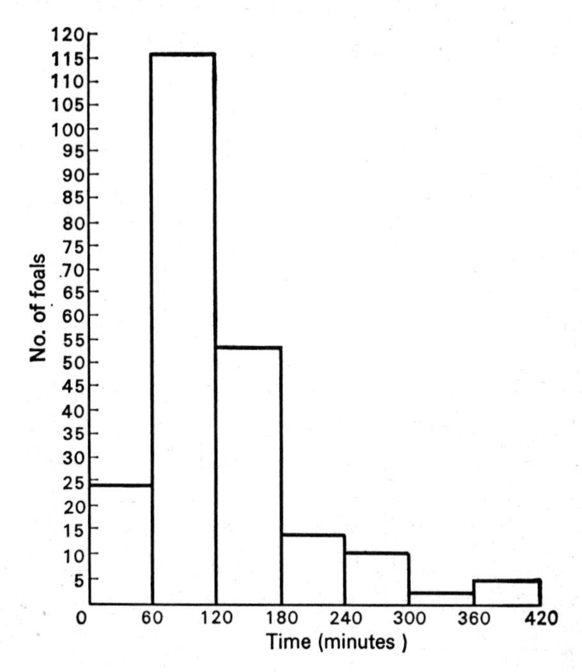

Fig. 5.10. The time taken to suck for the first time, as observed in Thoroughbred foals. (*After Rossdale 1967a*)

although normality of these activities can be judged only on a subjective basis; the ease with which they are performed, the strength of suck and successful draining of the mammary glands are cardinal signs of the foal's health status. Tyler (1972) observed New Forest ponies yawning, rubbing, rolling, nibbling, scratching, stamping and shaking often within hours of birth. They also showed the *Flehmen* posture and snapping expression.

Evacuation of meconium

Meconium consists of glandular secretions, digested amniotic fluid and cell debris. Before birth, meconium is propelled along the bowel by intermittent peristaltic movements (Morison 1970) and is stored in the colon, caecum and rectum; it is expelled before or during birth only under stressful conditions (notably asphyxia). The foal's meconium is brown, greenish-brown or black and occurs as hard pellets or a paste-like mass covered by a semi-viscous mucous layer. Mucosal enzymes, other than alkaline phosphatase, are found only in very small quantities despite the presence of large numbers of desquamated intestinal cells. Roberts (1975) suggests that this is due to the proteolytic action of meconium. The time taken by the newborn foal to void all its meconium varies considerably but it is usual for clearance – followed by the appearance of the yellowish 'milk dung' – to be complete by the fourth day post-partum. Jeffcott (1972) noted that pony foals showed signs of abdominal pain and straining within an hour (mean 145 minutes) of delivery. He states that 'in the next few hours the rest of the meconium was passed with little difficulty'. Retention of meconium as a clinical condition is a matter of painful signs rather than the length of time taken for evacuation and is discussed later. Jeffcott (1972) found that the mean time of first micturition in 17 pony foals was 8.5 hours (range 2.77–15 hours). Colt foals first urinated, on average, at 5.97 hours and fillies at 10.77 hours. The discrepancy is interesting, but unexplained. Passage of a continuous stream of urine has relevance to the diagnosis of ruptured (patent) bladder (see p. 342).

Pulmonary ventilation

Early in gestation the pulmonary air spaces are poorly developed and lined by cuboidal epithelium and the lungs are incapable of expansion (Fig. 5.11). This is known as the glandular stage and it is formed by branching and budding of the bronchial tree as it grows into the mesenchyme. Glycogen is usually present in the cells and traces of surfactant (a lipoprotein substance providing the alveoli with a surface film to oppose the effects of surface tension) may be found. Between Days 190 and 210 the architecture of the lung changes to the canalicular stage (Pattle et al. 1975). During this period the surface-active material (surfactant) increases but is not fully developed until about Day 300 or, in some foals, until after delivery (Figs 5.12, 5.13).

The cuboidal cell rosettes of the glandular stage develop into Type I cells of the adult lung, forming part of the blood–air barrier and Type II cells which have a phagocytic role. During the canalicular stage the blood–air barrier becomes more prominent and, simultaneously, an increasing number of lamellated osmiophilic bodies (LOPBs) develop. These represent intracellular surfactant. In the foal LOPBs and surfactant were present at Day 50 of gestation during the glandular stage. The main glandular to canalicular transition occurred between Days 190 and 210 and the reserves of surfactant are present at Day 250, the formation of a lining film is incomplete at 300 days and sometimes incomplete at full term. Confirmatory evidence that surfactant develops in the equine fetal lung at an early stage of gestation is shown by the significant increase in the concentration of total phospholipids in lung tissue and a concomitant rise in the amount of dipalmitoyl lecithin in amniotic fluid which occurs between 100 and 150 days of gestation (Arvidson et al. 1975).

The canalicular stage is succeeded by the post-natal 'alveolar' stage in which breathing stretches and thins the walls of the canaliculi. The alveoli continue to develop after birth (Reid 1967). Thus the equine fetus, as far as pulmonary development is concerned, is ready for extrauterine respiratory activity at 300 days of gestation, although full maturity may not be acquired until several weeks later.

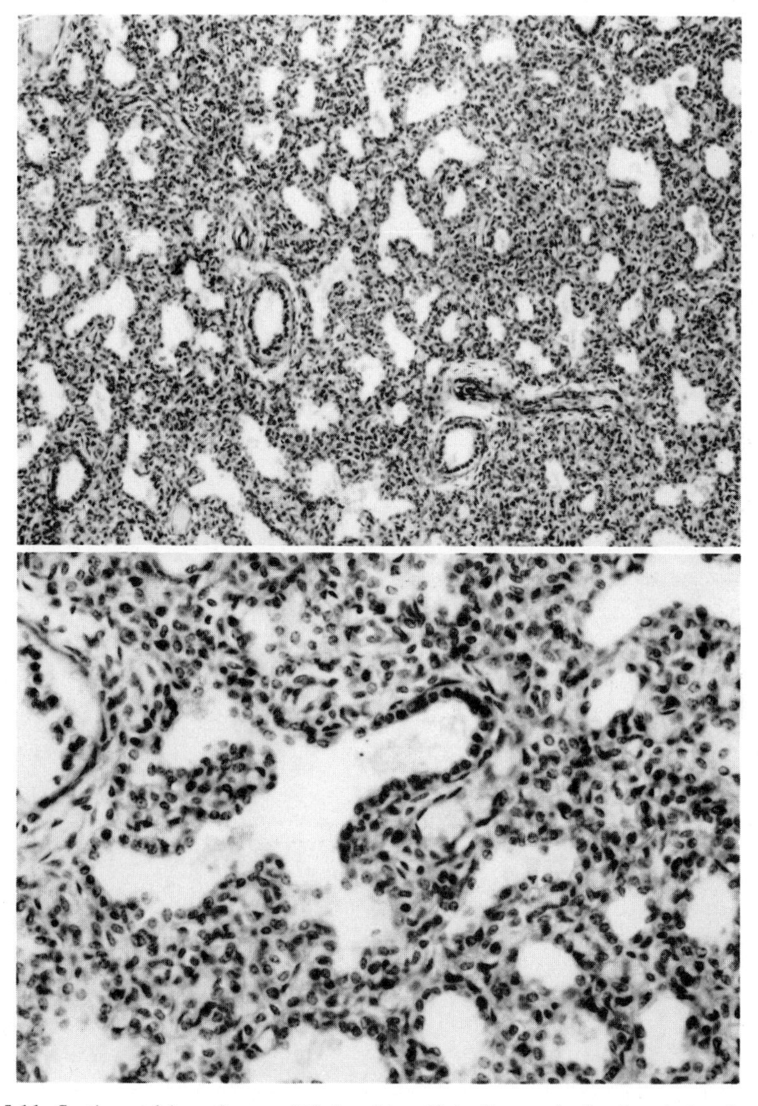

Fig. 5.11. Sections of lung from a 210-day fetus. Note the poorly developed alveoli and the presence of cuboidal epithelium lining the air spaces. H & E, above × 85; below × 260.

The newborn foal's lung has a low efficiency for gas exchange relative to that of the adult (Gillespie 1975) and the ratio of air/tissue interface area of the lungs to body surface area is three times greater in adults than in neonates (Dunhill 1962). In adults, end-expiratory volume or functional residual capacity (FRC) is probably set by the recoil of the relaxed chest wall outward opposing the recoil of the lung inward. When the adult lung is at FRC the pressures across the lung and chest are equal and opposite. This mechanism depends upon a stiff chest which resists change in shape and FRC is estimated at about 52% of total lung capacity. Foals have a relatively soft and compliant chest wall and FRC cannot be set at adult levels by

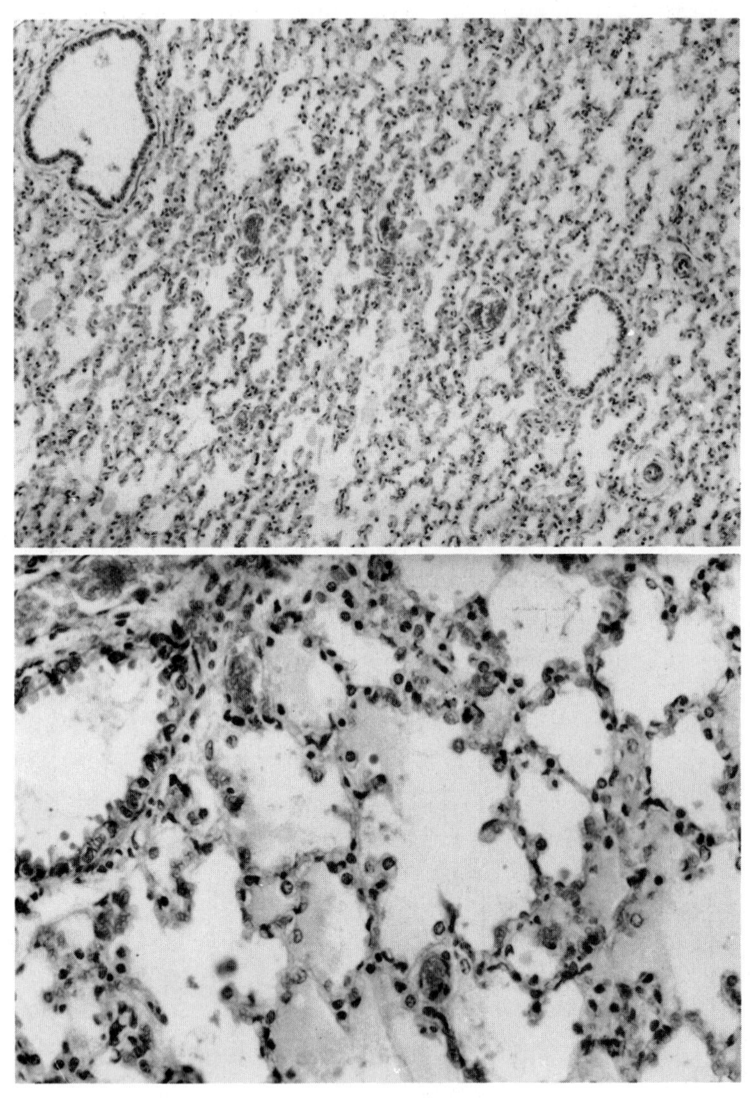

Fig. 5.12. Sections of lung from a 320-day still-born foal illustrating unexpanded but well developed alveoli containing fluid and only small amounts of cubodial epithelium. H & E, above × 85, below × 260.

the same mechanism. Gillespie estimates that the foal's FRC is low and that if the newborn is to avoid pulmonary atelectasis one of three mechanisms must operate: (1) dynamic expiratory air-trapping by stricture or closure of lower airways; (2) periodic expiratory narrowing or closure of the glottis; and/or (3) strong deflation mechanoreceptor reflexes. The newborn foal could achieve a higher end-respiratory volume by partly or completely closing the glottis during expiration and there is some evidence for this in the 'grunt' or 'bark' emitted by convulsing foals, but no evidence that healthy foals use this mechanism to maintain FRC. The Hering-Breuer reflex is present in all mammals and prevents deflated end-respiratory volumes by promoting strong inspiratory efforts and increased breathing frequency.

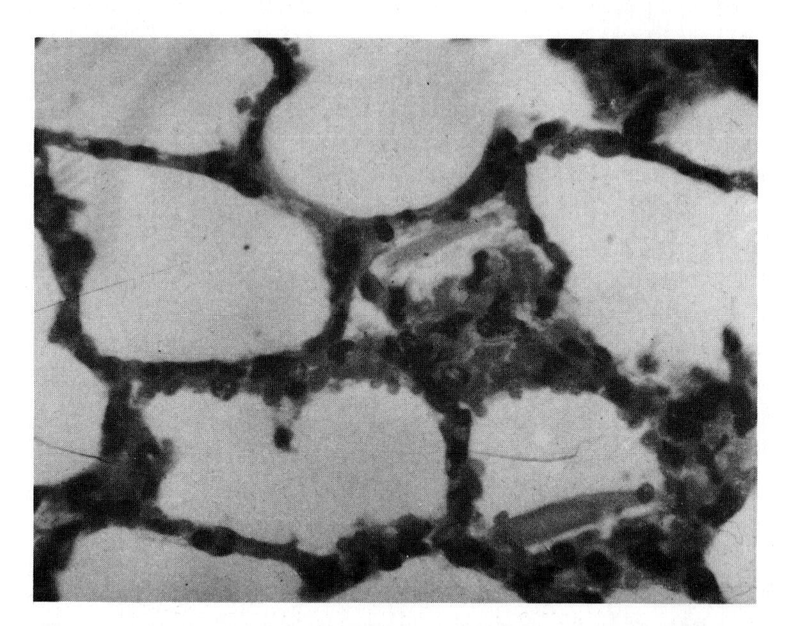

Fig. 5.13. A section of lung from a three-day foal which dies of a non-pulmonary condition. Two squames can be seen (middle and lower-right). H & E × 260.

The presence of a strong deflation reflex in newborn animals could defend FRC until the chest wall is stiffened with maturity. There is insufficient information at present on which of the mechanisms suggested by Gillespie contribute to the functional stability of the lung in the newborn foal.

The onset of breathing

There is evidence, in several species, that the fetus makes episodic breathing movements in utero (Dawes et al. 1972) associated with rapid eye movement sleep (REMS). The significance of this activity is unknown at the present time, but it may form part of neuromuscular preparation for extrauterine existence.

The stimuli for the first breath and subsequent rhythmic respiratory movements following delivery are tactile, cold and chemical (decreasing PaO_2 and increasing $PaCO_2$).

The foal may gasp as the chest is being delivered, but the onset of respiration and the establishment of rhythmic movements of the chest and abdomen is usually established within 30 seconds of the hips passing out of the birth canal.

Following the onset of a respiratory rhythm, the breathing rate declines from a mean of 75/minute to 50/minute at one hour and 34/minute by age 12 hours (Rossdale 1969*a*). Measurements of tidal volume (Vt)*, minute volume (V)† and maximal tidal volume (Vt_{max})‡ can be conveniently recorded using a Wright's respirometer (Wright 1959).

Recordings are made with the foal recumbent. The respirometer is connected to a mask which is placed over the foal's muzzle, the open end of the mask forming a seal between the nostrils and the eyes (Fig. 5.14). The foal is allowed to settle and ten respiratory movements timed (T) with a stop-watch and the amount (A) of air-flow measured with the respirometer. Respiratory rate ($10 \times 60/T$), tidal ($A/10$) and minute volumes can then be calculated. Vt_{max} is the highest respirometer reading obtained after the foal has been caused to struggle while restrained by rubbing it vigorously with the hand. Measurements from 70 Thoroughbred foals, between one and 48 hours post-partum, are summarized in Fig. 5.15. In this study (Rossdale 1969*a*) the respiratory rate and body weight of the foal were negatively correlated and the tidal volume and body weight positively correlated. The percentage increase in mean Vt_{max} was 69% over resting Vt.

Gillespie (1975) emphasized the apparent low efficiency of gas exchange in the newborn foal's lung; mean minute ventilation/kg body weight (Vm/kg) in foals was 498 ml/minute/kg compared to 161 ml/minute/kg in the adult horse (representing a decrease of 68%). He argues that functional residual capacity (FRC) in foals with a soft or compliant chest wall cannot be set at the adult levels of 50% of total lung capacity (TLC) and that the foal may therefore have difficulty in maintaining FRC and is consequently susceptible to pulmonary atelectasis and required to use increased energy to maintain alveolar expansion during the respiratory cycle (see p. 315).

Cardiac and circulatory status

Clinical methods of establishing cardiac and circulatory status are: (*a*) heart rate; (*b*) auscultation; (*c*) electrocardiography; (*d*) degree of venous engorgement and jugular pulse; (*e*) quality of the arterial pulse; and (*f*) colour of buccal and other mucous membranes.

The *heart rate* may be recorded by placing a hand over the heart on the left side of the chest and counting the beats for a half or full minute, measured with a stop-watch. The range immediately following normal delivery in healthy foals is 40–80 beats/minute (Rossdale 1967*b*). Foals suffering from pathological asphyxia (see below) initially suffer from bradycardia, i.e. less than 40 beats/minute,

* Tidal volume (Vt) is the amount of air moved during an inspiratory or expiratory movement at rest.

† Minute volume (V) is the tidal volume times respiratory movements per minute.

‡ Maximal tidal volume (Vt_{max}) is the amount of air moved during a forced expiratory or inspiratory movement, i.e. a movement from a position of maximal inspiration to maximal expiration (or the reverse). This measurement approximates vital capacity.

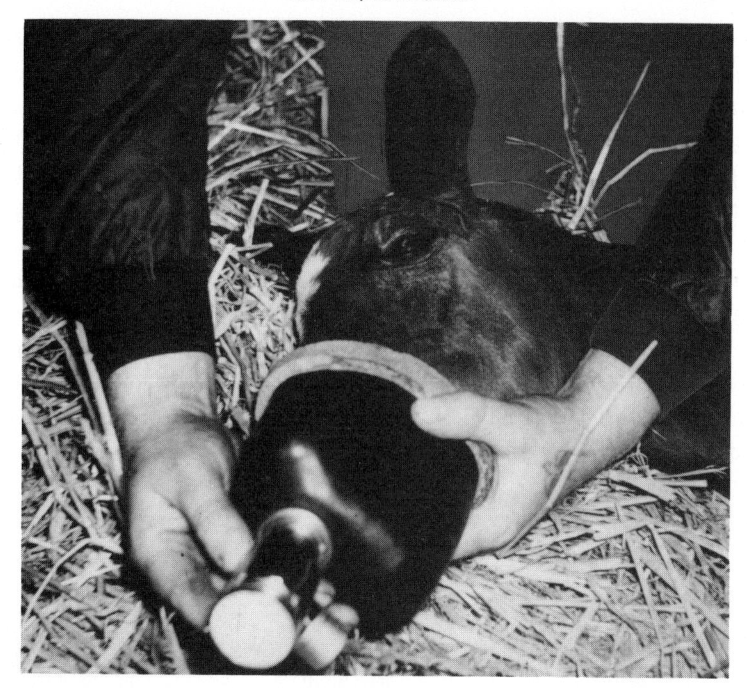

Fig. 5.14. The method of measuring pulmonary ventilation with a Wright's respirometer.

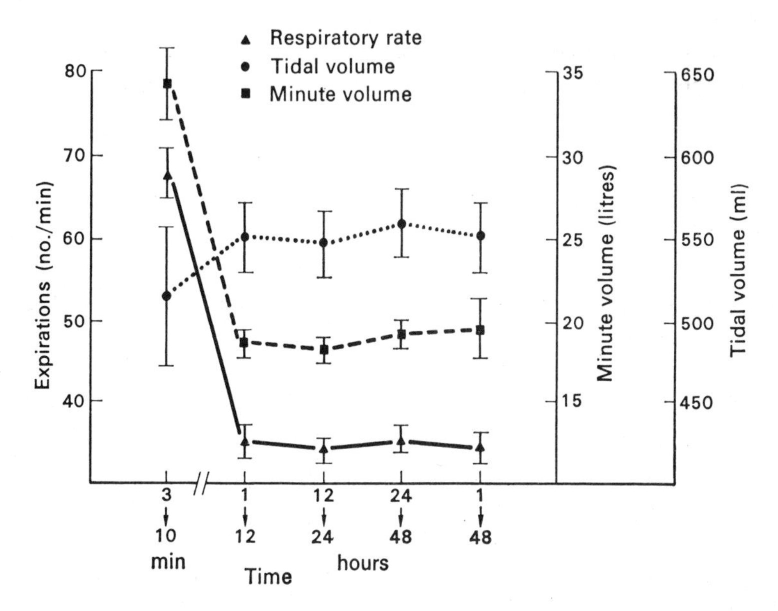

Fig. 5.15. Respirometer measurements (mean ± SE) of respiratory rate, tidal volume and minute volume in 70 Thoroughbred foals between the ages of three minutes and 48 hours. A significant fall occurred in rate and minute volume by 1 to 12 hours after birth. (*After Rossdale 1969a*)

followed by tachycardia (more than 150 beats/minute). Foals delivered in dystocia or with the mare standing may have a relative tachycardia (greater than 90 beats/minute). Colles et al. (1978) showed that the mean fetal rate decreases and mean maternal heart rate increases gradually from 150 days gestation to term. The fetal heart rate in the first stage of induced parturition was found to be related to the duration of first-stage labour: the shorter the period the higher the heart rate. Tachycardia was noted in all fetuses examined in the latter part of second-stage labour.

During the time the foal is trying to get to its feet for the first time, the heart rate increases to about 150 beats/minute. From age two hours the resting rate is 70–95 beats/minute. Some foals suffer from a sinus arrhythmia in the first few hours after birth and especially in the first half hour. There is no evidence that this type of arrhythmia is pathological except where it persists or is associated with other clinical signs.

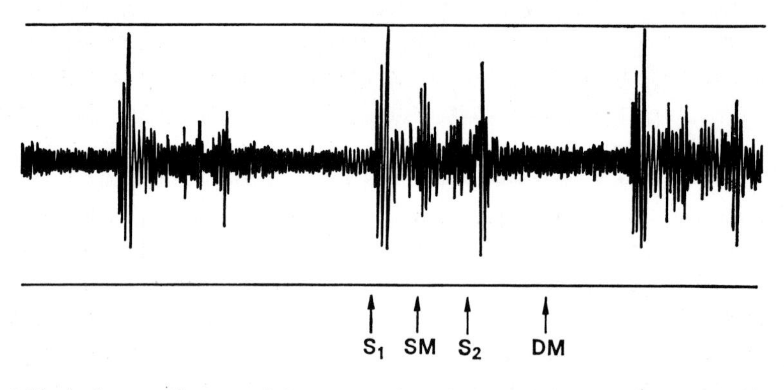

Fig. 5.16. A phonocardiogram of the murmur from ductus arteriosus in an 11-hour-old normal foal. The first and second heart sounds are arrowed S_1 and S_2 respectively. Systolic and diastolic components of the murmur are marked SM and DM. (*After Rossdale 1967b*)

A murmur (Fig. 5.16) can be detected on *auscultation* on the left side of the chest at the intersection of a line drawn horizontally from the shoulder joint and the posterior border of the triceps muscle, with the limb in the resting position. The area where the murmur can be detected radiates for about 5 cm from the point at which it is strongest. This point corresponds to the third intercostal space and lies immediately over the ductus vessel. The murmur can usually be detected in normal foals between two and 36 hours after birth and its intensity varies between Grade II and Grade IV. The murmur may be present by five minutes after delivery and usually disappears by age 90 hours.

The use of the *electrocardiogram* to investigate the foal's heart seems to have been neglected in clinical medicine. Knowledge of ventricular preponderance in conditions where the cardiovascular system is affected might be of considerable help in clinical diagnosis. In one study (Rossdale 1967*b*) the QRS vectors of normal foals tended to be different in direction from those recorded in yearlings, but individual variations in electrical axis due to rotation of the heart obviously limit the interpretation of vector analysis for clinical purposes. In view of the well known vulnerability of the foal's chest to birth trauma, we consider that electrocardiography coupled with pathological studies might form a rewarding field of study.

The foal's *arterial pulse* can be detected conveniently at the facial artery as it passes over the mandible, the brachial artery as it passes over the inner aspect of the elbow joint and the digital artery on either side of the posterior aspect of the fetlock joint. The normal pulse is only just detectable but can be felt. Its character may change markedly in stages of cardiovascular dysfunction, becoming abnormally full, bounding or hammer-like, or weak, thread-like and failing.

Jugular and subcutaneous veins of the head are not normally engorged and a consistent and obvious *jugular pulse* is not present in a healthy foal. Assessment of venous pressure is subjective without definite pressure measurements, but in describing conditions of maladjustment we shall postulate that a marked venous pulse or engorgement are signs of right heart failure.

During the terminal period of the second stage the *buccal mucous membranes* and tongue become purple and the jugular vein engorged. We believe that this is evidence of substantial circulatory stasis caused by temporarily restricted venous return during passage of the foal's chest through the maternal pelvis. Peak pressures of 200 mmHg have been recorded in the jugular vein at this stage, as the foal's head emerges from the vagina (Johnson & Rossdale 1975, Rossdale et al. 1976). Within a minute or two of complete delivery venous engorgement subsides and the colour of the buccal mucous membranes changes to pink. In the first two hours the membranes may be pale or greyish, but after this time they are normally pink and moist. If the gums are pressed with a finger they blanch but the blood returns rapidly and a healthy colour is restored. Capillary refill in the membranes is a subjective way to assess whether a foal is suffering from dehydration and failing circulation.

Rectal temperature

Rectal temperature may fall to 37°C immediately after delivery, but normally recovers to 38°C by age one hour (Rossdale 1968*b*). The normal range in the first four days post-partum is 37.2–38.3°C. The exact mechanism of thermoregulation in the foal is unknown but it is unlikely to differ fundamentally from other homeothermic species. The main sources of body heat are shivering (in the first three hours after birth), muscular activity associated with efforts to stand for the first time and, subsequently, active movements following the mare. Heat is lost by radiation, conduction, convection and evaporation. Non-shivering thermogenesis occurs in human infants, the newborn guinea-pig and rabbit, but the foal, like the lamb and piglet, shivers vigorously soon after birth. Brown adipose tissue is present in those species that do not shiver and absent in those that do.

Eye

Barnett (1975) has described the eye of the newborn foal as having a fundus similar to that of the adult horse. The optic disc is dull pink in colour with a darker border and clear outline, the edge being crossed by numerous fine retinal blood vessels.

The hyaloid artery is usually present and can be seen as a fine, dark, curving line passing through the vitreous from the centre of the optic disc to the back of the lens. The artery appears red at first but becomes dark in the first few days post-partum and eventually clears when the foal is about one week old. The pupils should be equal, large and circular in a day-old foal but become smaller and more oval by age one week, by which time the pupillary light reflex is much more active.

Immune status

Foals are born with insignificant circulating antibody and gammaglobulin levels in their blood but derive these in massive doses from the colostrum, the small intestine being permeable to protein for a brief period after birth, estimated at less than 36 hours (Brambell 1958; Hemmings & Brambell 1961; Rossdale 1966; Jeffcott 1971).

The immunoglobulin subclasses IgG, IgM and IgA have been identified in the horse (Weir & Porter 1966; Rockey 1967; Rouse 1971; Naylor 1979). In colostrum, IgG is predominant, whereas IgA is predominant in milk and is present in greater quantities than IgG at 16 days post partum (McGuire & Crawford 1973). IgG is absorbed more efficiently than the other immunoglobulins. Although serum concentrations rise rapidly after colostrum ingestion, circulating concentrations do not reach adult levels until four months of age, when active production has taken over (Jeffcott 1974). The half-life of IgG and IgG(T) is 23 days and 20 days respectively. Maternal IgM disappears from the serum of the foal much more rapidly. Colostrum-deprived foals remain almost completely agammaglobulinaemic for the first two weeks of life, after which immunoglobulin synthesis occurs and circulating levels are similar to those in colostrum-fed foals by five weeks of age.

It is known that mares immunized against tetanus and myxoinfluenza virus during pregnancy transmit specific antibodies to their foals in quantities which protect against early infection (Lemetayer et al. 1947; Chodnik et al. 1960; Rossdale & Scarnell 1961; Rossdale 1966).

Jeffcott (1971) has shown that the mechanism of colostral protein absorption is by pinocytosis by the epithelial cells of the small intestine and transfer through the lacteals to the systemic circulation (Fig. 5.17). The intestine is non-selective in its absorption of macromolecules and three hours after birth it will absorb 22% of a dose of labelled PVP, a synthetic polymer of similar molecular size to gamma-globulin.

Absorption declines with age to the lowest recorded levels at 20 hours and by 24 hours of life the intestinal epithelium is no longer permeable to marker antibody. Reilly and Macdougall (1973) studied the distribution and metabolism of IgG in seven newborn foals using ^{125}I-labelled IgG. They found an intravascular/extra-vascular ratio of 1/1. Colostrum contains certain substances capable of enhancing the efficiency of absorption of macromolecules. Thus absorption of macromolecules is reduced by 10% when foals are deprived of colostrum. Many factors seem to be involved in the process causing the loss of ability of absorption of macromolecules. Adrenal cortical hormones probably play an important role.

A marked transient proteinuria occurs in foals receiving colostrum in the first 24 hours post-partum. Urinary protein levels rise rapidly to a peak by six to 12 hours and then decline between 24 and 36 hours. The urinary protein consists almost exclusively of small-molecular-weight proteins, probably alpha-lactalbumin and beta-lactoglobulin. These small proteins are absorbed by the intestines together with the larger molecules and are selectively secreted in the urine due to their small size (Jeffcott 1975).

The practical implications of this passive transfer of immunity are that:

1. Foals should receive colostrum soon after birth.

2. The immunological status of the mare must be considered in relation to that of the newborn foal and therefore the foal should be reared in the prenatal environment until it is immunologically competent, that is by age two to three months.

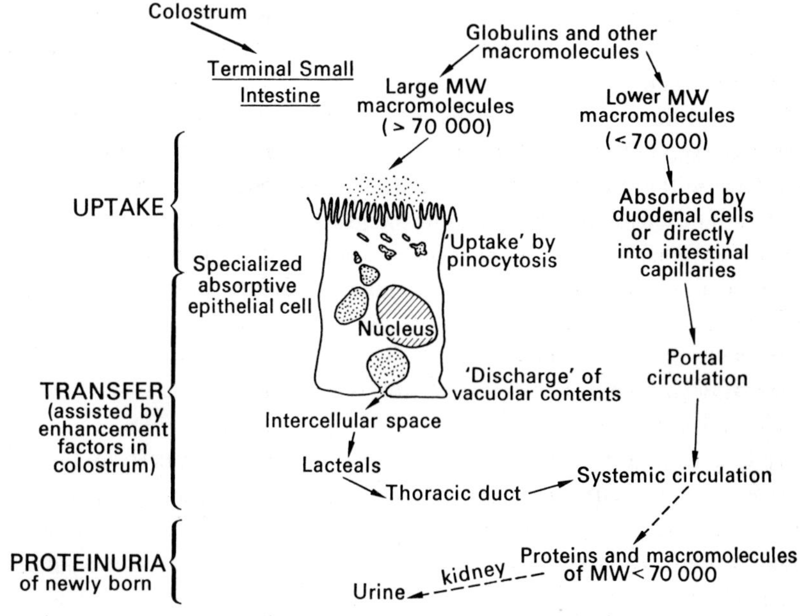

Fig. 5.17. Schematic representation of the absorption of globulins and other macromolecules from the small intestine of ungulates. (*After Jeffcott 1971*)

3. If a foal is deprived of colostrum, by the mare 'running' milk before parturition, donor colostrum should be given via artifical teat or stomach tube within 12 hours of birth. Colostrum may be stored deep-frozen for at least a year and a deprived foal should be fed as much as is available, up to about 500 ml.

Metabolic status

Information about the metabolic status of the foal is fragmentary owing to the limited interest of physiologists in this species during the first half of this century.

The abrupt transition at birth from dependence to independence is associated with numerous adaptive responses in physiological mechanisms. Survival depends on changes in the metabolic pool due to replacement of placental transference by gastrointestinal absorption.

Carbohydrate metabolism in young animals has been reviewed by Edwards (1964). Marked changes in the distribution of carbohydrates are known to occur in the fetus towards the end of gestation and at birth in a variety of species (Shelley 1961, 1964). Notable variations in carbohydrate enzyme systems and the deposition of glycogen in the liver mark the end of gestation. Rapid changes in the concentrations of various blood metabolites occur post-partum.

The level of blood glucose reflects the degree to which this metabolite is available for cellular use and the ratio of pyruvate to lactate represents the degree of anaerobic metabolism at any given time. Fructose is not utilized for energy and appears to be concerned solely with placental metabolism (Huggett 1961).

Goodwin (1957) studied one unsuckled foal in the first eight days after birth and found, contrary to experience in piglets, that starvation was not associated with hypoglycaemia. Blood sugar levels remained above 40 mg/dl for 230 hours. Fructose levels fell from 80 mg/dl to nearly zero by age 20 hours, which is consistent with findings in other fructogenic species such as the cow and the sheep.

In normal Thoroughbred foals mean whole blood glucose levels before sucking were between 2.8 and 3.8 mmol/litre and plasma glucose between 4.7 and 5.2 mmol/litre in the first hour after birth. The levels increase after feeding (Fig. 5.18). The levels are higher in plasma due to the relative impermeability of the erythrocyte cell membrane to glucose molecules at full term. In premature foals values in whole blood and in plasma are nearly equal. A decrease in mean blood fructose levels occurs from 95.81 ± 6.3 mg/dl at birth to 7.51 ± 3.13 mg/dl in the period 21–33 hours post-partum (Rossdale 1966).

Standard bicarbonate levels rise steadily over the period up to 36 hours after birth (Fig. 5.19).

Whole blood lactate levels rise immediately after birth and fall to adult levels by 36 hours (Fig. 5.20). The initial rise coincides with a fall in venous blood pH and may be due to changes in circulatory flow through muscle or to hypoxia in the interval between cessation of placental function and commencement of pulmonary ventilation.

The metabolic acidosis present after birth is corrected by 12 hours, but respiratory acidosis may persist into the second or third day post-partum (Rossdale 1968*a*). Arterial oxygen tensions rise steeply at the start of respiration but carbon dioxide tensions tend to remain high (45–50 mmHg) and pH is 7.30–7.38 (Fig. 5.21). Gillespie (1975) reported a lower range (41–47 mmHg) in three foals at age 24 hours and Littlejohn (1975), in a study of newborn foals 1300 m above sea level, found 39.6 mmHg and 38.4 mmHg at ages six to 60 hours and two to three weeks respectively.

Adrenal cortex hormones

In foals, a significant rise in plasma cortisol (from 5.25 to 8.3 μg/dl) occurs between birth and age 30 minutes. By six hours levels have fallen to near those of the adult (Fig. 5.22) (Rossdale et al. 1973). The picture of fetal and neonatal cortisol meta-

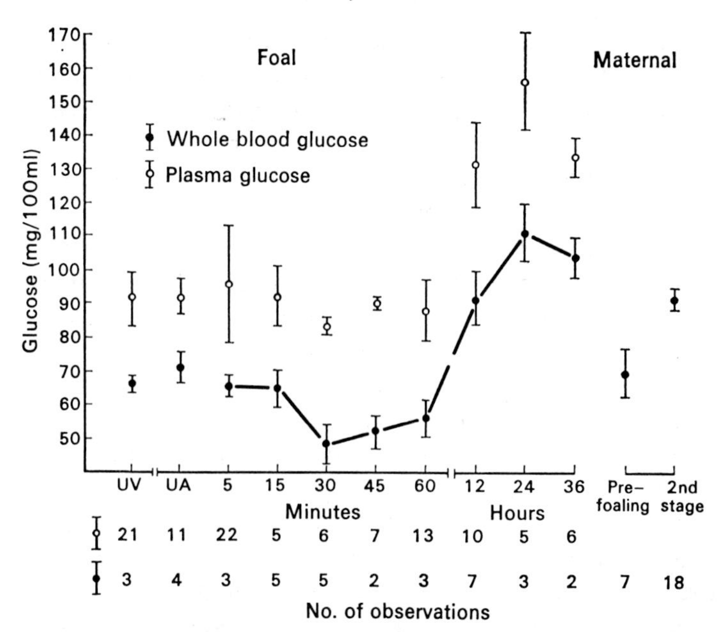

Fig. 5.18. Whole blood and plasma glucose levels (mean ± SE) in normal Thoroughbred foals between birth and age 36 hours. None of the foals had sucked before samples were obtained at age one hour, but all had sucked by age 12 hours. Maternal levels before foaling (at least one week before parturition) and during the second stage are also shown. Conversion factor: mg/100 ml × 0.0555 = mmol/litre.

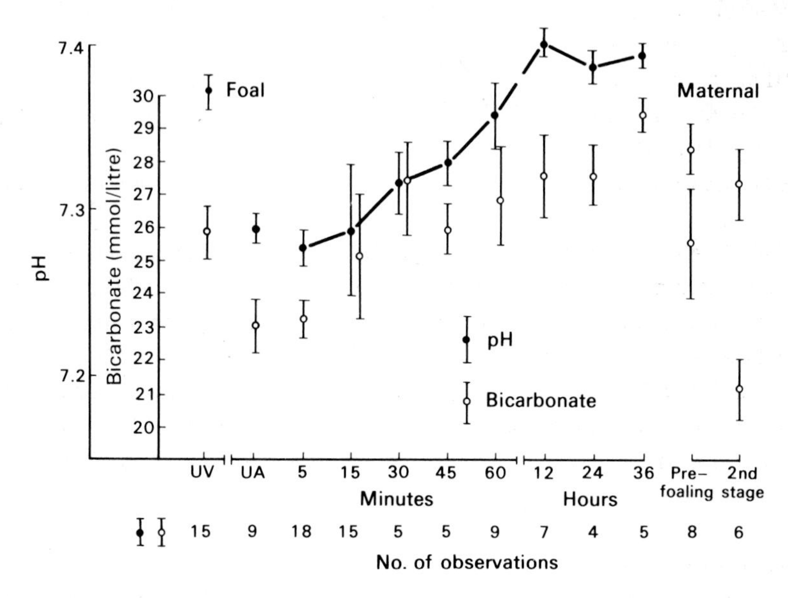

Fig. 5.19. Jugular venous pH and standard bicarbonate levels (mean ± SE) in 18 Thoroughbred foals between birth and age 36 hours. Maternal levels before foaling (at least one week before parturition) and during the second stage are also shown.

bolism (Nathanielsz et al. 1975) shows certain similarities with other species in which studies have been carried out on the activity of the adrenal cortex in the perinatal period. As in ruminants, there appears to be little placental transfer of cortisol in either direction, fetal plasma cortisol remains low throughout the last third of gestation and the post-natal values are highest immediately after birth. There is not sufficient evidence to say whether a prenatal cortisol surge occurs in the fetal foal and available evidence suggests that there is probably some increase in the adrenal activity near term, but that there is no spectacular rise as is seen in the

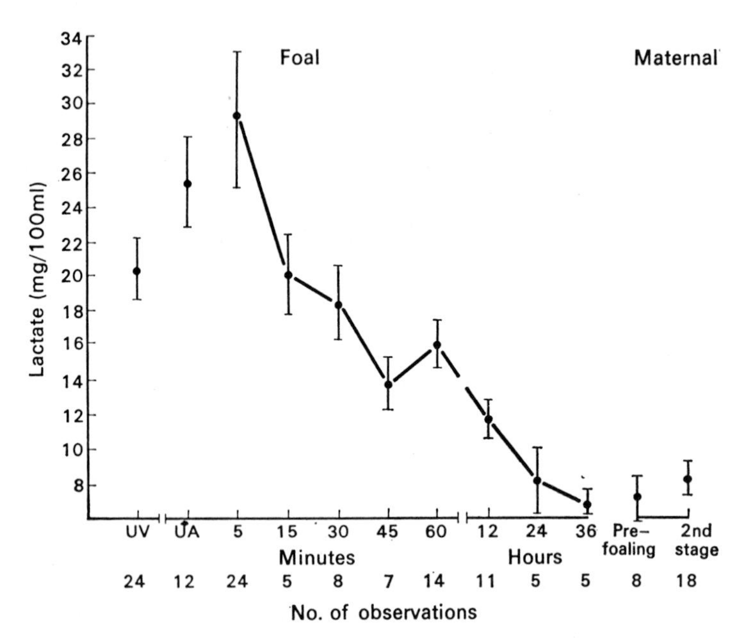

Fig. 5.20. Whole blood lactate levels (mean ± SE) in 24 Thoroughbred foals between birth and age 36 hours. Maternal levels before foaling (at least one week before parturition) and during the second stage are also shown. Conversion factor: mg/100 ml × 0.111 = mmol/litre

lamb just before birth (Nathanielsz et al. 1973). Plasma cortisol levels in two foals born before 320 days gestation were much lower than those in full-term foals and they did not show the characteristic rise and fall of cortisol in the immediate post-natal period. Very high plasma cortisol levels (125–300 mg/ml) were found in two foals that convulsed soon after birth. These findings in convulsant and premature foals are in marked contrast to those in normal full-term foals. They indicate that the maximum secretory capacity of the foal adrenal cortex may be very high in certain pathological conditions.

Laboratory assessment of metabolic status

Under ordinary field conditions the clinician can appreciate changes in the foal's metabolic status only by laboratory measurement of blood and plasma samples, but changes in various metabolite levels make measurements difficult to interpret.

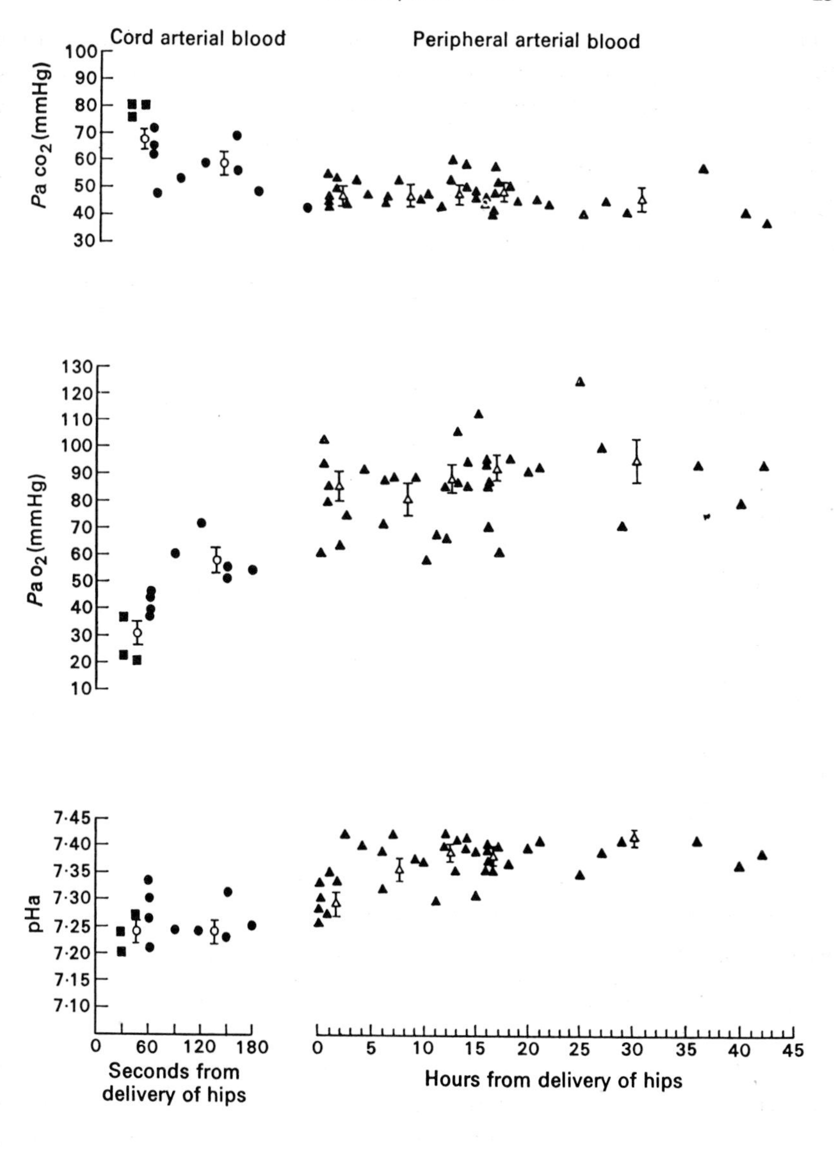

Fig. 5.21. Levels (mean ± SE) of pH, Po_2 and Pco_2 in umbilical and peripheral arterial blood during the first 42 hours after birth (50 samples from 38 foals). (*After Rossdale 1968a*)

Tables 5.1 to 5.4 are intended as a guide to the more common parameters for which laboratory techniques are available. These levels can be compared with results from clinical cases at various ages in the first four days; after this time the foal's metabolic processes are stabilized and usually resemble adult standards.

Haematological status

Packed cell volume, haemoglobin content and erythrocyte count. In the jugular blood these measurements may show an initial rise, but they subsequently fall

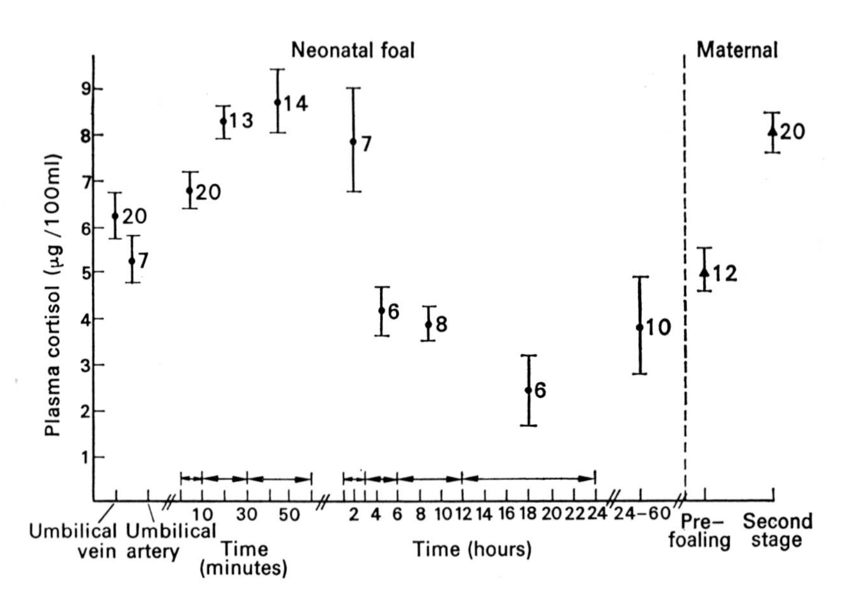

Fig. 5.22. Plasma cortisol levels in the fetus, neonatal and maternal horse during the perinatal period. Arrows indicate the time interval over which samples were taken. The number of samples for each mean figure is also given. Conversion factor: μg/100 ml × 27.59 = mmol/litre. (*After Rossdale et al. 1973*)

between one and 12 hours post-partum in Thoroughbreds (Rossdale 1966, 1973 unpublished) and ponies (Jeffcott 1971) (Fig. 5.23). The decrease in levels continues throughout the adaptive period, but the decline becomes more gradual. Immediate severance of the cord, depriving the foal of the 'placental' transfusion, accentuates the drop which starts, in these cases, in the first hour.

These changes indicate a degree of hydration, presumably brought about by a shift in fluid from extra- to intravascular compartments. In infants the shift appears in the reverse direction, packed cell volume and haemoglobin content rising in the first 12 hours postpartum (Gairdner et al. 1958). In the foal the reduced values may be a reversal of an increase brought about by birth stress, as fetal packed cell volume is in the range 0.3–0.4 litre/litre (Silver 1973, personal communication).

Leucocytes. Jeffcott (1971) reported an increase in total white cell count in the first 12 hours after birth due to an increase in polymorphonuclear leucocytes.

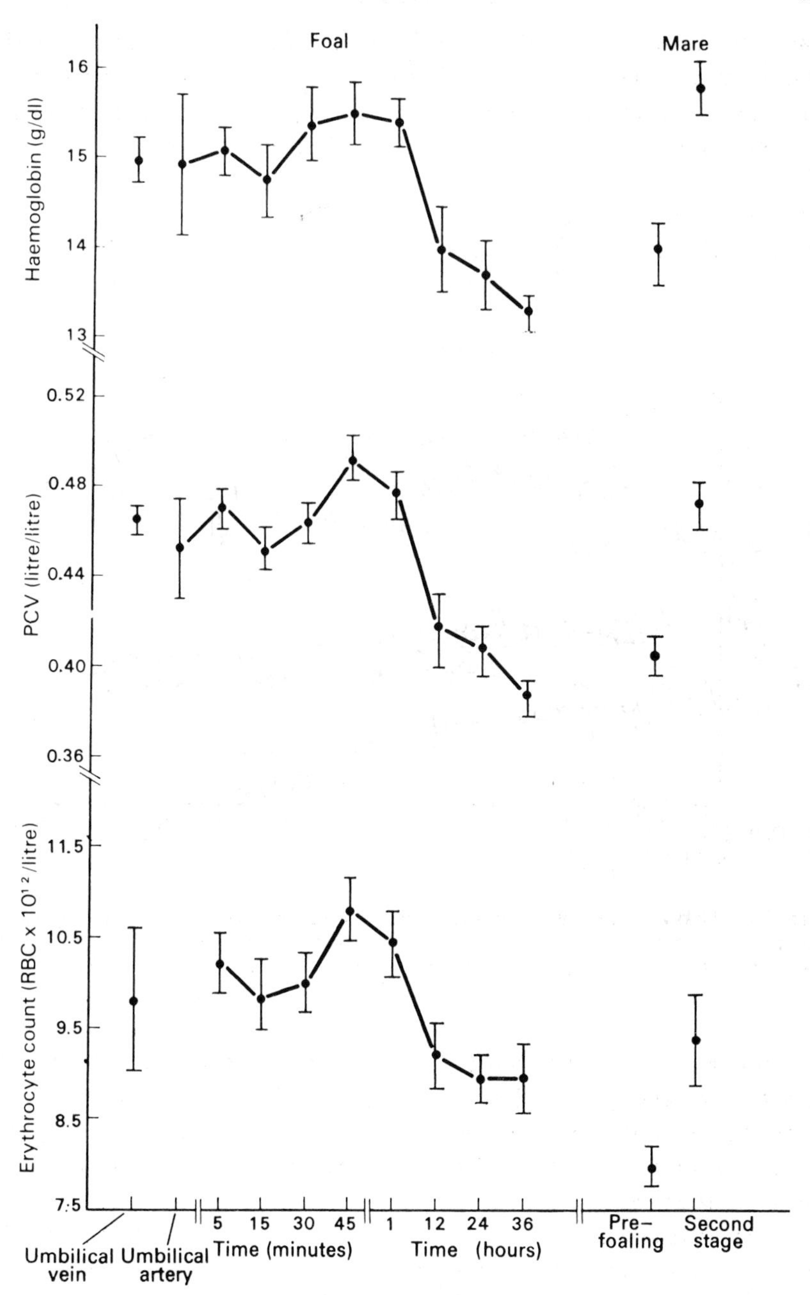

Fig. 5.23. Haemoglobin, packed cell volume and erythrocyte counts (mean ± SE) in the jugular blood of 29 newborn foals from birth to age 36 hours (*After Rossdale 1966*)

TABLE 5.1 PO_2, PCO_2, standard bicarbonate and lactate levels* in arterial and venous blood during the first 36 hours after birth

Age	*Source*	Po_2 (mmHg)	Pco_2 (mmHg)	pH	HCO_3 (mmol/litre)	*Blood plasma lactate* (mg/dl)
During second stage prior to delivery	Digital artery	22.6 ± 1.4	72.8 ± 2.21	7.172 ± 0.014	–	18.8 ± 2.63
0 to 60 seconds, some gasping	Umbilical artery	35.4 ± 3.86	69.1 ± 3.04	7.260 ± 0.018	23.06 ± 0.86	25.5 ± 2.66
90 to 180 seconds, respiration established	Umbilical artery	59.6 ± 3.24	57.6 ± 3.49	7.240 ± 0.014	–	–
12 hours	Facial and digital arteries	91.0 ± 3.3	48.4 ± 1.53	7.376 ± 0.016	27.50 ± 1.28	11.6 ± 1.11
5 minutes	Jugular vein	–	73.3 ± 4.29	7.277 ± 0.012	23.23 ± 0.58	29.22 ± 3.74
30 minutes	Jugular vein	–	72.1 ± 1.879	7.316 ± 0.019	26.90 ± 1.26	18.47 ± 2.28
1 hour	Jugular vein	–	61.4 ± 2.181	7.356 ± 0.02	26.94 ± 1.54	16.03 ± 1.47
36 hours	Jugular vein	–	57.0 ± 3.69	7.385 ± 0.0105	27.55 ± 0.914	8.160 ± 2.039
24 hours	Jugular vein	–	58.80 ± 2.29	7.392 ± 0.0065	29.30 ± 0.515	6.800 ± 0.815

*Mean ± SE. Data from Rossdale (1968*a* and unpublished).

TABLE 5.2 AST, SAP and CK levels in the jugular venous blood of 11 normal Thoroughbred foals between the ages of 12 and 96 hours

AST (IU litre)	*SAP* (IU litre)	*CK* (IU/litre)
71.5 ± 4.03	566.3 ± 20.64	52.3 ± 4.25

*Mean ± SE. Data from Rossdale and Ricketts (unpublished).

TABLE 5.3 Jugular venous protein content * before and after sucking for the first time

Age	*Total serum protein* (g/litre)	*Albumin* (g/litre)	*Total globulin* (g/litre)	*α-globulin* (g/litre)	*β-globulin* (g/litre)	*γ-globulin* (g/litre)
First hour before sucking	45†					
	45.8 ± 1.9‡	27.4 ± 1.7‡	18.4 ± 1.4‡			
	48.08 ± 1.6(12) §	33.25 ± 1.95(12) §	14.83 ± 1.74(12) §	5.1 ± 1.63(6) §	5.23 ± 0.71(6) §	0(6) §
12–96 hours after sucking	60†					
	54.4 ± 2.9‡	23.4 ± 1.3‡	31 ± 2.6‡			
	48.9 ± 1.43(29) §	28.24 ± 1.14(29) §	20.31 ± 1.63(29) §	6.59 ± 7.6(20) §	6.32 ± 5.6(20) §	8.1 ± 1.13(20) §

* Mean ± SE.
† Jeffcott (1972).
‡ Rossdale (1966).
§ Rossdale (unpublished date) from normal Thoroughbred foals. No. of samples in parentheses.

TABLE 5.4 Glucose, cortisol, sodium and potassium levels* in the jugular venous blood during the first 36 hours after birth

Age	*Whole blood glucose* (mmol/litre)	*Plasma glucose*† (mmol/litre)	*Plasma cortisol*‡ (nmol/litre)	*Serum sodium* § (mmol/litre)	*Serum potassium* § (mmol/litre)
10 minutes	3.6 ± 0.13	5.2 ± 0.33	6.75 ± 0.36	–	–
1 hour	3.1 ± 0.30	4.8 ± 0.44	8.70 ± 0.63	184.4 (5 samples) range 173.9–195.6	4.38 (5 samples) range 1.4–5.7
10 to 12 hours	5.0 ± 0.48	7.2 ± 0.69	3.75 ± 0.53	–	–
36 hours	5.7 ± 0.28	7.4 ± 0.33	3.75 ± 1.5	–	–

* Mean ± SE except where stated.
† Rossdale (unpublished data).
‡ Rossdale et al. (1973).
§ Rossdale and Ricketts (unpublished data).

TABLE 5.5 Erythrocyte count, haemoglobin content, packed cell volume and total and differential leucocyte count in jugular venous blood of 22 normal Thoroughbred foals from birth to 96 hours

Age	*Erythrocytes* ($\times 10^{12}$/litre)	*Haemoglobin* (g/dl)	*Packed cell volume* (litre/litre)	*Leucocytes* Total ($\times 10^{9}$/litre)	Polymorphs (%)	Lymphocytes (%)	Monocytes (%)	Eosinophils (%)
Birth	10.32 ± 0.213	15.07 ± 0.238	0.46 ± 0.007	6.83 ± 0.36	67 ± 2.34	32.5 ± 2.32	0.5	0
12 hours	9.20 ± 0.367	14.04 ± 0.567	0.41 ± 0.018	10.07 ± 1.02	74.4	24.2	1.4	0
24 hours	8.975 ± 0.2056	13.78 ± 0.358	0.40 ± 0.011					
36–96 hours	8.971 ± 0.3524	13.31 ± 0.20	0.38 ± 0.007	7.82	71.2	26.8	2	0

Rossdale and Ricketts (unpublished data).

TABLE 5.6 Plasma thyroxine and triidothyronine concentrations in the blood serum of foals and adult horses

Age	*Mean TT3* (ng/100 ml)	*Free T3* (%)	*Mean FT3* (ng/100 ml)	*Mean TT4* (μg/100 ml)	*Free T4* (%)	*Mean FT4* (ng/100 ml)
Cord	529 (5)	0.24 (4)	1.42 (4)	38.441 (8)	0.03560 (8)	13.499 (8)
1 to 10 hours	991 (4)	0.33 (2)	2.99 (2)	28.859 (11)	0.04490 (11)	12.122 (11)
1 to 3 days	940 (3)	0.42 (2)	4.34 (2)	28.026 (6)	0.03370 (6)	12.145 (6)
4 days	935 (2)	0.32 (2)	2.71 (2)	11.158 (6)	0.04450 (6)	5.896 (6)
5 to 11 days	631 (9)	0.42 (4)	2.40 (4)	7.447 (15)	0.05050 (15)	3.298 (15)
12 to 16 days	292 (5)	0.58 (5)	1.70 (5)	2.722 (4)	0.07258 (4)	1.925 (4)
22 to 90 days	192 (5)	0.69 (5)	1.33 (5)	2.572 (6)	0.06830 (6)	1.756 (6)
Adult	78 (100)	0.73 (48)	0.575 (48)	2.702 (100)	0.0920 (100)	2.581 (100)

After Irvine and Evans (1975).
No. of samples shown in parentheses.

In Thoroughbreds, the mean total count at birth was $6.83 \pm 0.357 \times 10^9$/litre and at age 12 hours $10.068 \pm 1.022 \times 10^9$/litre; polymorphs increased from mean 67% to 75% over the same period (Rossdale 1973, unpublished).

Table 5.5 shows haematological values which may be expected in normal foals during the first 36 days post-partum.

Thyroid hormones

Hormones from the thyroid which may be measured in blood serum include total thyroxine (TT_4), free thyroxine (FT_4), total triiodothyronin (TT_3) and free triïdothyronine (FT_3). Thyroid hormones regulate many functions affecting fetal and neonatal development and are concerned in energy metabolism, muscle and skeletal growth, neuromuscular maturation and thermogenesis through their energy-producing effect on the body tissues especially those such as brown fat through their potentiating action on catecholamines. Irvine and Evans (1975) reported levels of TT_4, FT_4, TT_3 and FT_3 in foal umbilical cord blood of, respectively, 14, five, seven and three times the concentrations of these hormones in adult horse blood (Table 5.6). He found that TT_4 levels declined rapidly to reach adult concentrations by Day 16 and FT_4 levels declined steadily during the first three months of life. TT_3 levels rose during the first ten hours after birth and thereafter declined although they were still two and a half times higher than adult levels at three months of age. Levels of FT_3 similarly increased after birth becoming eight times higher than adult levels at three days of age but declining after this time to about twice the normal adult level by three months of age.

It is the concentration of the three hormones which is physiologically significant because this is the form in which they cross the capillary wall and cell membranes (Irvine & Simpson-Morgan 1974). The very high levels of thyroid hormones in newborn foals may be responsible for their very marked ability to maintain their body temperature even against a very cold environment and for rapid pre- and postnatal growth rates of the musculoskeletal and nervous systems. The relationship between hypothyroidism and musculoskeletal defects in foals has been discussed by Baker and Lindsey (1968), Rooney (1972) and Gribble (1972) (see pp. 386 and 528).

DISEASES OF FIRST FOUR DAYS AFTER BIRTH

The relationship between neonatal conditions and the pre- and intranatal environment of the fetus is complex. Before birth the fetus may be affected by viral or bacterial infection, e.g. equid herpesvirus I (rhinopneumonitis) or *Actinobacillus equuli;* by developmental abnormality; or by placentitis due to hypoxia or idiopathic causes. These factors may cause retarded growth, malnourishment or functional immaturity of fetal organs. In these cases stresses normally imposed by birth and the newborn environment may become disproportionately great. Alternatively, birth may be abnormal and cause chemical or physical damage to a previously normal and well developed fetus. Pre- and intranatal disturbances account for non-infective conditions such as still-birth, 'prematurity' and 'immaturity', developmental abnormalities and states which we will describe under the neonatal maladjustment syndrome (i.e. barkers, wanderers, dummies and convulsive foals) (Fig. 5.24).

The term 'stress' defines abnormal changes in the environment of the fetus at any stage of gestation or birth. It may be acute or chronic according to the degree

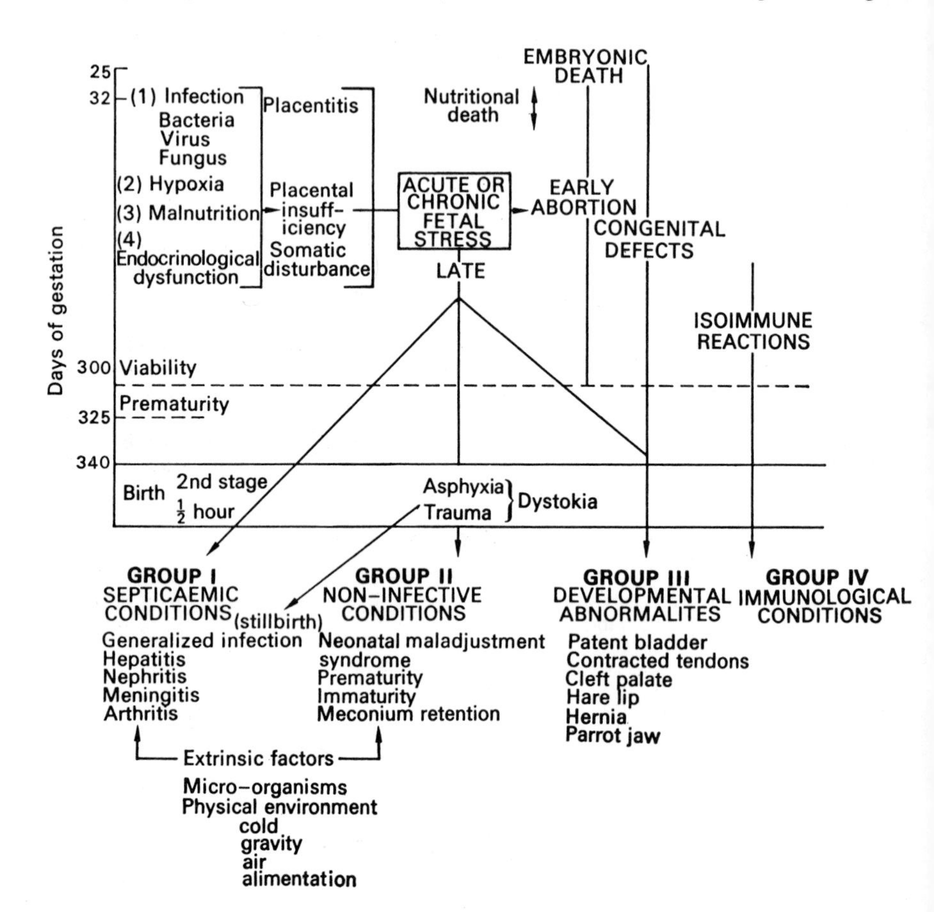

Fig. 5.24. Intrinsic and extrinsic factors which may affect fetal development and cause neonatal disease. (*After Rossdale 1972a*)

of interference produced in the physiological stability of the fetus. Acute stress early in gestation produces fetal death and abortion; in late gestation or during birth it causes still-birth, delayed onset of respiration, convulsions and other behavioural abnormalities.

Once delivered, the fetus is subjected to extrinsic factors, the most challenging of which are an air environment, gravity, relatively low surrounding temperature, the presence of micro-organisms and the need for alimentation and excretion unassisted by the placenta.

Classification of neonatal conditions

No table of conditions which have such a diverse, yet interrelated, aetiology can be more than a broad framework to which further definitions may be introduced as knowledge becomes available.

Infective conditions

Group I characterized by fever, lethargy and reduced strength of the suck reflex

Non-infective conditions

Group II characterized by gross disturbances in behaviour
Group III characterized by developmental abnormalities
Group IV characterized by immunological reactions between maternal and fetal tissues.

TABLE 5.7 Group 1: Bacteraemic, septicaemic and viraemic conditions

Condition	*Synonyms*	*Characteristics*	*Aetiology*
Generalized infections	Diarrhoea Scour Pleurisy Pneumonia Peritonitis	Fever to 39°C and persisting Diarrhoea Increased respiratory rate, with râles Dehydration, retraction of eyeballs	*Escherichia coli* *Streptococcus* spp.
Hepatitis	Virus abortion Rhinopneumonitis	Convulsions Lethargy Mild jaundice Leucopenia	Equid herpesvirus I Cytomegalovirus
Nephritis	Viscosum Shigellosis Sleepy foal disease Sleeper	Initial fever to 39°C, becoming subnormal Sleepiness Diminished strength of suck Diarrhoea, mild colic Convulsions Uraemia; protein, cells in urine Variable leucocytosis	*Actinobacillus equuli* (BVE)
'Meningitis'	Convulsions	Fever to 39°C and persisting Convulsions	*Streptococcus* spp. *Escherichia coli* *Actinobacillus equuli*
Encephalitis		Gross disturbances of behaviour Leucocytosis	
Infective arthritis	Joint ill Navel ill	Fever to 39°C and persisting Lameness	*Streptococcus* spp. *Salmonella typhimurium*
Tenosynovitis		Painful swelling round joints Increasing leucocytosis	*Staphylococcus* spp. *Escherichia coli*

Group I: Infective

Group I (Table 5.7) comprises infective conditions characterized by fever, lethargy and reduced strength of suck reflex. Synonyms are sleepy foal disease (Dimock et al. 1947; Belonje 1952; Leader 1952; Maguire 1958; Littlejohn 1959), septicaemia and meningitis.

Aetiology and incidence

Causal organisms include *Streptococcus zooepidemicus, Escherichia coli, Actinobacillus equuli* (*Bacterium viscosum equi, Shigella equirulus*), *Staphylococcus aureus, Salmonella typhimurium, Klebsiella aerogenes,* equid herpesvirus I (EHV-I) and cytomegalovirus, in approximate order of incidence. About 1% of foals are affected, but incidence varies according to geographical area, climate, management and the type and virulence of infecting organisms. In any particular locality the predominant challenging organisms may change from year to year. Miller (1950) reported that 50% and Platt (1973) 33% of foal mortality in the first seven weeks post-partum was caused by infection.

Neonatal foal disease associated with perinatal infection by equid herpesvirus I has been described by Bryans et al. (1977) and Dixon et al. (1978). This condition is postulated as representing a clinical entity, in addition to those of respiratory disease in young horses, abortion in mares and neurological disease. Some cases are ill at birth, presenting as weak foals, but the majority appear normal at that stage and receive their full complement of colostrum. Clinical signs become apparent during the first week of life and foals show a failure to nurse, lethargy and rapidly developing weakness. Rectal temperature may be normal, subnormal or elevated and pneumonia and/or diarrhoea may develop in most cases. Treatment with supportive and antibiotic therapy gives no significant improvement and most cases die. Haematological examinations reveal lymphopenia, sometimes a total leucopenia and hypogammaglobulinaemia. In treated foals, the course of the disease may vary from a few days to as long as two weeks. The foals may contract a variety of bacterial infections involving *E. coli, Str. zooepidemicus, Salmonella* sp. and *Bacillus piliformis.* Bryans et al. (1977) reported one foal with a virus-neutralizing titre of 1 in 40 for EHV-I.

Post-mortem findings reveal signs of secondary bacterial infection with their effects including bronchopneumonia, septicaemia, polyarteritis and enteritis as well as the more 'specific' lesions of splenic and thymic hypoplasia. The thymus and splenic lymphoid follicles are depleted of lymphocytes and may show areas of fibrosis and necrosis. The spleen is grossly small and abnormally dry on cut surface. Typical herpes intranuclear inclusion bodies are not seen in this disease, possibly because of their resolution by the immune response of the fetus to the viral infection which is acquired in utero, late in gestation. Bryans et al. (1977) suggest that the presence of intranuclear inclusion bodies in herpesvirus-infected tissues indicates an acute, productive viral infection. When abortion occurs relatively soon after infection, inclusion bodies are easier to detect. They speculate as to whether some of these 'recovered' cases may go on to present symptoms suggestive of the condition described as combined immunodeficiency disease (see p. 412).

Predisposing causes

Predisposing factors for Group I conditions are chronic endometritis, overcrowding and continual use of foaling boxes, prematurity, artificial severance and ligation of the cord, preparturient loss of colostrum and failure of immunoglobulin absorption mechanisms.

Transmission

Prenatal infection may occur by haematogenous spread or through the amniotic fluid and post-natal via the umbilicus or the alimentary tract. It is not usually possible to determine in any particular case whether infection occurred pre- or post-natally. Most causal organisms inhabit the alimentary or genital tract of the mare and are a cause of abortion and/or infection of the placenta. Acute signs of septicaemia may be present within 12 hours of birth and it is difficult to see in these cases how a fulminating infection could begin post-natally. However, to establish a prenatal origin of infection the organism must be recovered from the placenta and/or genital tract of the mare immediately after birth. Sources of post-natal infection are faeces-contaminated bedding, soil, mammary region of the mare, feeding utensils and the hands and clothes of attendants. Equine infectious anaemia (EIA) may be transmitted through the colostrum (Kemen & Coggins 1972).

Pathogenesis

Localization in various tissues depends on the nature of the causal organism. *Actinobacillus equuli* has a predilection for kidneys, adrenal glands and brain, and *Staph. aureus* and *S. typhimurium* for articular and periarticular structures including epiphyses. *Str. zooepidemicus, E. coli* and *Klebsiella aerogenes* are ubiquitous, occurring in lungs, peritoneum, pleura, joints and umbilicus. EHV-I and cytomegalovirus infect primarily liver and lung tissue. In practice it is rare to find complete localization and most cases are partially septicaemic. Traditional classifications have, however, been based on clinical signs and these are often related to the organs most severely affected, e.g. joint-ill, meningitis, diarrhoea and sleepy foal disease (nephritis). For this reason a summary of the predilection of causal organisms is presented in Table 5.7, together with a summary of predominant signs, but none of these subdivisions is likely to be found alone in any particular instance.

Clinical signs

Although many signs are related directly to the site of infection, most cases show lethargy, reduced strength of the suck reflex and inability to stand and hold the sucking position. Signs may appear at any time up to the end of the fourth day after birth but are most common on the second day. They start as slight dullness and a reluctance to feed. The reduced amount sucked from the mammary glands leaves the udder distended and milk may drip from the teats so that it stains the face and muzzle of the foal as it makes half-hearted attempts to suck. The rectal temperature at this stage may be normal or slightly raised to 38.6°C.

After several hours, depending on the severity of the condition, the foal becomes increasingly lethargic, is disinclined to suck and exhibits definite signs of illness. Rectal temperature may rise to 41°C, although in many cases it remains below 38.8°C, especially if the foal becomes comatose; terminally the temperature may become subnormal. Recordings should be made at least every six hours to establish the presence of transient rises which have diagnostic significance and may be missed by less frequent recordings. Buccal mucous membranes may become pale, injected or greyish. The conjunctiva may be pale or injected and the sclera tinged with jaundice.

Increasing heart and respiratory rates may be present and signs of dehydration include loss of mobility of the skin and retracted eyeballs. Convulsions, extensor rigidity and opisthotonus are common neurological signs; a foetid, evil-smelling diarrhoea may develop and be associated with signs of colic, such as rolling or lying in awkward attitudes, i.e. on the back, with the head turned backwards, or with a fore-leg hung over the poll. Lameness and painful swelling around the joints are associated with periarticular or articular infections and râles or dullness over the lung area can be detected in bronchitis and pneumonia.

It is possible to distinguish peracute, acute and chronic cases but premonitory signs are usually noted by watching carefully. In some instances, however, death occurs suddenly on the first day after birth.

Laboratory findings

Blood. A subnormal red cell count (5×10^{12}/litre) and haemoglobin content (10 g/dl) may be associated with reduced haemopoietic activity caused by bacterial toxins. There is a concurrent fall (0.36 litre/litre) in packed cell volume, but diarrhoea or dehydration may cause increases to about 0.45 litre/litre. The white cell count depends on the nature of the infecting organism and unknown factors associated with the body's response to infection. The count rises above 10×10^9/litre but sometimes not until some hours or days after the onset of the signs. Leucopenia (4×10^9/litre) occurs in viral or bacterial infections producing leucocidal substances. In general, a depressed white cell count indicates a poor prognosis.

Total serum protein is usually low (40 g/litre); globulin levels are less than 15 g/litre and gammaglobulin less than 3 g/litre.

In viral infections of the liver, serum bilirubin levels rise to 171 μmol/litre and give a direct Van den Bergh reaction. (In haemolytic disease levels approach 342 μmol/litre and always give an indirect Van den Bergh reaction.)

Nephritis causes blood urea levels, measured by the Urastat method, to rise above 20.7 mmol/litre.

Urine. The presence of epithelial cells, leucocytes and large amounts of protein in centrifuged samples of urine indicates nephritis, especially if associated with uraemia.

Bacteriology. Synovial, cerebrospinal, tracheal or peritoneal fluid, blood, faeces and urine can be cultured, although results are frequently negative or of no practical significance. Material should be collected before giving antibiotics and an attempt made to isolate the causal organisms. In *A. equuli* infection negative results may be due to the filter effect of the glomeruli which, on histological examination, can be seen to contain numbers of bacteria. Organisms can rarely be cultured from purulent synovial fluid, as they may be confined to the synovial membrane.

Diagnosis

Septicaemia should be suspected if a foal makes half-hearted attempts to suck and after a few swallows of milk lets its head fall down and, with eyelids half closed, allows milk to dribble from its mouth. The foal may also go lame, suffer from diarrhoea or show signs of dehydration. The rectal temperature is greater than 38.8°C. An increasing white blood cell count and blood urea, and the presence of protein in the urine, confirm the diagnosis, but a complete diagnosis can only be made when an organism is isolated from body tissues or fluids.

Treatment

Antibiotics should be given immediately infection is suspected, because delay may make this condition less amenable to treatment. For this reason all newborn foals should be observed hourly if managerial conditions allow. In the absence of laboratory isolation of the causal organism, the choice of a therapeutic agent is subjective. Neomycin sulphate, ampicillin, cloxacillin or trimethoprim and sulphadiazine may be used separately or in combination. For broad-spectrum cover chloromycetin, trimycetin or amoxycillin is recommended. Therapy must be evaluated against the response obtained and treatment should be continued for at least 48 hours after signs have subsided. Total daily dosage should be subdivided into two, preferably three, doses and given parenterally. The intrathecal route may be used in cases of meningitis; intra-articular administration is essential for infective arthritis and oral therapy for diarrhoea.

Dam's plasma (Fig. 5.25) should be administered intravenously and whole blood if the foal's packed cell volume is less than 0.35 litre/litre. Donor plasma should first be cross-matched against the foal's erythrocytes (see p. 546) and 100 ml can then be injected into one of the jugular veins using a syringe or transfusion apparatus. The dose may be repeated at three-hour intervals two or three times.

Prevention

Antibiotics can be given during the first three days after birth. The choice of drug and the length of time it should be given are subjective. A regimen of trimethoprim and sulphadiazine, intramuscular neomycin or oral framycetin, once daily for the first three to six days after birth, has been used in our practice with apparent benefit, but is recommended only where large numbers of foals are born each year on the same premises, if neonatal infective conditions are known to be prevalent or if the mare has 'run' milk before foaling. Platt (1977) reviewed the history of 2744 singleton and twin foals born alive in the course of a perinatal survey carried on an unspecified number of Thoroughbred stud farms during the years 1968–73 and

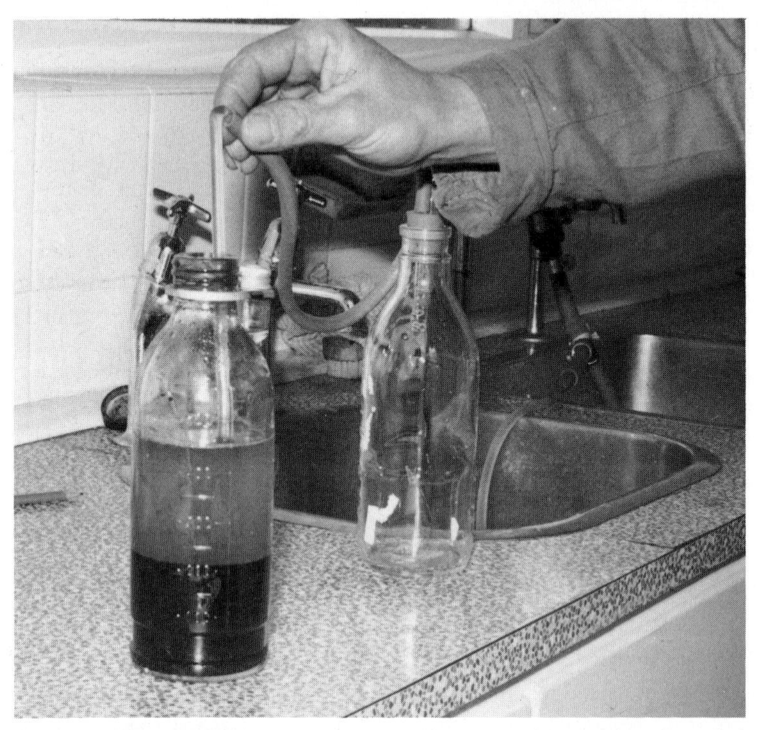

Fig. 5.25. Plasma for transfusion can conveniently be separated by suction after whole blood has been allowed to stand for one to two hours.

concluded that foals receiving neomycin (1 g/day) or framycetin (100 mg/day) orally for three days had significantly lower infection rates than foals not treated or given antibiotics on the first day only. Antibiotic therapy may be supplemented by about 200 ml of donor colostrum within two hours of birth. It can be fed from a bottle and artificial teat or by stomach tube. Selective administration of antibiotics or transfusion of dam's plasma is recommended if, in the period 6 to 24 hours after the first suck, gammaglobulin blood levels are below an arbitrarily defined level of 3 g/litre.

Pathology

Lesions vary with the type of organism and the site of infection. *Str. zooepidemicus* is associated with macroscopic abscessation, and with fibrinous or purulent exudates which may reach considerable quantities in both the peritoneal and pleural cavities.

E. coli infections are characterized by pleural and peritoneal effusions containing leucocytes and organisms but, unlike those of *Str. zooepidemicus*, not usually large amounts of fibrin. The carcass often possesses a characteristic sweet-smelling odour.

Actinobacillus equuli causes microscopic abscessation in many organs, particularly in the renal and adrenal cortices. Invariably, the organism may be cultured from the brain.

EHV-I infection causes microscopic foci of liver necrosis associated with intranuclear inclusion bodies. Cytomegalovirus presents a diffuse necrosis of the liver and pigmentation of cells without inclusion bodies.

TABLE 5.8 Group II: Non-infective conditions characterized by gross disturbances in behaviour

Condition	*Synonyms*	*Characteristics*	*Aetiology*
Neonatal maladjustment syndrome (NMS)	Barkers Wanderers Dummies Convulsives	Full-term gestation Onset within first 24 hours: often normal until onset Complete loss of suck reflex and ability to nurse Apparent blindness Convulsions, hypertonus, spasms Coma Hypothermia Acidaemia, hypercapnia	Asphyxia Birth trauma Fetal stress
	Respiratory distress	Low PaO_2 breathing air and 100% oxygen Respiratory rate and minute volume increased Tidal volume decreased	
Prematurity		300–320 days gestation Signs apparent at birth Weakness, delay in first standing Low birth weight Reduced strength of sucking, ability to suck and ability to maintain body temperature Tendency to colic after feeding 'Bedsores' Discolored tongue, silky skin PaO_2 low breathing air; increased breathing 100% oxygen	Fetal stress
Dysmaturity	Immaturity	More than 320 days gestation but appearance and signs of prematurity Emaciation, dehydration Diarrhoea Susceptibility to infection	Fetal stress Placentitis
Meconium retention	Stoppage Ileus	Signs from birth to third day Straining, colic, laying in awkward postures Generally not off suck and in good health Abdominal tympany	Unknown

The tongue may have a furry coating due to fungal or monilial infection after prolonged antibiotic therapy. Bacterial growth may be obtained from heart blood, lungs, liver, spleen or kidney, but cultures may remain sterile if the foal has had appropriate antibiotics before death.

Group II: Behaviour disturbances

Group II (Table 5.8) consists of non-infective conditions characterized by gross disturbances in behaviour. We recognize three categories: neonatal maladjustment syndrome (NMS), prematurity and dysmaturity (immaturity) and meconium retention (Table 5.8).

Neonatal maladjustment syndrome

Various other names for this syndrome are barkers (Reynolds 1930), wanderers, dummy or convulsive syndrome (Mahaffey & Rossdale 1957). The term neonatal maladjustment syndrome (NMS) has been coined to include both these conditions and respiratory distress. Future research will undoubtedly require the classification to be modified further, but for the present we consider it appropriate.

Aetiology and incidence

The causes are not fully understood, but hypoxia and circulatory disturbances are thought to be the predominant aetiological factors. Haemorrhages affecting the cerebral cortex and in some cases injury to the thorax suggest that birth trauma may be an exciting cause (see below). Incidence is about 0.75% of full-term births.

Pathogenesis

NMS is primarily a condition of disturbed stability of physiological mechanisms associated with the adaptive processes, especially the cardiopulmonary and nervous systems. Neurological signs include convulsions and loss of the suck reflex; pulmonary signs are associated with atelectasis and hypoxia; biochemical disturbances are characterized by acidaemia. The condition may end in right-heart failure.

A number of different pathways might account for the signs and pathology of the condition.

Cerebral oedema and haemorrhage. Vascular abnormalities have been found in the CNS in foals dying in the perinatal period (Haughey & Jones 1976) and ischaemic necrosis of the cerebral cortex and haemorrhage affecting the cerebrum, cerebellum and brain stem was observed at autopsy in foals that had suffered from the neonatal maladjustment syndrome (Palmer & Rossdale 1975, 1976). These findings suggest that cerebral hypoxia may precipitate the convulsive seizures, although blood gas analysis on cord blood prior to the onset of convulsions in four cases experienced by the authors revealed values within the normal range with no evidence of undue asphyxia having occurred during the birth process. Haughey has postulated that, because the brain, spinal cord and meninges are firmly anchored in the craniovertebral canal by dural attachments, blood vessels and nerves, the haemorrhages are evidences of shearing of sizeable vessels, due to differential movement of the skeleton and the CNS, generated by vigorous stage two labour. Another factor which may play a part is the raised fetal blood pressure during delivery (Rossdale et al. 1976). In nine foals peak pressures of 60–200 mmHg have been recorded in the jugular and digital veins during normal delivery. In one case carotid arterial pressure was measured from the time of emergence of the foal's neck from the birth canal and an initial pressure of 175/100 mmHg recorded, which fell to 100/50 mmHg by the time delivery was complete. Jugular venous and systemic arterial pressures in normal foals aged 12–48 hours were below 5 mmHg and 70/50 to 130/100 mmHg respectively.

Pulmonary and circulatory disturbances may be caused by compression of the thorax during passage through the maternal pelvis or severance of the cord immediately the foal is delivered and before respiratory rhythm has been established. As already described, this can deprive the foal of as much as a third of its circulating blood. Premature severance may be caused by obstetric procedures or, if the cord is relatively short, by the final expulsive efforts of the mare. Although depriving the foal of placental blood is probably unphysiological, it is not now thought to be a primary cause of convulsions because cases have occurred when the cord has remained intact (Millar & Bailey 1959; Rossdale 1969*b*).

Compression of the thorax and impeded venous flow during delivery may increase cranial pressure causing extravasation of fluid and blood in the cerebral cortex, followed by convulsions and gross disturbances in behaviour. In this context it may be significant that jugular venous pressure during second-stage delivery rises to 100 mmHg (Rossdale, unpublished).

Asphyxia may cause cerebral oedema and haemorrhage. Pre-, intra- or post-partum asphyxia may play a significant part in convulsions. Whatever the precipitating cause, a vicious circle of biochemical events supervenes in all but the mildest cases. Acidaemia may be profound (Rossdale 1969*b*), whether caused by convulsions or by hypoxia, and arterial pH falls to below 7.0, acidaemia causes increased pulmonary vascular resistance and arterial pressure, decreased power of the heart beat, profound changes in cerebral blood flow and ischaemia (Wyke 1963). Distortion of the pulmonary ventilation/perfusion ratio follows; atelectasis and/or right-heart failure contribute to the hypoxic state and hypoxia to cerebral oedema and haemorrhage.

Atelectasis and, in some cases, hyaline-membrane-like material (Fig. 5.26) in the alveolar ducts (Mahaffey & Rossdale 1959), absence of surfactant (Rossdale et al. 1967) and clinical evidence of respiratory distress (Rossdale 1970) has aroused interest because of similarities with hyaline membrane disease (respiratory distress syndrome) of newborn infants (Dunn 1972).

In the absence of conclusive experimental evidence, present indications suggest that NMS may be due to cerebral haemorrhage and oedema causing disturbed behaviour and convulsions. The convulsions result in a severe metabolic acidaemia and consequent cardiopulmonary dysfunction. Long periods of recumbency may predispose to pulmonary atelectasis due to reduced compliance of the chest wall (see p. 290) and a low functional residual capacity, leading to hypoxia and an

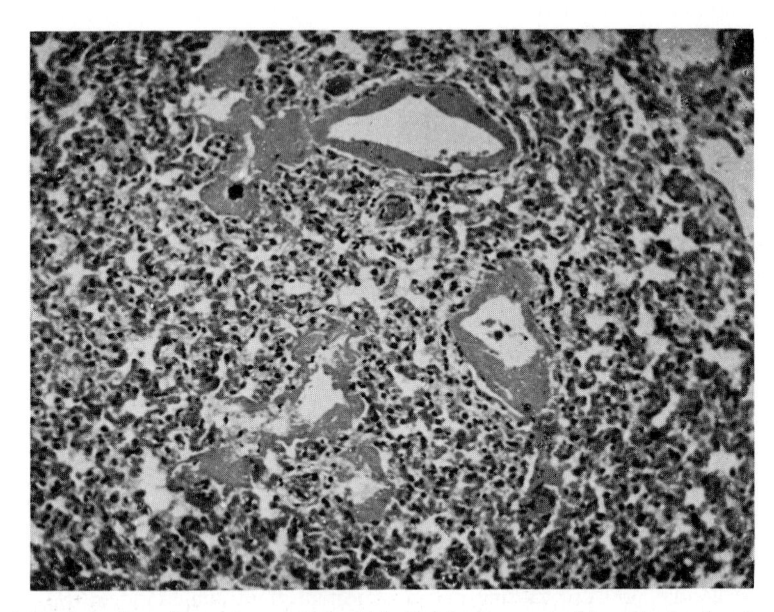

Fig. 5.26. A section of lung from a foal which died during a convulsive episode, showing atelectasis and hyaline-membrane-like material lining the alveolar ducts. H & E × 300.

increased acidaemia. Hypoxia and acidaemia add to the risk of cerebral haemorrhage and oedema, completing the vicious circle initiated by the primary cerebral condition caused by the birth process.

Clinical signs

Behavioural signs usually occur during the first 24 hours of life, most commonly during the first hours. The foal may appear normal at first, but becomes affected by convulsions of a jerky (clonic) or general type. There is a complete loss of the suck reflex and the ability to nurse, although both faculties have originally been present. The foal may be unable to stand or may make violent and aimless galloping movements with its limbs; at the same time it may dash its head against the floor. Opisthotonus and increased extensor tone may be present, the limbs extended and the tail held upright (Fig. 5.27).

Convulsions may be followed by, or may alternate with, periods of coma. Signs of irritability are manifest by continual chewing (Fig. 5.28), grinding the teeth, sneezing and wandering aimlessly round the box. When able to stand, the foal may appear blind and walk into or press against walls or other objects.

The affected foal may show exaggerated response to handling and restraint. Normal reflex behaviour may continue after stimulation has been removed and certain patterns of behaviour may become displaced. For example, a foal may suck a teat on a bottle whether or not it is receiving milk, and continue to suck until the teat is removed from its mouth, when it goes into a deep sleep. Some foals exhibit determined sucking motions with the head extended and directed

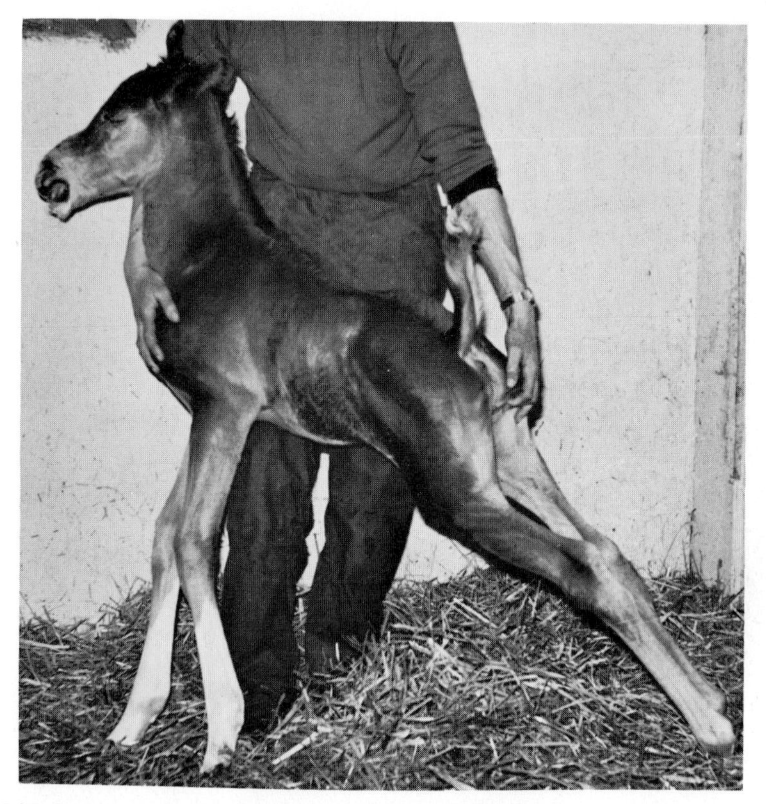

Fig. 5.27. Signs of cerebral haemorrhage and oedema include increased extensor tone, as seen in this foal after a convulsive episode.

downwards, but seem unable to adopt a sucking attitude under the mare and fight violently against being held in the position. Affected foals often lie in awkward positions and have a tendency to go into a deep sleep when laid on the ground.

Asymmetrical pupillary apertures are common, in some cases pinpoint on one side and fully dilated on the other. Petechial retinal haemorrhages are also seen, but these may be found in foals that show no other signs. Blood splashing of the sclera is sometimes found alone or with other optical signs. Some foals make abnormal vocal noises, described as 'barking', grunting or frantic whinnying.

Not every case is affected by all the behavioural signs described. Some foals do not convulse, but show loss of suck reflex and wandering; others may be able to suck at a bottle but lose the ability to suck from or even recognize their mothers.

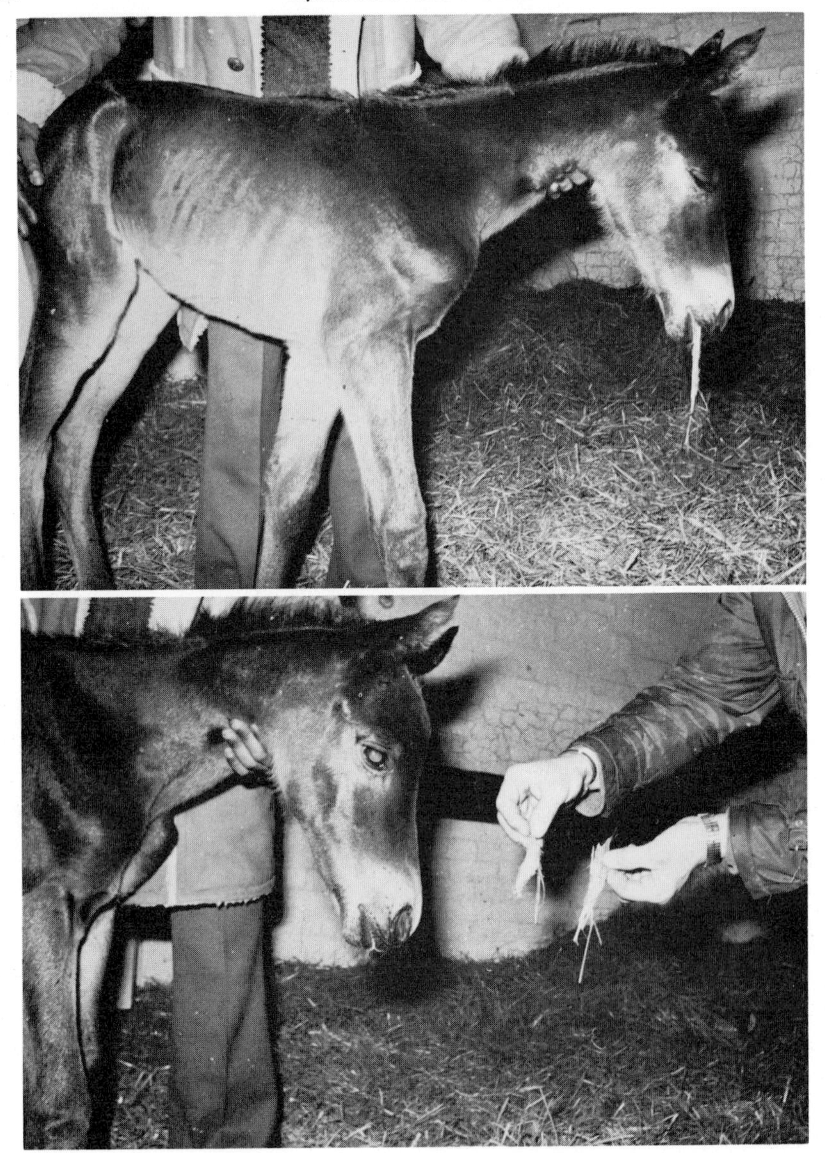

Fig. 5.28. Foals suffering from cerebral lesions often chew incessantly, and masses of chewed straw may be found in the buccal cavity. Its presence may stimulate further chewing.

The rectal temperature depends on the activity of the foal. It rises to 41.1°C and is accompanied by profuse sweating during convulsions and falls during coma to 35°C, remaining within normal limits in mild cases or during convalescence.

Cardiopulmonary function

Two distinct phases of pulmonary function exist in NMS (Rossdale 1969*b*).

Respiratory distress is characterized by increased respiratory rate (above 60/minute) and minute volume, decreased tidal (below 400 ml) and maximal tidal volumes (below 800 ml). During air or 100% oxygen inhalation, arterial blood gas tensions of less than 80 mmHg and less than 100 mmHg have been recorded (Rossdale 1970). Respiratory distress may be present at the onset of signs or appear during the illness and may be associated with hypercapnia (elevated arterial blood carbon dioxide tensions) or hypocapnia.

Râles and reduced air intake may be evident on auscultation, but because of the parallel position of each lung and the consequent transmission of sounds from one to the other, this method of clinical examination has limits. In addition, bronchial sounds may be transmitted through atelectatic areas and give the clinical impression of normal ventilation. In practice radiological examination is restricted by the lack of X-ray machines with sufficient kV to outline the pulmonary areas clearly enough to interpret them.

Foals suffering from acidaemia may present signs which simulate respiratory distress but which are related to increased ventilation activated by a compensatory drive to eliminate carbon dioxide. Tidal and maximal tidal volumes are within the normal ranges, that is about 500 ml and 1200 ml respectively; respiratory rate and minute volumes are increased; arterial blood carbon dioxide tensions are below 30 mmHg; arterial blood oxygen tensions of more than 80 mmHg and more than 200 mmHg are present during air and 100% oxygen inhalation respectively.

Cardiac dysfunction is suggested by rapid heart rate (above 120 beats/minute at rest), a jugular pulse and venous engorgement which is most readily seen in the head and neck. The arterial pulse may be imperceptible or hammer-like, probably reflecting a hypertensive state or high pulse pressure due to low diastolic and/or increased systolic pressures.

Course of condition

Signs of NMS may continue for several hours or for up to 30 days, before the foal is capable of sucking and following its mother. When recovery occurs it is usually complete. Convulsive foals recover in a definite sequence, exhibiting first coma and then the ability to get up and stand. Auditory and visual awareness returns before the ability to suck and recognize the mare.

Diagnosis

Pathognomonic signs of NMS are a sudden and complete loss of the suck reflex and loss of visual and other senses, including the ability to seek or follow the mare. Respiratory distress is defined by an increase in the respiratory rate, low maximal tidal volumes and low arterial blood oxygen tensions during air and oxygen inhalation.

Treatment

Symptomatic and supportive treatment is required, aimed at allowing time to re-establish somatic stability and conclude the adaptive process. Broad-spectrum antibiotic preventive therapy should be given during the course of the condition.

Behaviour and convulsions. Foals unable to get up or stand unaided should be kept under close observation with, if practicable, an attendant always in the box to prevent the foal from exhausting itself in its attempts to stand (Fig. 5.29). The attendant should sit with the foal's head resting on his lap, the animal being restrained in the recumbent position by placing a hand on the under-surface of its head, so that in periods of struggling the muzzle can be raised. At the same time

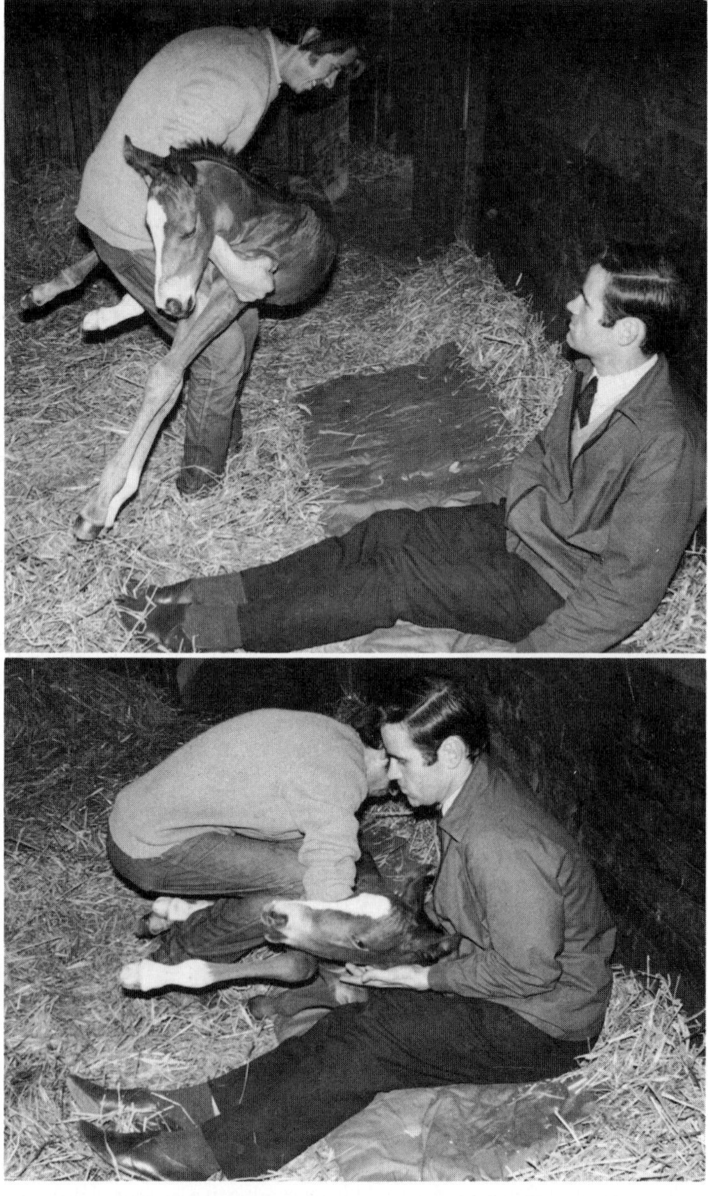

Fig. 5.29. Newborn foals should be handled very gently. These photographs show a convenient method of laying a foal on the ground to be 'nursed'.

the upper fore-leg is held so that the attendant can lean back and avoid being kicked by the hind-legs. It is helpful for a second person to grasp the tail of a foal which is convulsing or struggling violently, to keep the foal's body at right angles to the person at the head. The legs should not be held together since this may exacerbate the foal's struggling (Fig. 5.30).

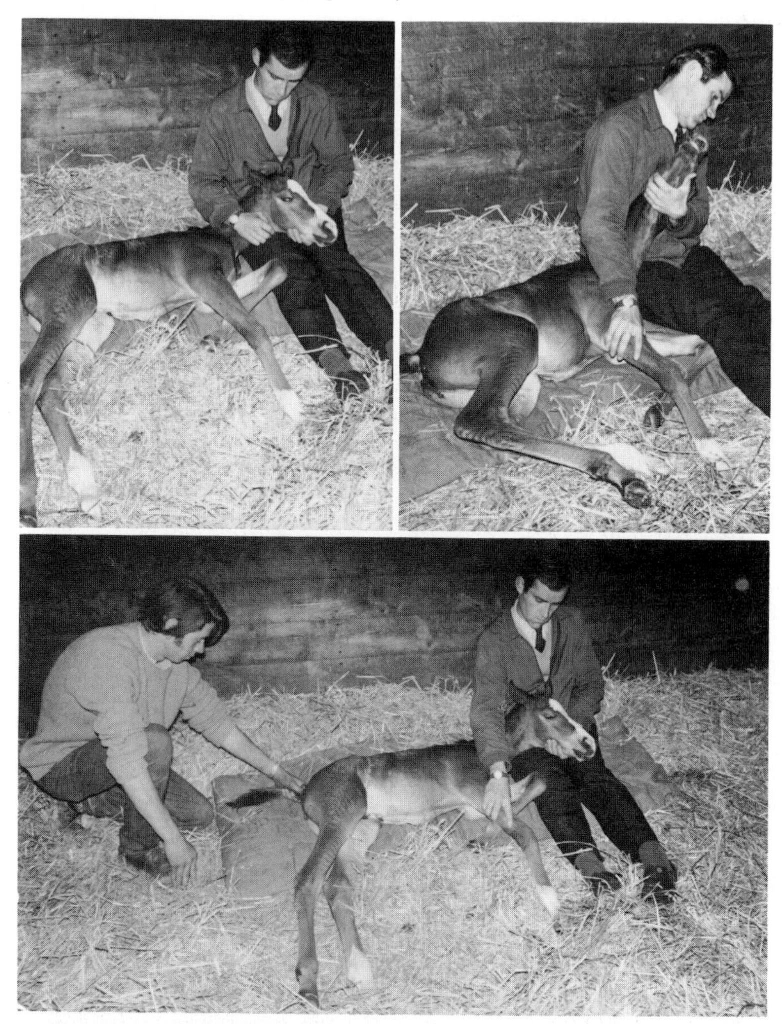

Fig. 5.30. Restraining a foal which is unable to stand or one which is convulsing.

Convulsions can be controlled by phenytoin administered intravenously, intramuscularly or orally at the rate of 5–10 mg/kg body weight followed by maintenance doses of 1–5 mg/kg body weight every two to four hours, reducing after 12 hours to every six or 12 hours, depending on the severity of the convulsions. Oral fluid appears to have a sedative effect. Primidone administered orally at a dose rate of 20–40 mg/kg may be used instead of, or in conjunction with, phenytoin sodium. Intravenous pentobarbitone sodium is very effective when used to control convulsions but because of its relative toxicity and depressant action on the CNS it has a much lower safety margin than phenytoin or primidone. However, it has the advantage of producing a relaxed state in a relatively short period and can be used to maintain semiconsciousness or light anaesthesia for many hours. The dose has to be computed against the reflex activity obtained during administration. About 8 ml of a solution of 60 mg/ml is usually sufficient to obtain appropriate

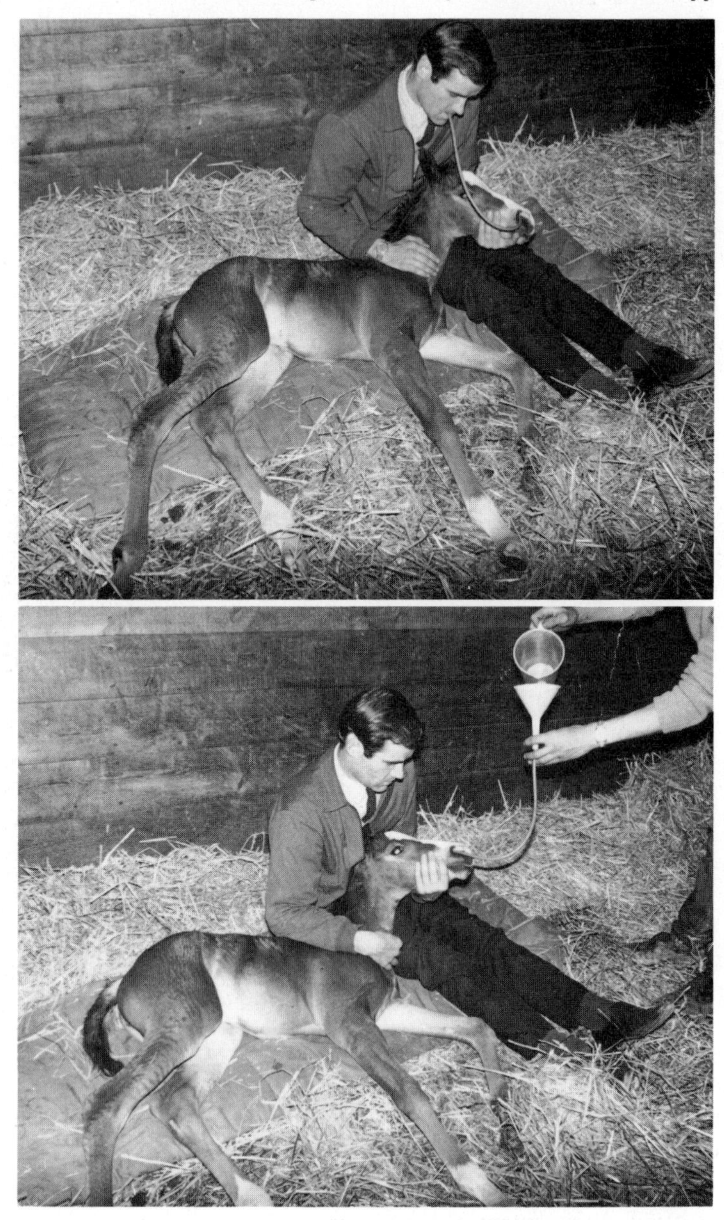

Fig. 5.31. Feeding a foal by stomach tube. The position of the tube is checked by feeling for a bolus of air as it is blown down the oesophagus.

narcosis in a 50 kg foal. In the initial convulsive state, immediate control can be obtained without the harmful struggling against restraint which is the feature of other methods. An in-dwelling catheter may then be sutured into position in the jugular vein for the convenient administration, over prolonged periods, of fluids, electrolytes and drugs.

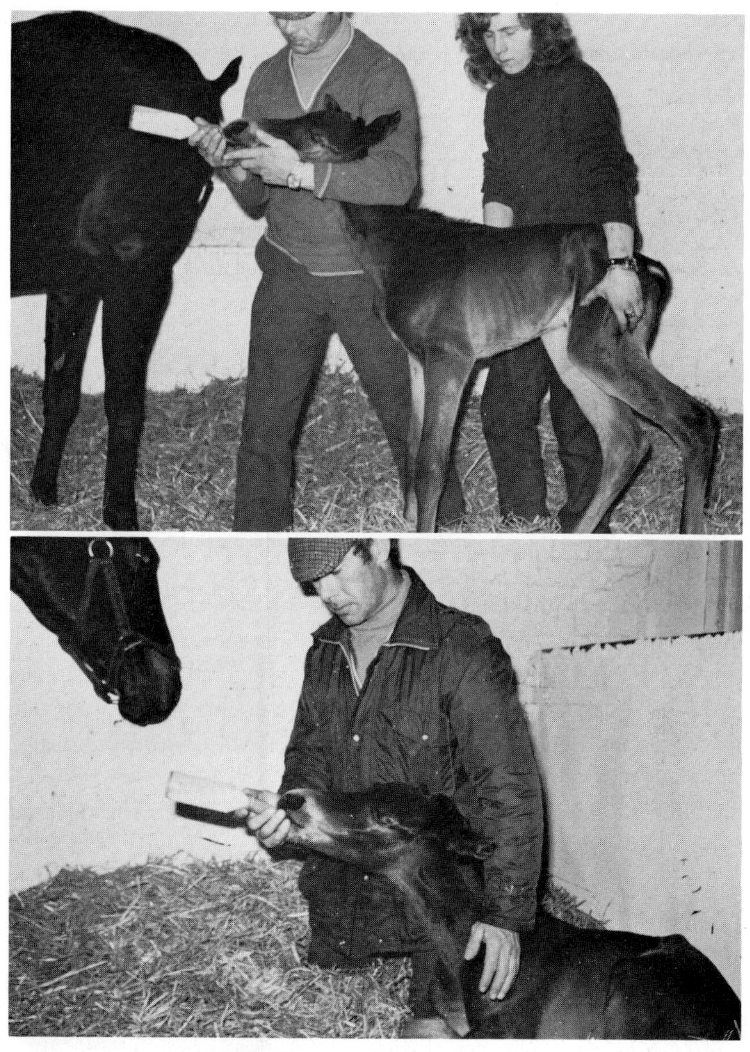

Fig. 5.32. Bottle-feeding a young foal.

Feeding. In the absence of a suck reflex the foal should be fed through a rubber or plastic stomach tube (Fig. 5.31) with outer diameter of about 1 cm and blunt distal end. The tube should be lubricated with water or liquid paraffin and may be passed with the foal either standing or recumbent. The end of the tube should not be passed beyond the entrance to the thorax. Before withdrawal it should be flushed with normal saline to avoid depositing milk in the nasal passages. A bottle with an artificial lamb's or calf's teat may be used if the suck reflex is present but the foal has lost the ability to suck from the mare (Fig. 5.32).

Clinical experience suggests that a foal up to one week old should be fed according to the following principles:

1. In the first three days after birth the quantity of fluid is more important than solid food.

2. Where a normal suck reflex is present the foal's appetite is a rough guide to the quantity of fluid necessary. If adequate quantities are given the foal should sleep readily after feeding and yet appear hungry at a subsequent feed.

3. Feeds may be of colostrum, mare's milk or dried milk. Mare's milk may be fed at the rate of 80–100 ml/kg body weight/day, divided into a minimum of ten equal feeds. A foal of 50 kg body weight would then be fed 4–5 litres/day. It has been found in other species that digestive upsets associated with the explosive growth of pathological coliforms are less serious when small feeds are given frequently. The dry matter of liquid diets should be somewhere between 15 and 20%, which is approximately double that of skimmed cow's milk. A number of proprietary dried milk preparations are available and these should be reconstituted using sufficient powder to provide 45 kilo-calories in 80 ml of water/kg body weight/day. At this rate a 50 kg foal receives 2250 kilo-calories (9417 kJ)/day.

4. Strict hygiene should be practised and it is important to feed at 38°C or below, but never above. For a further account of feeding orphan foals see p. 372.

Hypothermia. Body temperature represents the balance of heat produced by metabolism and heat lost by radiation, conduction, convection and evaporation. In the foal, the basis of heat production is shivering and muscular activity in movement. A normal foal can maintain its temperature against very low ambient temperatures, but one suffering from coma and hypoxia, which prevent normal oxygen consumption, requires special measures.

Mildly affected cases of NMS can be kept warm by fitting a woollen pullover over the body. Severely affected foals require ambient temperatures of 26.6–32.2°C. Radiant heat sources are the most effective, but if these are not available the foal may be covered by a washable electric blanket or rug. Hot air blowers have some effect, but they create draughts and thereby increase heat loss by evaporation.

As a general measure box walls, ceilings and windows should be adequately insulated to reduce loss by radiation. It has been estimated, in other species, that most heat is lost by this route (Oliver 1965).

Homeostasis. For clinical purposes it may be assumed that foals affected by convulsions, severe diarrhoea, or those that fail to establish a normal respiratory rhythm (see below), suffer from acidaemia. Depending on the severity of the condition, 5–10 ml/kg body weight of a 5% solution of sodium bicarbonate should be given intravenously through a 16G 3 cm hypodermic needle or a 15G intravenous catheter using a 50 ml syringe, or by gravity feed. This should be repeated two hours later if the acidosis seems still present, for example, if the convulsions or diarrhoea continue.

Oxygen may be administered through a mask or by a rubber tube inserted into one nostril at flow rates of about 10 litres/minute. The increment of arterial blood oxygen tensions is then similar to those obtained in closed circuit using a mask and Reuben's non-return valve (Rossdale, unpublished).

Foals suffering from convulsions, dehydration or coma, and with a packed cell volume above 0.5 litre/litre, should receive normal saline intravenously 10–20 ml/kg body weight every six hours until the packed cell volume has fallen below 0.5 litre/litre. Where signs of dehydration are severe and there is continual loss of fluid, as in diarrhoeic states, plasma should be given intravenously after cross-matching of foal's cells against donor plasma, at the rate of 250 ml for 15 minutes. The transfusion can be repeated after six hours if necessary. Administration should be slowed or stopped if there is a marked increase in heart or respiratory rate.

Blood sugar levels may be estimated and cases of hypoglycaemia (less than 16.6 mmol/litre whole blood glucose) treated by the intravenous or oral administration of glucose saline.

Cardiac failure. Cardiac embarrassment can be recognized by a heart rate greater than 120 beats/minute at rest, a marked jugular pulse and evidence of venous engorgement. The condition is relieved by 0.5 mg digoxin intramuscularly or intravenously followed by maintenance doses of 0.5 mg twice a day.

Cerebral haemorrhage. This can be diagnosed by examining the cerebrospinal fluid. It is most easily obtained by puncturing the foramen magnum with the foal under sedation and restrained in the recumbent position. There is little risk involved, but clinicians inexperienced in the technique may prefer to rely on the evidence of presenting signs, i.e. convulsions, unequal pupillary apertures and haemorrhagic splashing or petechiae on the sclera and retina. In these cases 10 mg of vitamin K1 intramuscularly initially and twice a day for two days may be helpful.

Adrenal malfunction. Premature foals have low plasma cortisol levels and despite the high levels reported in convulsive foals, corticosteroid therapy (e.g. 5–10 mg dexamethasone daily or twice daily) appears to provide definite clinical benefit in many cases. Treatment should not be started until some hours after the first feed of colostrum because cortisol may block the absorption of globulins through the intestinal mucosa.

Pathology

Macroscopic lesions are confined to the thorax and brain, although secondary infection may have caused pleurisy, pneumonia, peritonitis or furring of the tongue and pharynx. The lungs are blue and cut with the consistency of liver, presenting an airless appearance, and small portions sink in fixative solution. Oedema fluid may be seen in some cases oozing from the cut surface. The cerebral cortex may look congested or contain obvious areas of haemorrhage and/or ischaemic necrosis (Figs 5.33 to 5.36).

On microscopic examination there is evidence of atelectasis and congested alveolar capillaries with, in some cases, hyaline-membrane-like structures present in bronchioles and alveolar ducts. Reduced surfactant activity may be demonstrable (Rossdale et al. 1967), but is not a consistent feature. The pressure–volume relationship in excised lungs in four cases of NMS showed poor stability in two cases, a similar proportion to that found at autopsy in twins and foals classed as premature or dysmature (Rossdale & White 1975).

Cerebral lesions vary in nature and distribution. Most are confined to the cerebrum and occasionally the cerebellum (Palmer & Rossdale 1976) although Haughey and Jones (1976) reported a high frequency of meningeal lesions at autopsy in 26 foals drawn at random from obstetric and paediatric cases occurring on equine stud farms attended by the clinicians of the University of Sydney, New

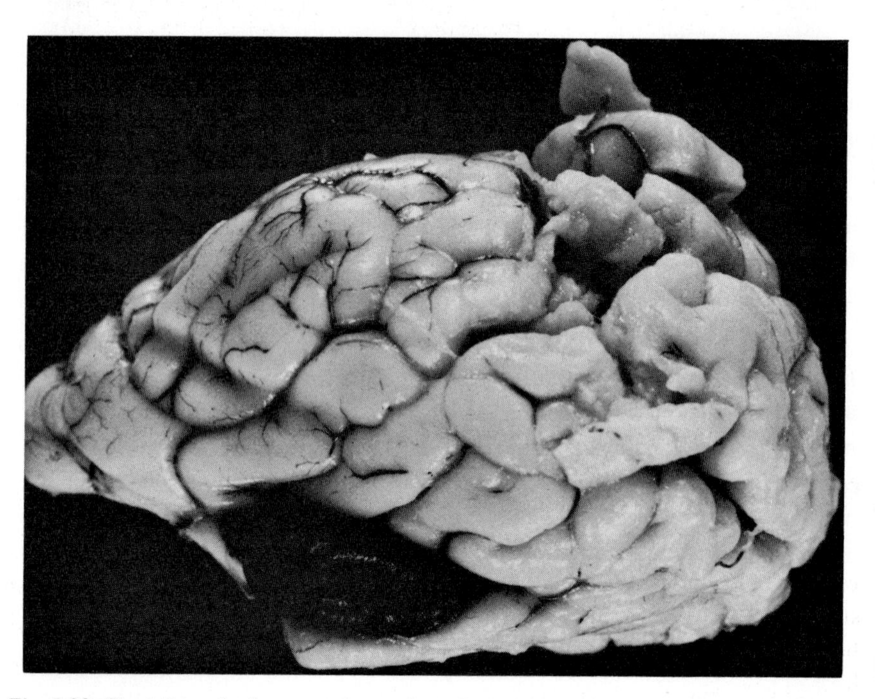

Fig. 5.33. The left cerebral cortex of a newborn foal which suffered convulsions and extensor rigidity. A haemorrhage is present in the cingulate girus. (*By kind permission of A.C. Palmer*)

South Wales. In Palmer and Rossdale's series, the neuropathological findings in 18 cases of foals affected with the neonatal maladjustment syndrome were compared with those in nine foals dying from other causes. Necrosis of the cerebral cortex of an ischaemic nature was found in nine of the NMS foals, frequently accompanied by local haemorrhage (Figs 5.35, 5.36). In three of this group there was also necrosis in the diencephalon and brain stem. In the brains of the nine other affected foals there was haemorrhage in the cerebrum and sometimes in the brain stem and cerebellum; in four there was also brain swelling or oedema. In the control group, significant haemorrhage in the brain was the only finding in two foals, one premature and one still-born, apart from minimal ischaemic damage in the latter.

Prevention

There are no specific measures which can be taken to prevent NMS. As far as possible, the cord should be left intact after birth until the placental circulation has

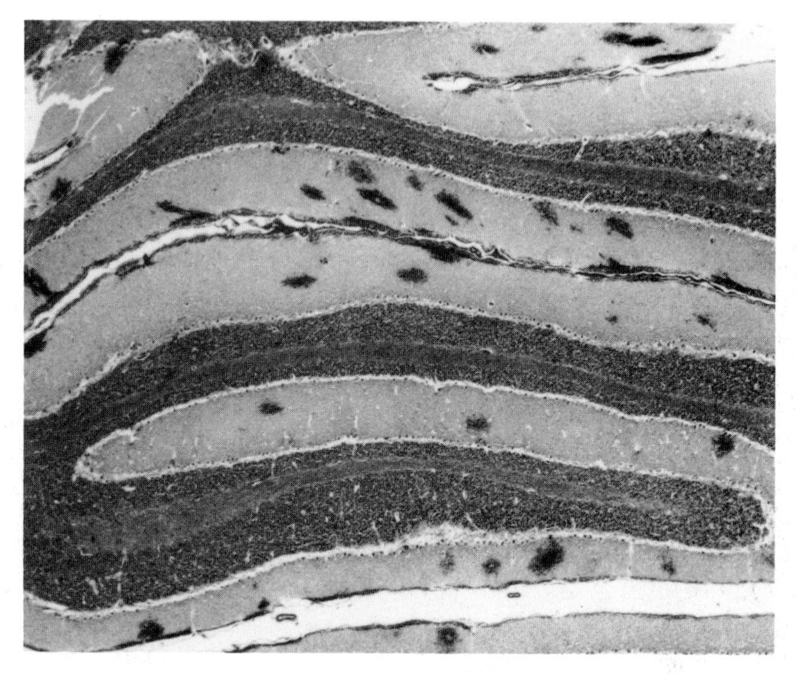

Fig. 5.34. Haemorrhages into the molecular layer of the cerebellum. H & E × 12 (*From Palmer & Rossdale 1976*)

ceased and a respiratory rhythm is established. Any action liable to place increased stress on the foal when it is getting to its feet and sucking for the first time should be avoided. During the first two hours post-partum, the foal should be handled as little as possible.

Fetal asphyxia

A comparison of published data (Table 5.9) from studies of blood $P\text{O}_2$, $P\text{CO}_2$, pH and lactate levels, in fetal pony and Thoroughbred foals before, during and immediately after delivery, suggest the foal normally suffers some degree of asphyxia (increase in arterial blood $P\text{CO}_2$ and decrease in $P\text{O}_2$ and pH) during birth. Comline and Silver (1970, 1973), using indwelling catheter techniques, found that before delivery, at full term the fetal foal's $P\text{O}_2$ and $P\text{CO}_2$ in umbilical arterial blood was 33.4 mmHg and 46.2 mmHg respectively. Fetal pH was 7.346 and lactate levels were in the range 10–22 mg/100 ml (Comline & Silver 1973). Compared with

TABLE 5.9 pH, PCO$_2$ lactate and PO$_2$ levels* in the fetus and normal foals during and immediately after birth

Source	pH	PaCO$_2$ (mmHg)	*Lactate* (mmol/litre)	PaO$_2$ (mmHg)
Fetal umbilical artery†	7.346 ± 0.009 (8)	46.2 ± 1.5 (8)	1.1 – 2.4	33.4 ± 0.9 (8)
Digital artery in second stage prior to respiratory movements‡	7.172 ± 0.014 (20)	72.8 ± 2.209 (18)	2.0 ± 0.22 (9)	22.6 ± 1.422 (17)
Umbilical artery, § gasping in some cases	7.26 ± 0.014 (7)	69.1 ± 3.04 (7)	2.4 ± 0.24	35.4 ± 3.84 (7)

* Mean ± SE. No. of samples shown in parentheses.
† Comline and Silver (1970 and personal communication).
‡ Rossdale (1972*c*).
§ Rossdale (1968*a* and unpublished data).

Comline and Silver's results, significantly lower PO_2 and pH and higher PCO_2 and lactate were recorded in blood samples obtained from the digital artery during second-stage and from the umbilical artery 0.30 seconds after delivery (Rossdale 1968*a*, 1972*c*).

A comparison of fetal and post-partum umbilical vein blood shows pre- and post-parturient values of pH 7.404 and 7.413, PCO_2 39 and 46.2 mmHg and PO_2 49

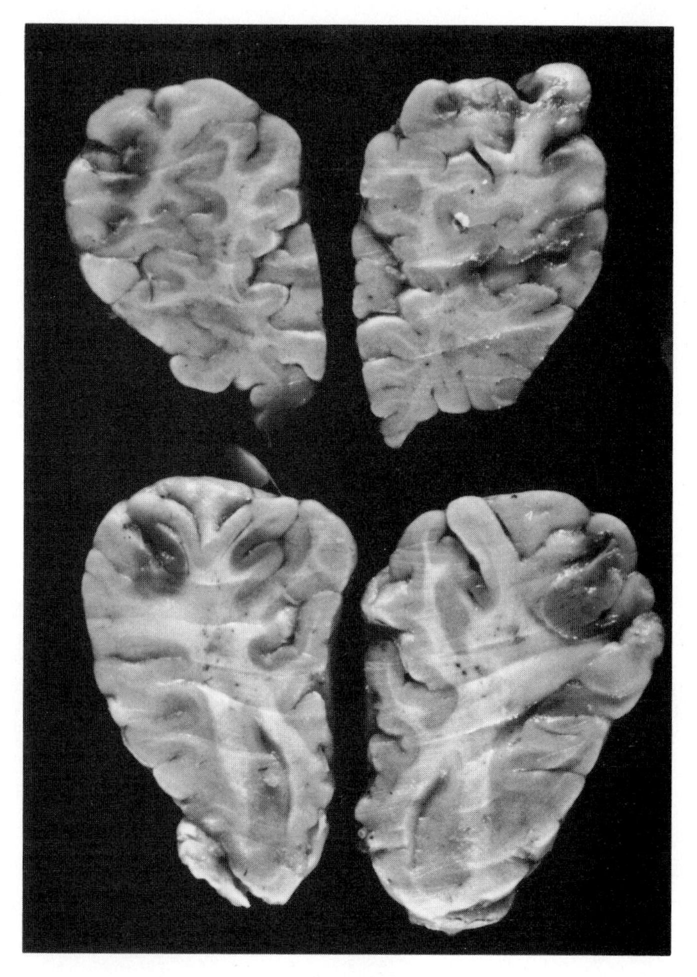

Fig. 5.35. Necrotic areas of the cortex visible as dark discoloration. (*From Palmer & Rossdale 1976*)

and 32.8 mmHg respectively. Although the studies were made under different conditions and any comparison must therefore be interpreted with care, the evidence sugests that asphyxial effects of birth may be due to reduced perfusion of the placenta or circulatory changes in the fetus associated with its passage through the maternal pelvis. It would be interesting to know if breed differences affect the degree of asphyxia suffered during the second stage.

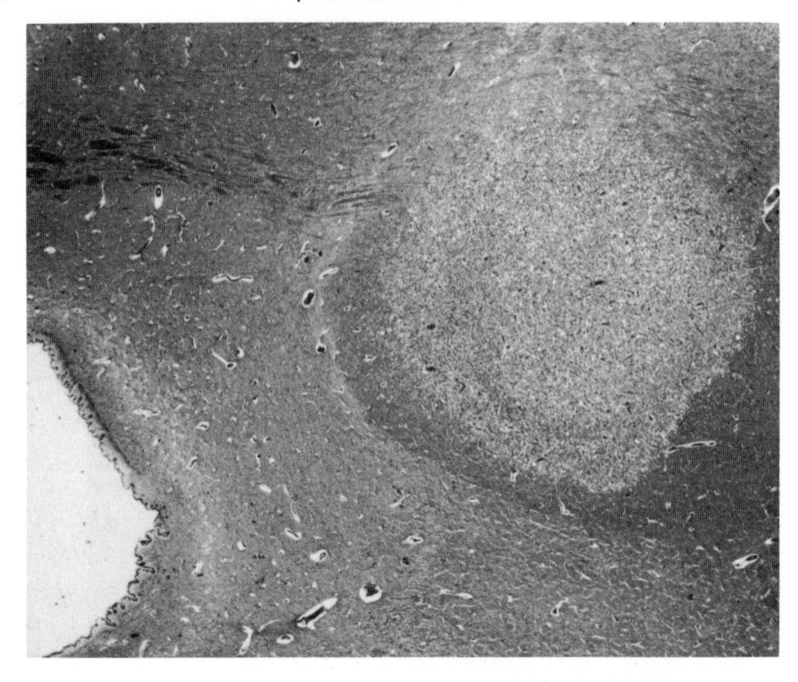

Fig. 5.36. Focal necrosis involving the inferior colliculus (*From Palmer & Rossdale 1976*)

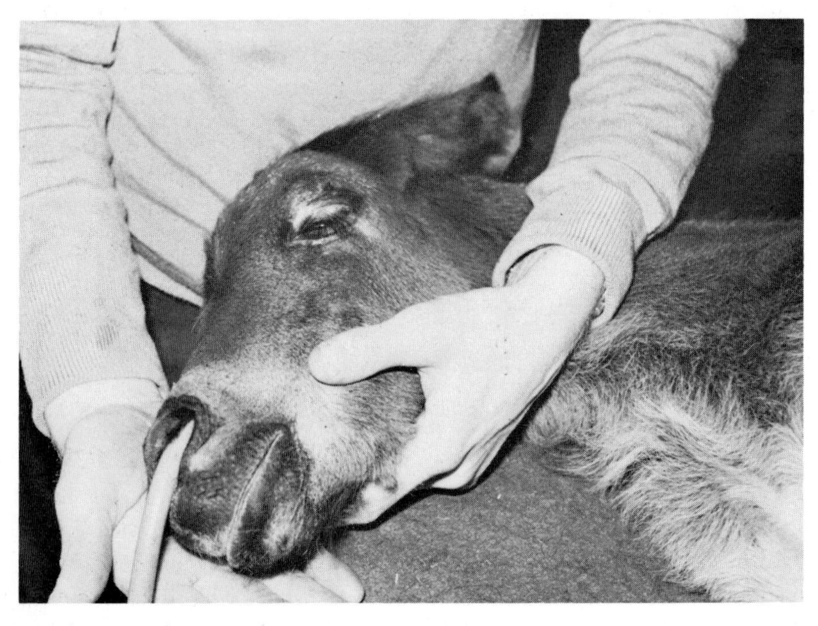

Fig. 5.37. To resuscitate a foal a tube is inserted into one of its nasal passages. For full details see text.

Alterations in blood gases may assume pathological proportions because of undue pressure on the umbilical cord during second-stage labour, before the thorax has been completely delivered. Pressure may be caused by (*a*) the cord becoming prolapsed so that a loop lies anterior to the umbilicus as the abdomen passes through the maternal pelvis; (*b*) posterior presentation; (*c*) tarsal flexion in which one or both hind-feet become lodged on the pubic brim; or (*d*) disproportion of the chest relative to the maternal pelvis. Other causes of pathological asphyxia are premature placentitis or prolonged manipulation to correct dystocia. In theory, changes in maternal uterine blood flow during birth might affect gaseous placental exchange to the detriment of the fetus, but as yet there is no evidence to support this. A further aspect which must be considered is that a fetus which has already been subjected to stress during development may be detrimentally affected by the usual asphyxial processes. These are physiological to a normal fetus.

Pathological asphyxia produces a period of gasping accompanied by clonic movements and bradycardia; this is followed by a primary period of apnoea and then a period of gasping which becomes weaker until it finally ceases and a secondary or terminal apnoeic period supervenes. If measures to resuscitate the foal are not applied, the heart beat declines in strength and frequency until death. The time from onset of asphyxia to the last gasp varies in different species. In newborn Rhesus monkeys primary apnoea occurs half a minute after the start of asphyxia, lasts for one minute and is followed by gasping for four to five minutes, after which terminal apnoea supervenes (Dawes 1968). The length of time to the last gasp is shortened by low arterial pH and increased by cooling. In the absence of experimental evidence, clinical experience suggests that the time intervals for foals are about the same as those quoted for the Rhesus monkey. Cerebral haemorrhage is also a sequela of pathological asphyxia and clinical signs after resuscitation are consistent with brain damage.

The newborn foal may be delivered in a state of primary apnoea but the gasping which follows will expand the lungs and, provided the airways are clear, spontaneous rhythmic breathing will be established. Respiratory stimulants are therefore unnecessary and all that is required is to ensure that the nostrils are not obstructed. In terminal apnoea, the respiratory centre does not respond to stimulants and resuscitation is essential. Since it is not possible to distinguish primary from secondary apnoea in a newly delivered foal, any individual that fails to establish a respiratory rhythm within 30–60 seconds should be resuscitated in the following manner:

1. The foal's head should be extended and the nostrils cleared of amnion and mucus.

2. The operator should kneel between the foal's head and fore-legs, placing the right hand under the foal's muzzle and inflate the lungs by (*a*) inserting a rubber tube attached to an oxygen cylinder into the upper nostril (Fig. 5.37) and allowing gas to flow at a rate of approximately 5 litres/minute or (*b*) applying the mouth to the upper nostril. In both cases the under nostril is closed with the right hand while

the left hand is free to seal the upper nostril around the rubber tube or mouth. The lungs are inflated by positive pressure but care must be taken not to over-inflate. It is necessary to move the chest only a perceptible amount to cause a substantial rise in $Pa\text{O}_2$. After inflating, both nostrils are released to allow exhalation of CO_2. This inflation should be maintained at the rate of about 25/minute until a spontaneous rhythm is established. Endotracheal intubation provides a more efficient means of lung inflation because it avoids accidental inflation of the stomach but, once the foal is conscious, the tube must be withdrawn to prevent excessive struggling.

3. As soon as possible after assisted respiration has been started, 200 ml of 5% sodium bicarbonate solution should be rapidly administered intravenously with a 100 ml syringe and large-bore needle. 250 mg phenytoin should be injected intravenously and a further 250 mg intramuscularly in anticipation of cerebral oedema or haemorrhage and to control consequent convulsions. 10 mg of vitamin K2 should be given intramuscularly as preventive therapy against cerebral haemorrhage. There is evidence that this therapy is helpful in haemorrhagic states of infants, but its efficacy has not been demonstrated in foals. Surrounding air temperatures should be raised to about 27°C and a rug or sacking placed over the foal to reduce heat loss.

4. Depending on the course of the condition, which is related to the amount of hypoxia, acidaemia and consequent cerebral damage, the foal should be further sedated and any convulsions controlled by further phenytoin and by gentle restraint. If the righting reflexes are intact and the foal is able to get to its feet after resuscitation these measures can be dropped. If behavioural disturbances develop, treatment should follow measures described for NMS on p. 319.

The following is an example of a foal resuscitated in practice at gestation age 338 days. Delivery was normal until the fetal hips became impacted against the maternal pelvis. The foal gasped, suffered apnoea and, after a further series of gasps, entered a state of terminal apnoea. After delivery insufflation was maintained with oxygen and 500 ml of 5% sodium bicarbonate were administered intravenously. A respiratory rhythm was established at age 12 minutes. The heart rate increased from 25 beats/minute to more than 150 beats/minute and during resuscitation a sluggish corneal reflex was present and the foal appeared flaccid and lifeless. At age 30 minutes, breathing air, systemic blood values were pHa 7.185, $Pa\text{O}_2$ 50 mmHg, $Pa\text{CO}_2$ 66 mmHg, whole blood lactate 11.5 mmol/litre (normal 1.7–3.9 mmol/litre, and glucose 3.9 mmol/litre (normal 2.8–3.9 mmol/litre). At age three hours, the foal suffered from respiratory distress and during 100% oxygen inhalation $Pa\text{O}_2$ was 65 mmHg and $Pa\text{CO}_2$ 70 mmHg; respiratory rate was 60/minutes (normal 30/minute), tidal volume 400 ml (normal 500 ml) and maximal tidal volume 500 ml (normal 1100 ml). The foal developed signs of opisthotonus, extensor rigidity and hypothermia (rectal temperature 36.3°C) but made a partial recovery and at age 24 hours it was able to stand and suck a bottle. $Pa\text{O}_2$ was then within normal levels, but at age 36 hours a relapse occurred and the foal was destroyed at 84 hours after convulsions and evidence of circulatory collapse. Post-mortem examination revealed oedema and ischaemic necrosis of the nerve cells of the cerebral cortex.

Many cases of still-birth are presumably the consequence of cord occlusion or placental dysfunction during second-stage labour causing the foal to be born in a state of terminal apnoea. In the absence of adequate measures of resuscitation death is recorded as a still-birth.

Prematurity, immaturity and dysmaturity

Considerable confusion surrounds the terminology of prematurity, dysmaturity and immaturity. In human medicine the term 'small-for-dates' has been used to recognize the fact that maturity is a relative state and that quality rather than length of gestation is the major factor. A pregnancy ending close to the average length may, in any species, result in an undersize, weak and at-risk individual. The term dysmaturity (Sjostedt et al. 1958: Gruenwald 1963) describes infants that are small-for-dates and suffering from deprivation due to placental dysfunction or insufficiency. Newborn maturity implies the ability to adapt to the extrauterine environment, but the definition must be qualified by the extent to which the environment can be artificially altered. Avery (1964) observed that, before extrauterine life is possible, organ maturation must evolve to a degree capable of function. But prematurity is not regarded as a disease in its own right (Morison 1970).

In equidae, the wide size variation between breeds – even within a breed – makes birth weight a somewhat unreliable parameter against which to measure maturity. Similarly there is a fairly wide distribution of gestational length about the mean of 340 days for Thoroughbreds and 333 days for small breeds. However, it is well recognized by clinicians that some foals born at full term or more than 340 days may be under-sized and show signs of prematurity, i.e. they are weak and smaller than expected. Thus the term prematurity may be used for foals with a gestational development shorter than the full term (95% range 325 to 355 days) but no longer than the pre-viable period which is generally regarded as being before the Day 300 of gestation. The signs of prematurity are weakness, such as delay in standing for the first time beyond the normal two hours, a low birth weight and in some cases an emaciated appearance, perhaps with meconium staining of the skin, a 'silky' feel to the coat and red or orange-red tongue and buccal mucous membranes.

Rossdale (1976) shows the mean (±SE) weight for full-term Thoroughbred foals to be 49.6 ± 0.45 kg. The mean birth weight of 144 normal Thoroughbred foals with a gestational age of more than 320 days was divided into 10-day periods and compared with the weights of 14 foals of 300–319 days gestation. The data indicated that mean birth weight was not affected by gestational age after 320 days but was significantly lower in the period 300–319 days ($P<0.05$). Of foals with a gestation period exceeding 320 days, first born foals had a significantly lower birth weight (mean 43.8 ± 1.15 kg) than foals born from multiparous mares (mean birth weight 50.6 ± 0.45 kg, $P<0.05$).

It must be accepted that the terminology is one of definition which for our purpose is as follows: prematurity in Thoroughbreds refers to a gestational length of less than 320 days but more than 300 days. Before this time birth is described as an abortion. The term dysmaturity (immaturity) is reserved for foals which have the signs of prematurity but are the result of a gestational length more than 320 days. There is usually evidence of gross or microscopic placental pathology in these cases. Chronic placental deprivation may be suspected in cases of low birth weight (more than 2 SD below the mean, i.e. 38.9 kg) and diminished crown-to-rump length (less than 95.5 cm). The influence of placental surface area on fetal size is illustrated by twin fetuses (see p. 177).

Aetiology and incidence

Premature birth and dysmaturity are related to endocrinological and placental dysfunction involving a general failure of physiological stability. A specific pathological definition has yet to be established. The incidence is about 1% in Thoroughbreds.

Signs and course of condition

The signs are of general weakness, characterized by delay in standing for the first time (in some cases extending to several days), low birth weight, reduced strength of suck and inability to achieve a normal relationship with the mare and to maintain body temperature. Signs of abdominal pain may develop due to tympany and failure to pass meconium. Paste-like faeces may accumulate in the large and small colon. Decubitus ulcers may develop over the angle of the hips and outer aspects of the shoulder and elbow joints. The tongue is often an unusual red or orange colour and the skin is silky. Pulmonary and cardiac function are normal by clinical standards although arterial blood gas oxygen tensions may be low (below 80 mmHg) when breathing air but usually increased to normal level (more than 200 mmHg) when breathing 100% oxygen.

Dysmaturity associated with placentitis is characterized by emaciation, dehydration and in many cases diarrhoea. Affected foals are unable to stand normally. They may make apparent progress during the first 24 hours after birth, but their condition deteriorates during the second and third day when they lose the righting reflexes, become comatose and exhibit extensor rigidity and opisthotonus resembling nervous symptoms displayed in cases of meningitis and NMS. The deterioration may be quite dramatic and so disappointing in view of the apparent improvement during the first day that it may be tempting to describe the deteriorating signs as the second-day syndrome. How far this is associated with an inability to establish renal and alimentary function in the presence of increasing quantities of dietary protein is a matter for speculation.

Diagnosis

There is no specific pathology associated with immaturity or prematurity. Affected individuals are small and under-weight, emaciated and dehydrated. Pericardial, pleural and peritoneal transudates are sometimes present. Cultures remain sterile on bacteriological examination of the main organs. Cloudy swelling of hepatic and renal cells may occur in dysmature foals; atelectatic lungs and pneumonitis are sometimes found but are usually secondary to a prolonged illness, especially in cases where the foal has been unable to stand.

Meconium retention

Aetiology and incidence

The aetiology is unknown, but there is some evidence to implicate a food deficiency, especially vitamin A, during the last third of gestation. Colt foals appear to be more commonly affected than fillies and it has been suggested that this may be due to a narrower pelvic outlet. Incidence is approximately 1.5%. Foals born after more than 340 days gestation appear to be more prone to the condition.

Pathogenesis

Meconium retention is a sign rather than a disease. From mid-gestation onwards faecal material accumulates in the caecum and large and small colon. It is not normally voided in utero but is passed when the foal is four to 96 hours old. Expulsion is not normally associated with tympany but in some cases the rectum becomes impacted with faecal pellets and gas accumulates behind the blockage. The site of impaction may extend far forward from the rectum. In other cases tympany is caused by fermenting colostrum and milk.

Clinical signs

Signs include straining, squatting, lifting the tail, rolling, looking round at the flanks, turning the head while recumbent and lying on the back or with a fore-leg over the head (Fig. 5.38). Affected foals may refuse to suck, but inappetence is not a feature. Bouts of colic often follow sucking. The eyelids and cornea may be injured by the straw bedding and there may be entropion of the lower eyelids.

Diagnosis

Meconium retention is diagnosed on the clinical signs and must be distinguished from a ruptured bladder, which is described under Group III.

Treatment

On most stud farms it is routine to treat meconium retention with enemas of soap and water or liquid paraffin. If this is not successful we recommend giving about 400 ml of warm liquid paraffin or paraffin emulsion by stomach tube. Emulsion has the advantage of passing more readily through a relatively narrow-bore tube.

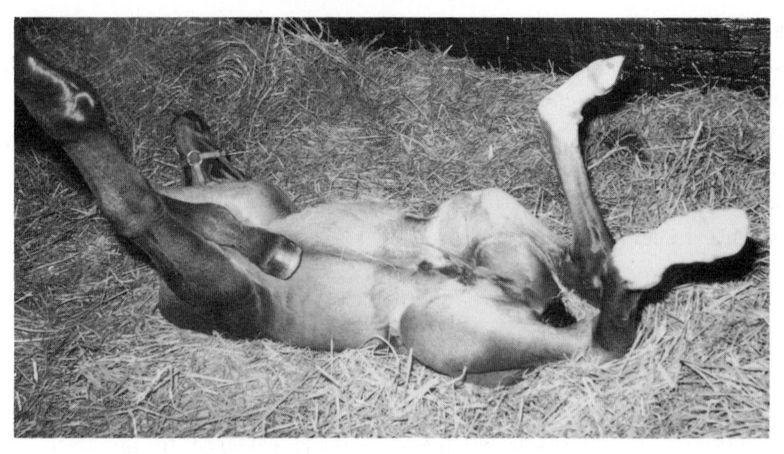

Fig. 5.38. Characteristic signs of colic in a foal suffering from meconium retention.

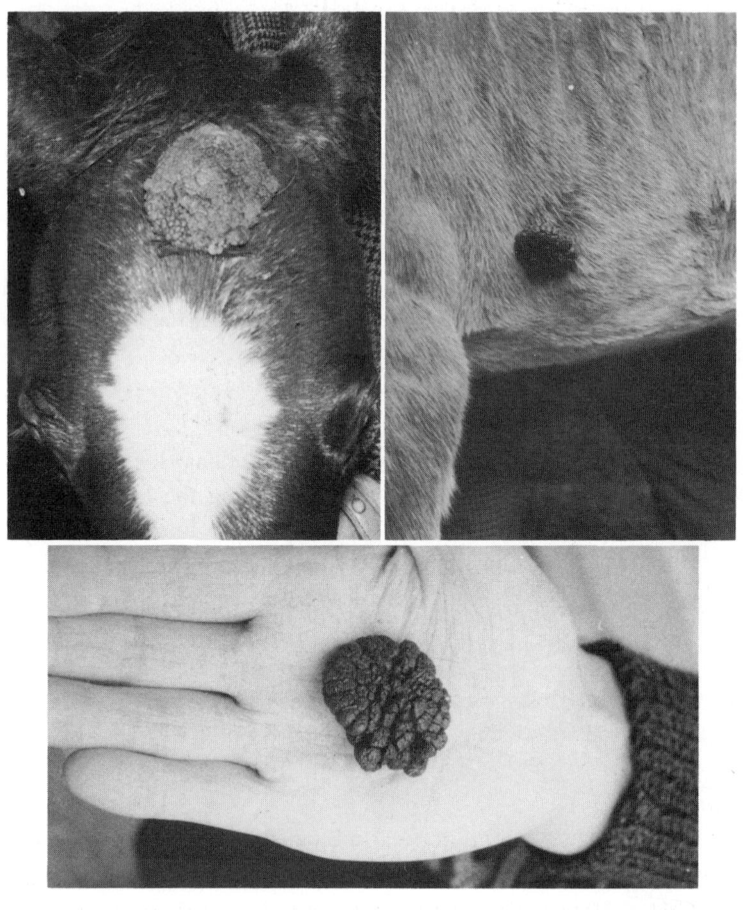

Fig. 5.39. Papillomatous growths on the forehead and flank of a newborn foal. These growths have a stalk and can be ligated easily for removal.

Foals that cease to nurse must be fed regularly by stomach tube. Pain may be relieved by intramuscular pethidine (5–10 ml of 5% solution) and foals must be attended so that they do not injure themselves (especially the periorbital region) when rolling. Removing faecal pellets from the rectum may alleviate a simple impaction, but in many cases the problem lies in the colon or caecum and over-zealous attempts to remove rectal faeces may exacerbate the condition by causing ballooning and atony of the rectal walls.

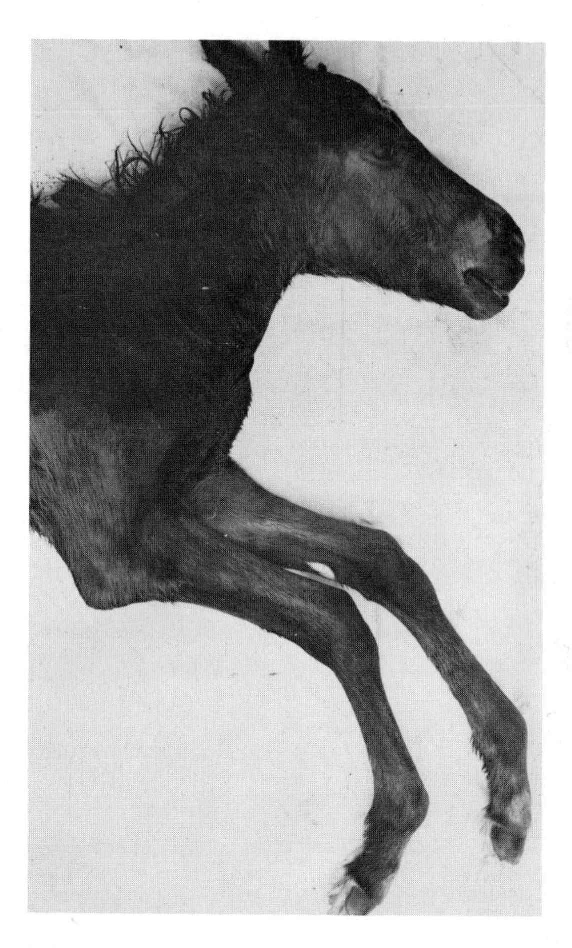

Fig. 5.40. Hyperflexion of the fore-legs is the most common developmental abnormality in Thoroughbred foals.

Pathology

Under the usual conditions of stud farm management in the British Isles, meconium retention rarely causes death. If it does, it is usually due to rupture of the rectum by manipulative instruments or enema tubes and the escape of faecal matter into the peritoneal cavity.

Group III: Developmental abnormalities

Some of the developmental abnormalities encountered in newborn foals; classed under Group III, are listed in Table 5.10. The incidence of development abnormalities is 3–4% of all foals born. Hyperflexion of the forelimbs is the most common abnormality, but incidence varies with the degree of knuckling-over defined as hyperlexion (Fig. 5.40).

TABLE 5.10 Developmental abnormalities found in foals and apparent in the first week of life

Conditions	*Synonyms*	*Characteristics*
Hyperflexion of limbs (Rooney 1966; Nemeth 1976)	Contracted tendons	Range from uprightness or fore- or hind-legs to knuckling over at the fetlock and/or inability to extend knee joints
Hypoflexion of limbs	Weakness Down on pasterns	Laxity of ligaments Muscle hypotonia
Parrot jaw	Over shot jaw Parrot mouth	Upper and lower incisors overlapping by degrees varying from 1 mm to 3 cm, molars also overshoot at front and back
Umbilical urachal fistula	Pervious urachus	Wet cord stump, maybe dripping Often necrotic tissue present on both sides of abdominal wall
Congenital abnormalities of genitourinary tract (Miller et al. 1966)		
Patent bladder	Ruptured bladder	Signs appear two to three days after birth: may be confused with meconium colic
Deviation and shortening of the maxillary bones and asymmetry of the mandibles	Squiffy face	Often the tongue is held to one side and the foal has difficulty in sucking
Atresia coli Anal agenesis (Gideon 1977; Lauwers & Devos 1966)	Incomplete alimentary tract	Signs of meconium colic becoming increasingly severe and unremitting
Cleft palate		Regurgitation of milk down nostrils soon after or during feeding
Microphthalmia	Button eyes	Blindness
Scrotal hernia		Soft swelling in scrotum due to descent of abdominal contents. Appears in first few days or immediately following birth; often resolves spontaneously but may become strangulated

Cardiac septal defects Persistent truncus (Greene et al. 1975)		Sudden death, fainting and/or respiratory embarrassment with rapid heart rate and murmurs
Hare lip		
Hydrocephalus		Excessively dome-shaped forehead
Omphalocele	Hernia	Open abdominal floor
Absence of urachus Megavesica (Dubs 1976)		Dystocia due to size of bladder. If delivered, foal may suffer from acute maladjustment, usually fatal
Ectopic lung (Rossdale, unpublished data)		Respiratory embarrassment if occurring in chest and swelling if on ventral aspect of neck

Aetiology and pathogenesis

The agents known to cause malformation and death in the young of domestic mammals have been listed by Woollam (1978) (Table 5.11). However, malformations are generally due to a subtle interplay between genetic and environmental factors and only rarely are they caused by genetic or environmental factors working alone.

TABLE 5.11 Hereditary conditions in horses with signs appearing with increasing age

Umbilical hernia	see p. 413
Cerebellar hypoplasia	see p. 410
Haemophilia and clotting defects	see p. 411
Combined immunodeficiency disease	see p. 412
Intersex	see p. 60
Gonadal dysgenesis	see p. 60

Entropion. Entropion of the lower eyelid may be caused by retraction of the eyeball into the orbit. This is often associated with septicaemia or rubbing on straw bedding. There is progressive damage to the cornea and the condition should be rectified without delay. Mild cases may be remedied by manipulation of the eyelid into its normal position, but where repeated entropion occurs surgery should be performed as follows:

The foal is restrained on the ground under tranquillization and a local anaesthetic injected subcutaneously at about four sites, approximately 0.5 cm from the rim of the eyelid; two or three mattress sutures of braided nylon or silk are inserted and tied so that the eyelid is everted just enough to avoid entropion. The surface of the eye should then be treated with a suitable ophthalmic ointment and tetanus antitoxin given. The sutures should be examined frequently to ensure that entropion has not recurred and they can be removed at about one week.

Teratogenic drugs. The passage to the fetus of drugs, chemical poisons and bacterial toxins depends on molecular size. Many drugs, including antibiotics, cross the placental barrier. The action of therapeutic and other agents on the embryo are reviewed by Woollam (1966).

The influence of teratogenic drugs on the fetus depends on its stage of development, its genetic susceptibility and, to a certain extent, the state of the mother. In general, the earlier in fetal life the drug is administered the greater the effects in terms of death or major malformation. There is a critical period for each organ during which normal development can be altered.

Susceptibility to drug action varies with the species and even within breeds or strains. Thalidomide, for example, produces obvious malformations in the rabbit, but none, apparently, in the rat, and variation in the cleft-palate-inducing effects of cortisone has been observed between strains of mice (Fraser et al. 1954).

A deficiency or an excess of nutritive material can modify a drug's teratogenic effects and either extreme can cause malformations. Woollam (1978) concluded: 'I have found that high dosage or exposure at a critical time of the dam to the teratogen leads to resorption. At a lower level I have seen dead deformed fetuses, at a lower level still, live deformed fetuses; and at the lowest level normal live fetuses. There is a gradual tendency to shift from normal fetuses through deformed to stillborn fetuses, often to abortions and resorptions as the dose goes up and the time at which the noxious agent is administered approaches the most critical time for the development of the fetus and placenta'. Pathological states of the mother, such as liver dysfunction, may alter the action of drugs and result in fetal damage.

Although there is no information on the teratogenic effects of drugs on the equine fetus, therapeutics in common use, such as corticosteroids, ACTH, phenylbutazone, anabolic steroids and tranquillizers, should be given with caution, especially in the first six weeks of gestation. After this time the effects on the fetus are likely to be less dramatic but in one case a mare kept on phenylbutazone from mid-pregnancy to term delivered a foal with atresia of the caecum and colon. This may, of course, have been a coincidence and another mare subsequently placed on a similar regimen bore a foal which was apparently normal and full term.

Infection. Mares are frequently infected with, or challenged by, a wide range of herpes and influenza viruses during pregnancy. Apart from abortions caused by EHV-I there are no reports of undesirable effects on the fetus. This may, however, reflect a lack of detailed study rather than lack of association. Bacterial, viral or fungal infection may cause abnormalities by interfering with placental function and disturbing the fetal environment. For example, errors of development late in fetal life, such as hypo- or hyperflexion of fore- or hind-legs, frequently coexist with placentitis and amnionitis. It is possible that teratogens act by depriving the fetus of one or both of its prime requirements, oxygen and glucose.

Genetic factors. Normally there is a hereditable component in parrot jaw conditions and some forms of limb hyperflexion and club foot. Despite the opportunity presented by a strictly controlled Stud Book entry for Thoroughbreds, no organized attempt has been made to investigate hereditable diseases and abnormalities.

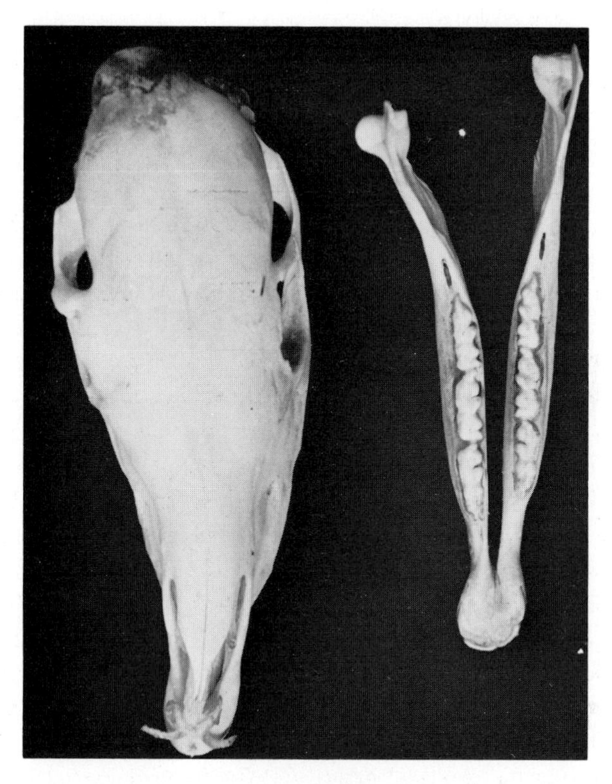

Fig. 5.41. Deviation and shortening of the maxillary bones and asymmetry of the mandibles in a newborn foal.

Hyperflexion of the limbs is a common cause of dystocia. Neonatal maladjustment depends on the extent of the developmental abnormality. Many cases can be corrected surgically or orthopaedically but it is not advisable to allow seriously inferior genetic material to survive.

Treatment

Each abnormality must be treated according to its position and severity. Hyperflexion of the limbs may be corrected with splints or appliances which aid the re-establishment of normal limb positions (Fig. 5.43). Surgical severance of fibres of the flexor muscles and tendons may be necessary in severe cases. Hypoflexion of the limb requires bandage support around the fetlocks and pastern joints and general nursing is required to help affected foals get up and suck.

Surgical interference is indicated in cases of patent bladder (see below) and open abdominal floor. Urachal fistulas that do not respond to antibiotics and astringents applied to the umbilicus may also require surgery. Cleft palates may be repaired, depending on the extent of the abnormality, but if the soft palate is involved the prognosis is poor.

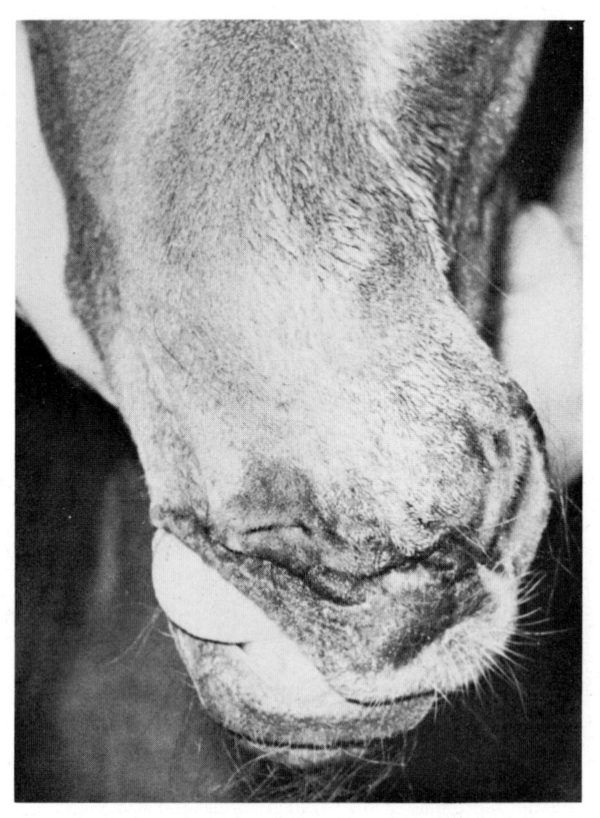

Fig. 5.42. Deviation of the muzzle due to congenital abnormality does not usually prevent a foal from sucking successfully.

Clinicians should consider carefully the justification for treatment in each case and weigh up the balance of likely future working and breeding soundness, the cost of therapy and the owner's particular interests.

Rupture (patent) bladder

The aetiology of this condition is obscure but is probably associated with birth trauma (Rooney 1972), especially passage through the maternal pelvis, rupture of a particularly tough umbilical cord when the force of traction is transmitted through the urachus to the bladder, developmental due to incomplete closure of the bladder wall (Wellington 1972) or a premature closure of the urachus causing overdistension during delivery (Whitwell, personal communication). The incidence is less than 0.5% of births (Rooney 1971).

Signs of this condition usually appear on the third day after birth. They simulate those of meconium retention; the foal strains and frequently adopts a crouching position. It may roll, lie in awkward postures and turn its head towards its flanks. The abdomen becomes distended with fluid but the condition can be distinguished from the much more common one of retained meconium by percussion. Urine may be passed in only small quantities, except where the tear in the bladder is small and

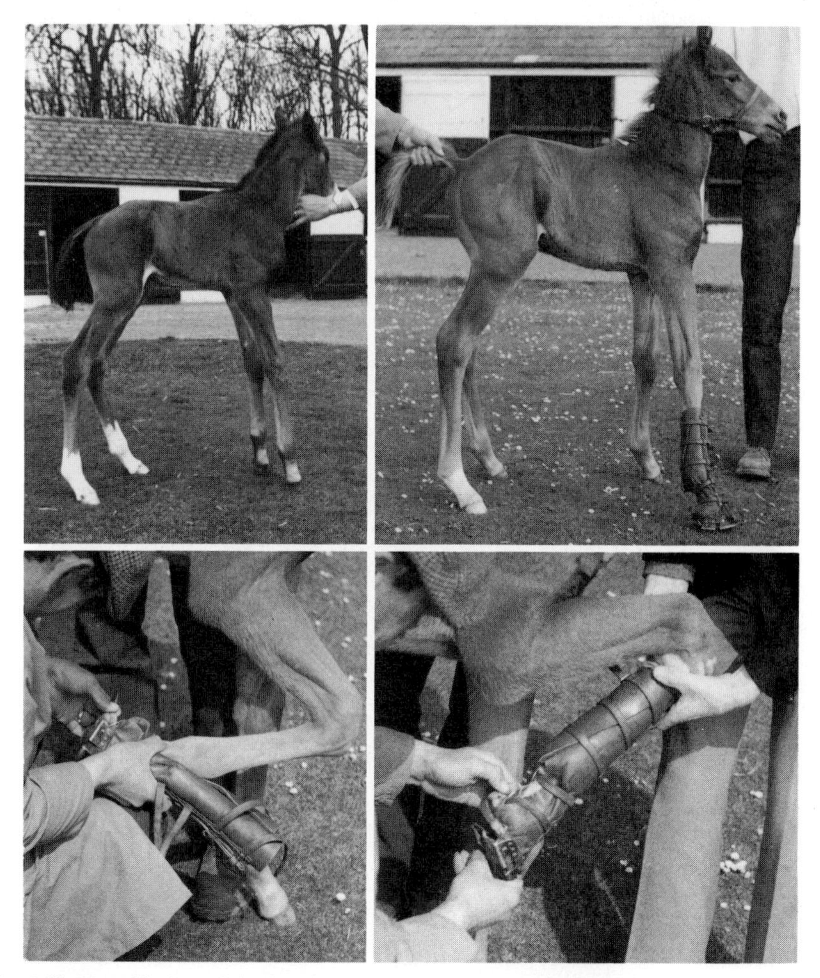

Fig. 5.43. Hyperflexion of the fore-leg, if not too severe, can be corrected by applying a boot with malleable metal strips on the anterior aspect. The lower figures show the method of application.

on the dorsal surface when almost normal quantities may be voided. Diagnosis is confirmed by paracentesis abdominis, when urine can be distinguished from ascitic fluid by its odour, high urea content (above 3 mmol/litre) and absence of fibrin. The state can be confirmed if necessary by introducing a dye such as fluorescein into the bladder and half an hour later withdrawing a sample of abdominal fluid to test for its presence.

Early surgical repair is indicated (Fig. 5.44). With the foal restrained in lateral recumbency, a small bleb of local anaesthetic should be placed under the skin of the abdominal midline, just in front of the umbilicus. A sterile cannula is carefully inserted into the peritoneal cavity and as much urine as possible is removed. This procedure considerably reduces the anaesthetic risk of the operative procedure itself. The whole procedure may be performed under local anaesthesia, with a cooperative patient, especially if the foal is considered to be a particular anaesthetic risk. In some cases, tranquillization with 10 mg acetylpromazine, by

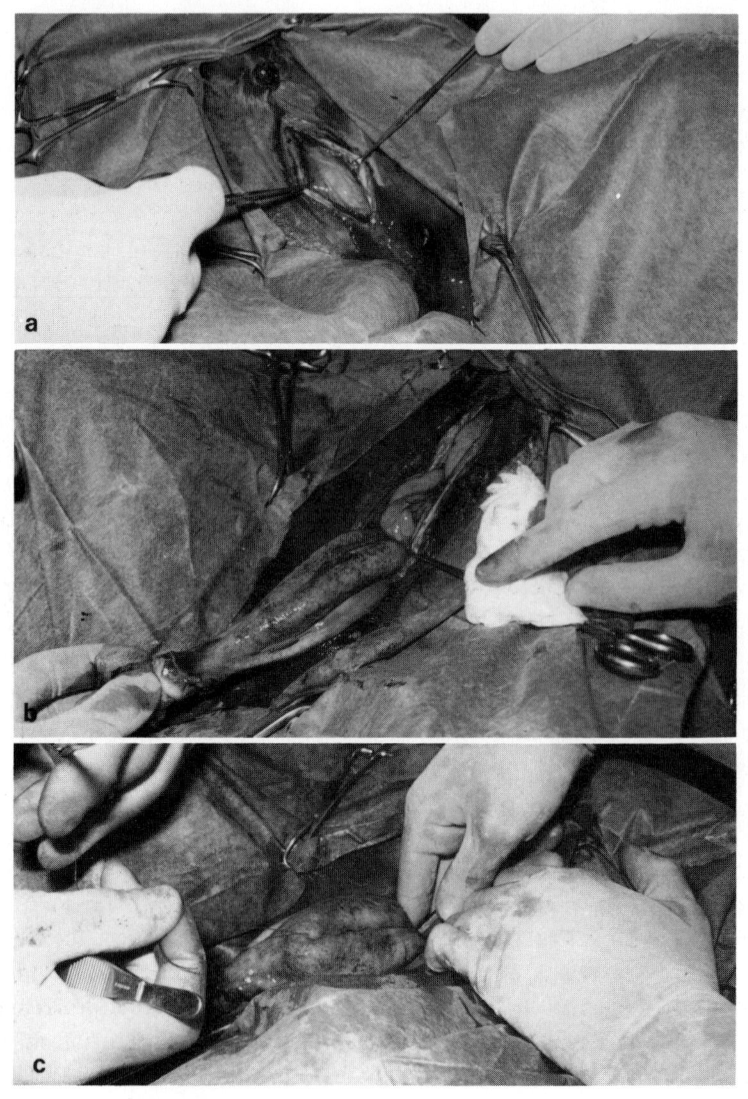

Fig. 5.44. A ruptured bladder can be repaired by surgery. (*a*) A midline incision is made from the umbilicus to the pelvic region in a filly (as here) or para-midline in a colt. (*b*) The bladder is freed from its umbilical attachment and brought outside the abdominal wounds. (*c*) The tear (in this case on the dorsal surface) is repaired by Lembert sutures.

intravenous injection, may be a considerable help. In other cases, general anaesthesia may be indicated. This may be accomplished using pentobarbitone sodium. Approximately 8 ml of a 60% solution, given slowly, intravenously, may be given 'to effect'. The plane of anaesthesia may be 'topped up' if necessary. General anaesthesia may be induced by the intravenous injection of thiopentone sodium at a dose rate of 0.25 g of a 5% solution per 10 kg body weight, 'to effect'. The foal may then be intubated and maintained by halothane and oxygen. Anaesthesia may be induced with halothane and oxygen, using a face mask, prior to intubation.

The foal is restrained in dorsal recumbency and the abdomen clipped and prepared using standard techniques. The operative technique has been described by Crowhurst (1970). A midline incision is made from just posterior to the umbilicus almost to the pubis. In colts, the incision deviates slightly so as to avoid the edge of the sheath, and in this case the subcutaneous tissues around the sheath must be separated to expose the true midline. The incision is then continued through the linea alba, exposing the peritoneum, which is then punctured. Remaining urine flows from the abdomen and should be either aspirated or swabbed out before proceding further. The bladder is exteriorized and the defect is identifed. The defect is closed with two layers of interrupted Lembert sutures using 0 chromic catgut. The bladder is replaced into the abdomen and any residual urine drained off. The peritoneum and linea alba are closed together with interrupted sutures using No. 1 chromic catgut. The subcutaneous tissues are coapted with interrupted or continuous sutures using 0 chromic catgut. In colt foals the sheath is incorporated in these sutures and stitched back into position. The skin is closed with interrupted sutures using monofilament nylon.

Crowhurst recommends draining the bladder via a urethral catheter as soon as the abdomen has been closed. He retains the catheter temporarily in place with a suture, which allows urine to drain until the foal regains consciousness and is able to stand. The catheter is withdrawn and urination occurs naturally.

The foal is given a course of prophylactic antibiotics for five days and the skin sutures are removed seven to ten days later.

Group IV: Immunological

Group IV includes immunological conditions characterized by a reaction between maternal and fetal tissues.

Haemolytic disease occurs naturally only in humans and equidae, although a similar disease has been induced in pigs and dogs. It was first recognized by Caroli and Bessis (1947) as being due to isoimmunization in mule foals, then later found to be wide-spread in Thoroughbred foals (Coombes et al. 1948: Cronin 1955). Fetal erythocytes escape into the maternal blood and, if they have an antigenic structure significantly different from those of the mother, stimulate production of antibodies. In foals signs occur only after the ingestion of colostrum, in contrast to the human infant in which the antibodies pass the placental barrier before birth. This is presumably because of a species difference in placental function. In the horse, antibodies rise to high levels in the blood at the end of pregnancy and become concentrated in the colostrum.

Incidence, aetiology and pathogenesis

The condition has a low incidence (below 0.5%) and high mortality rate. There is evidence that the incidence of subclinical cases, detectable only by blood examination, may be somewhat higher. The condition is rare in primigravid mares, but once a mare has foaled an affected individual she will probably do so in subsequent pregnancies.

The condition is based on differences of the inherited structure of fetal and maternal erythrocytes. The fetal cells contain antigens of the A, Q, R, S or E systems not present in the maternal cells (Scott 1972). A few fetal erythrocytes enter the mother's blood in the normal course of events due to capillary breakdown and their surface antigens provoke a strong antibody response in the maternal tissues. The antibodies become concentrated in the colostrum and are absorbed from the stomach after the first suck. They pass into the blood stream and attach themselves to the surface of the foal's erythrocytes, causing them to agglutinate and haemolyse. The ability of antibodies to be absorbed through the lining of the alimentary tract is limited to the first 12–24 hours after birth and ingestion of antibody after this time cannot cause the condition. This, as we will see later, forms the basis of preventive measures.

Once antibody has entered the foal's blood stream there is a continuing process of erythrocyte destruction causing profound anaemia and death.

Clinical signs

Foals become lethargic and may yawn repeatedly. If they are exerted or excited, their respiratory and heart rates increase markedly and a jugular pulse may be present. There is evidence of jaundice in the sclera and buccal and vaginal mucous membranes. The urine is discolored red. Signs may appear on the first, but more often the second, day post-partum. The severity of each case depends on the amount of erythrocyte damage and the speed at which it occurs. The first obvious sign in a peracute case is a collapsed and moribund state, although close observation may reveal earlier signs. Acute cases show obvious signs before the red cell count has fallen below 2×10^{12}/litre and 12–24 hours may elapse before it descends to a fatal level. Chronic or subclinical cases may or may not show signs and the red cell count does not fall below a critical level.

Diagnosis

The potential haemolytic case can be determined with reasonable accuracy by examining the mare's blood serum at weekly intervals from 320 days to full term. The serum is examined against a panel of red cells from six or more animals and a diagnosis made on the development of a titre during the last week. Positive titres rise to 1 in 40 or higher.

In cases where mares have been known to produce haemolytic foals the previous test may be supplemented or replaced by cross-matching umbilical cord blood erythrocytes with mare's serum collected at the time of foaling (see Cross-matching, p. 546).

Once a foal has sucked and its erythrocytes become coated with maternal antibodies, the agglutination test is no longer reliable and diagnosis depends on haematological examination. An erythrocyte count reduced to below 4×10^{12}/litre, a haemoglobin content less than 7 g/dl and a packed cell volume reduced to below 0.20 litre/litre are highly suggestive in a foal suffering from clinical signs. Ghost cells, yellow plasma (bilirubin levels approaching 342 μmol/litre and an indirect van den Bergh test) confirm the state. Jaundice due to infection or other causes can be distinguished by agglutination test of mare's serum against random samples of donor erythrocytes; in haemolytic disease a large number of those tested will agglutinate.

Treatment

Therapy, to be effective, must replace damaged erythrocytes and maintain circulating numbers above about 2×10^{12}/litre. Circulating antibodies will not destroy all the foal's red cells because some will be resistant. Therapy is aimed at supplementing these and maintaining sufficient numbers until the foal's bone marrow can replace those lost and restore the circulating number to normal levels. The process of replacement may take several weeks but once a decline has been arrested, recovery is usually uneventful.

Transfusion of donor erythrocytes is necessary when the count falls below 3×10^{12}/litre.

Some authorities (Osbaldiston et al. 1969) consider that the affected foal's dam is the best source of erythrocytes, but it is essential that they are washed free of plasma. This requires suitable facilities, notably a centrifuge capable of holding several hundred ml of blood. About 2 litres of dam's blood, collected into four flasks each containing 120 ml of sterile acid citrate dextrose, are centrifuged and the supernatant plasma removed by suction. The residual cells are mixed with normal saline and re-centrifuged. The supernatant saline is removed and the process repeated two or three times before the cells are safe to administer.

The supernatant saline is then removed and 1 litre of packed cells is given intravenously over one hour, using a 100 ml syringe and 16GA $\times$ 4 cm needle or 15G intravenous catheter inserted into the jugular vein. The quantity and number of subsequent administrations depend on the red cell count.

An alternative therapy is the exchange transfusion. A suitable donor is found by cross-matching foal's serum against donor erythrocytes. Donor blood is transfused into the jugular vein through a two-way tap and indwelling catheter by gravity feed or syringe. 50 ml of donor circulating blood are given and removed alternately and over one to two hours up to 3 litres of blood can be exchanged. The advantage of this method is that it removes a large quantity, although not all, of the antibody present in the foal's plasma. The disadvantage is that it takes longer than the administration of packed cells and needs prolonged restraint of a potentially weak foal. Restraint is helped by giving 5–10 ml of 5% pethidine intramuscularly. It may be impractical for those without adequate laboratory facilities to attempt therapy, but if the case is referred elsewhere involving a long journey, 500 ml of packed erythrocytes from a suitable donor should be transfused to help the foal survive the journey. In the absence of a suitable centrifuge apparatus, 1 litre of donor citrated blood should be allowed to stand at room temperature for one hour and the plasma removed by suction. The packed cells can then be administered.

After the first transfusion the quantity and number of others depend on the cell count. When this falls below 2×10^{12}/litre prognosis is grave, but should not be assumed hopeless. A foal may become acclimatized to levels of about 2×10^{12}/litre and, provided it is not subjected to undue exertion, will survive the critical period of two to three weeks before the losses are made good by erythropoietic activity. Under ordinary conditions the disease has a high mortality rate and

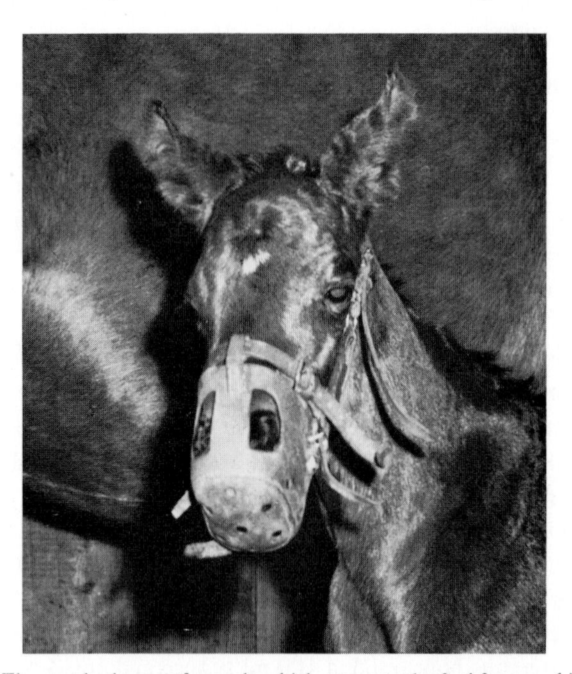

Fig. 5.45. The standard type of muzzle which prevents the foal from sucking its dam.

successful treatment depends on the continued monitoring of the erythrocyte count. All possible precautions should be taken to avoid exerting or exciting the foal and during convalescence it should not be turned loose in a paddock until the erythrocyte count is above 5×10^{12}/litre. Supportive treatment with vitamin C, vitamin B12 and antibiotics may help.

Prevention

Where a mare is diagnosed as having been sensitized to fetal erythrocytes her foal should be muzzled (Fig. 5.45) for 36 hours after birth and the mare's mammary glands stripped of colostrum. The foal should receive donor colostrum in the first feed and reconstituted dried milk in subsequent feeds until it is aged 36 hours. Broad-spectrum antibiotics should be given twice daily during the first week after birth.

DIFFERENTIAL DIAGNOSIS OF NEONATAL DISEASE

The age at which signs first appear (Table 5.12) is a useful basis for differential diagnosis. Further judgement relies on clinical signs (Table 5.13) and laboratory measurements (Table 5.14).

TABLE 5.12 Time of appearance of first signs

Condition	*Before 12 hours*	*12–24 hours*	*24–48 hours*	*48–72 hours*	*72–96 hours*
Group I					
Septicaemic conditions	+	++	+++	+++	+++
Group II					
NMS	+++	++	+	+	
Prematurity, immaturity	+++				
Meconium retention	+	+++	+++	+	+
Group III					
Patent bladder				+++	++
Congenital defects	+++	+ (Palate)			
Group IV					
Haemolytic disease			+	+++	++

After Rossdale (1972*b*).

Appearance of first signs

Neonatal maladjustment syndrome, prematurity and immaturity and developmental abnormalities are the most common signs to appear in the first 12 hours after birth. Congenital defects of the palate may be seen first when milk runs out of the foal's nose after it has sucked. Signs of septicaemia may develop between 12 and 36 hours, when colic from meconium retention is most likely. Signs of haemolytic disease develop on the second day and signs of patent bladder on the third.

Behavioural disturbances

Delay in standing for the first time is most commonly caused by prematurity, immaturity or septicaemia, but if a foal has trouble in standing after previously appearing normal in this respect it is usually a sign of NMS (especially if this develops suddenly and is associated with convulsions). Premature foals may gain

TABLE 5.13 Differential diagnosis: clinical signs

Sign	*Group I*		*Group II*		*Group III*	*Group IV*
	Septicaemia	NMS	Prematurity Immaturity	Meconium retention	Patent bladder	Haemolytic disease
Behavioural disturbances						
Inability to stand	+	++	++			
Loss of suck	+	++				
Weak suck			++	+		
Loss of affinity to mare	+	++				
Apparent blindness	+	++				
Convulsions						
Spasms (clonus)		++				
General (motor)	+	++				
Exaggerated extensor tone	+	++				
Irritability (wandering)	+	++		+		
Colic signs	+		+	++	+	
Rectal temperature	∧ >	∧ (convulsions) ∨ (coma)	>	>	>	>
Heart rate	∧ >	∧ > ∨	> ∨	>	>	∧
Jugular pulse	+	++ (cardiac embarrassment)				+
Respiratory rate	∧ >	∧ (RD) >	>	>	>	∧
Tidal volume	>	> ∨ (RD)	>	>	>	>
Minute volume	∧ >	∧ (RD) >	>	>	>	∧
Maximum tidal volume	>	> ∨ (RD)	>	>	>	>
Respiratory sound		++				
Other diagnostic signs	Intensity of signs gradually increases	Cerebral haemorrhage: asymmetrical pupil diameter and extensor rigidity	Low birth weight	Crouching	Crouching, swelling of abdomen with fluid	Jaundiced membranes, red urine

After Rossdale (1972*b*).
+ Sometimes present
> Normal
> Above normal
RD, respiratory distress

TABLE 5.14 Differential diagnosis: laboratory measurements

Measurement	*Group I*		*Group II*		*Group III*	*Group IV*
	Septicaemia	NMS	Prematurity Immaturity	Meconium retention	Patent bladder	Haemolytic disease
Packed cell volume	∧ > ∨	∧ >	∨	>	>	∨
Haemoglobin	∧ >	∧ >	∨	>	>	∨
Red cell count	∧ >	∧ >	∨	>	>	∨
White cell count	∧ ∨	>	> ∨	>	>	>
Blood glucose	>	∧ >	> ∨	>	>	>
Blood lactic acid	>	∧ >	> ∨	>	>	>
Blood protein						
Albumin	>	>	∨	>	>	>
Globulin	> ∨	>	∨	>	>	>
Venous blood pH	> ∨	∨	>	>	>	>
PaO_2	>	∨	> ∨	>	>	>
$PaCO_2$	>	∧ ∨	>	>	>	>
PaO_2 breathing 100% O_2 increases to 200–400 mmHg	>	> ∨ (RD)	>	>	>	>

After Rossdale (1972*b*).
> Normal
> Above normal
> Below normal

RD, respiratory distress

strength provided they receive adequate help, but foals suffering from septicaemia generally lose strength.

Suck reflex

Sudden loss of the suck reflex is a pathognomonic signs of NMS and gradual loss is associated with septicaemia. Foals suffering from meconium retention may go off suck temporarily.

Affinity for the mare

Complete loss of the foal's ability to seek and find the mare is pathognomonic of NMS. In premature and septicaemic conditions the foal's directional instincts are weakened.

Neurological signs

Spasmodic contractions (jerks or clonus), wandering and restlessness, jaw champing or chewing, exaggerated extensor tone, motor convulsions (aimless limb movements), loss of postural tone and righting reflexes are typical of NMS and often associated with cerebral haemorrhage or oedema. Some foals suffering from septicaemia and others with meconium retention may show 'wandering' signs. The examination of cerebrospinal fluid samples (see Chapter 8) may be useful (Tables 5.15, 5.16). Creatinine kinase (CK) protein levels and leucocyte counts may be above normal in foals suffering neurological signs.

Opthalmic signs

Asymmetrical pupillary apertures, scleral splashing, retinal petechiae and nystagmus indicate cerebral haemorrhage.

Colic

Abdominal pain is commonly associated with meconium retention. Symptoms include frequent rolling, lying on the back, rotation of the head, and lying in unusual positions. Some of these symptoms may be seen in patent bladder, prematurity or septicaemia, especially that caused by *E. coli* and *A. equuli.*

Rectal temperature

Rectal temperature is not such a reliable guide to infection as in the older animal. In NMS it may fluctuate between 32.2 and 40.6°C depending on the muscular activity, i.e. in coma it falls, in convulsion it rises. Transitory rises may occur in septicaemic conditions.

Heart rate

Bradycardia (less than 50 beats/minute) immediately after birth followed by tachycardia (more than 150 beats/minute) indicates asphyxia. Tachycardia also occurs in foals suffering from convulsions and in septicaemia associated with

TABLE 5.15 CSF analysis in 12 foals showing no evidence of neurological signs

Foal	*Breed*	*Age at sampling* (hours)	*RBC* (× 10^{-6}/litre)	*WBC* (× 10^{-6}/litre)	*Total protein* (g/litre)	*Albumin* (g/litre)	*Globulin* (g/litre)	*Creatine kinase* (IU/litre)
2/77	Pony	10	2	1	1.5	0.5	1	22
3/77	Pony	14	1	0	1.6	–	–	4.0
11/77*	Pony	27	3280	0	–	–	–	39.6
12/77*	Pony	36	1	0	0.9	0.7	0.2	28
18/77	Mule	108	30	0	–	–	–	7.0
16/78	Pony	6	–	–	1.7	0.9	0.8	26.4
18/78†	Pony	10 min	70	25	1.3	1.3	0	23.3
22/78†	Pony	15 min	55	0	2.5	1.3	1.2	18
29/78	Pony	12	0	0	1.3	1.0	0.3	6.0
13/78‡	TB	24	150	20	1.2	–	–	13.6
15/78‡	TB	96	–	–	1.6	0.5	1.0	19.4
25/78‡	TB	14	125	10	0.9	0.3	0.6	9.5
Mean ± SE					1.45 ± 0.15	0.81 ± 0.13	0.64 ± 0.15	18.1 ± 3.1
Mean + 2 SD					2.37	1.57	1.50	39.3

After Rossdale et al. (1979).
* Foaling induced with fluprostenol.
† Induced by manual dilatation of cervix and rupture of allantochorionic membrane.
‡ Slaughtered within 24 hours because of limb deformity or other abnormalities.

TABLE 5.16 CSF analysis in 10 foals exhibiting neurological signs

Foal	Age at sampling (hours)	RBC (× 10⁻⁶ /litre)	WBC (× 10⁻⁶ /litre)	Total protein (g/litre)	Albumin (g/litre)	Globulin (g/litre)	Creatine kinase (IU/litre)	Neurological signs	Outcome
Neonatal maladjustment syndrome									
4/77	32	8	0	1.5	–	–	7	'Wandering'	Died 12 days
	59	75	1	1.5	–	–	22	24 hours post convulsions	
	71	10	0	1.5	–	–	22	Convulsions	
	155	3	0	–	–	–	8	Sucking from mare	
	179	1530	0	1.7	–	–	9	Sucking from mare	
	288	463	1	1.2	–	–	7		
13/77	12	1200	0	1.9	–	–	7	Convulsions	Died 48 hours
	48	1235	3	2.8*	–	–	120		
7/78	4	30	0	1.9	1.8*	0.1	9.3	Convulsion	Recovered
	40	40	0	1.4	1.0	0.4	9.1	Quiet	
	120			1.6	1.4	0.2	166*	Minor convulsions	
	144	35	5	2.5*			33	Severe convulsions + 'barking'	
	168	40	0	2.3	1.8*	0.5	5.2	Sucking from mare	
Asphyxia neonatorum									
32/78	10	120	0	2.5*	1.5	0.8	17.6	Comatose	Died 60 hours
	30	–	–	–	–	–	15	Comatose	
Dysmature									
1/77‡	18	2	0	0.4	0.1	0.3	38	Comatose	Died 18 hours
3/78	39		–	1.5	1.3	0.2	7.2	Convulsions at 32 hours	Died 60 hours
17/78	45 min	325	50	2.1	1.4	0.7	2.5	Weakness	Died 48 hours
	22	550	50	1.8	1.3	0.5	7.0	Convulsions	
	48	230	20	2.0	1.3	0.7	4.3	Postmortem sample	
24/78	72	12 000	200	1.4	0.8	0.6	8.4	Collapse	Died 96 hours
28/78†‡	12 min	14 500	150	2.2	0.9	1.2	94.3*	'Wandering'	Recovered
	48	1,250	2	2.3	1.2	1.1	44.8*	Normal	
2/78	12	–	–	1.3	0.9	0.4	27.6	Weakness: postmortem sample	Died 12 hours

After Rossdale et al. (1979).
*Values > 2 SD above mean for control subjects.
†Pony, remainder Thoroughbred.

fever. Bradycardia (less than 50 beats/minute) usually occurs during coma and convalescence from NMS. A rapid heart rate with forceful beat may be observed through the thoracic wall and jugular vein engorgement and pulse wave occurs in haemolytic disease and in foals suffering from cardiac failure due to NMS or septicaemia.

Respiratory rate

Increased respiration rates in foals over two hours of age may be due to (*a*) respiratory distress, i.e. reduced pulmonary function associated with atelectasis; (*b*) metabolic acidaemia involving the compensatory process of increased ventilation; (*c*) hyperthermia; or (*d*) pneumonia.

Differentiation of these states requires measurement of ventilatory capacity and arterial or venous blood gas chemistry.

In respiratory distress tidal volume (Vt) and maximal tidal volume (Vt_{max}) are reduced (below 400 ml and below 600 ml respectively). Respiratory rate and minute volume (V) are increased (above 60/minute and above 40 litres respectively).

Expiratory sounds of 'barking', grunting or high-pitched whinnying occur during convulsive episodes and are probably associated with biochemical or neurological disturbances.

Other diagnostic signs

The intensity of signs in Group I conditions gradually increases over the course of illness and their nature depends on the site of the infecting agent. The eyeballs often sink into the orbits in septicaemia and diarrhoea.

Emaciation is seen in cases of prematurity and in immaturity associated with placentitis due to infection and other causes.

Clinical diagnosis of haemolytic disease rests on yellow mucous membranes, a reddish urine and laboratory diagnosis on erythrocyte count below 4×10^{12}/litre, haemoglobin below 7 g/dl and packed cell volume below 0.20 litre/litre, the presence of ghost cells, bilirubin levels greater than 340 μmol/litre and an indirect van der Bergh reaction. Serological tests on the dam's plasma and foal's erythrocytes complete the diagnosis.

Laboratory measurements

Packed cell volume. Foals suffering from diarrhoea or convulsions have increased packed cell volume (above 0.44 litre/litre). Reduced levels (below 0.35 litre/litre) are experienced in septicaemia, inflammatory conditions of the fetal membranes and prematurity. In haemolytic disease the packed cell volume falls to below 0.20 litre/litre.

Haemoglobin and erythrocyte counts usually follow packed cell readings, ranging from above 17 g/dl and 9×10^{12}/litre respectively in diarrhoea and below 7 g/dl and 4×10^{12}/litre respectively in haemolytic disease.

White cell count. A leucocytosis (more than 14×10^9/litre) occurs in most septicaemic conditions, although to establish a diagnosis it may be necessary to carry out serial determinations over 48 hours. However, a leucopenia (less than 4×10^9/litre) may be present if the infecting agent produces leucocidal substances, and low white cell counts are often found in premature foals and those associated with placentitis.

Blood glucose. Levels rise about 1.67 mmol/litre after feeding. Hyperglycaemia (whole blood glucose greater than 8.32 mmol/litre occurs during convulsions and reduced levels (whole blood glucose less than 1.67 mmol/litre in prematurity. Hypoglycaemia is usually symptomless in the neonatal period.

Blood lactic acid. A significant increase (above 8.9 mmol/litre) in blood lactic acid occurs in foals suffering from respiratory distress or convulsions because of anaerobic metabolism and exaggerated muscular activity.

Serum proteins. Low levels of serum proteins occur in prematurity and subnormal globulin levels are often present in septicaemia.

Venous blood pH. Acidaemia (pH below 7.10) occurs in foals that do not establish an initial respiratory rhythm and those suffering from convulsions. Low levels (pH below 7.30) occur in diarrhoeic foals.

Arterial blood gas tensions. Low oxygen tensions (below 70 mmHg) are a feature of NMS and premature foals. In NMS, however, increments of oxygen tensions during oxygen inhalation may not increase to normal levels (above 200 mmHg). Carbon dioxide tensions may rise in cases of respiratory distress, but are reduced (below 30 mmHg) in metabolic acidaemia provided pulmonary ventilation is normal.

Urine. Heavy deposits of protein in the urine suggest nephritis, although a positive reaction may be expected in the first 36 hours of life due to the presence of low molecular weight milk proteins. Leucocytes and bacteria in smears made from centrifuged deposits or grown on culture are diagnostic of infective nephritis.

PERINATAL MORTALITY

In modern medical usage, *perinatal deaths* refer to still-births and babies dying within seven days of birth (Butler & Bonham 1963). By *perinatal mortality* we refer to equine fetal death just before, during or in the first week of life in the viable period, i.e. more than 300 days' gestation. Bergin (1969) defined perinatal mortality as loss between Day 30 of gestation and 30 days post-partum. In reviewing the literature he pointed out the absence of universally accepted criteria to form a reliable basis of comparison. Platt (1973) refers to perinatal mortality as death between Day 299 of pregnancy and the end of the second month of post-natal life. From a survey of 2242 pregnancies (which included twin deliveries) the still-birth rate was 2.3% and the post-natal mortality rate 1.8% in the first week and

1% in the second to eighth week. Excluding twin deliveries, in which the death rate was substantial, the still-birth rate was 1.2% and death in the first week 1%. Merkt and Von Lepel (1971) calculated a loss of 5% from death in the first four weeks after birth. Rossdale and Leadon (1975) reported a mortality rate of 3.6% on two stud farms in the Newmarket area in a survey conducted over a ten-year period based on cases that showed signs in the first week, irrespective of the age at which death occurred.

TWINS

Thoroughbred twins are of particular concern because of the economic loss incurred. Mahaffey (1958) quoted a survey from Russia in which, of 266 twin pregnancies, only 16 pairs and 13 single foals could be reared. Of the rest, 199 aborted both fetuses, 21 produced both foals still-born and 17 had two weak foals, one or both of which soon died.

Jeffcott and Whitwell (1973) reported an incidence of 1–2% in the General Stud Book between 1929 and 1968. They found that relatively few cases presented before seven months' gestation and that 72.6% were seen between eight months and term. The outcome of the twin pregnancies was that in 64.5% both aborted, in 21% one was born alive and in 14.5% both were born alive. Of a possible 124 fetuses, the total number born alive was 31 and only 18 survived to two weeks of age.

Rossdale (1966) found a mean weight of 50 kg in a group of 32 singleton Thoroughbred foals and only 20 kg in six live surviving twins with gestational ages of 325–335 days. Jeffcott and Whitwell (1973) recorded a mean weight of 31 kg in seven of the largest twins in their series. The smallest weighed 1.5 kg. Twins may be considered as a naturally induced situation of dysmaturity because the competition between the two placentae causes damage to both (see p. 177).

References and further reading

Arvidson, G., Astedt, B., Ekelund, L. & Rossdale, P.D. (1975) Surfactant studies in the fetal and neonatal foal. *J. Reprod. Fert.*, Suppl. **23**, 663.

Avery, M.E. (1964) *The Lung and Its Disorders in the Newborn Infant*, p. 3. Philadelphia and London: W.B. Saunders.

Baker, H.J. & Lindsey, J.R. (1968) Equine goiter due to excess iodide. *J. Am. vet. med. Ass.*, **153**, 1618.

Barnett, K.C. (1975) The eye of the newborn foal. *J. Reprod. Fert.*, Suppl. **23**, 701.

Belonje, C.W.A. (1952) Some diseases associated with breeding of horses. Part II. Post-natal deaths. Diseases of foals. *J. S. Afr. vet. med. Ass.*, **23**, 27.

Bergin, W.C. (1969) A survey of embryonic and perinatal losses in the horse. *Proc. 15th ann. Conv. Am. Ass. equine Practnrs*, 121.

Brambell, F.W.R. (1958) The passive immunity of the young mammal. *Biol. Rev.*, **33**, 488.

Bryans, J.T., Swerczek, T.W., Darlington, R.W. & Crowe, M.W. (1977) Neonatal foal disease associated with perinatal infection by Equine Herpesvirus I. *J. equine Med. Surg.*, **1**, 20.

Butler, N.R. & Bonham, D.G. (1963) *Perinatal Mortality*. Edinburgh and London: Livingstone.

Caroli, J. & Bessis M. (1947) Sur la cause et le traitement de l'ictere graves des muletone nouveaunes. *C. r. hebd. Seanc. Acad. Sci., Paris*, **224**, 969.

Chodnik, K.S., Jull, D.J. & Addison, I.A. (1960) The transmission of immunity to tetanus from ewe to lamb. *Vet. Rec.*, **72**, 277.

Colles, C.M., Parkes, R.D. & May, C.J. (1978) Foetal electrocardiography in the mare. *Equine vet. J.*, **10**, 32.

Comline, R.S. & Silver, M. (1970) pO_2, pCO_2 and pH levels in the umbilical and uterine blood of the mare and ewe. *J. Physiol., Lond.,* **209**, 587.
Coombes, R.R.A., Crowhurst, R.C., Day, F.T., Heard, D.H., Hinde, I.T., Hoogstraten, J. & Parry, H.B. (1948) Haemolytic disease of newborn foals due to isoimmunisation of pregnancy. *J. Hyg., Camb.,* **46**, 403.
Cronin, M.T.I. (1955) Haemolytic disease of newborn foals. *Vet. Rec.,* **67**, 479.
Crowhurst, R.C. (1970) Abdominal surgery in the foal. *Equine vet. J.,* **2**, 22.
Dawes, G.S. (1968) *Foetal and Neonatal Physiology.* Chicago: Medical Publishers.
Dawes, G.S., Fox, H.E. & Leduc, B.M. (1972) Respiratory movements and rapid eye movement sleep in the foetal lamb. *J. Physiol., Lond.,* **220**, 119.
Dimock, W.W., Edwards, P.R. & Bruner, D.W. (1947) Infections of fetuses and foals. *Bull. Ky agric. Exp. Stn,* 509.
Dixon, R.J., Hartley, W.J., Hutchins, D.R., Lepherd, E.E., Fielen, C., Jones, F.F., Lore, D.N., Sabine, M. & Wells, A.L. (1978) Perinatal foal mortality associated with a herpesvirus. *Aust. vet. J.,* **54**, 103.
Dubs, B. (1976) Megavesica due to congenital absence of urachus in a r. wborn foal. *Schweizer Arch. Tierheilk.,* **118**, 393.
Dunhill, M.S. (1962) Postnatal growth of the lung. *Thorax,* **17**, 329.
Dunn, P.M. (1972) Human 'barkers'. *Equine vet. J.,* **4**, 128.
Edwards, A.V. (1964) Resistance to hypoglycaemia in the newborn calf. *Proc. J. Physiol.,* **171**, 46.
Fraser, F.C., Kalter, H., Walter, B.E. & Fainstat, R.D. (1954) Experimental production of cleft palate with cortisone and other hormones. *J. cell. comp. Physiol.,* Suppl. **43**, 237.
Gairdner, D., Marks, J., Roscoe, J. & Brettell, R. (1958) The fluid shift from the vascular compartment immediately after birth. *Archs Dis. Childh.,* **33**, 489.
Gideon, L. (1977) Anal agenesis with rectourethral fistula in a colt (a case report). *Vet. Med. small Anim. Clin.,* **72**, 238, 240.
Gillespie, J.R. (1975) Postnatal lung growth and function in the foal. *J. Reprod. Fert.,* Suppl. **23**, 667.
Goodwin, R.F.W. (1957) The concentration of blood sugar during starvation in the newborn calf and foal. *J. comp. Path. Ther.,* **67**, 289.
Greene, H.J., Wray, D.D. & Greenway, J.J. (1975) Two equine congenital cardia anomalies. *Irish vet. J.,* **29**, 115.
Gribble, D.H. (1972) The endocrine system. In *Equine Medicine and Surgery,* ed. E.J. Catcott & J.F. Smithcors, 2nd ed., p. 433. Wheaton, I11.: American Veterinary Publishers.
Gruenwald, P. (1963) Chronic fetal distress and placental insufficiency. *Biol. Neonat.,* **5**, 215.
Haughey, K.G. & Jones, R.T. (1976) Meningeal haemorrhage and congestion associated with the perinatal mortality of foals. *Vet. Rec.,* **98**, 518.
Hemmings, W.A. & Brambell, F.W.R. (1961) Protein transfer across the foetal membranes. *Br. med. Bull.,* **17**, 96.
Huggett, A. St. G. (1961) Carbohydrate metabolism in the placenta and foetus. *Br. med. Bull.,* **17**, 122.
Irvine, C.H.G. & Evans, M.J. (1975) Postnatal changes in total and free thyroxine and triiodothyronine in foal serum. *J. Reprod. Fert.,* Suppl. **23**, 709.
Irvine, C.H.G. & Simpson-Morgan, M.W. (1974) Relative rates of transcapillary movement of free thyroxine, protein-bound thyroxine, thyroxine-binding proteins and albumin. *J. clin. Invest.,* **53**, 156.
Jeffcott, L.B. (1971) Perinatal studies in Equidae with special reference to passive transfer of immunity. Ph. D. Thesis, University of London.
Jeffcott, L.B. (1972) Observations on parturition in crossbred pony mares. *Equine vet. J.,* **4**, 209.
Jeffcott, L.B. (1974) Studies on passive immunity in the foal, 1. Gammaglobulin and antibody variations associated with maternal transfer of immunity and the onset of active immunity. *J. comp. Path.,* **84**, 93.
Jeffcott, L.B. (1975) The transfer of passive immunity to the foal and its relation to immune status after birth. *J. Reprod. Fert.,* Suppl. **23**, 727.
Jeffcott, L.B. & Whitwell, K.E. (1973) Twinning as a cause of foetal and neonatal loss in the Thoroughbred mare. *J. comp. Path.,* **83**, 91.
Johnson, P. & Rossdale, P.D. (1975) Preliminary observations on cranial cardiovascular changes during asphyxia in the newborn foal. *J. Reprod. Fert.,* Suppl. **23**, 695.
Kemen, M.J. & Coggins L. (1972) Equine infectious anaemia: transmission from infected mares to foals. *J. Am. vet. med. Ass.,* **161**, 496.

Lauwers, H. & Devos, N.R. (1966) Atresia coli and hydrocephalus in a foal. *Vlaams Diergeneesk. Tijdschr.*, **35**, 505.
Leader, G.H. (1952) The clinical aspect of some diseases met with in young Thoroughbred foals. *Vet. Rec.*, **64**, 241.
Lemetayer, E., Nichol, L., Jacob, L., Girard, O. & Corvazier, R. (1947) Immunité anti-toxique transmise de la jument au penlain, cas particulier de l'immunité des juments vaccinées contre le tetanes. *Annls Inst. Pasteur, Paris,* **73**, 297.
Littlejohn, A. (1959) Sleepy foal disease in Natal. *J.S. Afr. vet. med. Ass.*, **30**, 143.
Littlejohn, A. (1975) Aspects of respiration in anaesthetized newborn foals. *J. Reprod. Fert.*, Suppl. **23**, 681.
McGuire, T.C. & Crawford, T.B. (1973) Passive immunity in the foal: measurement of immunoglobulin classes and specific antibodies. *Am. J. vet. Res.*, **34**, 1299.
Maguire, L.C. (1958) The role of *B. viscosum equi* in the causation of equine disease. *Vet. Rec.*, **70**, 989.
Mahaffey, L.W. (1958) Foetal deaths. *Br. Racehorse,* September.
Mahaffey, L.W. & Rossdale, P.D. (1957) Convulsive and allied syndromes in newborn foals. *Vet. Rec.*, **69**, 1277.
Mahaffey, L.W. & Rossdale, P.D. (1959) A convulsive syndrome in newborn foals resembling pulmonary syndrome in the newborn infant. *Lancet,* **2**, 1223.
Merkt, H. & Von Lepel, J.D. (1971) Report on the Autumn 1970 examinations of West German Thoroughbreds (bloodstock). *Vollblut,* **34**, 26.
Millar, R. & Bailey, K.C. (1959) Clinical cases of convulsive syndrome in the newborn foal. *Aust. vet. J.*, **35**, 489.
Miller, R.M., Kind, R.E. & Rick, R.W. (1966) Congenital anomalies of the abdominal musculature and urogenital tract in a foal. *Vet. Med. small Anim. Clin.*, **61**, 652.
Miller, W.C. (1950) Foal disease – two years' survey. *Br. Racehorse,* **2**, 391.
Morison, J.E. (1970) *Foetal and Neonatal Pathology,* 3rd ed. London: Butterworths.
Nathanielsz, P.W., Rossdale, P.D., Silver, M., Comline, R.S. & Hall, L.W. (1973) Plasma cortisol in the foal during the late foetal and early neonatal period. *Res. vet. Sci.*, **15**, 395.
Nathanielsz, P.W., Rossdale, P.D., Silver, M. & Comline, R.S. (1975) Studies on fetal, neonatal and maternal cortisol metabolism in the mare. *J. Reprod. Fert.*, Suppl. **23**, 625.
Naylor, J.M. (1979) Colostral immunity in the calf and the foal. *Vet. Clins N. Am. lge Anim. Pract.*, **1**, 331
Nemeth, F. (1976) Contracted tendons in the foal. *Prakt. Tierarzt,* **57**, 3.
Oliver, T.K., (1965) Temperature regulation and heat production in the newborn. *Pediat. Clins N. Am.*, **12**, 765.
Osbaldiston, G.W., Coffman, J.R. & Stowe, E.C. (1969) Equine isoerythrolysis–clinical pathological observations and transfusion of dam's red blood cells to her foal. *Can. J. comp. Med.*, **33**, 310.
Palmer, A.C. & Rossdale, P.D. (1975) Neuropathology of the convulsive foal syndrome. *J. Reprod. Fert.*, Suppl. **23**, 691.
Palmer, A.C. & Rossdale, P.D. (1976) Neuropathological changes associated with the neonatal maladjustment syndrome in the Thoroughbred foal. *Res. vet. Sci.*, **20**, 267.
Pattle, R.E., Rossdale, P.D., Schock, C. & Creasey, J.M. (1975) The development of the lung and its surfactant in the foal and in other species. *J. Reprod. Fert.*, Suppl. **23**, 651.
Platt, H. (1973) Etiological aspects of perinatal mortality in the Thoroughbred. *Equine vet. J.*, **5**, 116.
Platt, H. (1977) Joint-ill and other bacterial infections on Thoroughbred studs. *Equine vet. J.*, **9**, 141.
Reid, L. (1967) The embryology of the lung. In *Development of the Lung,* ed. A.V.S. de Renck & R. Porter. London: Churchill.
Reilly, W.J. & MacDougall, D.F. (1973) The metabolism of IgG in the newborn foal. *Res. vet. Sci.*, **14**, 136.
Reynolds, E.B. (1930) Clinical notes on some conditions met with in the mare following parturition in the newly born foal. *Vet. Rec.*, **10**, 277.
Roberts, M.C. (1975) The development and distribution of mucosal enzymes in the small intestine of the fetus and young foal. *J. Reprod. Fert.*, Suppl. **23**, 717.
Rockey, J.H. (1967) Equine antihapten anitbody, the sub units and fragments of anti-beta-lactoside antibody. *J. exp med.*, **125**, 249.
Rooney, J.R. (1966) Contracted foals. *Cornell Vet.*, **56**, 172.
Rooney, J.R. (1971) Rupture of the urinary bladder in the foal. *Vet. Path.*, **8**, 445.
Rooney, J.R. (1972) The musculoskeletal system. In *Equine Medicine and Surgery,* ed. E.J. Catcott & J.F. Smithcors, p. 489. Wheaton, I11.: American Veterinary Publishers.

Rossdale, P.D. (1966) A clinical and laboratory assessment of the health status of the newborn foal. Fellowship thesis, Royal College of Veterinary Surgeons.

Rossdale, P.D. (1967*a*) Clinical studies on a newborn Thoroughbred foal. 1. Perinatal behaviour. *Br. vet. J.*, **123**, 470.

Rossdale, P.D. (1967*b*) Clinical studies on the newborn Thoroughbred foal. II. Heart rate auscultation and electrocardiogram. *Br. vet. J.*, **123**, 521.

Rossdale, P.D. (1968*a*) Blood gas tensions and pH values in the normal Thoroughbred foal at birth and in the following 42 hours. *Biol. Neonat.*, **13**, 18.

Rossdale, P.D. (1968*b*) Clinical studies on the newborn Thoroughbred foal. III. Thermal stability. *Br. vet. J.*, **124**, 18.

Rossdale, P.D. (1969*a*) Measurements of pulmonary ventilation in normal newborn Thoroughbred foals during the first 3 days of life. *Br. vet. J.*, **125**, 157.

Rossdale, P.D. (1969*b*) Clinical studies on 4 newborn Thoroughbred foals suffering from convulsions with special reference to blood gas chemistry and pulmonary ventilation. *Res. vet. Sci.*, **10**, 279.

Rossdale, P.D. (1970) Some parameters of respiratory function in normal and abnormal newborn foals with special reference to levels of p_aO_2 during air and oxygen inhalation. *Res. vet. Sci.*, **11**, 270.

Rossdale, P.D. (1972*a*) Modern concepts of neonatal disease in foals. *Equine vet. J.*, **4**, 117.

Rossdale, P.D. (1972*b*) Differential diagnosis and treatment of equine neonatal disease. *Vet. Rec.*, **91**, 581.

Rossdale, P.D. (1972*c*) A clinical assessment of perinatal respiration in the foal. *VII int. Kongr. Tier. Fortpfl. Munchen,* 605.

Rossdale, P.D. (1976) A clinician's view of prematurity and dysmaturity in Thoroughbred foals. *Proc. R. Soc. Med.*, **69**, 631.

Rossdale, P.D., Falk, M., Jeffcott, L.B., Palmer, A.C. & Ricketts, S.W. (1974) A preliminary investigation of cerebrospinal fluid in the newborn foal as an aid to the study of cerebral damage. *J. Reprod. Fert.*, Suppl. **27**, 593.

Rossdale, P.D., Jeffcott, L.B. & Palmer, A.C. (1976) Raised fetal blood pressure and haemorrhage in CNS of newly born foals. *Vet. Rec.*, **99**, 111.

Rossdale, P.D. & Leadon, D. (1975) Equine neonatal disease: a review. *J. Reprod. Fert.*, Suppl. **23**, 685.

Rossdale, P.D., Pattle, T.E. & Mahaffey, L.W. (1967) Respiratory distress in a newborn foal with failure to form lung lining film. *Nature, Lond.*, **215**, 1498.

Rossdale, P.D. & Scarnell, J. (1961) Immunisation of the newborn foal against tetanus. *Vet. Rec.*, **73**, 184.

Rossdale, P.D., Silver, M., Comline, R.S., Nathanielsz, P.W. & Hall, L.W. (1973) Plasma cortisol in the foal during the late foetal and early neonatal period. *Res. vet. Sci.*, **15**, 395.

Rossdale, P.D. & White, S. (1975) Studies on pressure volume relationships in excised equine lungs. *J. Reprod. Fert.*, Suppl. **23**, 673.

Rouse, B.T. (1971) The immunoglobulins of adult equine and foal sera. A quantitative study. *Br. vet. J.*, **127**, 45.

Scott, A.M. (1972) Red cell groups of horses. In *Equine Infectious Diseases,* ed. H. Gerber & J.T. Bryans, 3rd ed., p. 384. Basel: Karger.

Shelley, H.J. (1961) In *Ciba Symposium on Somatic Stability in the Newly Born,* ed. G.E.Q. Wolstenholme & M. O'Connor, p. 12, London: Churchill.

Shelley, H.J. (1964) Carbohydrate reserves in the newborn infant. *Br. med. J.*, **1**, 273.

Silver, M., Steven, D.H. & Comline, R.S. (1973) Placental exchange and morphology in ruminants and mare. In *Fetal and Neonatal Physiology: Proceedings of the Sir Joseph Bancroft Centenary Symposium.* Cambridge: Cambridge University Press.

Sjostedt, S., Engleson, G. & Routh, G. (1958) Dysmaturity. *Archs Dis. Childh.*, **33**, 123.

Tyler, S.J. (1972) The behaviour and social organisation of the New Forest ponies. *Anim. Behav. Monogr.*, **5**, 2.

Weir, R.C. & Porter, R.R. (1966) Comparison of the structure of the immunoglobulins from horse serum. *Biochem. J.*, **100**, 63.

Wellington, J.K.M. (1972) Bladder defects in newborn foals. *Aust. vet. J.*, **48**, 426.

Woollam, D.H.M. (ed.) (1966) Advances in teratology. *Adv. Teratol.*, **1**, 2.

Woolam, D.H.M. (1978) The long search for the causes of congenital malformation in mammals. *Equine vet. J.*, **10**, 43.

Wright, B.M. (1959) *Symposium on Pulmonary Ventilation,* ed. R.P. Harbord & L. Woolmer. Altricham: John Sherratt.

Wyke, B.W. (1963) *Brain Function and Metabolic Disorders.* London: Butterworths.

The Older Foal and Yearling 6

The foal, once established in its new environment, leaves behind the dramatic physiological events of the adaptive period. Development and growth are more leisurely now and the problems of survival less acute. Clinically the foal can be considered a replica of the adult, although immunologically less competent and prone to the diseases of 'youth', especially those of bone.

The clinician must recognize certain differences in this formative stage, such as changes in behaviour as the foal develops towards complete independence and changes in diet – milk, to milk plus fibre and then fibre only. Further, growing bone is susceptible to damage by injudicious management and immature tissues are challenged by micro-organisms.

In this chapter we are concerned with recognizing the special physiology and disease to which the older foal and yearling are heir. Our account is therefore confined to aspects peculiar to the period and not general to equine medicine. We start with the clinical appraisal of normality.

HEALTH

Behaviour forms the basis of clinical interpretation, yet it is only recently that the study of equine ethology has received the attention necessary to raise it from a subjective art to an objective science. One of the most important aspects in such a study is to compare behaviour under various forms of management with wild or feral states. Such a comparison provides a basis for beneficial changes in management. We cite two methods of weaning in support of this contention. In the traditional method foals are removed from the 'herd' and isolated for several days; in the method which more nearly simulates natural conditions the dams are withdrawn, leaving the foals with their fellow herd members. This is less disturbing to the foal and reduces the risk of a serious setback in condition and health. An understanding of equine relationships is also essential in arranging the fostering of orphan foals.

Relationship with other herd members

There have been few studies of feral horses. In a report on the behaviour and social organization of New Forest ponies Tyler (1972) found that day-old foals showed a strong tendency to follow any large moving object and frequently followed mares other than their own dam. By the second day they followed only their dam, but some foals showed attachment to a fixed object such as a tree. Most day-old foals nibbled at grass or chewed leaves but did not swallow them. The amount of time spent nibbling or grazing gradually increased with age from a mean of 12 minutes/hour by 12 weeks to 40 minutes/hour at 36 weeks. The amount of time young foals rested decreased from half the daylight hours up to the third month, to roughly one-fifth at six months. Foals stood for a greater proportion of their resting time after age 13–16 weeks.

Mares that have recently lost their own foal may sometimes 'poach' another. Even barren mares and those with a young foal at foot may show poaching behaviour, but the phenomenon is rare and mares usually exhibit strongly hostile attitudes to the approach of a foreign foal.

On Thoroughbred stud farms in the northern hemisphere mares foal in loose boxes and are usually confined for several days before being turned out with other mares and foals. The foal–dam relationship is by then firmly established and the risks of poaching are minimal. In some instances a foal may develop a strong instinct to approach and suck from a mare other than its own dam and may establish a dual relationship with another member of the herd, whose own foal may thus be deprived of some of its dam's milk. In these cases the mare and 'poaching' foal should be placed in separate paddocks. Such a relationship was observed by one of us (P.D.R.) over a period of two weeks at a stud farm in Newmarket, England (Fig. 6.1). Two two-month-old foals played together and one was able to suck from the other's dam at will, provided her own foal was not in the sucking position, in which event the mare showed the usual antagonistic behaviour towards the 'foreign' foal.

In the southern hemisphere where foals are born out of doors, other members of the herd may interfere with the foal–dam relationship. But as Tyler (1972) observed in New Forest ponies the curiosity of older herd members soon wanes and yearlings show the greatest interest in newborn foals.

Sucking behaviour

A foal moves in front of its mother to stop her before it approaches the mammae. The mare usually cooperates by ceasing to graze, standing still and flexing the hind-leg on the side away from the foal. Mares hinder sucking and bring the sucking bout to an end by moving away, kicking or biting at the foal. Tyler (1972) found that the mother ended 40% of the bouts in the first week of the foal's life but by three months the proportion was below 25%. Although mares cooperated more with older foals, these foals sucked infrequently compared with young ones; sucking was often the only contact between dam and an older foal. The natural path to weaning is thus a gradual one in which both dam and offspring play a positive role in diminishing the contact. The mean frequency of sucking bouts in Tyler's study decreased from four per hour in the first week of life to two per hour in the sixth week, one per hour in the sixth month and 0.5 per hour in the eighth month. Length of

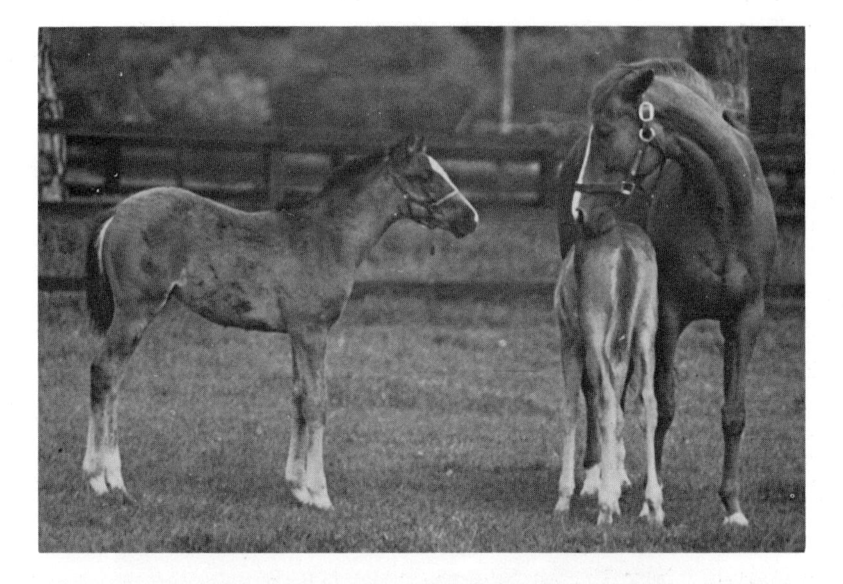

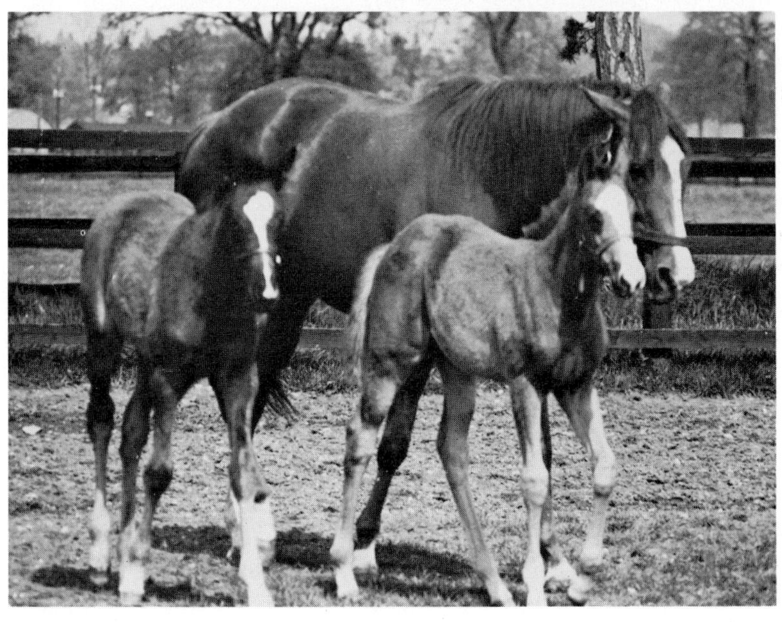

Fig. 6.1. Two foals develop a close play relationship at Herringswell Manor Stud, Newmarket. The mare allowed both foals to suck from her and was antagonistic to the 'poaching' foal only when her own foal was sucking.

sucking bouts varied from seconds to several minutes (mean 70 seconds) in the first week and a significant decrease in bout length occurred by the fourth month.

Coprophagia

Frances-Smith and Wood-Gush (1977) observed the behaviour of four Thoroughbred foals. They were seen to eat part of the fresh faeces deposited by their own dams on some 40% of the occasions when the mare was observed to defaecate, between the second and fifth week post-partum. They did not eat faeces before or after this period. This behaviour was thought to be a feeding pattern which formed a normal part of the foal's development. It may introduce bacterial flora into the foal's gut and supply certain vitamins which the foal is unable so synthesize.

Play

Tyler (1972) noted a close relationship between mare and foal for more than a year following birth. The time a foal spent within 5 yards (5 m) of its mother gradually declined and the time 5–25 yards (5–20 m) away increased, but even at five months old foals spent less than 10% of time more than 50 yards (40 m) from their dams.

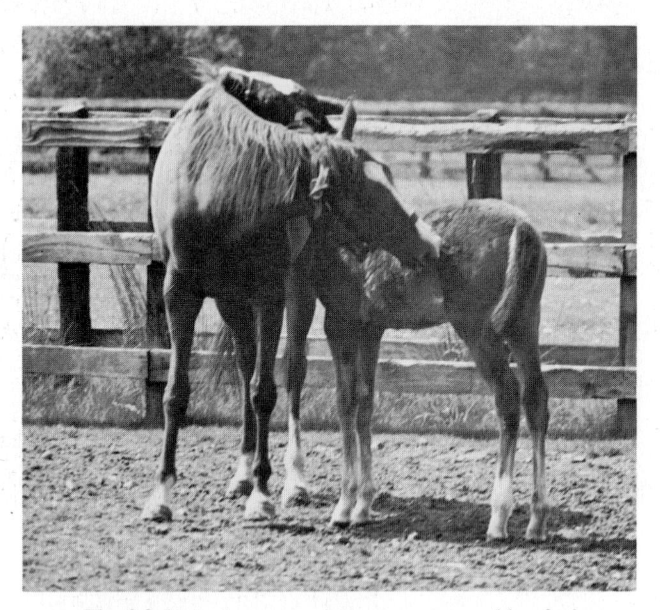

Fig. 6.2. Mutual grooming between a mare and her foal.

Play is characterized by patterns of moving, eating, aggressive, grooming and sexual behaviour. (For definitions of play in mammals see Loizos 1966.) From their first day foals show interest in their mothers' bodies, nibbling at their legs, mane and tail and kicking at or jumping on them. Mares are tolerant of this early play which gives way, at two to three weeks, to mutual grooming (Fig. 6.2).

Galloping round the mare (Fig. 6.3) is common after the first week and the distance increases with age, but according to Tyler (1972) this behaviour decreases as interactions with other foals becomes more numerous. The percentage of hours in which foals played on their own or around their mothers decreased from 56% in their first week to 7.4% in their seventh and eighth weeks. Interactions with other foals however increased from 2.6% to 50% over the same period (Fig. 6.4).

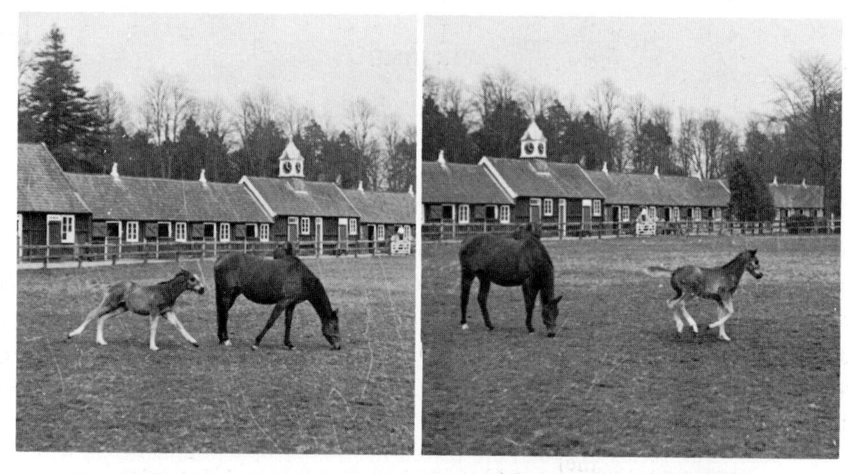

Fig. 6.3. The distance at which foals play by circling the mare increases with age.

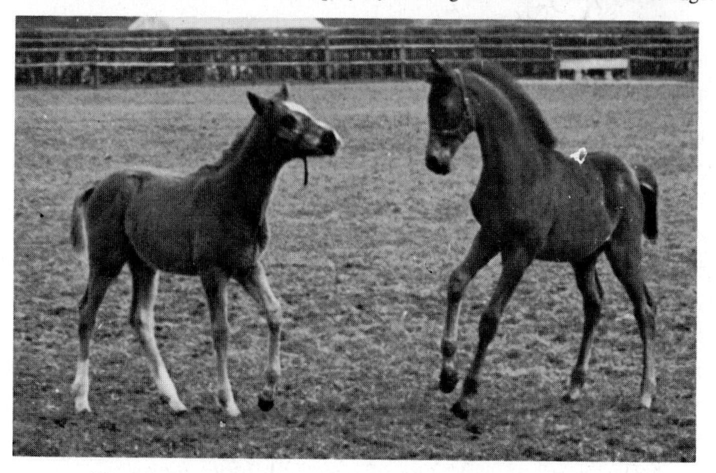

Fig. 6.4. The time spent by foals in play increases with age.

Tyler found that the play of colts older than four weeks became markedly different from that of fillies. Colts spent long periods play-fighting together in pairs. Play between colts and fillies usually consisted of mutual grooming bouts but the colts became rough and gripped their partners' necks and bit at their heads and fore- and hind-legs.

Precocious sexual behaviour, when colts sniff at their mothers' hind-quarters and vulva and show *Flehmen* posture and penile erection, may occur as early as three months, although mounting behaviour of a playful nature (i.e. without erection or obvious sexual intent) occurs in the first four weeks. Copulation before age 18 months is rare but colts, because of their roughness, should be separated from fillies by age nine months old. Sperm is present in the testes at about 13 months (Nishikawa 1959) and ejaculation of sperm can occur in most colts at 16–20 months (Cole & Cupps 1959).

WEANING

Under feral conditions weaning occurs at about one year, a few days or weeks before the mare gives birth to a new foal or, if the mare is barren, at up to two years (Tyler 1972). In modern stud farm management foals are weaned at five to six months. The traditional method is to confine a group of foals of similar age to their loose boxes while removing the mares to a part of the stud farm where they are out of earshot. The foals are left with the box doors closed and windows boarded until they have settled, which usually takes three to six days, and are then turned into a well fenced paddock. During this period the foal often eats little and some individuals may develop habits of weaving and box-walking. Injuries to the head may be caused by the foal dashing at the stable door.

On some stud farms the foals are placed in pairs or in adjoining boxes with an aperture through which they can see and smell one another. This reduces the immediate effects of weaning but may cause a further period of disturbance when the 'paired' foals are finally separated. There is little doubt that vices and other behavioural problems of riding horses stem from experiences at weaning, although no objective study of the relationship has yet been reported.

Free-range weaning (Fig. 6.5) is now practised in many breeding centres and gaining popularity. In this method mares and their foals of comparable ages are brought together in a well fenced and secluded paddock and allowed to familiarize themselves with one another and with the paddock environment for at least a week and preferably longer. They may be housed at night or remain in the paddock all the time, depending on climatic conditons and managerial preferences.

On the first day one or two mares are removed from the group as they are being turned out in the morning, or, if out day and night, at a convenient time in the morning. The weaned foals may become restive and call out but they are not usually seriously disturbed, continue to play with other foals and do not approach other mares. In the evening if the group is housed at night, the weaned foals are returned to the same loose boxes which they shared with their dams. The top door may be closed but this is a precaution rarely necessary as the foals usually eat normally and are little if at all distressed. The following morning the weaned foals are returned to the paddocks. Another mare is removed from the group after two or three days and the process continued until only one mare remains with up to 15 foals (the optimum group size is about eight). This mare may be taken away or left with the foals for several weeks. In the southern hemisphere it is customary to leave an old mare or gelding with weaned foals and yearlings as it is argued that this has a quietening effect.

Free-range weaning carries little risk of injury. Any mare that is known to be vicious or one that is inclined to cause a disturbance by galloping or 'paddock-walking' should be one of the first removed.

After weaning the mares may be placed in a paddock without any special precautions, except that they should be out of hearing distance of their foals. The mammary glands become distended but it is not usually necessary to treat them.

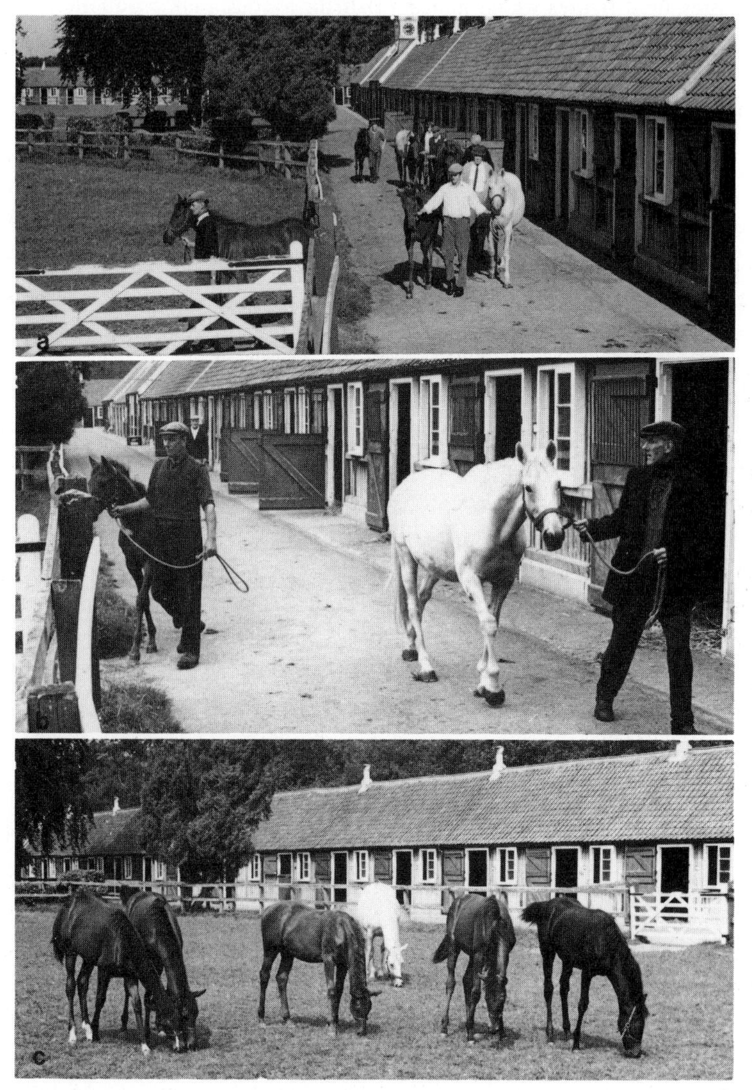

Fig. 6.5. Free-range weaning. (*a*) Mares and their foals, together with a weaned foal, are turned on to the paddock at Cheveley Park Stud, Newmarket. (*b*) The act of weaning. The mare is led away as her foal is turned on to the paddock with the other members of the herd. (*c*) Weaned foals are left with one mare in the paddock.

LACTATION

The quantity of mammary secretion which continues until weaning has not been documented. In the first two weeks post-partum 4–8 litres/24 hours can be obtained from a Thoroughbred mare. Jeffcott (1973, personal communication) collected 2–4 litres/24 hours from small pony mares in the first week. These values are a fair reflection of secretory capacity at this particular time but do not provide a reliable basis to calculate the quantity of milk produced before weaning. Tyznik (1972) presented figures which indicate that the average milk production for mares rises in the first three months after foaling from 15.4 kg/day in heavy breeds and 10.3 kg/day in pony breeds to 18.2 kg/day and 12.5 kg/day respectively. The quantity then falls, by five months, to below post-foaling levels. Neseni et al. (1958) reported that light breed foals obtained 221 g of milk at each nursing.

TABLE 6.1 Proteins in mares' colostrum

Protein	*Amount*	
Total serum proteins (g/litre)	Mean	135
	Range	56 to 216
Albumin (g/litre)	Mean	29
	Range	13 to 57
Globulin (g/litre)	Mean	106
	Range	27 to 187
Alpha (g/litre)	Mean	31.55
	Range	3.7 to 91.7
Beta (g/litre)	Mean	34.28
	Range	7.68 to 66.4
Gamma (g/litre)	Mean	40.15
	Range	10.1 to 79.8
Alpha (%)	Mean	27.4
	Range	4.87 to 60.0
Beta (%)	Mean	33.1
	Range	10.8 to 55.9
Gamma (%)	Mean	39.5
	Range	8.8 to 69.5

Figures are unpublished data from Rossdale and Ricketts.

There is more information on the quality of milk: colostrum is very high in protein (Table 6.1). Ullrey et al. (1966) studied Arabian and Quarterhorse mares and reported a steep fall in gross energy, specific gravity, total solids and protein within 12 hours of birth and a steady fall from this age to four months. Lactose concentration and lipids increased over the same period (Figs 6.6, 6.7). These authors found that phosphorus concentration rose from bith to 48 hours post-partum and then declined, whereas calcium content dropped for 12 hours, rose to a peak at eight days and then declined. Levels of magnesium, potassium and sodium fell over the first four months post-partum (Figs 6.8, 6.9).

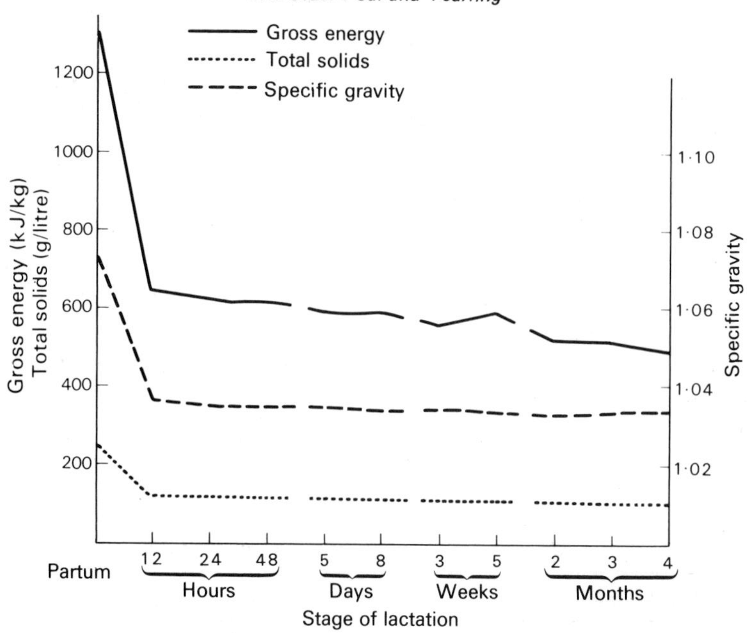

Fig. 6.6. Changes in the specific gravity and concentration of gross energy and total solids in mares' milk at various stages of location. (*After Ullrey et al. 1966*)

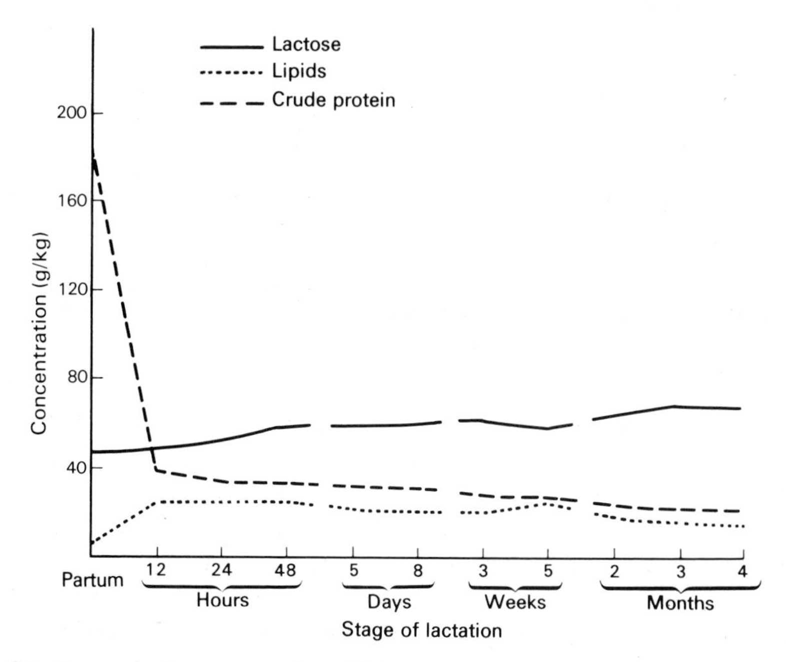

Fig. 6.7. Changes in the concentration of lactose, crude protein and lipids in mares' milk at various stages of lactation. (*After Ullrey et al. 1966*)

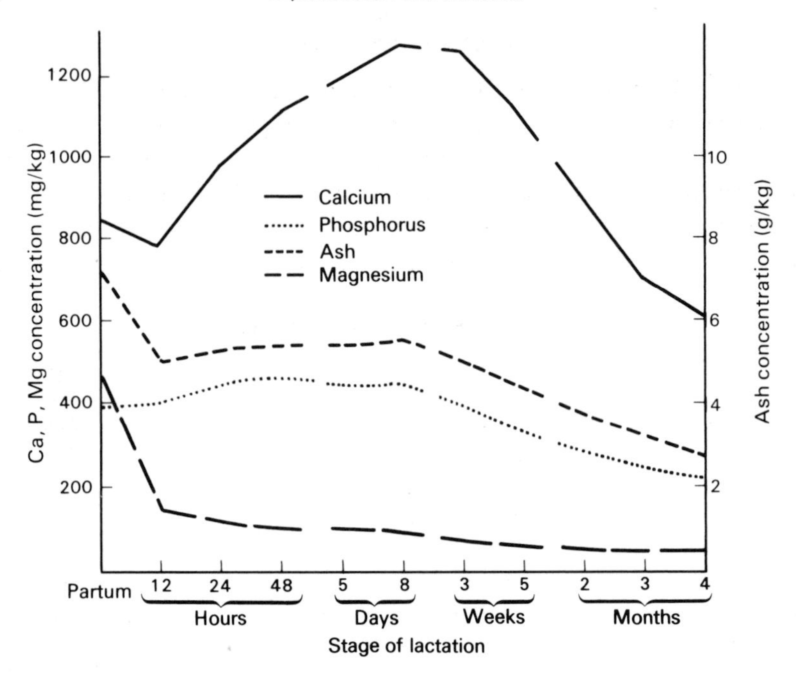

Fig. 6.8. Changes in the concentration of ash, calcium, phosphorus and magnesium in mares' milk at various stages in lactation. (*After Ullrey et al. 1966*)

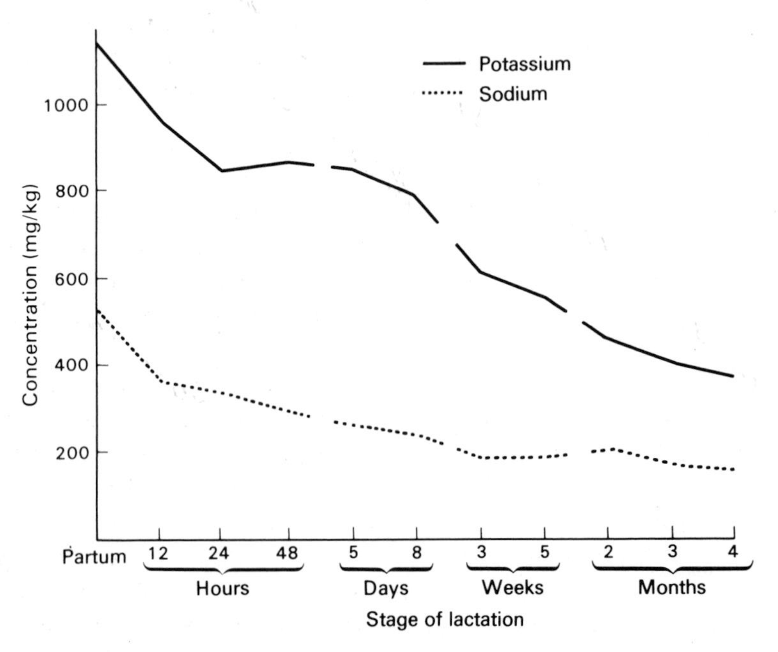

Fig. 6.9. Changes in the concentration of potassium and sodium in mares' milk at various stages of lactatation. (*After Ullrey et al. 1966*)

Supplementary feeding

The most rapid physical growth rate occurs during the first few months (see p. 382). Protein requirement for growth is high and milk supply may fall short of supplying adequate proteins to allow maximal potential growth, either for genetic or environmental reasons or because peak production has been passed. Thus supplementary feeding is usually practised, making use of 'creep' feeders either inside the box or in the paddock (Tyznik 1975). Supplemented rations for foals should

TABLE 6.2 Recommended creep ration

	Constituent	%
187.0	Corn	37.4
165.0	Soya bean meal	33.0
115.0	Oats	23.0
2.5	Brewers' yeast	0.5
15.0	Molasses	3.0
5.0	Dicalcium phosphate	1.0
5.0	Limestone	1.0
5.0	TM salt	1.0
0.5	Vitamin A and D	0.1
500.0		

After Tyznik (1975).

contain a minimum of 20% protein in highly digestible form. Many suitable pelleted rations are available and soya bean meal appears to be a useful high protein source. Tyznik recommends the creep ration shown in Table 6.2. Frape (1973, personal communication) considers that foals should consume 0.5 kg of concentrate cubes per day by two months old and weaning should be possible at four months.

Mastitis

Mastitis is rare in mares, compared with cows. It may occur at any stage of lactation and is sometimes seen in non-sucking mares. It occasionally affects mares in the post-weaning phase of 'drying-off'. *Str. zooepidemicus* is the most commonly isolated organisms (Reese & Lock 1978) but other organisms may be involved, e.g. *Corynebacterium ovis* (Addo et al. 1974).

Signs of mastitis are a hot, swollen, painful mammary gland with oedematous swellings extending anteriorly along the abdomen and posteriorly into the perineal fold between the hind-legs. The affected mare may suffer stiffness and inappetence. The mammary secretion is thick and contains numerous polymorphonuclear leucocytes. The contents of an intramammary tube of antibiotics, as used in cattle, should be squeezed into the gland on two or three consecutive days, after draining the contents of the udder, if this is possible. Parenteral antibiotic treatment is recommended in addition, or alone if local treatment is not possible. The teat ducts of mares are sometimes very small and some mares with mastitis object violently to handling.

ORPHAN FOALS

A foal may be 'orphaned' because of its dam's death, antagonistic behaviour or inadequate milk. Alternative means of maintenance may therefore be required at any time from birth to five months. Fostering an 'orphan' foal (under age 12 weeks) onto a suitable milking mare is usually considered the best way of promoting growth and normal development; but foals have been successfully reared from birth by artifical feeding or by fostering onto a cow or goat (Fig. 6.10).

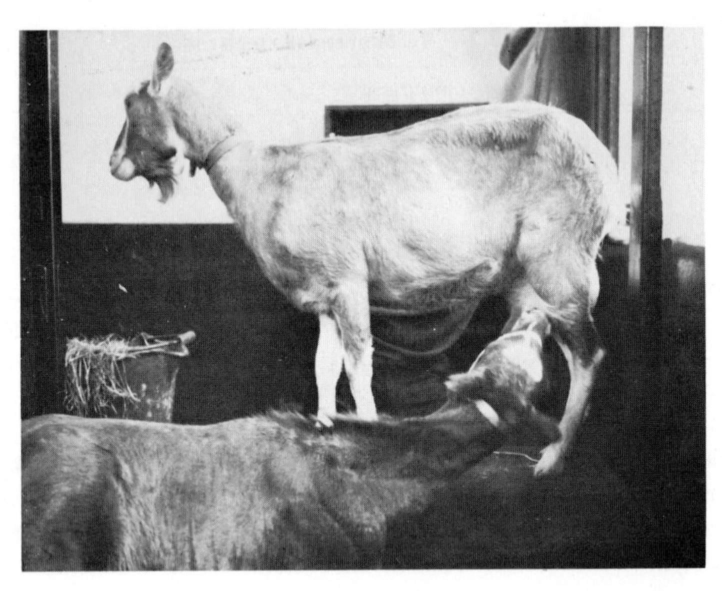

Fig. 6.10. An orphan foal fostered by a goat at Hadrian Stud, Newmarket.

No critical study has been reported by which one method of 'fostering' foals can be evaluated against another.

Fostering

In our experience successful fostering depends on a number of variables affecting the mare–foal relationship.

Whichever method is used to introduce the orphan foal to the foster mare – several methods are possible – the major factors affecting a successful fostering are:

1. The lactational age of the foster mare. Mares who have had still-born foals, or which have not been suckled, less readily accept a 'foreign' foal.

2. The period between the death of the foster mare's foal and introduction of the orphan. The longer the time, the less the chance of success.

3. The discrepancy in size between the foster mare's foal and the orphan. If it is great, acceptance is less likely.

4. The orphan foal's sucking behaviour. If the foal has been reared artificially for several weeks or has never sucked from a mare, it gradually loses the instincts

necessary for successful fostering. It may be frightened by the presence of the foster mare and this may occur if the foster mare kicks the foal, irrespective of the time of separation from its natural dam.

5. The mare's strength of 'mothering' instinct. The degree to which this is due to genetic factors or to past experience is unknown. Some individuals accept a 'foreign' foal reluctantly but without obvious hostile actions. These 'sullen' mares are the most difficult because they usually accept the foal while attendants are present and reject it as soon as they have gone. Other mares show extreme hostility but once they accept a foal they are usually the best mothers. It seems they have strong maternal instincts.

Methods of fostering

All methods rely on the confusion of the maternal instinct. This is achieved by:

1. Placing a strong-smelling ointment in the mare's nostrils.

2. Removing the mare from the box where she has been with her own foal for long enough to allow a weakening of her 'knowledge' of her foal.

3. Disguising the orphan foal. This may be achieved by covering it with the foster mare's amnion or foal's skin (Fig. 6.11). A mare recognizes her foal by sight, smell and taste. After the mother–foal bond has been established sight is important at a distance and smell in contact (Tyler 1972). Auditory cues may be less important.

4. Blindfolding the mare and putting her in a solid-sided wooden crush with an opening near the mammary region, so that the foal can suck. Strong-smelling ointment is put in the nostrils. After three to four days the mare is freed and usually accepts the foal.

5. Tranquillizers may help to reduce antagonistic response in the vital period of introduction.

The following description of one method of fostering which we have found successful is presented as a guide to what we feel is as much a matter of the mare's instinctive mothering capacity as of good judgement on the part of those introducing the orphan foal.

The foster mare should be placed in a loose box with her own foal, its skin or amnion. She is then led away and the orphan foal, which should have been starved for at least two hours, is put into the box. The skin or amnion of the foster mare's foal should be tied over the orphan foal (Fig. 6.11) so as to cover as much as possible of the body, neck and hind-legs.

The foster mare is then returned to the box and held by a bridle with her hind-quarters towards a corner. A tranquillizer may be given to help handling.

The foal is held by an attendant and the mare allowed to smell its covered parts (Fig. 6.11b). The foal is then encouraged to suck from the mare (Fig. 6.11c). After about 30 seconds it is led away from the mare who is allowed to follow round the box and again to come into contact with the covered parts. This process of sucking, smelling and movement should be repeated at intervals and two attendants should stay in the box until the mare shows signs of acceptance. This may

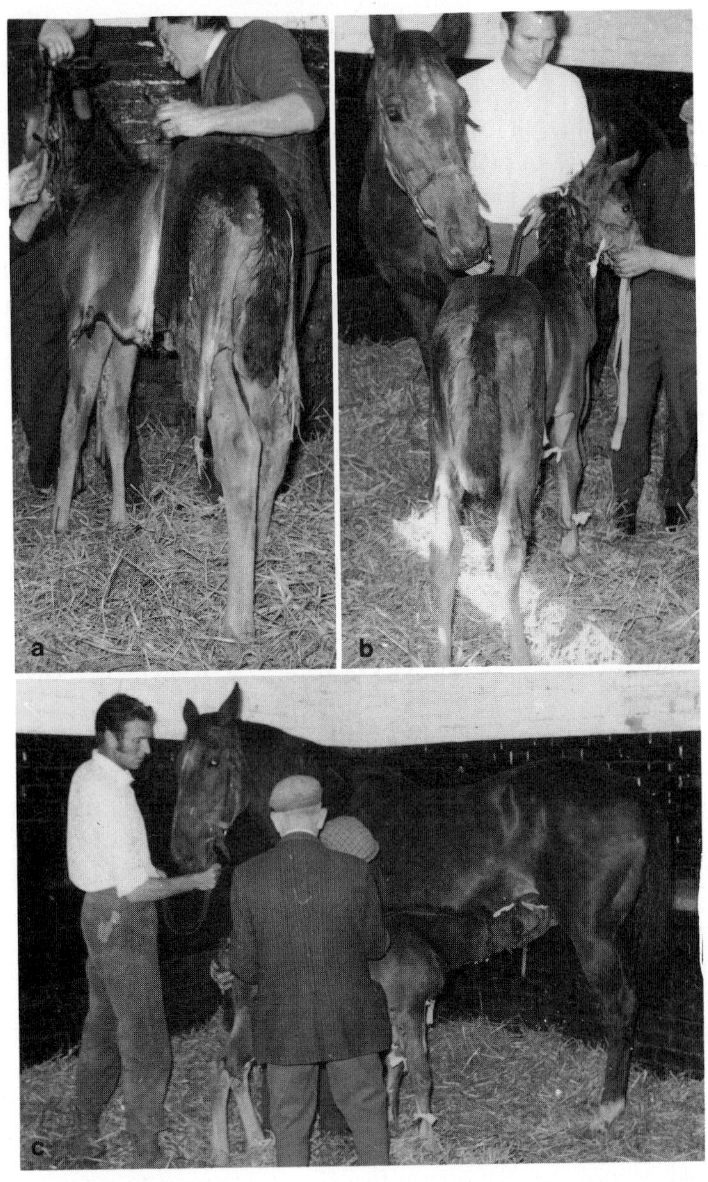

Fig. 6.11. (*a*) An orphan foal is draped in the skin of the foster-mother's foal. (*b*) It is the introduced to the potential foster-mother. Note the position of the attendants at the head o the mare and foal. (*c*) Close control of mare and foal is necessary at the first suck.

occur up to 12 hours after introduction of the foal. Signs include nickering to th foal and readily letting down milk during sucking bouts. If the mare shows n signs of accepting the foal after 12 hours the chances of success are small, althoug after a period of separation the foal may be reintroduced and a successful relation ship established at a second or even a third attempt.

When the mare has accepted the foal an attendant should remain in the box or close at hand for two to three hours to ensure that the mare does not develop antagonistic behaviour (Fig. 6.12). The amnion or skin should be removed 12–24 hours after a successful relationship has been established. The foal should receive prophylactic antibiotic injections for three to five days.

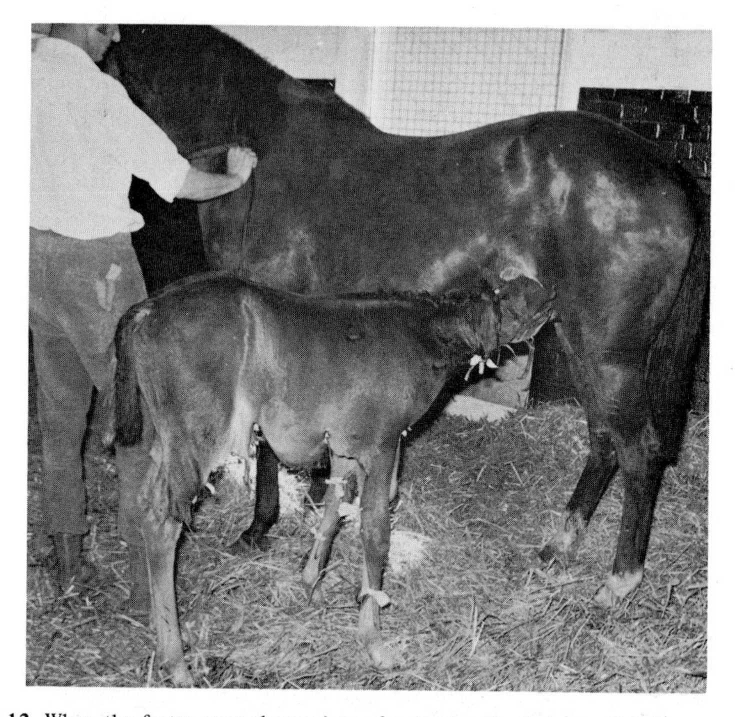

Fig. 6.12. When the foster mare shows signs of accepting the foal one attendant stays in the box until the mare/foal relationship is complete.

If the skin or amnion of the foster mare's foal are not available odoriferous ointment should be smeared on the mare's nostrils and over the orphan foal's buttocks, hind-quarters and head. The ointment should be renewed at frequent intervals. The process of introduction is similar to that described above. In some practices this method is prferred to that in which the skin is used and the chances of success are said to be as good.

Artificial diets

A wide range of proprietary milk substitutes and regimens of feeding practices have been found successful in rearing orphan foals. In the absence of critical trials it is difficult to evaluate each particular method. The end point is also a matter of subjective assessment, although obesity and stunted growth are obvious errors found in hand-reared foals at age six to 12 months. Here we present data from various authors by which the practitioner may judge a particular diet.

Frape (1973, personal communication) recommends that to ensure successful rearing of orphan foals it is essential to give colostrum within 12 hours of birth. Hygiene of the highest order should be maintained, particularly during the first 72 hours. The foal should be reared in clean, fresh quarters which have not been occupied for two or three weeks and in which there has been no incidence of enteric disease.

To avoid diarrhoea, the processing of the protein in the milk substitute must not cause a loss in the basic amino acids. An excess of liquid milk substitute at any one meal can swamp the digestive enzyme system, the acidity control in the stomach, and cause rapid proliferation of pathogenic enteric organisms.

A proposed feeding scale for foals up to 16 weeks old using a cow's milk substitute is given in Table 6.3. This must be interpreted so that small breeds receive less than large ones. Approximately 105 ml/kg body weight/day is a reasonable rate of feeding. The composition of the food received by the foal should differ from that of the calf, because mare's milk contains less protein and more lactose (Table 6.4).

TABLE 6.3 Scheme for feeding orphan foals up to 16 weeks old

Age of foal	*Warm water* (litres/day)	*Spillers high fat Calflacton* + 15% *glucose* (kg/day)	*Solids* (approx. %)	*Feeds* (minimum no./day*)
3 days	2.5	0.145	18	4
4 days	3	0.60	20	4
5 days	4.5	0.80	18	4
6 days	6	1.10	18	4
7 days	7	1.40	20	4
2nd week	8.5	1.70	20	4
3rd week	10.0	1.90	19	3
4th week	11.0	2.30	21	3
5th week	10.0	2.50	25	2
6–8 weeks	9.0	2.50	28	2
9–12 weeks	8	2.40	30	2
13–14 weeks	6	1.70	28	2
15–16 weeks	5	1.30	26	1

* If studmen are available then up to eight feeds per day, especially during the first and second weeks, are advised.

TABLE 6.4 Distribution of kilojoules in cows' and mares' milk

	Cows' milk	*Mares' milk*
Total gross kJ (per 100 g solids)	2199	1931
kJ from protein (%)	20	20
kJ from fat (%)	50	30
kJ from carbohydrate (%)	30	50

Proprietary mare's milk substitutes (Equilac, Horsepower) are available. The manufacturers include feeding schedules but experience has shown that constipation and dehydration usually occur if they are not fed at greater dilution than recommended for the first few weeks. Nevertheless, if used carefully, we have found them very useful and convenient products.

Utensils used for feeding should be kept clean and no liquid milk should be allowed to stand for long before consumption. The foal should be taught as soon as possible to drink directly from a bucket or bowl. Its muzzle is pushed into the bucket with the middle fingers in the mouth. Obstinate individuals may need a teat in the mouth for the first few days while the head is pushed into the bucket. Older

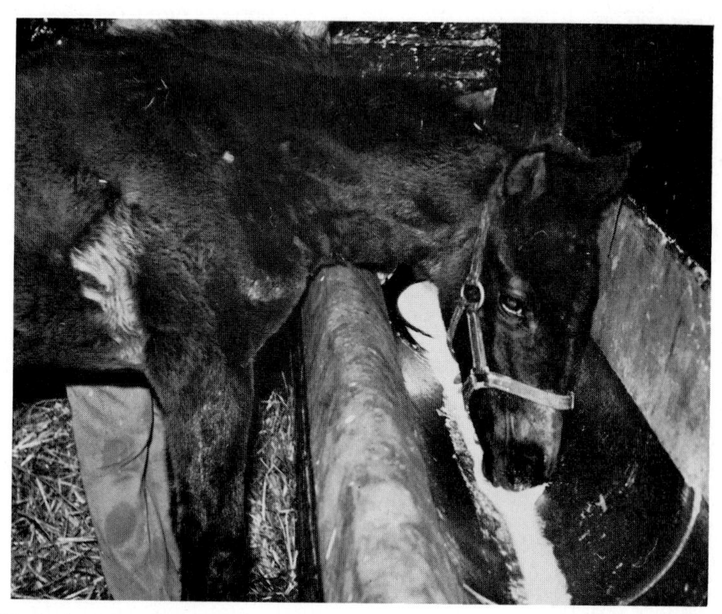

Fig. 6.13. A three-month-old Throughbred foal, recently orphaned, drinks milk substitute from a manger.

foals may prefer to feed from a manger (Fig. 6.13). The liquid should be approximately 37.5°C. If diarrhoea occurs, the milk substitute should be withdrawn and replaced by a solution of 50 g of glucose in 500 ml of water for one or two days and then the foal gradually returned to milk feed. The greater the number of feeds per day with the same total daily consumption, the less the likelihood that the foal will succumb to diarrhoea.

It may be safe to provide fresh, clean water, although in some instances this will make the foal reluctant to consume its normal ration of milk. By two or three weeks old, the foal should have access to hay and concentrates or feeding cubes. The foal should not be weaned from the liquid milk until it is eating adequate amounts of dry food (see p. 371); the changeover should be allowed to occur gradually, giving the digestive enzymes time to adapt. If sudden changes are instituted, digestive upsets may occur and there would be a depressed growth curve at this time. In the early stages, artificial rearing may be especially difficult with foals not born at term, but care and patience can overcome this.

Monson (1968) described a dried substitute for mare's milk containing: protein 20.2%, fat 14.4%, fibre 0.2%, lactose 52.6%, ash 7.2% calcium 0.9%, phosphorus 0.8%. Gross energy: 869 kilo-calories/kg; digestible energy: 782 kilo-calories/kg.

Three foals were reared from two days with this substitute and four foals allowed to remain with their dams as controls. Similar growth was found in orphaned foals and controls at age five months. Monson recommended a dilution of 20% solids/80% water and feeds were provided four times in 24 hours to provide 5380 digestible kilo-calories (22 488 kJ) at age up to two weeks rising to 10 230 kilo-calories (42 761 kJ) by age six weeks and 16 000 (66 880 kJ) by age 14 weeks. The foals were induced to drink from a bucket.

Drummond et al. (1973) successfully reared gnotobiotic foals using evaporated milk diluted with twice its volume of sterile water to produce a content of protein fat and sugar of 2.6, 2.8 and 4.1 g/100 ml respectively. Sugar was added to approx imate an analysis of 2.7, 1.6 and 6.1 g/100 ml respectively which conforms tc mares' milk (Linton 1931).

The quantity of milk fed depends on the foal's size, appetite and quantity of other nutrients available. As a rule a foal requires about 100 ml/kg body weight day of fluid, i.e. a 100 kg foal consumes about 10 litres a day. This may be offerec in regular feeds at two- to three-hour intervals or ad lib to older foals. It is importan that orphan foals should receive adequate exercise to avoid obesity.

Glendenning (1974) described a method of rearing foals using an automati calf feeding machine; 22 foals were given three different milk substitute powder and adverse signs included constipation and obesity. She recommended that foal reared by this method should have the company of other foals.

Supplementary feeding

If a mare produces too little milk, it may be possible to supplement intake, using a artificial rearing diet similar to the ones described above, while the foal is bein suckled. Methods used to try to increase milk production in such a mare includ the injection of oxytocin and β-carotene and the provision of good lush green gras and lucerne. These methods may be successful in some cases, but in others there is n alternative but to use a teat and bottle or, if the foal is young enough, foster the foa

HAEMATOLOGICAL STANDARDS

During the first three weeks post-partum the erythrocyte count, haemoglobi content, packed cell volume, mean corpuscular volume and neutrophil coun decrease, while total leucocyte, lymphocyte and eosinophil count increase; bas phils and eosinophils do not appear until after age seven days (Medeiros et a 1971). Jeffcott (1971) studied eight pony foals and found that the erythrocyt count declined to age ten days, followed by a rise to a peak at age two months an then gradual fall to mean 8.63×10^{12} litre at one year. The same author reported that haemoglobin content decreased steadily over the first three months from mean 16 g/dl at birth to 11.2 g/dl at 12 weeks rising to 12 g/dl at 12 months. Packed cell volume fell to 0.31 litre/litre at nine months and then increased. Total white cell count fell from 14.9×10^9/litre at seven months to 11.6×10^9/litre at one year.

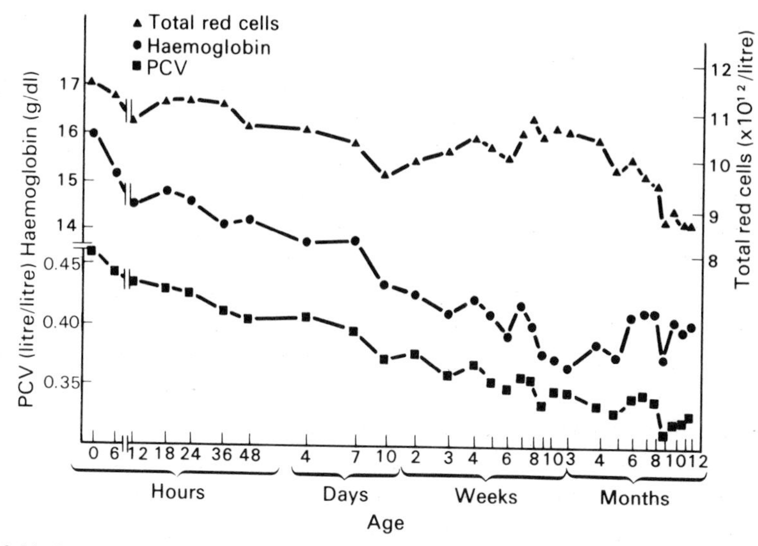

Fig. 6.14. Total red cells, haemoglobin and packed cell volume (mean values) in eight pony foals from birth to one year. (*After Jeffcott 1971*)

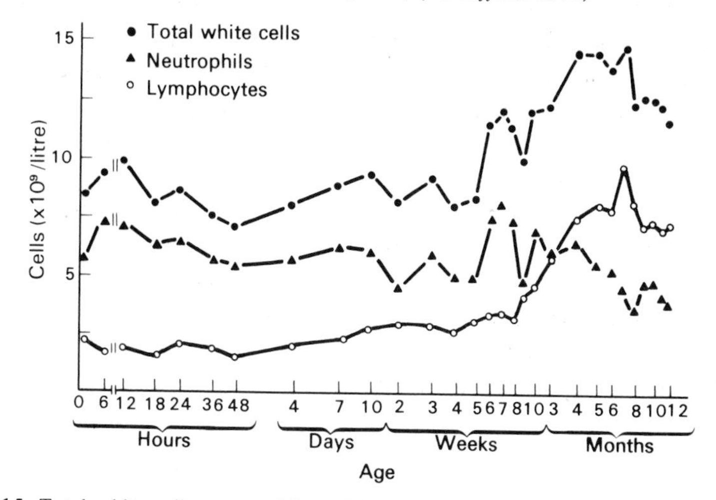

Fig. 6.15. Total white cells, neutrophils and lymphocytes (mean values) in eight pony foals from birth to one year. (*After Jeffcott 1971*)

Neutrophils increased to 8.2×10^9/litre at seven weeks followed by a fall to 4×10^9/litre at 12 months. Lymphocytes increased to a peak of 9.7×10^9/litre at seven months, eosinophils to a peak of 0.58×10^9/litre at five months (Figs 6.14, 6.15, 6.16).

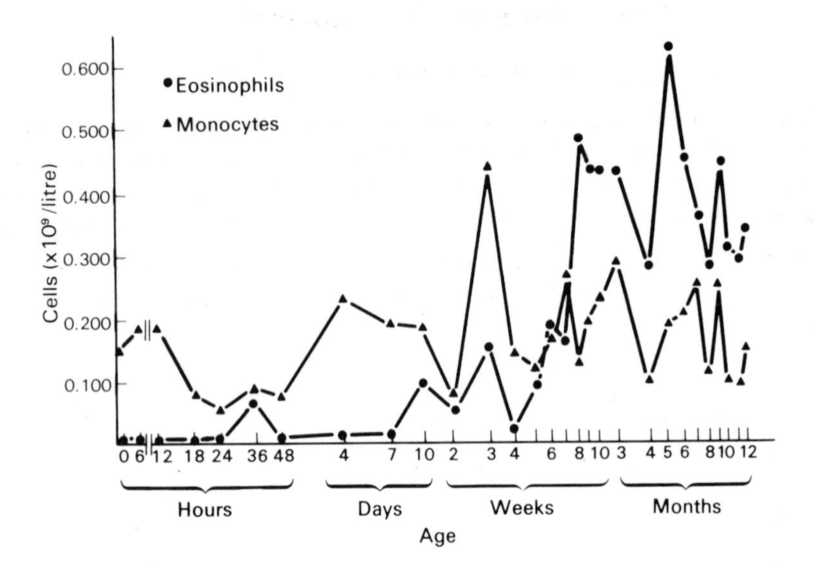

Fig. 6.16. Eosinophils and monocytes (mean values) in eight pony foals from birth to one year. (*After Jeffcott 1971*)

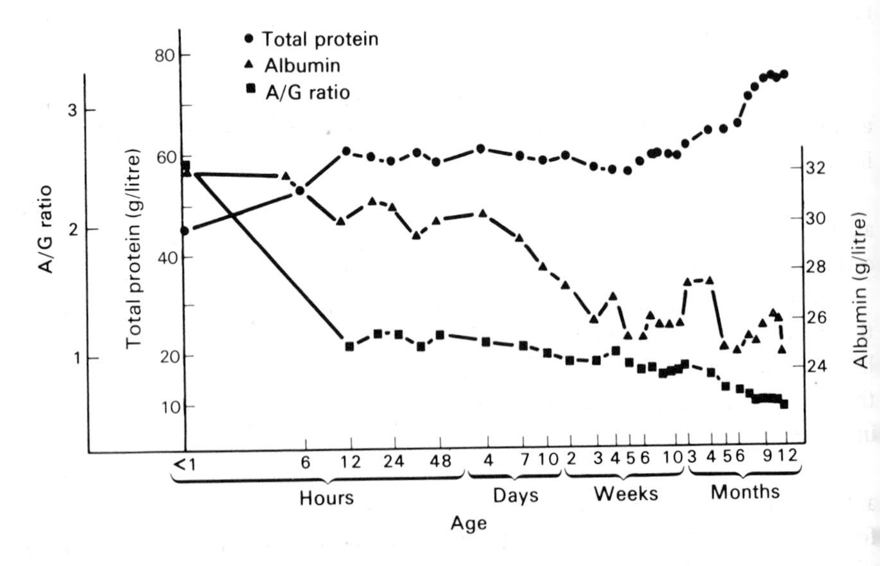

Fig. 6.17. Total serum protein, albumin and albumin/globulin ratio in eight pony foals from birth to one year. (*After Jeffcott 1971*)

BIOCHEMICAL STANDARDS

Serum protein values to age one year

Jeffcott (1971) established levels of serum protein in eight pony foals from birth to one year. He found mean values for total serum protein at birth of 45 g/litre, which rose by 33% after the ingestion of colostrum. Peak values of 60 g/litre were recorded by age four days and these fell by 5 g/litre at five weeks, gradually rising to 73 g/litre at one year. Serum albumin was highest before sucking and levels fell after the ingestion of colostrum and continued to fall to age six months (Figs 6.17, 6.18).

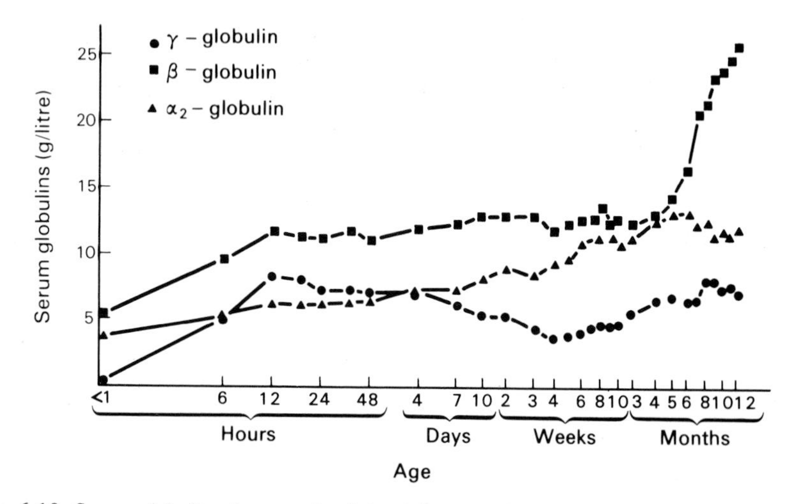

Fig. 6.18. Serum globulins (mean values) in eight pony foals from birth to one year. (*After Jeffcott 1971*)

The albumin/globulin (A/G) ratio continued to fall over the neonatal period and a more marked drop occurred at three months old when serum globulins began to increase.

The α-globulin did not alter significantly throughout the first year of life but all other globulins showed a marked rise after the ingestion of colostrum. The α-globulin increased steadily to peak levels of 13 g/litre at four to six months. Before the ingestion of colostrum only one band of β-globulin was detectable, the β_1 peak. The concentration of β-globulin was doubled in the first 12–48 hours of life, with the appearance of the β_2 peak. From five months to one year, there was a sharp increase in the β-globulin concentration, due mainly to an increasing β_1 peak.

All the foals were agammaglobulinaemic at birth. After absorption of passive antibody the γ-globulin values rose to a peak of 8.2 g/litre at 12 hours. There followed a gradual decline in these levels to the lowest recorded mean levels of 3.8 g/litre at four to five weeks. No significant rise in γ-globulin appeared until three months of age when the level rose fairly steeply to seven to eight months. This level approximated the peak values recorded after birth and was maintained to 12 months old.

Serum calcium, phosphorus and alkaline phosphatase levels

Serum phosphorus levels decline from about 2.26 mmol/litre in the first month post-partum to 1.9 mmol/litre at six months and 1.6 mmol/litre at 18 months. Serum calcium levels are 3–3.5 mmol/litre throughout this period. Serum alkaline

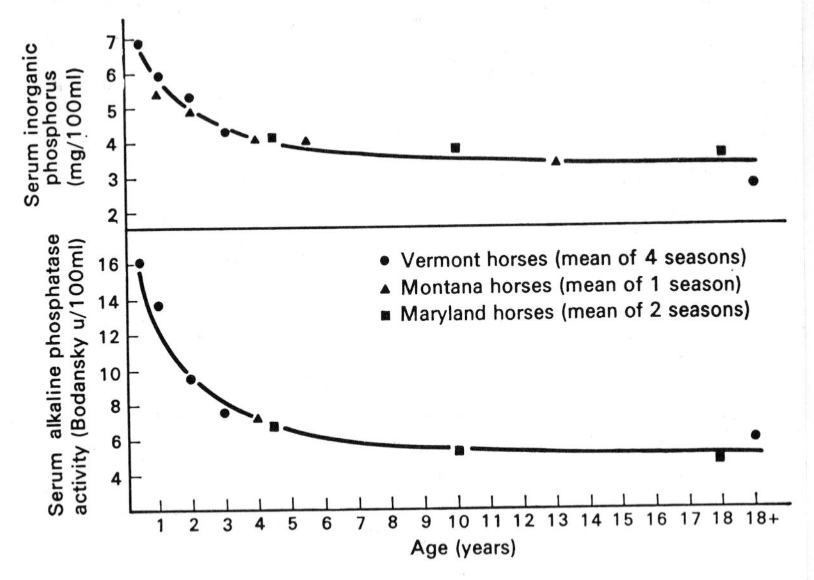

Fig. 6.19. Serum inorganic phosphorus and serum alkaline activity in groups of horses of different horses at different ages. Conversion factors: SIP mg/100 ml × 0.323 = mmol/litre; SAP: direct comparison between Bodansky and SI units is not possible, but Bodansky units × 15 ≙ mmol/litre. (*After Earle & Cabell 1952*)

phosphatase activity falls steeply over the first three years (Earle & Cabell 1952) (Fig. 6.19).

GROWTH

Growth is the multiplication and, to a lesser extent, enlargement of cells in various tissues of the body. In the context of equine stud farm medicine the growth of bone is of primary concern because this controls height and the relative conformation of the limbs which have a direct bearing on athletic performance.

Objective studies of growth rate in young horses have been reviewed by Green (1961), who suggests that periods of intensity of growth are similar under different climatic conditions. The most rapid growth is during the first month after birth with a second intense phase between six and 12 months and a third phase after puberty (Figs 6.20, 6.21).

Green (1969) made monthly measurements of the girth, the height at the withers and the circumference of the metacarpal bones just below the knee. He found that bone measurement for colts was 0.9 cm greater than for fillies at birth and this differential was maintained throughout the first 12 months of life. The relationship of height to girth changed at four months; before this age height exceeded girth but afterwards girth exceeded height. In the first three months gains in height and girth were only slightly less than the gains recorded during the whole

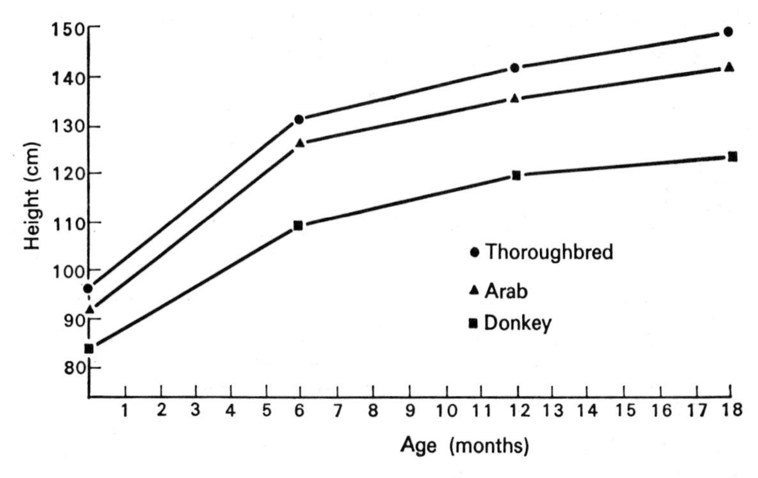

Fig. 6.20. Comparative growth curves for Thoroughbred horses, Arabs and donkeys from birth to 18 months at remount depots in Pakistan. (*After Green 1961*)

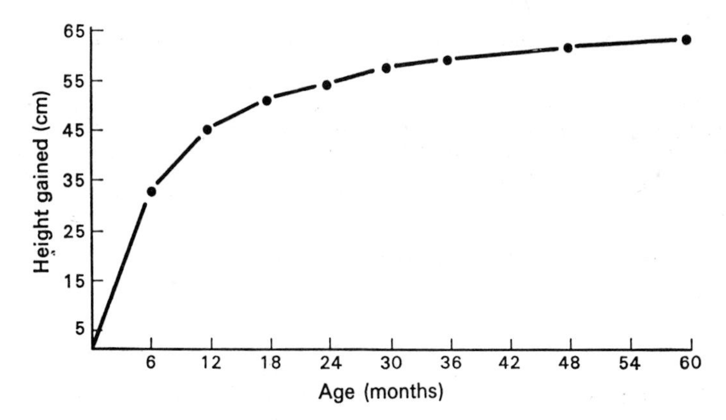

Fig. 6.21. The growth curve for Budennyi colts at the S.M. Budennyi Stud in Russia from birth to five years. (*Data from Scekina 1950; after Green 1961*)

of the next nine months. This intense growth in the first three months has been reported in other breeds.

Hintz et al. (1979) obtained measurements of weight, height at withers and front cannon bone circumference at the mid-point of 1991 Thoroughbred foals at a Canadian stud farm between 1958 and 1976. At birth, colts were heavier and taller and had larger cannon bones than fillies and differences increased with age. Dams under seven or over 11 years had foals of lighter weight, which were also shorter and had smaller cannon bones than foals of mares of 7–11 years of age. These differences persisted at 510 days of age. The authors suggest that smaller foals are probably related to the decreased ability of the younger dams to provide nutrients to the fetus. Foals born in April, May or June were heavier and taller and had larger cannon bones than foals born in January, February or March. Diet was probably not a factor because none of the mares was turned out to pasture until the end of May. The mares with late spring foals had a gestation period about three days shorter than mares with early foals. The size difference in the foals may have been related to hormonal responses to changes in daylight length. This factor is known to influence the reproductive cycle of the mare. At the latitude of the stud farm concerned, the difference between the longest and shortest days was six hours. Year of birth influenced all three measurements; the authors could make no conclusions as to why this should have occurred. Many factors such as weather, management practices, food supply and health conditions may have been involved. Extrapolating from the measurements obtained and the average mature weights, heights and cannon bone sizes of Thoroughbred horses, these authors calculated that Thoroughbred foals attain about 46, 67 and 80% of their mature weight and 83, 90 and 95% of their mature height at 6, 12 and 18 months respectively. Foals gained 110 kg during the first 90 days after birth, 75 kg during the second 90 days, 60 kg during the third 90 days and only 45 kg during the fourth 90 days. This demonstrates that the greatest amount of bone elongation takes place during the first few months of life and that proper nutrition during this period is obviously of great importance.

Hintz and Schryver (1976) reviewed the nutritional factors which influenced bone development, growth and disease in the horse and considered that ten essential requisites for proper bone development are energy, protein, calcium and phosphorus, vitamin A, vitamin D, zinc, manganese, copper and iodine. The nutritional role of these requisites and problems associated with their deficiencies, imbalances and excesses were described. The relative economic and nutritional merits of different hays, pasture grasses and grains were examined. Routine weighing, measuring and observation was found to be essential when regulating the diet and good quality hay was found to be the key to simplified horse feeding. Adequate amounts of the essential amino acid lysine were found to be essential and legume hay, dry skimmed milk and soya bean meal were all good sources.

Pasture management is of vital importance to the health and growth of young horses and Archer (1978) has described studies of producing and maintaining balanced pastures.

Green (1976) measured the height, girth and cannon bone circumference of yearlings and two-year-olds on six separate stud farms: 45 colts and 59 fillies were measured. In the yearlings, a period of intense active growth was seen during the spring and early summer, slowing down in later summer. An exception to this pattern was seen in the yearlings being prepared for the autumn sales and fed on a high plane of nutrition, when significant increase of girth measurements were found. Growth rates in the yearlings in training stables during the months October to March were more variable and irregular growth phases were seen. There was a notable increase in height of both colts and fillies in the autumn and early winter months. The excess weight resulting from preparation for the sales was soon shed as animals were put into work, so that only small increases in girth resulted over this six-month period.

Ellis and Lawrence (1978*a, b, c*) showed that restricted nutrition in a group of pony foals, over the winter period, caused retardation in growth, as measured by live weight gain. Although they have not conclusively proved it, these authors suggest that there would have been little difference in the mature live weight attained. There appeared to be a similar compensation in conformation, which indicated that permanent stunting had not been induced. The measured food intake of the restricted group, following the end of the experiment, was greater than that of the control group. The results also showed that the onset of oestrus was delayed by retarding growth between approximately 6 and 12 months of age. In addition it appeared that the cycle number and length were less than in the control group.

The clinician is mainly concerned with bone growth as it affects the epiphyseal plates and centres of ossification. For a description of the general principles of bone

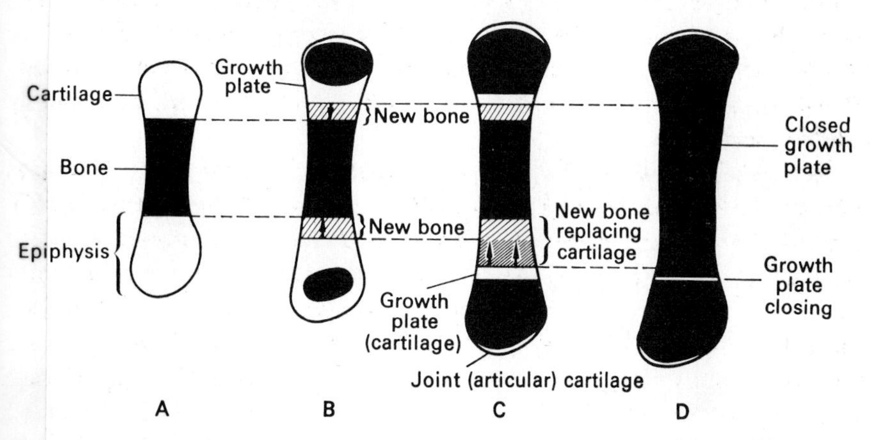

Fig. 6.22. The growing life of a typical lone bone in the body (left to right). If we suppose that it represents the fore-arm bone (radius), which extends from the elbow to the knee-joint in the horse's fore-leg, then A represents the state of the bone before the foal is born. B represents the condition at birth; C at about 18 months old; and D at 2 to 2½ years.

development the reader is referred to Ham and Leeson (1965). Long bones grow by means of laying down new bone in cartilaginous growth at either end (Fig. 6.22). Adams (1966) describes the age of epiphyseal closure based on Quarterhorse and Thoroughbred breeds:

> First phalanges 6 to 9 months; distal metacarpal (metatarsal) 9 to 12 months; radius proximal 12 to 18 months and distal 24 to 30 months; humerus, medial epicondyle 9 to 12 months, distal 12 to 18 months; olecranon 24 to 30 months; proximal tibial 24 to 30 months; distal 18 to 24 months; femur and os calcis 24 to 30 months.

In practice, the areas of growth which most concern us are those at the distal extremities of the radius, the tibia, the third metacarpal bone (MC3), third metatarsal bone (MT3) and proximal extremity of the proximal phalanx (P1) (Brown & MacCallum 1976).

MUSCULOSKELETAL DISORDERS

Epiphysitis

Epiphysitis consists of swelling of the distal end of MC3 or MT3 in the foal and at the distal end of the radius in the yearling. These swellings are sometimes hot and painful in the acute phase and the animal may be lame. The epiphyses on the medial aspects of the limb are usually affected (Fig. 6.23).

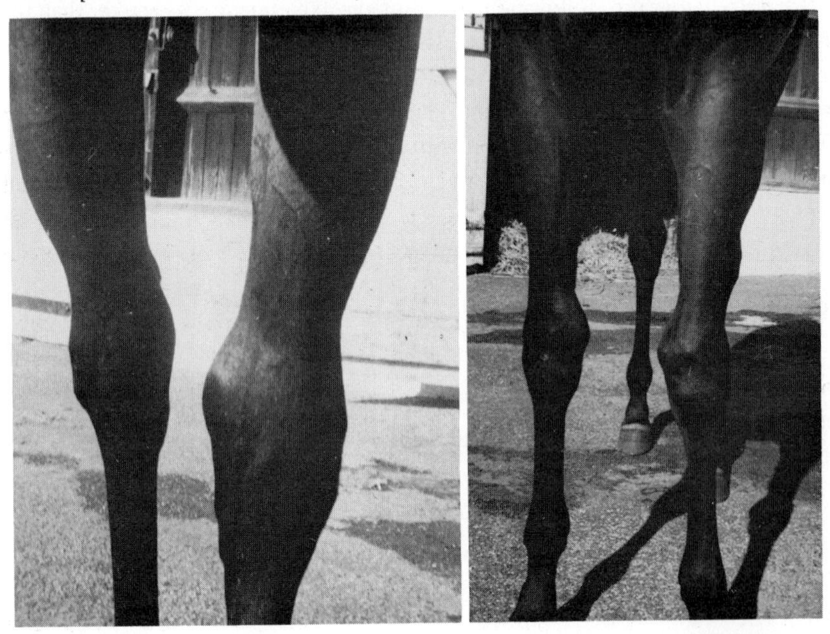

Fig. 6.23. Enlargements on the inner aspects of the hock and knee due to epiphysitis.

The condition sometimes results in angular deformity of the limb (Fackelman et al. 1975; Ellis 1976; Vaughan 1976; Campbell 1977). Rooney (1969) stated that the epiphyseal cartilage is crushed and thin on the involved side and that clinical observations support the hypothesis that epiphysitis is a compression lesion of the cartilage. Brown and MacCallum (1976) examined 26 cross-bred foals of Quarterhorse, Belgium, Percheron and other heavy breeds. Their epiphyses were examined both radiologically and histologically and varied in age from 52 to 104 days at the time of disposal and examination. The observations made were very similar to those described for overt 'epiphysitis', including irregularity and thickening of the growth plate, bridging of the plate by bony spicules, distortion of the plate adjacent to foci of fusion and metaphyseal lipping. The authors questioned whether these were normal foals or had subclinical 'epiphysitis'. They suggested that 'epiphysitis' is perhaps a misnomer and propose 'dysplasia of the growth plate' as a preferable term. This may be the correct term in those foals showing no clinical symptoms and epiphysitis for those with signs of swelling associated with heat, pain and lameness.

Brown and MacCallum (1976) report that suggested causes are improper nutrition, faulty conformation and hoof growth, muscle imbalance, overweight, malpositioning of the fetus in utero, radial paralyses and compression of the growth plate which may inhibit endochrondral ossification and acceleration of fusion. There is no doubt that, in practice, one sees the condition most frequently in the well grown, fast-growing, 'heavy topped' foals during the summer months when the ground is dry and hard and on stud farms where the calcium/phosphorus ratio in the diet shows imbalance. One must conclude that all these factors may play a part.

Treatment consists of reducing food intake to reduce body weight or at least growth rate, confined exercise in a yard or a large, well ventilated loose box on 'soft going' (peat moss, deep straw, shavings or sand), making sure that the feet are carefully and frequently trimmed and correcting the diet if necessary. The calcium/phosphorus ratio should be adjusted to 1.6 : 1 and protein content limited to less than 10% of dry matter. In general terms bran should not be fed and di-calcium phosphate or bone flour (10–30 g daily) should be added to the diet. Vitamin D supplements by oral or parenteral routes are indicated. An oral calcium and vitamin D combined supplement is available.

As a preventive measure the older foal or yearling which is over-fat or 'heavy topped' should be watched carefully for clinical signs, especially when the ground is hard and dry. When these conditions prevail it is wise to cut down food rations and restrict exercise.

Angular limb deformities

If retarded bone growth or fusion occurs eccentrically on the growth plate, angulation deformities may occur (Brown & MacCallum 1976). These deformities are quite commonly seen in Thoroughbred foals (Ellis 1976). The condition may be present at birth or may appear in older foals following 'epiphysitis' or when a healthy limb bears excessive weight due to prolonged lameness on the opposite limb. The condition is usually seen as a lateral angulation of the limb from the carpus (Fackleman et al. 1975; Vaughan 1976; Campbell 1977) (Fig. 6.24).

Ellis (1976) reports that most angular deformities correct themselves without treatment. Regular trimming of the feet and limitation of exercise may be of value in some cases. Splinting of the leg is only recommended in very young foals where the angle of deformity may be straightened by passive manipulation. Cases should be observed regularly so that surgical treatment, if indicated, may be carried out in good time.

The principle of the surgical treatment is to insert a rigid implant across the growth plate on the convex side of the curvature, in order to retard growth on that side and allow the opposite side to grow level (Vaughan 1976). The desired effect may take several weeks so it is essential to begin treatment well before plate closure occurs. At the carpus and hock it should be performed by 15 months and at the fetlock by six months. Ellis suggests that if progress following conservative treatment is not satisfactory by three months, surgery should be performed and that it may be wise to operate on badly deviated fetlocks as early as two months of age.

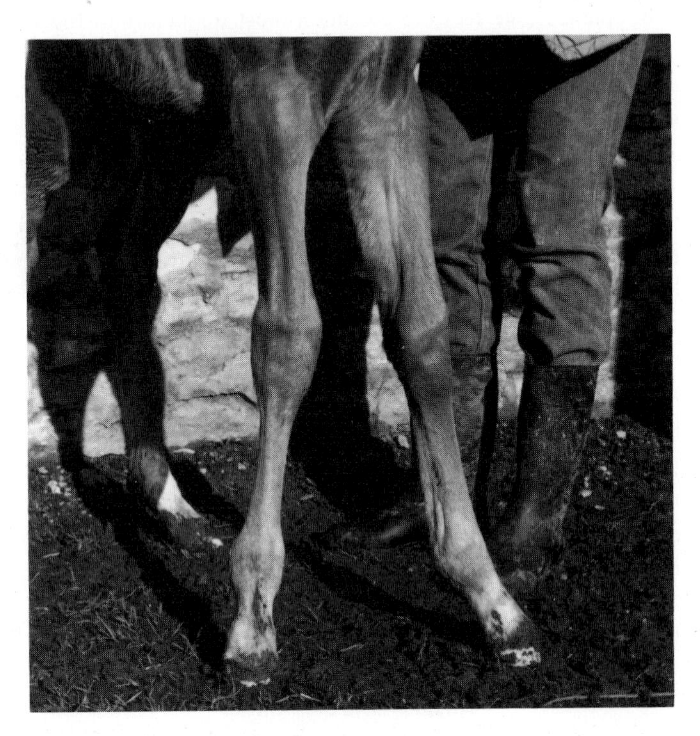

Fig. 6.24. A seven-day-old Thoroughbred foal showing lateral angulation of the fore-limb from above the carpi. The foal improved to normality without surgical interference.

Campbell (1977) and Turner and Fretz (1977) have reviewed the different methods of surgical treatment described in the literature. These include the use of a plate and screws (Delahanty & Gibbens 1953), epiphyseal stapling (Heinze 1966; Vaughan 1976) and the use of compression wire around screw heads (Fackleman et al. 1975). Adams (1966) described the technique for epiphyseal stapling as follows:

> The foal is anaesthetized by a standard method. The convex side of the distal end of the tibia or distal end of the radius is clipped and shaved and prepared for aseptic surgery. A skin incision is made longitudinally over the convex surface of the bone. The epiphysis is identified by its prominence or by radiographs and 3 staples are placed so that one leg of the staple is below the epiphyseal line and one above it. The legs and body on the staples are approximately 2.5 cm (1 in) long. 3 staples are ordinarily used in the tibia or a radius.

The staples can easily be made from Steinman intermedullar pins. They are approximately 2 mm ($\frac{5}{64}$ in) in diameter, and the ends are sharpened with a file. They are driven into the bone by use of a bone hammer. Special apparatus for holding the pins while driving them is available (Heinze 1963 & 1965). Readymade staples are also available. The subcutaneous tissue is closed over the pins with a 00 catgut suture. The skin is then closed with a non-capillary type suture with simple interrupted pattern. A pressure bandage is kept in place over the incisions for approximately 2 weeks. Exercise should be limited for 60 days.

Campbell (1977) reports that staples and fixation by plate and screws have the following disadvantages:

1. Compression of the growth plate is not immediate but is produced by continued growth at the epiphyseal line.
2. The effect of compression extends along the arms of the staple and is not concentrated at the outer aspect of the bone curvature.
3. The position and angulation of both arms of the staple have to be considered and controlled simultaneously.

To try to overcome this problem, Campbell tried a compression plate but found it unsatisfactory. It produced rapid ossification and epiphyseal closure before the angulation was corrected. Campbell suggests that the advantages of two bone screws and heavy gauge stainless steel compression wire are:

1. Screws are fixed only with relation to one another, at the surface of the bone, and are able to move apart at the tips.
2. Immediate compression is applied at the area of greatest curvature, promoting more rapid return to normal.
3. The screws can be inserted independently, at convenient sites, after the location and direction of the growth plate has been determined.

Under suitable general anaesthesia, and after preparation of the leg, an incision is made through the skin and fascia over the area of greatest curvature. Two radiographs at right angles are taken with a radiopaque probe in the growth plate, to confirm the position of the growth plate, and to ascertain the direction in which the epiphyseal screw must be inserted to avoid penetration of the growth plate or joint surface. A stab wound is made through the fascia, collateral ligament etc. over the area chosen for insertion. A hole is drilled, in the previously determined direction, to the required depth, the hole is tapped and the screw inserted for about 90% of its length. The use of AO orthopaedic equipment is recommended. Screws of the length required to achieve satisfactory grip are chosen. A second screw is then inserted in the metaphysis, well clear of the growth plate and still on the line of greatest curvature of deviation. A piece of heavy (18 gauge) stainless steel wire is applied around the screws and tightened on both sides alternately by means of a loop twist (Fig. 6.25) until satisfactory compression is achieved. The screws are then driven fully home, but increasing still further the degree of compression. Catgut sutures are inserted in the fascia and routine closure of the skin carried out. A padded elastic dressing is applied for seven to ten days, after which the skin sutures are removed.

Following straightening of the limb the area is re-exposed, the wire is identified within its bed of fascia and cut and the screws are removed. The wound is treated as before.

Ellis (1976) reports least satisfactory results with stapling in cases with rotational as well as angular deformity of the epiphysis and when surgical treatment has been delayed.

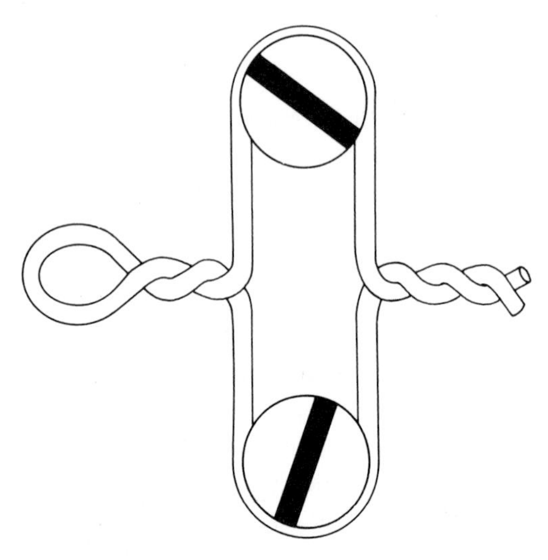

Fig. 6.25. Method of applying compression wire and round screw heads. (*After Campbell 1977*).

Epiphyseal injuries

Vaughan (1976) has used the classification of Salter and Harris (1963) to describe epiphyseal injuries in the foal (Fig. 6.26).

Type 1, separation without fracture. After realignment, healing is rapid and the prognosis is good. Femoral head detachment is the exception because if the epiphyseal vessels are damaged, avascular necrosis of the caput follows.

Type 2, involving fracture of a triangular piece of metaphysis. With accurate reduction, the prognosis is good.

Type 3 occurs towards the end of growth. The prognosis is good.

Type 4 involves transepiphyseal fracture. Unless the fragments are precisely realigned, union may occur between the epiphysis of one piece and a metaphysis of the other, causing premature fusion and resulting in angulation and shortening.

Type 5 results from a crush injury to one area of the plate and is most likely near hinge joints. Diagnosis is difficult initially because displacement is rare. Premature fusion, with resultant deformity and shortening, is inevitable.

Type 6 results from a blow to the periosteum and perichondral ring. A bridge forms, closing a segmental area and leading to angulation.

Types 1 to 4 are not commonly seen but usually present as acute joint sprain. Diagnosis can only be made radiographically and these examinations should be

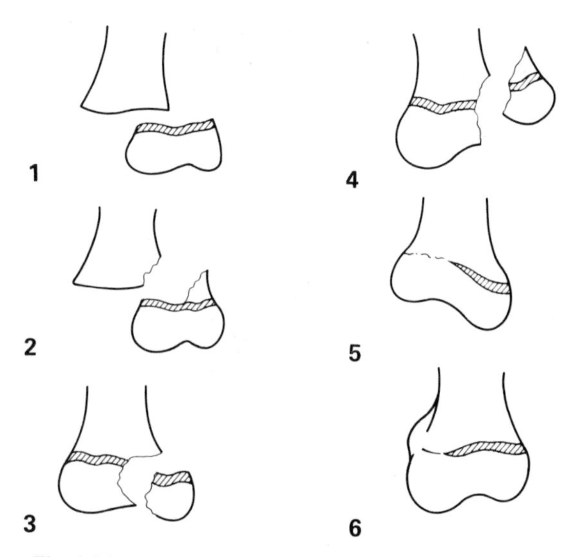

Fig. 6.26. Types of epiphyseal injury. (*After Vaughan 1976*)

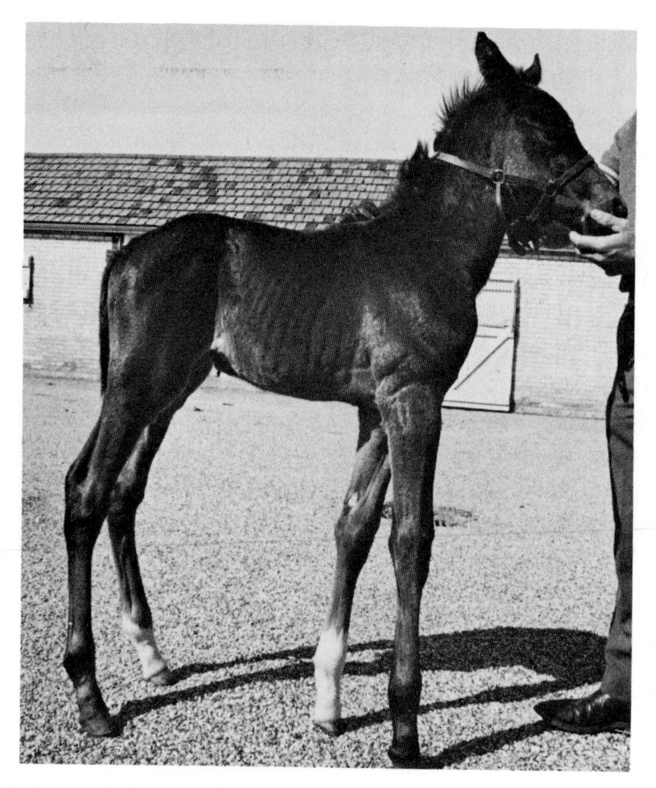

Fig. 6.27. A four-week-old Thoroughbred foal showing early signs of hyperflexion in both fore-legs and, to a lesser extent, in the hind-legs.

performed in all cases of joint enlargement in young foals. Prompt and accurate replacement of the epiphyses is required, followed by external support with a cast or splint to maintain alignment. Compression screws are sometimes useful. If bone growth has been disturbed, limb angulation often follows and may be treated as described above.

Hyperflexion of the coronopedal (P2/P3) joint

Owen (1975) reports that this condition is seen in Thoroughbred, Hunter, Arabian and pony foals and involves both sexes (Fig. 6.27). The onset is usually between May and June and often involves rapidly growing foals in very good condition. The onset of symptoms is rapid, the heel rising off the ground within 24–48 hours.

Owen et al. (1978) discount the possible causes of concussion, calcium and phosphorus nutritional imbalance, muscular dystrophy and genetics and postulate that lush grass between May and June and the high concentrate rations often fed cause mares to produce large volumes of milk and as a result the foals will grow fast and fat. Under these conditions the foals do not exercise to the required degree. This compounds the problem. Owen suggests that tendons do not 'contract' but simply fail to grow at the same rapid rate as the bones. The flexor tendon pull overcomes that of the extensors, which stretch, and the foal goes 'over on its toes'.

Treatment suggested is for the foal to be provided with grass and water only and turned out at all times. Heels should be rasped down twice weekly. Using this form of treatment Owen reports that some cases return to normal within one month.

In the yearling, Owen suggests that the suspensory ligament does not stretch, as in the foal, so that the heel stays on the ground and the pastern becomes straight.

As with many other problems seen in veterinary medicine, this 'ballerina' syndrome may be multifactorial. At Newmarket, we see cases in foals which are turned out at pasture day and night, on ground which is dry and rock hard, sparsely covered with grass which is far from lush. These foals may nevertheless be 'doing well', because of supplementary feeding, but some cases appear to demonstrate pain in the feet, possibly associated with exercise on very hard ground. These often respond, if diagnosed early, to restricted exercise with the provision of 'soft going' with peat moss, deep straw, shavings or sand and a short course of pain-relieving drugs, e.g. phenylbutazone.

In all cases, careful trimming of the feet is essential. Damage and excessive wear to the toe may be prevented by the use of a small shoe or 'tip'. In cases that do not respond rapidly to conservative treatment, a tip may have the added bonus of increasing the strain on the flexor tendons to try to bring the heel down. This tension may be increased by rasping the heels and fitting a tip with a forward extension. Where these measures are needed, cases that have been put on soft going should be removed to a small yard or loose box with a concrete floor and no bedding, or the benefits of the tips will be lost.

The prognosis is unfavourable where a response to treatment is not seen fairly rapidly or where the condition causes knuckling over. Plaster casts and corrective boots may be applied to very young foals but are seldom successful in older ones.

In these cases, partial desmotomy of the flexor tendons or complete inferior check ligament desmotomy (McIlwraith & Fessler 1978) may be performed but, in our experience, surgical procedures have seldom been successful. In cases that fail to respond to treatment euthanasia should be considered on humanitarian grounds. Rupture of the common digital extensor tendon has been seen in severe cases (Myers & Gordon 1975).

Recently, a yearling who suddenly developed typical signs of bilateral vertical front pasterns with both heels on the ground; after unsuccessful conservative treatment, a bilateral superior check ligament desmotomy was performed (Peace, personal communication). Under general anaesthesia, with the yearling in lateral recumbency, an area approximately 10 × 10 cm, just above the carpus on the medial aspect of the forearm, was clipped and prepared for surgery. A 5 cm longitudinal skin incision was made, just above the carpus and just behind the distal radius. The subcutaneous tissues were separated and the distal extremity of the flexor carpi radialis muscle retracted caudally to expose the radial head of the superficial digital flexor tendon (superior check ligament), which was completely transected. The subcutaneous tissues were closed with interrupted chromic catgut sutures and the skin with interrupted monofilament nylon sutures. The yearling was turned over and the operation was repeated on the other leg. Immediately on recovery from anaesthesia, the angles of the front pasterns were markedly improved. Aftercare consisted of daily wound cleansing and the application of antibacterial wound powder. Systemic antibiotic cover was maintained for five days postoperatively. Four months later, the yearling has apparently normal front leg conformation and shows no signs of lameness or gait abnormality.

Nutritional muscular dystrophy (NMD)

Nutritional muscular dystrophy has been reported in Australia (Gabbedy & Richards 1970), New Zealand (Dodd et al. 1960), the Netherlands (Kroneman & Wensvoort 1968), the UK (Baker 1969), Norway (Schougaard et al. 1972) and the USA (Wilson et al. 1976). The incidence is low and the condition occurs in all breeds and both sexes but mainly in young horses. The cause is thought to be vitamin E and selenium deficiency.

Clinical signs include stiffness, lethargy and painful subcutaneous swellings on the nuchal crest or abdomen. Affected foals may have difficulty in standing and swallowing. AST and serum CK enzyme levels rise. Acute cases die from exhaustion and circulatory failure. Muscular lesions cause a generalized pallor or white streaks. Subcutaneous oedema is often present and fat may have a brown discoloration.

Schougaard et al. (1972) described two foals that died showing typical muscular pathology; three other foals on the same premises had raised AST and ALT which, returned to normal after treatment with vitamin E and selenium.

Recommended treatment is two injections of sodium selenite 10–20 mg a week apart and oral vitamin E 1000 mg daily for three to five days. On farms where cases occur, parturient mares should be injected with 20–30 mg selenium a month before the due date of birth and the newborn foal given 10 mg (Dodd 1972).

Fracture of the proximal sesamoid bones

Ellis (1979) describes 18 cases of fracture of the proximal sesamoid bones in Thoroughbred foals. Most cases occurred under two months of age, in the front legs, and commonly followed a period of exhaustive exercise in the paddock. Clinical signs were enlargement of the fetlock, with variations in degree of lameness, but pain on pressure over the fracture site was always present.

Diagnosis is by radiographic examination. Ellis found that the type of fracture varied but a simple base fracture of the medial sesamoid bone was most frequent. Six foals sustained a fracture of more than one sesamoid bone and one foal fractured all four proximal sesamoid bones in the front legs. With conservative treatment of confinement to the loose box and pressure bandaging the prognosis for chip, fissure and simple fractures, without displacement of the fragments, is good. Where there is displacement of the fracture, remodelling of the bone is poor and the prognosis is bad. In these cases Ellis recommends surgical removal of the displaced fragment.

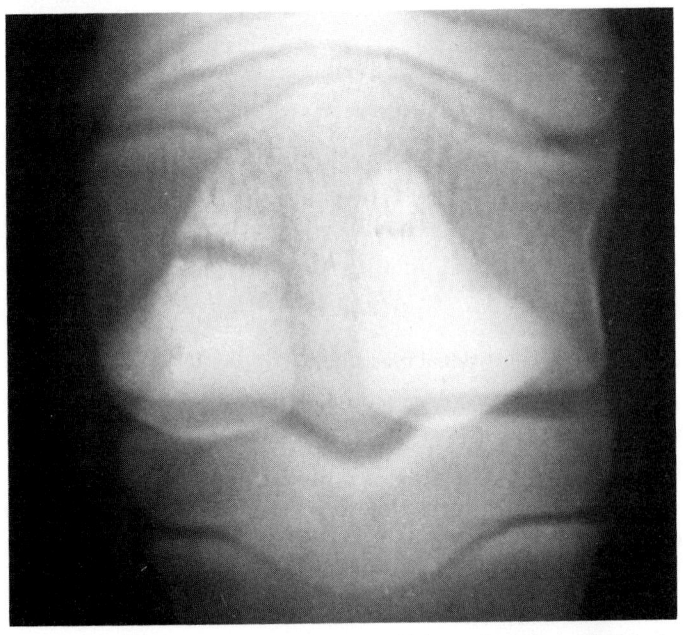

Fig. 6.28. Apical fractures of both promixal sesamoid bones in a young foal (anteroposterior view).

Following the induction of suitable general anaesthesia and preparation of the leg a skin incision is made about 5 cm in length extending from the apex of the sesamoid bone, parallel to the caudal border of the metacarpal bone, to the medial tuberosity of the first phalanx. The fascia and underlying collateral sesamoidean ligament are incised to expose the joint capsule which is incised and extended distally to meet the collateral ligament of the fetlock joint. The joint is flexed to bring the basal fragment of the seasmoid bone into view. The fragment is dissected free from its attachments and removed from the joint. The joint capsule and collateral sesamoidean ligament are closed with simple interrupted catgut sutures and the skin closed with monofilament nylon. The fetlock joints are bandaged for three weeks following surgery and the foal confined to a loose box for one month. It is then allowed into a small yard or paddock, daily, for gradually increasing periods.

Prevention should include the provision of small nursery paddocks and care and supervision of mares and foals at exercise, especially when first turned out after foaling. In cases where exercise has been delayed owing to adverse weather conditions or foal illness, the mare should be allowed to exercise on her own at first. This must be done with care or the mare may suffer from azoturia or 'tying-up'.

Osteochondrosis

Defects in endochondral ossification and associated abnormalities in cartilaginous growth may occur at various periarticular sites. The aetiology and pathogenesis of this condition are incompletely understood but genetic and nutritional factors,

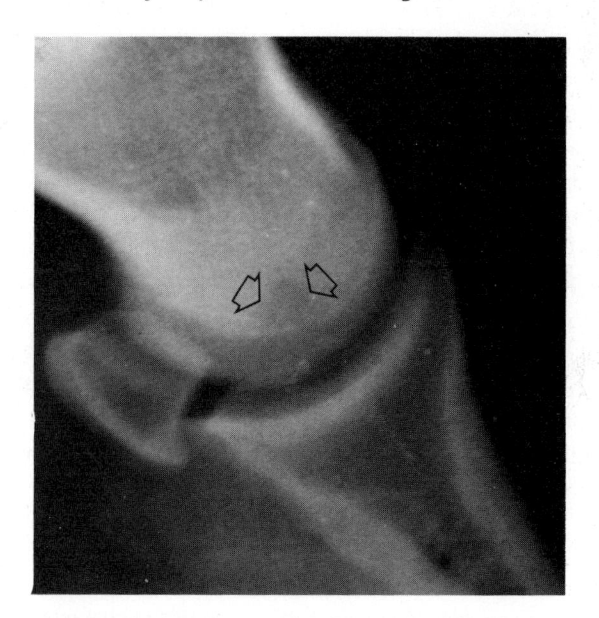

Fig. 6.29. Subchondral 'bone cyst' (arrowed) at the distal end of the second phalanx of an eight-month-old Thoroughbred filly foal who was lame.

leading to ischaemic necrosis, may be involved. The condition usually presents in foals or yearlings in the form of intermittent lameness which varies in degree. After localization of the site of pain by clinical examination and the use of local anaesthetic nerve blocks, careful radiographic examinations may reveal irregularities of the radiographic joint silhouette with scalloping or fragmentation. This has been reported at the head of the humerus (Meagher et al. 1973; Mason & Maclean 1977) and at the lateral trochlear ridge of the femur (Moore & McIlwraith 1977). In other cases, osseous cyst-like lesions (sometimes called subchondral bone cysts) (Fig. 6.29) are seen (Petterson & Reiland 1968; Reid 1970). Petterson and Reiland described mostly phalangeal lesions whereas Reid described 64 individual cases of varying age, breed and type with lesions at a variety of sites. These were radius three, accessory carpal one, radial carpal three, intermediate carpal one, ulnar carpal seven, third carpal two, third metacarpal ten, proximal sesamoids five, first phalanx six, second phalanx four, third phalanx five, navicular six, femur 12, tibia two, tibial tarsal one and fourth tarsal one. Identification of the joint involved is sometimes helped by the obvious distension of the joint capsule with excessive synovial fluid. Cytological and bacteriological examinations of the fluid reveal no evidence of acute inflammation or infection (Moore & McIlwraith 1977).

The prognosis in all cases must be guarded. Some foals and yearlings with this condition have been known to show no further signs of lameness after six to 12 months, during which time they have received no specific treatment and no appreciable change in management. In some cases, restricted exercise appears to have been successful. Reid (1970) warns that some of these cases may become lame again when they are put into work. Some veterinarians in Standardbred practice have claimed success following a prolonged course of strenuous exercise under the influence of pain-killing drugs such as phenylbutazone.

Mason and Maclean (1977) have described a surgical approach to the shoulder joint. On opening the joint, the indented lesion is exposed and a curette used to remove all the undermined cartilage and devitalized bone. The joint is irrigated by introducing a flexible catheter to its deepest point and flushing, under pressure, with physiological saline containing aqueous penicillin. Closure is by standard methods. This operation was performed on two foals. Both showed no signs of lameness at the walk and trot, but were slightly lame following more severe exercise, up to one year after the operations were performed. The authors state that both cases were destined to be used for breeding purposes. Stromberg (1979) believes that the condition has a definite genetic basis and questions the ethics of breeding from confirmed cases.

Infective arthritis (joint-ill, navel-ill)

This condition of foals aged five days to four months is characterized by painful swellings of the joints and associated structures. It may be caused by a number of opportunist organisms, e.g. *Str. zooepidemicus, Staph. aureus, E. coli, Salmonella typhimurium* or *Actinobacillus equuli.* Polyarthritis caused by a chlamydial infection has been described by McChesney et al. (1974) and *Mycoplasma* organisms were isolated from an arthritic foal by Moorthy et al. (1977).

Organisms may enter through the umbilicus or the alimentary tract. Abscesses in the umbilical vein may act as a reservoir of infection. The reason why bacteria pass to certain sites in joint tissue is unknown, although local conditions and trauma may be responsible (Rooney 1962). Organisms may become ‘trapped’ in the complex vascular bed of the epiphyses and spread to the synovial membrane may occur from this site (Fig. 6.30). We have isolated *Corynebacterium equi* from three such cases. The metaphyseal blood vessels link towards the growth plate where they ramify. The terminal capillaries communicate with large sinusoids in which the blood flow is particularly slow and ideal for the localization of pathogenic bacteria

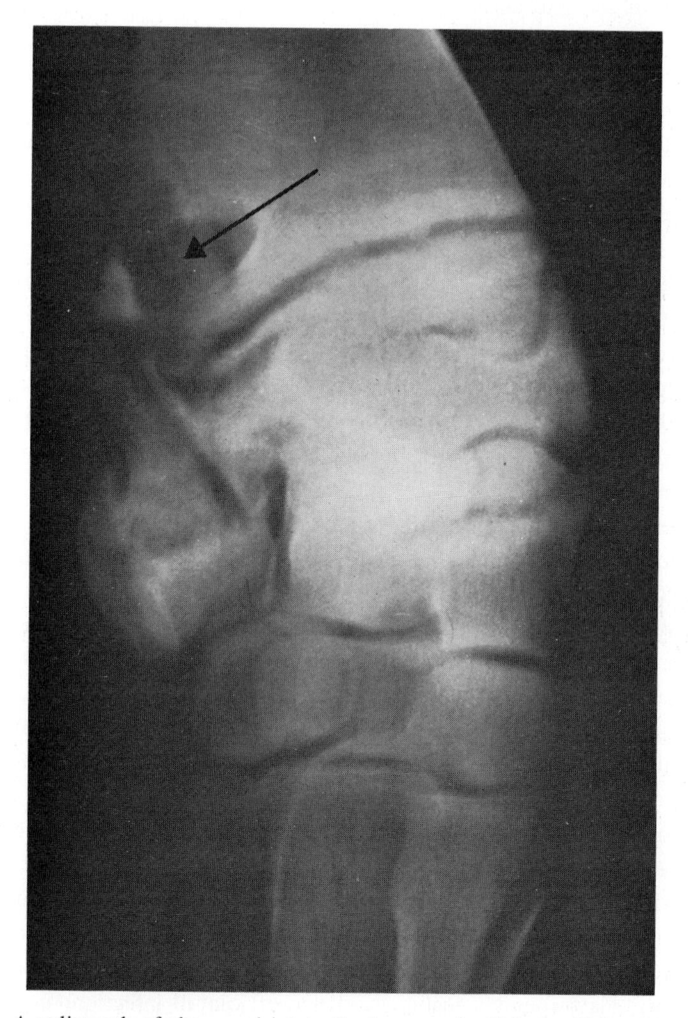

Fig. 6.30. A radiograph of the carpal joint of a four-month-old foal suffering from arthritis. The condition started as an abscess caused by *Staphylococcus aureus* in the epiphyseal region.

and/or emboli (Bennett 1978; Van Pelt & Riley 1969). Infective tenosynovitis can develop from an area of infection adjacent to the tendon sheath and spread to the joint capsule or in a reverse direction.

Lameness and fever (38.5°C) are cardinal signs of infective arthritis. One or more joints may be involved. The fetlock, stifle, hip and elbow joints are the most commonly affected. Local signs include synovial distension, oedema of periarticular tissues, thickening of the joint capsule and pain on movement. Leucocytes ($1-50 \times 10^9$/litre) are present in the synovial fluid of affected joints. Clinical signs and the presence of leucocytes in the synovial fluid are diagnostic. Radiographic examination should be made to establish the extent of damage to articular and periarticular structures. Diagnosis of coxofemoral involvement is hindered by the relative inaccessibility of this particular joint.

Intra-articular injections of 0.25 g of neomycin sulphate are recommended daily until the cell count of synovial fluid has reduced to less than 1×10^9/litre and signs have abated. Corticosteroids should be administered sparingly and used only once or twice. Parenteral antibiotics may be given to prevent metastatic spread and to treat epiphyseal abscesses. In order to try to prevent extensive damage to hyaline cartilage, early treatment with oral sodium salicylate and vitamin C may be helpful (Simmons & Christman 1965).

Treatment by saline lavage (Norrie 1975) may be helpful in some cases. Following induction of suitable general anaesthesia and preparation of the leg, two 1 cm skin incisions are made for the placement of two 12 gauge needles into the joint. If possible they should be placed on either side of the joint but depending on the joint involved, this may not always be possible. Sterile saline solution, warmed to body temperature, is connected to the uppermost needle and a stopcock is attached to the draining needle. During lavage, the drainage needle is closed and the saline administered under pressure so that the joint capsule becomes fully distended. The stopcock is then opened to allow drainage. Norrie recommends the use of 6 litres of saline by this method. On completion of the lavage, the administration needle is removed, the remaining saline expressed from the joint and the drainage needle removed. The skin is closed by standard methods and the joint is bandaged during recovery from anaesthesia.

Some cases do not respond to treatment and euthanasia is indicated on humanitarian grounds. Post-mortem examinations reveal varying degrees of erosion and ankylosis of the articular surfaces, deformation of the epiphyses and adhesions between the joint capsule and overlying structures. Cases associated with epiphyseal abscesses appear to have a particularly bad prognosis. Platt (1977) followed foals which survived joint-ill infections until they were rising four years old and classified them according to their racing performances using the Time Form system. Only 37% of the foals with joint-ill subsequently raced, as compared with over 60% of normal foals. Platt found a higher incidence of joint-ill infections in foals with other perinatal abnormalities and in foals in which the receipt of colostrum had been delayed. There was a higher incidence of the disease in foals from mares who had suffered prenatal lactation and whose colostrum was thus deficient in antibody. There was a significant reduction in the incidence of disease in foals given a course of prophylatic antibiotics.

Prevention must be concerned with making sure that foals receive sufficient good quality colostrum as early as possible post-partum. Deep-frozen colostrum should be stored at stud farms to supplement those foals who are considered in need. Postnatal prophylatic antibiotic programmes and the measurement of serum globulin levels 36–48 hours post-partum (see p. 311) are recommended.

Idiopathic tenosynovitis

Tenosynovitis presents with signs of inflammation, pain on palpation and distension of tendon sheaths due to excessive synovial effusions (Van Pelt 1969). The condition is apparently non-infective but responds to intrathecal injection of hydrocortisone acetate and antibiotics.

OTHER DISORDERS

Zinc and lead poisoning

Lead poisoning may result from the ingestion of concentrates or grass contaminated by paint or the effluent of lead works. Most of the lead absorbed from the alimentary tract passes via the portal circulation to the liver. Signs include loss of weight, swelling of the limbs, gradual paralysis of the head and a characteristic shortness of breath or roaring caused by paralysis of the laryngeal muscles (Garner 1957). Continuous ingestion of lead over a long period may cause a blue/black line in the gums.

Zinc poisoning may occur in animals grazing near iron works and brass foundries. Large doses of zinc salts produce acute signs of metal poisoning, i.e. purging, abdominal pain and collapse.

Willoughby et al. (1972) fed rations containing lead, zinc or a combination of these minerals. All the animals given lead and zinc died in ten days to ten weeks. Those fed lead developed pharyngeal and laryngeal paralysis; those fed zinc or zinc and lead also developed stiffness and lameness caused by epiphysitis of the long bones. The animals that received zinc lost weight and developed anaemia but these signs were not apparent in foals that received only lead. Foals that received lead and zinc suffered symptoms which resembled zinc poisoning and the hepatic and renal tissues contained lead levels twice as high as those fed only lead. The authors suggest that the findings indicate that toxic amounts of zinc mask typical signs of lead poisoning in young horses.

Respiratory tract infections

Foals and yearlings are particularly prone to upper respiratory tract infections (snotty nose, stable cough) (Fig. 6.31) and to a lesser extent pneumonia. These conditions are caused by various herpesviruses, adenoviruses and rhinoviruses followed by secondary bacterial infection, particularly streptococci, staphylococci and *E. coli.* Viral conditions are described in Chapter 7, together with other infectious diseases which affect horses of all ages.

Upper respiratory tract infections in young horses are often recorded as distinct entities because of their prevalence and characteristic signs, despite their multiple aetiology. A serous nasal discharge becoming profuse, mucopurulent and persistent is common among young stock at studs and training stables. Coughing and fever are sometimes present and occasionally an acute or chronic penumonia develops.

The conditions have nuisance value in that they cause unsightly nostrils as the nares become lined with dried discharge and purulent matter, which is also smeared on the coat and on stable walls. But infection also gives the young horse a level of immunity. Contact with stud mares is valuable since it serves as a 'natural' vaccine

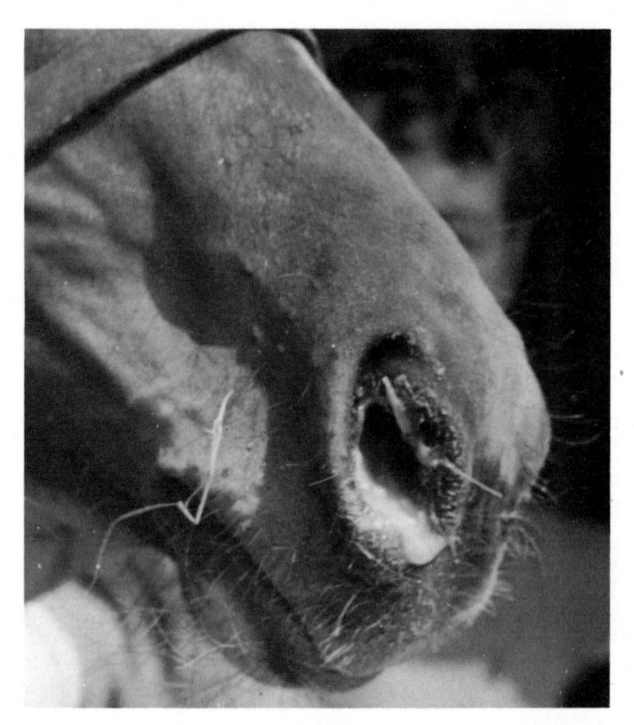

Fig. 6.31. Herpesvirus infection causes 'scalding' of the nostrils, followed by mucopurulent nasal discharge.

by providing a recurring challenge of equid herpesvirus I infection. The infection assumes serious proportions only when it causes acute or chronic bronchopneumonia or, in the case of equid herpesvirus I infection, when associated with outbreaks of abortion (see p. 200) or the neurological form of the disease (see p. 425). Influenza virus and adenovirus (McChesney & England 1975; Henry & Gagnon 1976) may cause an acute proliferative pneumonia in young foals. Signs include dyspnoea and fever. Death may occur in 24–72 hours although some cases become chronic and may recover, in which event differential diagnosis from other respiratory infections may remain in doubt. For a further discussion of viral pneumonia see Chapter 7. *Bordetella bronchiseptica* infection has been reported as a cause of foal pneumonia in Argentina (Monteverde et al. 1972) and in adult horses in Britain (Miller 1965).

In cases of pneumonia and excessive or persistent mucopurulent discharge, antibiotic therapy is indicated and should be continued until signs abate. Some cases appear more refractory to treatment than others and with these cases there is a risk of chronic pulmonary damage and sometimes abscess formation. To try to avoid these unfortunate sequelae, early treatment with the mucolytic agent bromhexine (0.5 mg/kg daily by intramuscular injection) and the nicotinic acid derivative isoniazid (6 mg/kg orally daily) (Roberts 1971) may be helpful. For a further discussion of upper respiratory tract infections see p. 424. Foals should be vaccinated against equine influenza, from three months of age, as a routine prophylactic measure.

Corynebacterium equi infection

This infectious disease of young foals, two to three months of age or older, is characterized by suppurative bronchopneumonia, mediastinal lymphadenitis and occasionally alimentary tract involvement (Magnusson 1938; Mahaffey 1962; Bain 1963; Rooney 1966; Linton & Gallagher 1969; Cimprich & Rooney 1977; Roberts & Polley 1977).

Corynebacterium equi is a Gram-positive bacillus, forming mucoid pale pink colonies on blood agar. Biochemically the organism is inactive and does not ferment carbohydrates. The disease occurs in most countries. It is sporadic in the UK but may reach epidemic proportions in Australia (Bain 1963). The condition may be restricted to particular farms and the mortality rate is high. The organism is thought to survive in soil and, although the mode of transmission is unknown, entry is presumably by ingestion or inhalation. It has been suggested that migrating parasitic larvae carry the infection through the body. The lymphatic system and blood are other possible routes of spread. Suppurative foci develop in many organs, particularly the lungs. Mahaffey (1962) found the organism in the mesenteric lymph nodes and mandibular lymph nodes of apparently normal foals. Woolcock et al. (1980), using a selective medium, cultured the organism from the faeces of a large variety of healthy and diseased horses in Australia. They suggested that *C. equi* is widespread in that country and may be part of the 'normal' equine faecal flora.

The condition is generally insidious in onset and the pulmonary changes are usually well advanced before signs appear. A rapid respiratory rate with dyspnoeic breathing, a marked pleuritic line and double phase expiratory movements are characteristic features. Coughing and mucopurulent nasal discharge are evident early and fever of 39–41°C is consistent. Cases with alimentary involvement (Cimprich & Rooney 1977; Roberts & Polley 1977) may show an extremely insidious onset, with dullness and loss of condition. Signs of abdominal pain may be present but not all cases show obvious diarrhoea. Spinal lesions causing paralysis of the limbs have been reported (Rooney 1966). In our own experience, the most frequent isolation of this organism has been in foals with joint-ill associated with epiphyseal abscesses.

The respiratory condition may develop rapidly and death occurs within about ten days of the first signs. Other cases run a protracted course of several weeks but it is generally accepted that recovery is rare once the condition has become established. It is possible, however, that some undiagnosed cases respond to antibiotic treatment for non-specific pneumonia.

Persistent high temperature and signs of pneumonia which fail to respond to antibiotic treatment suggest *Corynebacterium* infection. Positive diagnosis rests on recovery of *C. equi* from nasal discharge or tracheal aspiration. Isolating the causal organism is extremely difficult in practice although it should be attempted. Tracheal aspiration (see p. 539) may prove a more reliable technique than nasal swabbing. There is extensive abscessation of lung parenchyma and mediastinal lymph nodes. The causal organism is present in large numbers in the creamy pus contained in thick-walled abscesses.

C. equi is usually sensitive to penicillin and high dose rates are recommended every eight or 12 hours. But once it is established it seems the antibiotic does not penetrate to organisms in abscesses and treatment usually has little effect on the course of the condition.

Diarrhoea

Diarrhoea is encountered in horses of all ages but its incidence in foals up to five months is very high. Most foals show signs once or more before weaning.

Aetiology

Managerial, nutritional, bacterial, viral, fungal and parasitic factors have been incriminated or suggested as causes of diarrhoea in foals. The aetiology of each case is usually unknown; even in epidemics the causal agent is rarely diagnosed.

Nutritional disturbances include those caused by ingestion of oestrous milk and of poor quality feeds, such as mouldy hay or grass in rapid growth phase. The foal-heat scour is well recognized and regarded by many veterinarians as being physiological. Changes in milk composition, overloading of the foal's digestive tract, ingestion of genital discharge, straw, faeces, grass and other foreign material have been suggested as causes of the foal-heat scour. Johnston et al. (1970) studied milk volume, pH, oestrogen content, bacterial contamination and fat, lactose, ash, crude protein, casein and total solids for possible fluctuations associated with foal-heat scour. They concluded that milk was not a factor in foal-heat scouring. But there is little doubt that under certain conditions, such as the existence of epidemic diarrhoea, oestrus-induced scours predispose foals to more serious and prolonged attacks of diarrhoea.

The salient feature of the gastrointestinal tract of the newborn foal is the relatively narrow calibre and small bulk of the caecum and large colon (Dyce 1960).

Fibre is necessary for development of the large intestine. Although little is known of the way in which bacterial seeding of the colon and caecum takes place, it is presumed that some digestive disturbances are associated with increasing quantities of fibrous material and with changes in the bacterial flora of the large intestine.

Roberts (1975*a*) suggests that the continued ingestion of lactose may be detrimental to foals suffering from severe diarrhoea. Acute or chronic enteritis will damage the small intestinal epithelium, causing depression of brush-border disaccharidase levels which in turn results in a transient malabsorption of sugars. Roberts

(1975*b*) suggests that the oral lactose tolerance test (OLTT) may be useful in such cases. A change to a non-lactose diet together with supporting therapy may produce a marked clinical improvement.

Escherichia coli infection is a common cause of diarrhoea in calves and piglets and of septicaemia in young foals. Pathogenic *E. coli* serotypes in foals have not been determined (Davies 1978) but many cases of diarrhoea in foals are probably the result of infection with this organism. *Salmonella* spp. are a cause of diarrhoea in foals, yet they are rarely encountered (see p. 000).

Campylobacter spp. have recently been isolated from the faeces of diarrhoeic foals (Atherton 1980, personal communication).

Rotavirus injection. The isolation of rotavirus (reovirus) particles from diarrhoeic foals during the first few weeks of life has been reported by Flewett et al. (1975), Bass and Sharpee (1975), Kanitz (1976), Studdert et al. (1976) and Tzipori and Walker (1978). The virus ranges in diameter between 60 and 66 nm and possesses characteristic morphology from which it gets its name. Isolations have been made from neonates of a variety of species including man.

The signs include pyrexia, dullness, abdominal pain and sometimes a craving to lap water. Diarrhoea may not always be seen immediately but usually follows within 24 hours of the onset of illness. The diarrhoea is a frequent watery discharge which is often passed without lifting the tail.

Most cases recover spontaneously, or with symptomatic treatment, within 48–72 hours. Cases that are complicated by bacterial enteritis and/or by an 'upset' in the intestinal bacterial flora may take longer.

The epidemiology of this disease is not completely understood but it appears from serological studies that the virus is wide-spread in the environment and the majority of newborn animals are challenged within the first few weeks of life. Only a small proportion show signs of abnormality and diarrhoea and one imagines that environmental or other factors may play a complicating role. Epidemics of diarrhoea in young foals, associated with the isolation of this virus, have been reported (Kanitz 1976).

Mycotic infection is a cause of diarrhoea in many species but has not yet been incriminated with certainty in the foal. Profuse growths of fungus are occasionally recovered from the faeces of diarrhoeic foals, especially after prolonged antibiotic therapy. *Candida* spp. may be associated with 'furring' of the tongue frequently encountered in foals suffering from acute diarrhoea.

Infestation with small strongyles and ascarids may cause diarrhoea because the parasites irritate and ulcerate the alimentary tract. Parasitic disease is a major cause of intestinal abnormality and ill-thrift in foals and yearlings. A detailed discussion of parasitic problems is included in Chapter 7.

Coccidiosis is rarely recorded in horses. Sheahan (1976) described the occurrence of *Eimeira (Globidium) leuckarti* in a two-month-old Thoroughbred foal which died following an acute illness characterized by massive intestinal haemorrhage.

In summary, diarrhoea may be caused by a number of aetiological agents acting singly or together.

Clinical signs

Diarrhoea is but one clinical sign of alimentary disturbance. Associated signs depend on the causal agent and the amount of fluid and electrolytes lost in the faeces.

The diarrhoeic faeces may be watery, cow-like or pasty. In the latter event they are often grey; in other cases they may be brown, black, green, yellow or (occasionally) red. Colour has little diagnostic significance except for green, which is often associated with grass, and black or red, which may indicate the presence of blood. The faeces may have a foetid or foul smell.

The rectal temperature may be raised to 39–40°C, but apparently normal or subnormal readings may be unreliable because of the relaxed state of the rectum.

Conjunctival and buccal mucous membranes may be injected, brick-red, purple or normal, depending on severity. The tongue may be coated with a white or greyish slough-like membrane. Pulse rate and quality varies with the amount of body fluid loss and toxaemia. In severe cases the pulse becomes weak and imperceptible.

The general condition of the foal may deteriorate and dehydration develop, or it may remain good, despite a continuing and profuse diarrhoea. Signs of dehydration are loss of skin pliability, eyeballs retracted into their orbits and a stary coat.

An affected foal may continue to suck vigorously, suck indifferently or go completely 'off suck'. Some foals develop an insatiable thirst and remain for hours with their muzzles in or close to the water manger or bucket. Peristaltic sounds are usually increased and tympanitic noises heard. Flatus is passed in severe cases and the abdomen may become distended.

In severe forms the foal may show signs of colic or excessive straining. Recovery may be spontaneous or death may occur 24–48 hours after onset. Young foals are more vulnerable to acute diarrhoea than older ones and the course of the condition, if left untreated, is usually shorter. Some individuals develop chronic diarrhoea which continues for weeks or even months. They continue to pass liquid faeces but retain their condition and continue to suck the mare. Other foals, especially those passing grey, pasty faeces, continue to feed but do not suck the mare's mammary glands dry.

Venous blood pH, $P\text{CO}_2$ and bicarbonate levels are a reliable guide to the severity of the condition (Rossdale & Mullen 1970). Standard bicarbonate blood levels below 20 mmol/litre indicate a poor prognosis unless the case is suitably treated.

The voiding of diarrhoeic faeces usually but not always occurs. Some cases show paste-like faeces and a marked reluctance to feed. Other cases show signs of marked abdominal pain which may, in many cases, be followed 24 hours later by signs of diarrhoea. A rectal swab for bacteriological examination should be taken as a routine diagnostic measure, before antibiotic treatment, to look for evidence of salmonellosis.

Treatment

Many cases recover spontaneously. Many appear to recover quickly following a course of treatment with oral framycetin. Excessive treatment with oral antibiotics may, however, exacerbate the condition. Treatment must be based on an assessment of the severity of each case. In the presence of fever, loss of condition, inappetence or signs of dehydration, antibiotics should be administered intramuscularly. Neomycin, sulphonamide-type drugs or trimethoprim are antibiotics of choice as they have a wide range of bacteristatic or bactericidal activity. If the case does not respond to this treatment intravenous or intramuscular chloramphenicol may be used. Intestinal absorbents such as kaolin, aluminium hydroxide and carbon may be useful. Hyoscine *N*-butylbromide may be useful to relieve pain.

Many cases of diarrhoea in young foals that do not resolve quickly following a course of oral framycetin respond rapidly to a single dose of antibiotic-resistant *Lactobacillus acidophilus* by stomach tube. One must assume that in these cases an 'upset' in the normal intestinal bacterial flora has occurred and that the *Lactobacillus* helps to correct this.

Fluid replacement is important if signs of dehydration occur. Rossdale and Mullen (1970) studied 21 Thoroughbred foals with diarrhoea and treated those with venous pH and bicarbonate levels below 7.35 and 24 mmol/litre with 500 ml of 5% sodium bicarbonate solution intravenously. A rapid improvement in general condition and desire to suck was noted. Normal saline and dam's plasma given intravenously are also helpful in severely affected foals. Bicarbonate solution and plasma may be mixed in equal quantities before injection.

Foals should not be prevented from drinking water and it is advisable to include a balanced electrolyte mixture in the water. Physiological fluids should be administered to foals that are dehydrated and 'off suck' at two-hour intervals. The quantity of fluid is an arbitrary decision in the absence of an exact estimate of fluid loss. As a guide, 100 ml/kg body weight in 24 hours is recommended. Administration may be intravenous or through a stomach tube.

Anthelmintics should be given to foals over two months old if they are not already included in a regular parasite control programme (see pp. 444 and 448).

Salmonellosis

This zoonosis may be a specific cause of diarrhoea in foals and yearlings. It may be diagnosed by isolating the causal organism by faecal culture on McConkey or DCA agar and submitting the growths to serological tests. Swabs or faecal samples may be incubated in selenite enrichment broth for 18–24 hours before culture on solid media. Suspicious growths may be further examined by biochemical sugar tests and slide agglutination tests with specific antisera. *S. typhimurium* and

S. enteritides are the most common pathogenic types present in epidemics of foal diarrhoea (Smith et al. 1978).

Signs include fever up to 42°C, rapid respiratory rate, anorexia, thirst, colic and teeth-grinding. A profuse watery and blood-stained diarrhoea usually develops. The condition may be sudden in onset and end in rapid death or continue for several days. Most cases are fatal but recovery can occur if treatment with a suitable antibiotic is started soon after the first signs. In one case (Mahaffey 1952) 3 g of chloramphenicol were given orally at six-hour intervals but death occurred about 48 hours after onset of signs. At post-mortem there was an intense haemorrhagic colitis with enlarged haemorrhagic caecal and colic lymph nodes from which *S. typhimurium* was recovered.

Carter et al. (1979) reported two outbreaks of acute salmonellosis on stud farms in New Zealand. Morbidity and mortality rates amongst the foals were high. *Salmonella typhimurium* was the predominent serotype isolated and epidemiological studies suggested that the organisms were capable of surviving in soil for at least nine months. This could be a problem in carrying the infection over from one stud season to another. A bacterin was prepared, from an isolate from a foal which died, and used to vaccinate mares and foals. Although changes in management practices and hygiene measures were introduced at the same time, the authors believe that the vaccination programme was helpful. They also imply that this disease is a particular risk on stud farms which are badly managed and over-stocked.

Eugster et al. (1978) and Tzipori and Walker (1978) describe outbreaks of concurrent rotavirus and *Salmonella* infection in foals, some of which died.

Goitre

Enlargement of the thyroid gland may be associated with hyper-, hypo- or euthyroidism. Baker and Lindsay (1968), Drew et al. (1975) and Driscoll et al. (1978) have reported hyperthyroidism and leg weakness in foals born to mares fed high iodine supplements in late pregnancy. In one case, a seaweed product was to blame and in another a compounded feed nut was found to be particuarly high in iodine content. In the case of Drew et al. (1975), two of the four foals affected died within 18 hours of birth. The other two subsequently recovered.

Rooney (1963) described two cases of equine congenital goitre in which hypothyroidism was associated with defective ossification, leading to collapse of the central and third tarsal bones. The foals had palpable enlargement of both thyroid glands, dry hair coats and flabby muscles. Shaver et al. (1979) described two foals with degenerative changes involving the tarsal bones and clinical, histopathological and post-mortem changes suggestive of hypothyroidism.

Foreign body obstruction of the small intestine

Like other young growing animals, foals may investigate, bite, chew and sometimes swallow a variety of foreign bodies if given the chance. Baker et al. (1974) have described an acute obstruction of the proximal small intestine in a five-month-old Thoroughbred filly. The foal was showing all the recognized signs of acute colic and shock (see p. 462) without significant response to tranquillization and intestinal spasmolytic treatment. During exploratory laparotomy under general anaesthesia, an obstruction caused by a bundle of string from hay bales was found in the proximal small intestine, forming a concertina-like segment of bowel. Following surgical removal, the foal made an uneventful recovery.

Tyzzer's disease

Tyzzer's disease is a fatal hepatitis caused by a long slender intracytoplasmic spore-bearing bacillus (*Bacillus piliformis*) which was first seen in a colony of laboratory Japanese waltzing mice. The disease has since been recorded in foals by Swerczek et al. (1973), Hall and Van Kruininger (1974), Pulley and Scheveley (1974), Harrington (1975, 1976) and Swerczek (1977) in the USA, by Whitwell (1976) in the United Kingdom and by Thompson et al. (1977) in Canada.

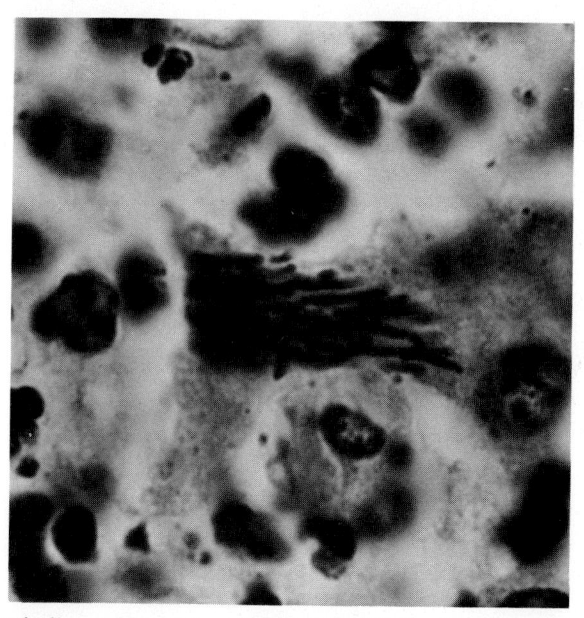

Fig. 6.32. Tyzzer's disease. Many intracytoplasmic bacilli (*Bacillus piliformis*) in the centre of an hepatic focal necrotic lesion from a 24-day-old Thoroughbred foal. Warthin–starry silver × 1000.

Typically, the foals appear normal prior to a short terminal illness or being found dead. The sick foals show depression, collapse, recumbency, pyrexia (up to 46.6°C) and sometimes convulsions.

Post-mortem examinations reveal a grossly enlarged mottled liver and pale foci may be seen. Histologically there are multiple focal necrotic areas with surrounding inflammatory cell infiltration (Fig. 6.33). Special stains, e.g. Giemsa, Levaditti and Warthin–starry silver, may show the characteristic intracytoplasmic bacilli.

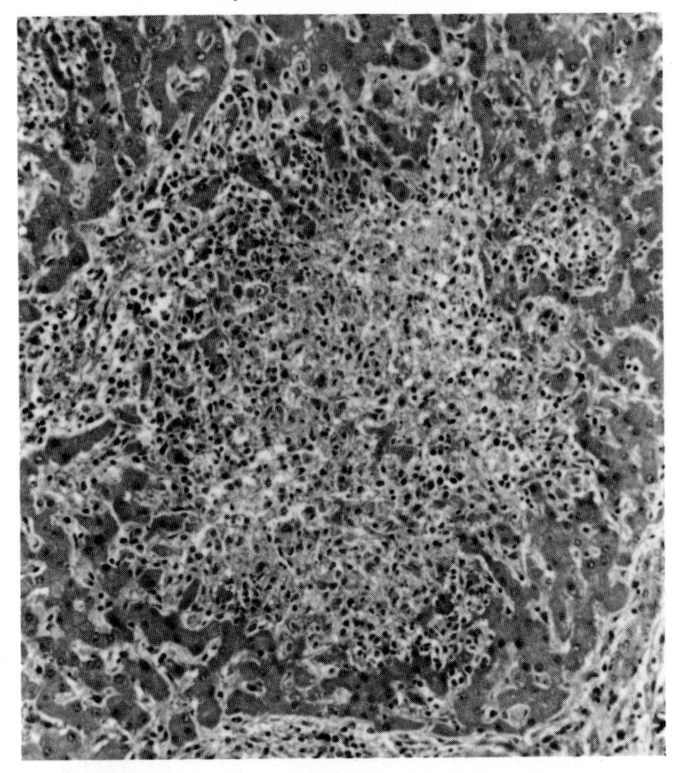

Fig. 6.33. Tyzzer's disease. Hepatic focal necrosis in a three-week-old Thoroughbred foal that was found dead. H & E × 100.

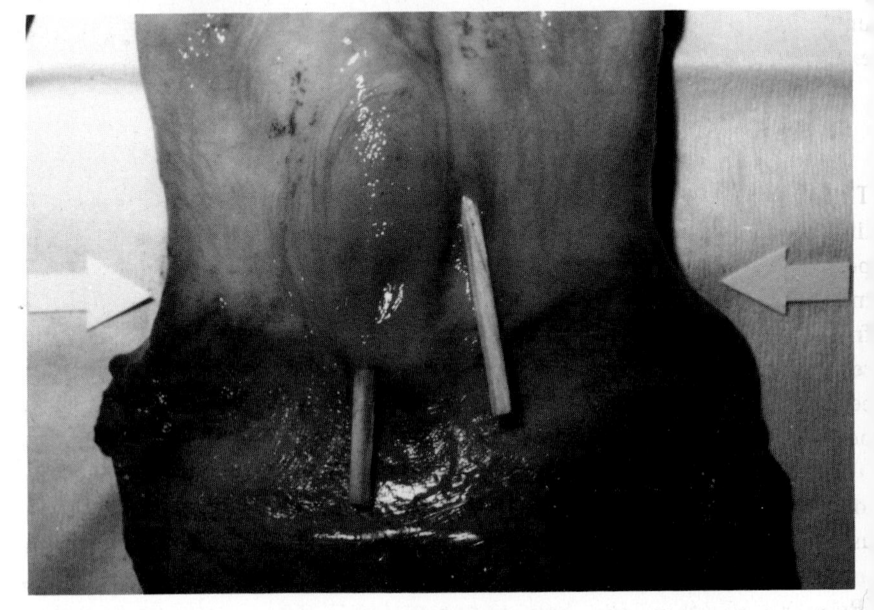

Fig. 6.34. Ectopic ureter in a two-year-old Thoroughbred filly with a history of urinary incontinence since birth. Arrows show the level of the bladder neck. Matchsticks are placed in the openings of the ureters.

In contrast to the disease in mice, in foals Tyzzer's disease is sporadic. Although infection via contact with the environmental rodent population cannot be ruled out, Whitwell (1976) suggests that dams of affected foals may be carriers.

Generalized steatitis

Platt and Whitwell (1971) described a condition of pony and donkey foals in which fever, accelerated respiration, coughing, inappetence and depression were the main clinical signs. Subcutaneous tissues became inflexible, oedematous and tender and ill-defined plaque-like areas appeared. Blood cholesterol levels increased from 7.74 mmol/litre at onset to 23.22 mmol/litre terminally. All cases ended fatally and the pathology included deep yellow firm fat deposits and degenerative changes in the adrenal cortex.

Ureteral ectopia

Ordidge (1976) has described ureteral ectopia (Fig. 6.34) in a five-month-old Standard bred filly which had showed signs of urinary incontinence since birth. On post-mortem examination the left ureter extended caudally beyond the neck of the bladder. We have seen a similar case in a two-year-old Thoroughbred filly who had also been incontinent since birth. Urine dribbled freely from the vulva at all times and extensive 'scalding' of the hind-legs was present. Methylene blue dye was injected by catheter directly into the bladder after removing as much urine as possible. After removal of the catheter, the dribbling of colourless urine continued until voluntary urination occurred, producing blue-dyed urine. At post-mortem examination, one ureter extended caudally beyond the neck of the bladder.

Shaker foal

The condition has been reported in Kentucky between the third and eighth week of life (Rooney & Prickett 1967) as affecting Thoroughbreds, Standardbreds and ponies. The clinical signs and pathology vary. There is a sudden onset of severe muscular weakness. The foal is unable to stand for long and, although able to suck from the mare, it soon begins to tremble and suddenly drops to the ground. While recumbent it appears bright, but on standing the trembling recurs. Complete cessation of peristalsis is a prominent sign but fever is not characteristic and death occurs in about 72 hours due to respiratory failure.

Treatment is unrewarding in most cases. Recent research suggests a neurophysiological problem at the sympathetic ganglion level and neostigmine therapy has been used with varying results.

A case resembling the Kentucky condition has been reported from Newmarket (Rossdale & Mullen 1969). These authors found an extreme metabolic acidaemia and a pathology of hepatic necrosis and other changes suggesting enterotoxaemia.

Cerebellar hypoplasia and degeneration

A form of cerebellar hypoplasia in pure and half-bred Arabian foals has been described by Dungworth and Fowler (1966), Frazer (1966), Sponseller (1967), Palmer et al. (1973) and Beech (1976). The disease appears in the first four months of life and is characterized by ataxia of all four legs, especially the hind ones. There is hypermetria of the fore-legs (an exaggerated, over-reaching gait) and over-reaching and circumduction of the hind-legs. The foal may adopt a base-wide stance and hold its neck high. There is a characteristic head tremor. When standing still with the head raised, the foal tends to collapse backwards and, conversely, if the head is lowered tends to collapse forwards. Affected animals have a close family relationship and it seems possible that an hereditary factor, probably an autosomal recessive gene, plays an aetiological role (Palmer et al. 1973). Affected foals may show signs at birth or may appear healthy for up to nine months. The fine nodding head movement is most marked when an intentional movement is made. Blindfolding may accentuate the clinical signs.

Cerebellar lesions consist of widespread loss of Purkinje cells and of neurones of the granular layer. Some Purkinje cells appear to be in the process of degeneration The width of the molecular and granular cell layers is decreased so that individual cerebellar folia appear atrophied (Palmer et al. 1973).

Severe progressive ataxia occurring at four to eight weeks in the Oldenberg breed (Koch & Fischer 1950) and which is invariably fatal has similarities with, but according to Palmer is not identical to, the condition in the Arabian breed.

Cerebellar hypoplasia has been reported in Swedish Gotland ponies (Bjorck et al. 1967). Most ponies showed signs of ataxia soon after birth, but in some signs were not obvious until age four to six months.

'Wobbler' disease

This condition of young, predominantly male, horses causes ataxia involving especially the hind-legs (Dimock & Errington 1939; Fraser & Palmer 1967; Beech 1976; Falco et al. 1976).

The onset of clinical signs is usually sudden and signs are generally bilateral Incoordination of the hind-limbs is the principal sign but in some cases (depending on the site of the lesion) the fore-legs may also be involved. At slow gaits and when the horse is brought to a sudden halt from the trot, it cannot control its hind quarters, which sway or collapse, almost causing a fall. On tight turning, the outer hind-limb swings at the foot (circumduction) and on backing the hind-legs are used awkwardly and the horse may fall.

Post-mortem examinations reveal cervical cord compression with diffuse degeneration of the white matter, axonal swelling and secondary wallerian degeneration extending anteriorly and posteriorly from the site of the damage. This compression is caused by a variety of abnormalities of the cervical vertebrae forming the spinal canal (Rooney 1963).

Much debate has occurred regarding the aetiology of the condition. Despite widely held impressions of a genetic basis, Falco et al. (1976) analysed a series of 67 horses showing signs of wobbler disease and 67 control horses for both simple and complex modes of inheritance, using a computer, and found no evidence of a genetic basis. It appears probable that this is a clinical syndrome with multifactorial pathogenesis. One imagines that injury or damage to the cervical vertebrae as well as developmental malformation may result in a narrowing of the spinal canal. Falco et al. (1976) found no evidence of a single mare producing more than one affected offspring. We have, among our patients, a mare who has produced two confirmed 'wobblers' by different sires and who herself retired early from training due to an incoordination problem.

The disease can usually be confirmed on clinical neurological grounds but in some cases radiology of the cervical vertebrae may be helpful (Beech 1976; Jeffcott & Whitwell 1976). Another very useful diagnostic test is the endoscopic 'slap' test (Greet et al. 1980). With the horse restrained for examination (see p. 512) the larynx is viewed by endoscope. The horse is slapped manually on either side of the withers in turn. In the normal horse, the vocal cords on the opposite side to the slap adduct quickly following each slap, but in a case of wobbler disease adduction of the cords on one or both sides may be absent.

Tympany of the guttural pouch

This condition is most frequently seen unilaterally and causes tympanitic swelling of the area of the guttural pouch (Wheat 1962; Gibbons 1964; Johnson & Raker 1970; Cook 1971; Milne & Fessler 1972; Forbes & Bennett 1975; McAllister 1977).

An abnormality of the mucosal flap on the guttural pouch side of the naso-pharygeal orifice acts as a one way valve. As the orifice opens and closes, air is trapped in the guttural pouch. Sometimes the swelling may be quite large, causing dysphagia and even respiratory distress. In some cases infection occurs and guttural pouch empyema may complicate the picture.

Diagnosis is by percussion of the air-filled pouch and quick relief either by passing a catheter through the nasopharygeal opening or by needle aspiration through Viborg's triangle (the branches of the carotid artery and the posterior angle of the jaw).

Provided that the abnormality is unilateral, the condition may be corrected by surgical fenestration of the medial septum of the two pouches (Cook 1966). If the condition is bilateral, the abnormal mucosal flaps may be surgically trimmed to provide decompression (Wheat 1962). The fenestration operation may be done through an incision in the lateral wall of the guttural pouch, through Viborg's triangle or using electrocautery introduced through the nasopharygeal orifice of the guttural pouch (Cook 1971, 1974).

Haemophilia

True haemophilia, an inherited defect in the blood-clotting mechanism, due to a deficiency of factor VIII or antihaemophilic globulin (AHG), has been reported in Thoroughbred and Standardbred horses (Archer 1961; Sanger et al. 1964; Hutchins et al. 1967; Archer & Allen 1972). The condition in horses is probably similar to that seen in man (Archer & Allen 1972). The character for haemophilia occurs as a sex-linked recessive on the X chromosome.

Affected foals are apparently normal at birth, but within a few days show a number of small subcutaneous haematomas along the back and in other areas where the mare may nibble the coat. Later, swellings may appear over the hind-quarters and hocks and haemorrhage may occur into joints causing swelling and pain. A secondary normocytic anaemia develops (Archer & Jeffcott 1977).

Treatment with antihaemophilic globulin of bovine or porcine origin may be beneficial but only temporarily (Nossel et al. 1962). The majority of cases are fatal or require euthanasia on humanitarian grounds.

Combined immunodeficiency disease (CID)

A condition resulting in a functional lack of B and T lymphocyte systems is seen as a genetic defect in the Arabian and part Arabian horse (McGuire & Poppie 1973 McGuire et al. 1974, 1975*a*, *b*).

Affected foals appear normal at first and those that receive adequate colostral immunoglobulins continue to appear normal for several days to a month or more. When passive maternal antibody levels decline, the foals are immunodeficient and highly susceptible to a variety of infectious diseases, e.g. adenovirus and *Pneumocystis carinii* (McGuire et al. 1975*b*), cryptosporidiosis (Snyder et al. 1978) and listeriosis (Clarke et al. 1978).

The abnormality is apparently transmitted by an autosomal recessive character since parents are unaffected. Male and female offspring are affected in equal numbers and do not live to breeding age (McGuire et al. 1975*b*).

Laboratory diagnosis is based on a severe lymphopenia in the peripheral blood ($< 1.0 \times 10^9$/litre) and the absence of IgM. Lymph-node biopsy or post-mortem examinations reveal the absence of germinal centres and primary follicles from the lymph-nodes and spleen. Periarteriolar lymphocytic sheaths are absent from the spleen. Plasma cells are absent in both organs. Extreme thymic hypoplasia occurs with very few lymphoid cells visible. The lymphocyte defect has been characterized by the absence of in vivo and in vitro responses to phytohaemagglutinin, the absence of 'natural' antibodies to rabbit erythrocytes, the failure to produce specific antibody after antigenic stimulation and failure to mount a specific delayed hypersensitivity reaction, after attempted sensitization (McGuire et al. 1975*b*). The prevalance of this abnormality in Arabian and part-Arabian foals may be as high as 3%.

Perryman et al. (1977) describe the treatment or maintenance for experimental purposes of foals with CID. Treatment is directed at the prevention and control of secondary infection by bacteria, adenovirus and *Pneumocystis carinii.* The control of respiratory tract infections is the biggest obstacle. Their procedure was as follows at birth, a blood sample was taken and the umbilicus was disinfected with iodine. The foal was assisted in nursing if necessary. A tentative diagnosis of CID was made on a low total lymphocyte count and confirmed by the demonstration of the absence of IgM in serum. Affected foals were placed in semi-isolation, with their dams, to minimize contact with other horses. A second serum sample was obtained at 36–48 hours of age and the adequacy of transfer of colostral immunoglobulin determined by quantitation of IgG. Foals with CID that failed to receive adequate colostral immunoglobulin developed infections within the first few weeks of life and died before the effects of tissue transplantation or other experimental procedures could be adequately evaluated. Intravenous hyperimmune plasma was given twice a week, the first dose at five to seven days of age, and was continued for the life of the foal; 125–175 ml were given each time, depending on the size of the foal treated and the adenovirus antibody titre of the plasma used. This regimen usually maintained the serum IgG concentrations in the foal at 4–14 g/litre. Although the control of adenovirus infection was the main purpose of the hyperimmune plasma, it also provided antibodies directed against other microbial agents to which the foal was exposed. When bacterial infections developed, the foals were initially treated with gentamicin sulphate and later given other antibiotics, if indicated by the results of culture and antibiotic sensitivity test.

Perryman et al. (1977) reported that the treatment of *P. carinii* infection still remained the major unsolved problem. Pentamidine isothionate had been used against the protozoan with partial success. The availability of the drug, however, is limited. The authors suggest that potentiated sulphonamides may be useful and attempts are being made to prepare hyperimmune antisera against an in vitro growth of *P. carinii* for prophylactic and therapeutic use.

Umbilical hernia

An extended swelling (Fig. 6.35) appears at the umbilicus at about age six weeks and steadily increases in size depending on the diameter of the umbilical ring, which varies from 2 to 6 cm. The swelling may be differentiated from an abscess, which is not reducible, by squeezing it gently. The contents of the hernia will return to the abdomen and the edges of the ring can be identified.

Hernias are unsightly but usually regress spontaneously, as the ring closes, by age nine to 18 months. Occasionally the contents may become strangulated, causing inappetence, dullness and increasing evidence of abdominal pain. Diagnosis is confirmed by the presence of a hot, painful non-reducible swelling at the umbilicus.

Surgery is essential in cases of strangulation and is the procedure of choice if the hernia is to be eliminated for cosmetic reasons. In the latter case, the operation is performed under general anaesthesia when the foal is three to four months old, before weaning. As foals of this age are often affected by respiratory infection, a careful preoperative clinical examination should be made and the operation delayed if the foal shows signs of pneumonia or bronchiolitis. The technique is as follows (Fig. 6.36).

1. With the foal in dorsal recumbency the skin over the hernial sac and surrounding area is clipped and sterilized for surgery. Two incisions each of 2 cm are made at the base of the hernial sac in the midline, cranially and caudally.

2. A communication is made by blunt dissection with scissors either side of the hernial sac, between the two incision lines.

3. The skin between the two is incised and the underlying fascia separated. The umbilicus with skin attached is retracted and dissected away by blunt dissection.

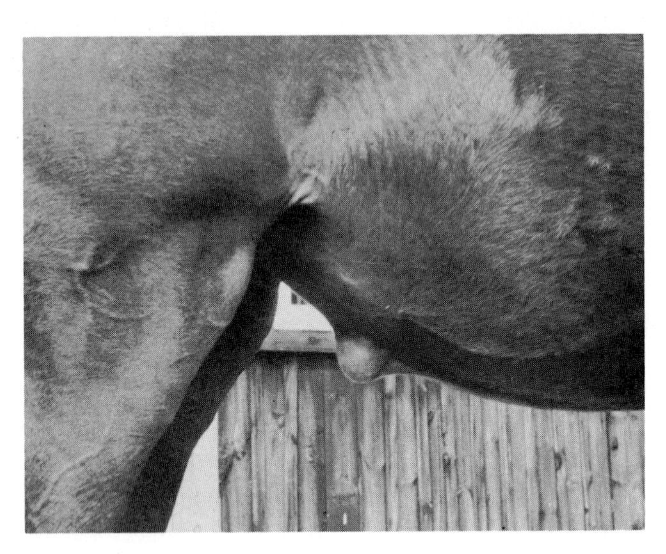

Fig. 6.35. An umbilical hernia in a five-month-old Thoroughbred foal.

4. The hernial sac is exposed and surrounding fascia dissected to clearly show the hernial ring.

5. The sac is pushed into the abdomen and three preplaced horizontal mattress sutures of double-stranded No. 4 chromic catgut are inserted.

6. The sutures are pulled tight with the sac inside and securely tied. The subcutaneous tissue and skin are closed in a routine manner.

In the case of small hernias (up to 3 cm) in which there is no evidence of strangulation, treatment with Elastrator elastic bands may be a simple method of repair, avoiding the use of general anaesthetic. For this method the foal may be tranquillized (with up to 10 mg acetylpromazine intravenously) and should be held against a loose box wall with its hind end backed into a corner. The hernial sac may then be grasped and twisted tightly with thumb and forefingers. This procedure makes sure that the contents of the hernial sac are reduced into the abdomen. One rubber ring is then placed carefully around the twisted sac, as close to the abdominal wall as possible, using the spring-loaded four-pronged Elastrator applicator. Two more rings may then be placed, in a similar fashion, above the first one. The hernial sac is observed daily and antiseptic powder applied locally until the avascular sac separates from the abdominal wall.

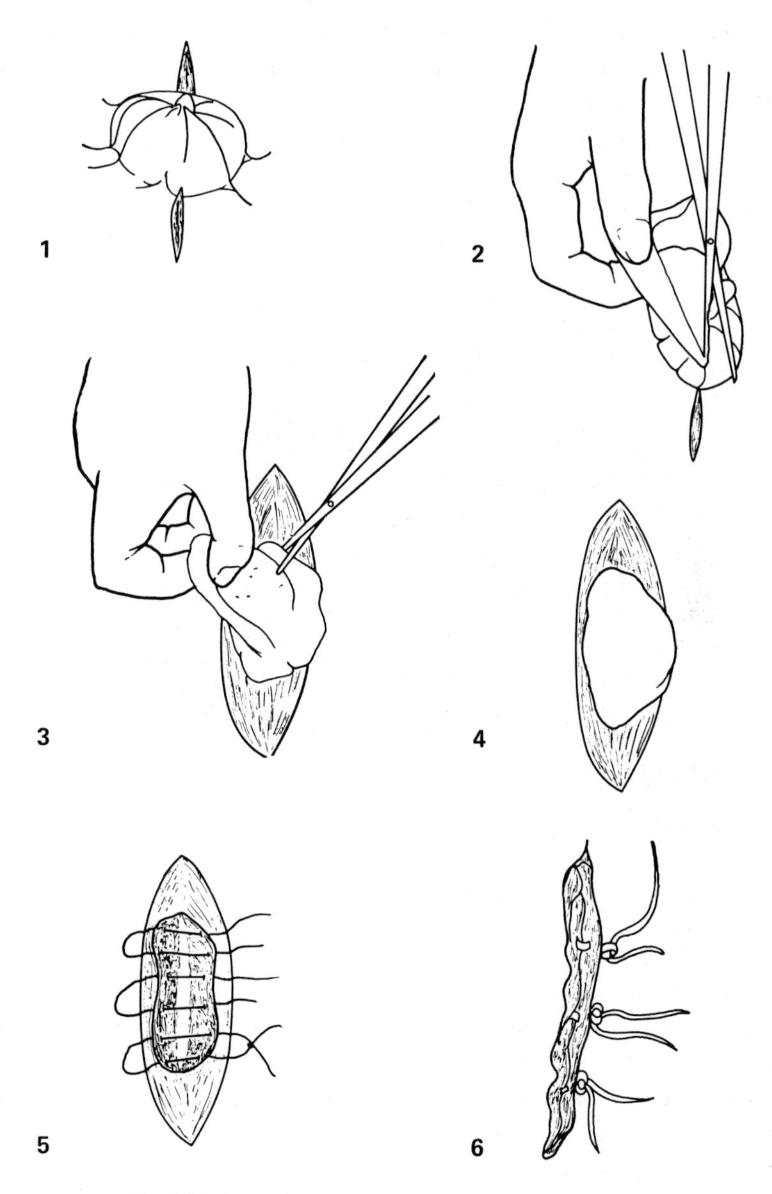

Fig. 6.36. Surgical repair of umbilical hernia. For details see text.

There appear to be two risks with this procedure. Separation of the hernial sac may occur before adequate closure of the linea alba. This may be avoided by using the procedure only on small hernias and by instructing owners and handlers never to try to hasten the separation of the sac. The separation procedure often takes four or five weeks but the major local swelling reaction is usually over within seven to ten days. Presumably, the maintenance of the abdominal contents inside the peritoneal cavity allows the linea alba to close and seal with encouragement from a local inflammatory reaction. The production of an area of necrotic tissue, in a site which may be contaminated by soiled bedding and faeces, may be ideal for bacterial infection, e.g. tetanus. In an attempt to prevent non-specific bacterial infection, a course of oral sulphamethazine (28 g orally daily for seven days) may be given to the foal on the day before and immediately after the application of the rings. As this procedure is often performed prior to tetanus vaccination, double doses of tetanus antitoxin at the time of ring application and at two weekly intervals, until the tissue separates, are recommended.

References and further reading

Adams, O.R. (1966) *Lameness in Horses,* 2nd ed. Philadelphia: Lea & Febiger.

Addo, P.B., Wilcox, G.E. & Taussig, R. (1974) Mastitis in a mare caused by *C. ovis. Vet. Rec.,* **95**, 195.

Archer, R.K. (1961) True haemophilia (haemophilia A) in a Thoroughbred horse. *Vet. Rec.,* **73**, 338.

Archer, M. (1978) Studies in producing and maintaining balanced pastures for studs. *Equine vet. J.,* **10**, 54.

Archer, R.K. & Allen, B.V. (1972) True haemophilia in horses. *Vet. Rec.,* **91**, 655.

Archer, R.K. & Jeffcott, L.B. (1977) *Comparative Clinical Haematology.* Oxford: Blackwell Scientific Publications.

Bain, A.M. (1963) *Corynebacterium equi* infections in the equine. *Aust. vet. J.,* **39**, 116.

Baker, G.L., Dodman, N.H. & Clayton, H.M. (1974) Foreign body obstructions of the small intestine of a foal. *Vet. Rec.,* **95**, 293.

Baker, H.J. & Lindsay, J.R. (1968) Equine goitre due to excess dietary iodide. *J. Am. vet. med. Ass.,* **153**, 1618.

Baker, J.R. (1969) Muscular dystrophy in the horse. *Vet. Rec.,* **84**, 488.

Bass, E.P. & Sharpee, R.L. (1975) Coronavirus and gastroenteritis in foals. *Lancet,* **2**, 822.

Beech, J. (1976) Cerebellar hypoplasia. *Proc. 22nd ann. Conv. Am. Ass. equine Practnrs,* 77.

Bennett, D. (1978) Pathological features of multiple bone infections in the foal. *Vet. Rec.,* **103**, 482.

Bjorck, G., Everz, K.E., Hansen, H.J. & Henricson, B. (1967) Cerebellar hypoplasia in the Gotland pony breed. *18th Wld vet. Congr., Paris.*

Brown, M.P. & MacCallum, F.J. (1976) Observations on growth plates in limbs of foals *Vet. Rec.,* **98**, 443.

Campbell, J.R. (1977) Bone growth in foals and epiphyseal compression. *Equine vet. J.,* **9**, 116.

Carter, M.E., Dewes, H.E. & Griffiths, O.V. (1979) Salmonellosis in foals. *J. equine Med. Surg.,* **3**, 78.

Cimprich, R.E. & Rooney, J.R. (1977) *Corynebacterium equi* arteritis in foals. *Vet. Path.,* **14**, 95.

Clarke, E.G., Turner, A.S., Boyson, B.G. & Rouse, B.T. (1978) Listeriosis in an arabian foal with combined immunodeficiency. *J. Am. med. Ass.,* **172**, 363.

Cole, H.H. & Cupps, P.T. (1959) *Reproduction in Domestic Animals.* New York and London: Academic Press.

Cook, W.R. (1966) Clinical observations on the anatomy and physiology of the equine upper respiratory tract. *Vet. Rec.,* **78**, 396.

Cook, W.R. (1971) Diseases of the ear, nose and throat in the horse. *Vet. Ann.,* **12**, 12.

Cook, W.R. (1974) Some observations on diseases of the ear, nose and throat of the horse and endoscopy using a flexible fibreoptic endoscope. *Vet. Rec.,* **94**, 533.

Davies, M.E. (1978) Some studies of equine strains of *Escherichia coli. Equine vet. J.,* **10**, 115.

Delahanty, D.D. & Gibbens, R. (1953) Traumatic epiphysitis in a young foal with metacarpas vara. *J. Am. vet. med. Ass.,* **123**, 31.

Dimock, W.W. & Errington, E.J. (1939) Incoordination of equidae: wobblers. *J. Am. vet. med. Ass.,* **95**, 261.

Dodd, D.C. (1972) Nutritional myopathy (nutritional muscular degeneration, white muscle disease). In *Equine Medicine and Surgery,* ed. E.J. Catcott & J.R. Smithcors, 2nd ed., p. 592. Wheaton, Ill.: American Veterinary Publications.

Dodd, D.C., Blakely, A.A., Thornbury, R.S. & Dewes, H.F. (1960) Muscle degeneration and yellow fat disease in foals. *N. Z. vet. J.*, **8**, 45.
Drew, B., Barber, W.P. & Williams, D.G. (1975) The effect of excess dietary iodine on pregnant mares and foals. *Vet. Rec.*, **97**, 93.
Driscoll, J., Hintz, H.F. & Schryver, H.E. (1978) Goitre in foals caused by excessive iodine. *J. Am. vet. med. Ass.*, **173**, 858.
Drummond, A.J., Trexler, P.C., Edwards, G.B., Hillidge, C. & Cox, J.E. (1973) A technique for the production of gnotobiotic foals. *Vet. Rec.*, **92**, 555.
Dungworth, D.L. & Fowler, M.E. (1966) Cerebellar hypoplasia and degeneration in a foal. *Cornell Vet.*, **56**, 17.
Dyce, K.M. (1960) Observations upon the gastro-intestinal tract of the living foal. *Br. vet. J.*, **116**, 241.
Earle, I.P. & Cabell, C.A. (1952) Blood chemistry of equidae – some variations in inorganic phosphorus, alkaline phosphatase activity, calcium, and magnesium in blood serum of horses. *Am. J. vet. Res.*, **13**, 330.
Ellis, D.R. (1976) Growth plate defects in foals. *Vet. Rec.*, **98**, 225.
Ellis, D.R. (1979) Fractures of the proximal sessamoid bones in thoroughbred foals. *Equine vet. J.*, **11**, 48.
Ellis, R.N.W. & Lawrence, T.L.J. (1978*a*) Energy under-nutrition in the weanling filly foal. 1. Effects on subsequent liveweight gains and onset of oestrus. *Br. vet. J.*, **134**, 205.
Ellis, R.N.W. & Lawrence, T.L.J. (1978*b*) Energy under-nutrition in the weanling filly foal. 2. Effects on body conformation and epiphyseal plate closure in the forelimb. *Br. vet. J.*, **134**, 322.
Ellis, R.N.W. & Lawrence, T.L.J. (1978*c*) Energy under-nutrition in the weanling filly foal. 3. Effects on heart rate and subsequent voluntary food intake. *Br. vet. J.*, **134**, 333.
Eugster, A.K., Whiteford, H.W. & Mehr, L.E. (1978) Concurrent rotavirus and *Salmonella* infections in foals. *J. Am. vet. med. Ass.*, **173**, 857.
Fackelman, G.E., Reid, C.F., Leitch, M. & Cimprich, R. (1975) Angular limb deformities in foals. *Proc. 21st ann Conv. Am. Ass. equine Practnrs*, 161.
Falco, M.J., Whitwell, K. & Palmer, A.C. (1976) Investigations into the genetics of 'wobblers' disease in Thoroughbred horses in Britain. *Equine vet. J.*, **8**, 165.
Flewett, T.H., Bryden, A.S. & Davies, H. (1975) Virus diarrhoea in foals and other animals. *Vet. Rec.*, **96**, 477.
Forbes, J.R.S. & Bennett, D.G. (1975) Tympany of the guttural pouch in a foal. *Aust. vet. J.*, **51**, 164.
Frances-Smith, K. & Wood-Gush, D.G.M. (1977) Coprophagia as seen in thoroughbred foals. *Equine vet. J.*, **9**, 155.
Fraser, H. (1966) Two dissimilar types of cerebellar disorder in the horse. *Vet. Rec.*, **78**, 608.
Fraser, H. & Palmer, A.C. (1967) Equine incoordination and wobbler disease of young horses. *Vet. Rec.*, **80**, 338.
Gabbedy, B.J. & Richards, R.B. (1970) White muscle disease in a foal. *Aust. vet. J.*, **46**, 111.
Garner, R.J. (1957) *Veterinary Toxicology*, pp. 89–97, 121–4. London: Baillière, Tindall & Cox.
Gibbons, W.J. (1964) Tympanities of the guttural pouch. *Mod. vet. Pract.*, **45**, 66.
Glendenning, S.A. (1974) A system of rearing foals on an automatic calf feeding machine. *Equine vet. J.*, **6**, 12.
Green, D.A. (1961) A review of studies on the growth rate of the horse. *Br. vet. J.*, **117**, 181.
Green, D.A. (1969) A study of growth rate in Thoroughbred foals. *Br. vet. J.*, **125**, 539.
Green, D.A. (1976) Growth rate in thoroughbred yearlings and two year olds. *Equine vet. J.*, **8**, 133.
Greet, T.R.C., Jeffcott, L.B. & Whitwell, K.E. (1980) The slap test for laryngeal adductory function in horses with suspected cervical spinal cord damage. *Equine vet. J.*, **12**, 127.
Hall, W.C. & Van Kruininger, H.J. (1974) Tyzzer's disease in a foal. *J. Am. vet. med. Ass.*, **164**, 1187.
Ham, A.W. & Leeson, T.S. (1965) *Histology*, 5th ed. Philadelphia: Lippincott.
Harrington, D.D. (1975) Naturally occurring Tyzzer's disease (*Bacillus piliformis* injection) in horse foals. *Vet. Rec.*, **96**, 59.
Harrington, D.D. (1976) *Bacillus piliformis* infection (Tyzzer's disease) in two foals. *J. Am. vet. med. Ass.*, **168**, 58.
Heinze, C.D. (1963) Epiphyseal stapling. *Proc. 9th ann. Conv. Am. Ass. equine Practnrs*, 203.

Heinze, C.D. (1965) Orthopaedic panel, epiphyseal closure and stapling. *Proc. 11th ann. Conv. Am. Ass. equine Practnrs,* 273.

Heinze, C.D. (1966) Epiphyseal stapling in the horse. *Mod. vet. Pract.*, **47**, 40.

Henry, J.N. & Gagnon, A.N. (1976) Adenovirus pneumonia in an arabian foal. *Can. vet. J.*, **17**, 220.

Hintz, H.F., Hintz, R.L. & Van Vleck, L.D. (1979) Growth rate of Thoroughbreds. Effect of age of dam, year and month of birth, and sex of foal. *J. Anim. Sci.*, **48**, 480.

Hintz, H.F. & Schryver, H.F. (1976) Nutrition and bone development in horses. *J. Am. vet. med. Ass.*, **168**, 31.

Hutchins, D.R., Lepherd, E.E. & Crook, J.G. (1967) A case of haemophilia. *Aust. vet. J.*, **43**, 83.

Jeffcott, L.B. (1971) Perinatal Studies in Equidae with Special Reference to Passive Transfer of Immunity. Ph. D. thesis, University of London.

Jeffcott, L.B. & Whitwell, K.E. (1976) Fractures of the thoracolumbar spine of the horse. *Proc. 22nd ann. Conv. Am. Ass. equine Practnrs,* 91.

Johnson, J.H. & Raker, C.W. (1970) The relationship of the guttural pouch to upper respiratory conditions. *Proc. 16th ann. Conv. Am. Ass. equine Practnrs,* 267.

Johnston, R.H., Kamstra, L.D.& Kohler, P.H. (1970) Mares' milk composition as related to 'foal heat' scours. *J. Anim. Sci.*, **31**, 549.

Kanitz, C.L. (1976) Identification of an equine rotavirus as a cause of neonatal foal diarrhoea. *Proc. 22nd ann. Conv. Am. Ass. equine Practnrs,* 155.

Koch, P. & Fischer, H. (1950) Die Oldenburger Fohlenataxie als Erbkrankheit. *Tierarztl. Umsch.*, **5**, 317.

Kroneman, J. & Wensvoort, P. (1968) Muscular dystrophy and yellow fat disease in Shetland Pony foals. *Neth. J. vet. Sci.*, **1**, 42.

Linton, J.A.M. & Gallaher, M.A. (1969) Suppurative bronchopneumonia in a foal associated with *Corynebacterium equi. Ir. vet. J.*, **23**, 197.

Linton, R.G. (1931) The composition of mares' milk. *J. agric. Sci., Camb.*, **21**, 669.

Loizos, C. (1966) Play in mammals. *Symp. zool. Soc. Lond.*, **18**, 1.

McAllister, E.S. (1977) Guttural pouch disease. *Proc. 23rd ann. Conv. Am. Ass. equine Practnrs,* 251.

McChesney, A.E., Becerra, V. & England, J.J. (1974) Chlamydial polyartheritis in a foal. *J. Am. vet. med. Ass.*, **165**, 259.

McChesney, A.E. & England, J.J. (1975) Adenoviral infections of foals. *J. Am. vet. med. Ass.*, **166**, 83.

McGuire, T., Banks, K.L. & Poppie, M.J. (1975*b*) Immunodeficiency disease in foals. *Proc. 1st int. Symp. equine Haemat.*, 190.

McGuire, T.C. & Poppie, M.J. (1973) Hypogammaglobulinaemia and thymic hypoplasia in horses: a primary combined immunodeficiency disorder. *Infect. Immunol.*, **8**, 272.

McGuire, T.C., Poppie, M.J. & Banks, K.L. (1974) Combined (B- and T-lymphocyte) immunodeficiency: a fatal genetic disease in Arabian foals. *J. Am. vet. med. Ass.*, **164**, 70.

McGuire, T.C., Poppie, M.K. & Banks, K.L. (1975*a*) Hypogammaglobulinemia predisposing to infection in foals. *J. Am. vet med. Ass.*, **166**, 71.

McIlwraith, C.W. & Fessler, J.F. (1978) Evaluation of inferior check ligament desmotomy for treatment of acquired flexor tendon contracture in the horse. *J. Am. vet. med. Ass.*, **172**, 293.

Magnusson, H. (1938) Pyaemia in foals caused by *Corynebacterium equi. Vet. Rec.*, **50**, 1459.

Mahaffey, L.W. (1952) *Salmonella typhimurium* in foals in Western Australia. *Aust. vet. J.*, **28**, 8.

Mahaffey, L.W. (1962) Respiratory conditions in horses. *Vet. Rec.*, **74**, 1295.

Mason, T.A. & Maclean, A.A. (1977) Osteochondrosis dissecans of the head of the humerus in two foals. *Equine vet. J.*, **9**, 189.

Meagher, D.M., Pool, R.R. & O'Brien, T.R. (1973) Osteochondrosis in the shoulder joint of the horse. *Proc. 19th ann. Conv. Am. Ass. equine Practnrs,* 247.

Mederios, L.O., Ferri, S., Barcelos, S.R. & Miguel, O. (1971) Hematologic standards for healthy newborn Thoroughbred foals. *Biol. Neonate,* **17**, 351.

Miller, W.C. (1965) Equine virus rhinopneumonitis. *Proc. 4th Br. equine vet. Ass. Congr.*, 32.

Milne, D.W. & Fessler, J.F. (1972) Tympanities of the guttural pouch in a foal. *J. Am. vet. med. Ass.*, **161**, 61.

Monson, W.J. (1968) Nutrition of the young foal–including orphaned foals. *Borden Bull.*, **IX**, 3.

Monteverde, J.J., Monteverde, H.J. & Chialvo, E.J. (1972) Bordetella bronchiseptica en neumonia de potrillos (English summary). *Revta Med. vet. B. Aires,* 77, 81.

Moore, J.N. & McIlwraith, C.W. (1977) Osteochondrosis of the equine stifle. *Vet. Rec.,* **100**, 133.

Moorthy, A.R.S., Spradbow, P.B. & Eisler, M.E.D. (1977) Isolation of mycoplasmosis from an arthertic foal. *Br. vet. J.,* **133**, 320.

Myers, V.S. & Gordon, G.W. (1975) Ruptured common digital extensor tendons associated with contracted flextor tendons in foals. *Proc. 21st ann. Conv. Am. Ass. equine Practnrs,* 67.

Neseni, R., Flade, E., Heidler, G. & Steger, H. (1958) Milcheistung und Milchzusammensetzung von Stuten im Verlufe der Laktation. *Arch. Tierheilk.,* **1**, 91.

Nishikawa, Y. (1959) *Studies on Reproduction in Horses.* Tokyo: Japan Racing Association.

Norrie, R.D. (1975) The treatment of joint disease by saline lavage. *Proc. 21st ann. Conv. Am. Ass. equine Practnrs,* 91.

Nossel, H.L., Archer, R.K. & McFarlane, R.G. (1962) Equine haemophilia: report of a case and its response to multiple infusions of hetero-specific AHG. *Br. J. Haemat.,* **8**, 335.

Owen J.M. (1975) Abnormal flexion of the coronopedal joint or 'contracted tendons' in unweaned foals. *Equine vet. J.,* 7, 40.

Owen, J.M., McCullagh, K.G., Crook, D.H. & Hinton, M. (1978) Seasonal variations in the nutrition of horses at grass. *Equine vet. J.,* **10**, 260.

Ordidge, R.M. (1976) Urinary incontinence due to unilateral ureteral ectopia in a foal. *Vet. Rec.,* **98**, 384.

Palmer, A.C., Blakemore, W.F., Cook, W.R., Platt, H. & Whitwell, K.E. (1973) Cerebellar hypoplasia and degeneration in the young Arab horse. Clinical and neuropathological features. *Vet. Rec.,* **93**, 62.

Perryman, L.E., McGuire, T.C. & Crawford, T.B. (1977) Maintenance of foals with combined immunodeficiency: causes and control of secondary infection. *Am. J. vet. Res.,* **39**, 1043.

Petterson, H. & Reiland, S. (1968) Periarticular subchondral 'bone cysts' in horses. *Proc. 14th ann. Conv. Am. Ass. equine Practnrs,* 245.

Platt, H. (1977) Joint ill and other bacterial infections on Thoroughbred studs. *Equine vet. J.,* **9**, 141.

Platt, H. & Whitwell, K.E. (1971) Clinical and pathological observations on generalized steatitis in foals. *J. comp. Path.,* **81**, 499.

Pulley, L.T. & Scheveley, J.N. (1974) Tyzzer's disease in a foal: light and electon microscopic observations. *Vet. Path.,* **11**, 203.

Reese, G.L. & Lock, T.F. (1978) Streptococcal mastitis in a mare. *J. Am. vet. med. Ass.,* **173**, 83.

Reid, C.F. (1970) Radiographic diagnosis and appearance of osseous cyst-like lesions in horses previously reported as periarticular subchondral bone cyst. *Proc. 16th ann. Conv. Am. Ass. equine Practnrs,* 185.

Roberts, M.C. (1975*a*) The development and distribution of mucosal enzymes in the small intestine of the foetus and young foal. *J. Reprod. Fert.,* Suppl. **23**, 717.

Roberts, M.C. (1975*b*) Carbohydrate digestions and absorption studies in the horse. *Res. vet. Sci.,* **18**, 64.

Roberts, M.C. & Polley, L.R. (1977) Corynebacterium equi infections in a thoroughbred foal. *Equine vet. J.,* **9**, 159.

Roberts, W.D. (1971) Isoniazid in equine therapy. *Proc. 17th ann. Conv. Am. Ass. equine Practnrs,* 33.

Rooney, J.R. (1962) Joint-ill. *J. Am. vet. med. Ass.,* **141**, 1259.

Rooney, J.R. (1963) Equine incoordination. 1. Gross morphology. *Cornell Vet.,* **53**, 411.

Rooney, J.R. (1966) Corynebacterial infections in foals. *Mod. vet. Pract.,* **47**, 43.

Rooney, J.R. (1969) *Biomechanics of Lameness in Horses.* Baltimore: Williams & Wilkins.

Rooney, J.R. & Prickett, M.E. (1967) 'Shaker' foal syndrome. *Mod. vet. Pract.,* **48**, 44.

Rossdale, P.D. & Mullen, P.A. (1969) Muscular tremors in an unweaned foal suffering from metabolic acidaemia. *Vet. Rec.,* **85**, 702.

Rossdale, P.D. & Mullen, P.A. (1970) Alterations to whole blood pH, pCO_2 and plasma bicarbonate index values during a metabolic acidosis occasioned by neonatal diarrhoea in Thoroughbred foals. *Br. vet. J.,* **126**, 82.

Salter, R.B. & Harris, W.P. (1963) Injuries involving the epiphyseal plates. *J. Bone Jt Surg.,* **45A**, 587.

Sanger, V.L., Mairs, R.E. & Trapp, A.L. (1964) Haemophilia in a foal. *J. Am. vet. med. Ass.,* **144**, 259.

Sčekina, E.S. (1950) Development of young on the S.M. Budennyi stud. *Horsebreeding, Mosk.*, **20**, 24.

Schougaard, H., Basse, A., Gissel-Nielsen, G. & Simesen, M.G. (1972) Nutritional muscular dystrophy in foals (In Danish with English summary). *Nord. VetMed.*, **24**, 67.

Shaver, J.R., Fretz, P.B., Doige, C.E. & Williams, D.M. (1979) Skeletal manifestations of suspected hypothyroidism in two foals. *J. equine Med. Surg.*, **3**, 269.

Sheahan, B.J. (1976) *Eimeria leukarti* infections in a thoroughbred foal. *Vet. Rec.*, **99**, 213.

Simmons, D.P. & Christman, O.D. (1965) Salicylate inhibition of cartilage degeneration. *Arthritis Rheumatism*, **8**, 960.

Smith, B.P., Reinagnerra, M. & Hardy, A.J. (1978) Prevalence of epizootiology of equine salmonellosis. *J. Am. vet. med. Ass.*, **172**, 353.

Snyder, S.P., England, J.J. & Crain, C. (1978) Cryptosporidiosis in immunodeficient arabian foals. *Vet. Path.*, **15**, 12.

Sponseller, M.L. (1967) Equine cerebellar hypoplasia and degeneration. *Proc. 13th ann. Conv. Am. Ass. equine Practnrs*, 123.

Stromberg, B.R.G. (1978) Ostechondosis in the horse: pathology and clinical and radiographic signs. Paper given at BEVA Congress, York.

Studdert, M.J., Mason, R.W. & Pattern, B.E. (1978) Rotavirus diarrhoea of foals. *Aust. vet. J.*, **54**, 363.

Swerczek, T.W. (1977) Multi-focal hepatic necrosis and hepatatis in foals caused by *Bacillus piliforms* (Tyzzer's disease). *Vet. Ann.*, **17**, 130.

Swerczek, T.W., Crowe, M.W., Prickett, M.E. & Bryans, J.T. (1973) Focal bacterial hepatitis: preliminary report. *Mod. vet. Pract.*, **54**, 66.

Thompson, G.W., Wilson, R.W., Hall, E.A. & Physik-Sheerd, P. (1977) Tyzzer's disease in the foal: case reports and review. *Can. vet. J.*, **18**, 41.

Turner, A.S. & Fretz, P.B. (1977) A comparison of surgical techniques and associated complications of transphyseal bridging in foals. *Proc. 23rd ann. Conv. Am. Ass. equine Practnrs*, 275.

Tyler, S.J. (1972) The behaviour and social organization of the New Forest ponies. *Anim. Behav. Monogr.*, **5**, 2.

Tyznik, W.J. (1972) Nutrition and disease. In *Equine Medicine and Surgery*, 2nd ed., ed. E.J. Catcott & J.R. Smithcors, p. 239. Illinois: American Veterinary Publications.

Tyznik, W.J. (1975) Feeding the foal. *The International Stockman's School Stud Manager's Handbook*, vol. 11, p. 54. Agriservices Foundation.

Tzipori, S. & Walker, M. (1978) Isolation of rotavirus for foals with diarrhoea. *Aust. J. exp. Biol. med. Sci.*, **56**, 453.

Ullrey, D.E., Struthers, R.D., Hendricks, D.G. & Brent, B.E. (1966) Composition of mares' milk. *J. Anim. Sci.*, **25**, 217.

Van Pelt, R.W. (1969) Idiopathic tenosynovitis in foals. *J. Am. vet. med. Ass.*, **155**, 510.

Van Pelt, R.W. & Riley, W.F. (1969) Clinicopathological findings and therapy in septic arthritis in foals. *J. Am. vet. med. Ass.*, **155**, 1467.

Vaughan, L.C. (1976) Growth plate defects in foals. *Vet. Rec.*, **98**, 165.

Willoughby, R.A., MacDonald, E., McSherry, B.J. & Brown, G. (1972) Lead and zinc poisoning and the interaction between Pb and Zn poisoning in the foal. *Can. J. comp. Med.*, **36**, 348.

Wilson, T.M., Morrison, H.A., Palmer, N.C., Finly, G.B. & Van Dreumel, A.A. (1976) Myodegeneration and suspected selenium/vitamin E deficiency in horses. *J. Am. vet. med. Ass.*, **169**, 213.

Wheat, J.D. (1962) Tympanities of the guttural pouch of the horse. *J. Am. vet. med. Ass.*, **140**, 453.

Whitwell, K.E. (1976) Four cases of Tyzzer's disease in foals in England. *Equine vet. J.*, **8**, 118.

Woolcock, J.B., Mutimer, M.D. & Farmer, A.M.T. (1980) Epidemiology of *Corynebacterium equi* in horses. *Res. vet. Sci.*, **28**, 87.

General Medicine 7

In this chapter we are concerned with diseases which the clinician may encounter in stud farm practice, but which are not particular to the problems of reproduction or growth. Our account is necessarily abridged since our primary purpose has been to discuss reproductive phenomena. We therefore include references and suggestions for further reading. For further reading on this general subject we recommend Blood et al. (1979), Catcott and Smithcors (1972). Bruner and Gillespie (1966) and Lapage (1968).

INFECTIOUS CONDITIONS

Viruses

Considerable progress has been made in the study of the fundamental character of viruses in recent years and although the extent of our knowledge is not yet sufficient to warrant the use of a Linnaean binominal nomenclature it is possible to group viruses according to some of their outstanding properties. For a detailed investigation of the subject the reader is referred to Huck (1964), Cruickshank (1965), Andrews et al. (1978) and, with particular reference to equine virus infections, Scott (1971).

Scott (1971) summarized virus classification as follows:

> Viruses are unique because they contain only one type of nucleic acid whereas all other forms of life contain two. The type of nucleic acid is the cornerstone of virus taxonomy; it may be either deoxyribonucleic acid (DNA) or ribonucleic acid (RNA). Viruses, thereafter, are further differentiated by physical and morphological features.

Scott (1971) reviewed the literature concerning equine viral infections and part of his review is reproduced here.

> *DNA Viruses*
> DNA viruses fall into five groups [Table 7.1]. At least twelve viruses affecting horses are DNA viruses; one or perhaps two are Papovaviruses, namely equine papilloma and equine sarcoid; at least one is an Adenovirus (Mayr, Pette and Pape, 1966), seven are Herpesviruses [Fig. 7.1] and perhaps three are Poxviruses, horse pox, grease and papular dermatitis. Horse

pox characterised by the development of typical pocks on the lips and oral mucosa and grease characterised by dermatitis of the pasterns and heels may be different clinical manifestations of infection by the same virus. Papular dermatitis, on the other hand, is unlikely to be a variant of horse pox (McIntyre, 1949).

The seven herpesviruses are equine herpes 1 (Plummer and Waterson, 1963) commonly called equine rhinopneumonitis virus and often implicated in upper respiratory tract infections, and abortions, herpes 2 (Plummer and Waterson, 1963) isolated from the respiratory tract of a colt within rhinitis, CEO virus (Kono and Kobayashi, 1964) isolated in Japan spontaneously from cultures of equine kidney and bone marrow cells, herpes 3 (Karpas, 1966) isolated from the kidneys of an apparently healthy foal, equine cytomegalovirus (Hsuing, Fischman, Fong and Green, 1969) isolated from lesions on a stallion, and Iowa leukocyte virus (Kemeny and Pearson, 1970) isolated from the leukocytes of 71 out of 80 apparently normal Iowa horses. The antigenic relationships of the Iowa leukocyte virus to the other equine herpesviruses has yet to be established.

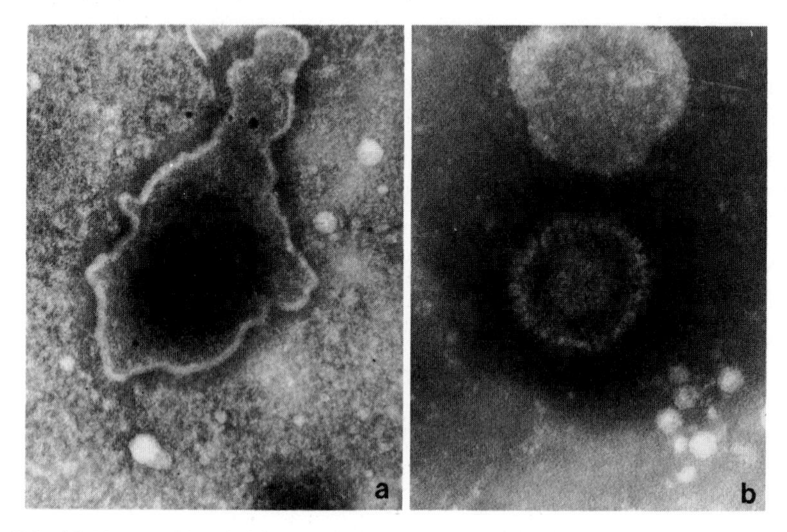

Fig. 7.1. (*a*) Herpes virion in tissue culture material inoculated with nasal washings from a two-year-old Thoroughbred colt with rhinitis. (*b*) A higher magnification of the virion from the same preparation, which shows inner icosahedral nucleocapsid and outer envelope. Sodium phosphotungstate preparation. Instrument magnification × 91 000 (*a*) and × 150 000 (*b*) (*Reproduced by kind permission of Dr J. Nagington and Mrs M. Rose*)

TABLE 7.1 DNA viruses affecting the horse

Group	*Virus*
Picornavirus	–
Papovavirus	Equine papilloma
Adenovirus	Equine adeno
Herpesvirus	Herpes I (rhinopneumonitis)
	Herpes II (slow growing)
	Herpes III (coital exanthema)
Poxvirus	Horse pox
	Grease
	? Papular dermatitis

After Scott (1971).

RNA Viruses

RNA viruses have either cubic, helical or unknown symmetries. There are two groups of cubic RNA viruses, Picornavirus and Reovirus, four groups of helical RNA viruses, Myxovirus, Rhabdovirus, Paramyxovirus and Coronavirus, and two groups with unknown symmetries, Arbovirus and Oncornavirus [Table 7.2]. Three Picornaviruses infect horses, namely rhino 1 (Plummer, 1962), rhino 2 (Ditchfield and Macpherson, 1965) and aborted foal virus (Bohm, 1964). African horse sickness virus is believed now to be a Reovirus (Ozawa, 1968). Three Myxoviruses, influenza A (Heller, Espmark and Viriden, 1956), influenza B (Ditchfield, Macpherson and Zbitnew, 1965) and influenza C (Ditchfield *et al.*, 1965) and three Rhabdoviruses, rabies, vesicular stomatitis and cocal viruses, infect horses. Serological evidence (Ditchfield *et al.*, 1965) incriminates parainfluenza-1 and parainfluenza-2 viruses belonging to the Paramyxovirus group.

In addition, parainfluenza-3 virus has been isolated from horses with upper respiratory tract infections (Ditchfield, Zbitnew and Macpherson, 1963). There is possibly one Coronavirus affecting horses; Ditchfield (1969) isolated a virus from a Thoroughbred with undifferentiated respiratory disease and found that it possessed a morphology similar to that of infectious bronchitis virus of poultry, the type-virus of the Coronavirus group.

TABLE 7.2 RNA viruses affecting the horse

Group	*Virus*
Picornavirus	Rhino 1
	Rhino 2
	Aborted foal
Reovirus	African horse sickness
Myxovirus	Influenza A
	Influenza C
Paramyxovirus	Parainfluenza 3
Rhabdovirus	Rabies
	Vesicular stomatitis
Coronavirus	Rotavirus
Arbovirus	Eastern encephalitis
	Western encephalitis
	Venezuelan encephalitis
	West Nile
	Japanese B encephalitis
	Murray Valley encephalitis
Oncornavirus	Equine infectious anaemia
Ungrouped	Infectious arteritis

After Scott (1971).

There are more than 200 Arboviruses and at least 27 affect horses. Equine infectious anaemia virus probably belongs to the Oncornavirus group, i.e. the RNA tumour viruses. Infectious arteritis virus (Doll, Bryans, McCollum and Crow, 1957), on the other hand, is known to be a RNA virus but it is as yet ungrouped. Recent electronmicroscopic studies revealed a morphology like that of the Arboviruses (Breese and McCollum, 1969).

Unclassified Viruses

Three diseases of horses, Borna disease (Zwick and Witte, 1929), Near East equine encephololomyelitis (Daubeny and Mahlau, 1957) and Nigerian horse staggers (Porterfield, Hill and Morris, 1958) are caused by viruses as yet unclassified and it is possible that the three diseases are caused by the same virus. Finally there are at least three other alleged viral diseases, serum hepatitis (Theiler, 1919), grass sickness (Obel, 1955) and virus diarrhoea (Rooney, 1969).

Already 50 viruses are known to affect horses and half of these are responsible for clinical disease. The other half are incriminated only by the detection of specific antibodies in horse sera. Here we shall confine ourselves to a description of the common infections which affect horses at stud.

Equine influenza

This acute infection of the upper respiratory tract is characterized by coughing, fever and mild malaise. The condition is caused by myxovirus (influenza A/equi 1 and 2) (Beveridge et al. 1965; Bryans et al. 1967). It is enzootic in most countries and epidemics tend to occur every four years. Spread is explosive; Gerber (1966) reported that 98% of 634 horses in a remount depot become infected within eight days of the first signs of the disease.

Clinical signs include fever of 39–41°C lasting one to four days, a slight serous nasal discharge and dry, deep cough lasting five to ten days.

Bacterial complications are rare. Gerber (1966) reported a moderate normochromic anaemia and a decrease in leucocyte count due to reduced lymphocyte content followed by an increasing monocytosis.

Although the condition lasts on average for a week and sequelae are rare, infection among foals or horse populations which have had little exposure to the virus may lead to more serious illness and, especially in foals, death. Mahaffey (1966) described pathological findings in foals which died of A/equi 2 infection in Newmarket. The foals suffered signs of pneumonia with increasing dyspnoea and at post-mortem there was consolidation due to cellular proliferation involving mononuclear cells, presumably associated with the immune response evoked by the virus. Mares affected during this epidemic sometimes showed signs of distress, dyspnoea and colic, but they usually recovered in three to four days.

Influenza can be diagnosed by viral isolation or by the examination of acute and convalescent sera, i.e. sera obtained at the onset of signs and ten days to two weeks later. Sera are examined by complement-fixation and haemagglutination-inhibition tests and a rising titre is considered positive.

Treatment is seldom necessary but affected horses should be confined to stables that are well ventilated. Rest is essential for at least ten days after signs have abated. Mares and foals should be turned on to paddocks and confined to loose boxes only where necessary for climatic reasons. When secondary infection occurs antibiotics may be administered and, in cases of dyspnoea and distress, small doses of corticosteroids are sometimes helpful. Gerber (1969) has noted an association with chronic pulmonary disease due to asthmatic bronchitis.

Infection with influenza virus may produce secondary organic damage including myocarditis and hepatic changes (Gerber 1969). Oedema of the legs has occasionally been reported following infection and may be a sequel of cardiac and hepatic damage (Powell 1975). Sufficient convalescence and rest from strenuous exercise is thus essential.

Inactivated influenza virus vaccines are highly efficacious in preventing the disease (Bryans et al. 1966). Rose et al. (1974) isolated influenza A/equi 1 during an outbreak of coughing which occurred among unvaccinated horses in 1973.

Vaccinated horses maintained a high level of antibodies against both subtypes of equine influenza virus and escaped infection. Similarly, Powell and Felmingham (1977) reported outbreaks of influenza A/equi 1 in unvaccinated horses. Recently, outbreaks of influenza A/equi 2 have been seen in vaccinated horses in Great Britain. It is not yet clear whether antigenic variants occurred. It has been suggested that insufficiently frequent booster vaccinations in these horses may have been a relevant factor. Recently it has been suggested that booster vaccinations should be given every three or four months to obtain a satisfactory level of immunity. With pregnant mares, booster vaccinations may be given in the last month of pregnancy to produce maximal colostral immunity. Foals should receive their primary vaccinations at two and three months of age.

Equid herpesvirus I infection

Four clinical manifestations of this disease have now been recognized:

1. Upper respiratory disease in foals, yearlings and horses in training (Rose et al. 1974; Powell 1975; Thompson et al. 1976) (see also p. 399).
2. Sporadic or epizootic abortion in mares (Dimock & Edwards 1933; Dimock et al. 1942; Doll 1952) (also see p. 200).
3. Neonatal foal disease (Bryans et al. 1977; Dickson et al. 1978) (also see p. 308).
4. Neurological disease with paralysis (Saxegaard 1966; Little et al. 1974; Thorsen & Little 1975; Charlton et al. 1976; Dinter & Klingborn 1976; Jackson et al. 1977; Moyer & Rooney 1972; Greenwood 1979).

Several, if not all, types may be seen in a particular outbreak (Greenwood 1979) and it is debatable whether the type of disease seen is influenced by strain differences or by environmental and immunological factors. Burrows and Goodridge (1975) suggest that the epidemiology of the disease in Britain indicates that differences in virulence occur between different strains of the virus. Their in vitro studies indicated that strains isolated from an aborted fetus had a wider tissue culture host range and grew better in organ cultures of equine tissue than did most strains isolated from respiratory disease.

The respiratory disease, abortion and neonatal foal disease have been described previously. Here we are concerned with the neurological form of the disease, which has been reported from Scandinavia (Saxegaard 1966; Dinter & Klingborn 1976), Canada (Little et al. 1974), the USA (Jackson & Kendrick 1971; Moyer & Rooney 1972) and recently England (Greenwood 1979).

Affected horses show marked posterior ataxia, often with tail paralysis, absence of anal reflex and urinary incontinence. Some cases have shown impaired cranial nerve function with tongue or pharyngeal paralysis. In many cases, the respiratory form of the disease has been seen concurrently with dullness, slight inappetance, watery or mucopurulent nasal discharge and a temperature rise to 38.9–39.5°C in mares and 39.2–40°C in foals. In some reports, equid herpesvirus I abortions have occurred on the same or adjacent premises within a month of the first neurological case.

Most reports record haematological and blood biochemical findings within normal limits but Greenwood (1979, personal communication) reports a marked monocytosis in most cases, as high as 25% in some.

Pathological findings reported are a marked adventitial accumulation of mononuclear cells, predominantly histiocytes (Dinter & Klingborn 1976) and a heavy perivascular infiltration of mononuclear cells and leucocytes, some perivascular oedema, necrosis of neurones and malacia in the immediate vicinity of the infiltrated vessels, involving the basal ganglia with only slight changes in the corpora quadrigemina and the thalamus (Moyer & Rooney 1972). These authors also reported one case with marked haemorrhagic infiltration of the cauda equina and slight wallerian degeneration in the ventral portions of the cervical, thoracic and lumbar portions of the spinal cord.

Most reports have been able to demonstrate a serological response to equid herpesvirus I and in some cases the virus has been grown from nasal swabs and post-mortem tissues. Jackson and Kendrick (1971) and Little et al. (1974) have reproduced the condition in horses inoculated experimentally with virus, which was, in the latter report, isolated from the nervous tissue of a paralysed horse.

Dinter and Klingborn (1976) debate whether the CNS lesions are caused by direct action of the virus or are mediated immunologically following the formation of virus–antibody complexes. Their clinical and virological findings and their calculated incubation period of about seven days lead them to conclude that the 'acute disseminated post-infectious encephalomyelopathy' may be due to an early immunological reaction. They suggest that there is an accelerated response of sensitized or primed immunocytes, reaching high levels in a few days following reinfection, which appears serologically to account for most of the cases of paresis. They suggest that the virus strain involved in paralytic outbreaks must be a virulent one, otherwise similar cases of paresis should occur occasionally with attenuated strains following vaccination, which in 'primed' horses resembles reinfection. These authors also debate whether their epidemic was due to a rapid spread of reinfection with an exogenous virus strain or an accumulation of recurrent infection provoked by some common but unknown factor or factors. A fact that seems to support the theory of an early immunological reaction is that, in some cases, the early administration of very large doses of corticosteroids may help (Greenwood & Simson 1980). On the other hand, the facts that, in the Newmarket outbreak, the disease did spread to in-contact mares on other premises, and that Mumford and Edington (1980) were able to induce paresis experimentally in a Welsh pony mare with EHV-I isolate obtained from an ataxic Thoroughbred, suggest direct action by an exogenous virus. Owing to the risk of disease spread, control must be based on early identification and isolation of cases and direct contacts. Individual treatment can be only symptomatic and supportive. Slings may be valuable but unfortunately many horses will not tolerate or cooperate with them. The early use of large quantities of corticosteroids may be helpful, assuming that an immunological mechanism is involved. Many cases progress to a state where euthanasia is indicated on humanitarian grounds.

Other equid herpesvirus infections

Plummer and Waterson (1963) isolated herpesvirus II from a foal out of a mare called Lady Kells suffering from catarrh. For some time this was known as the LK virus. It is serologically distinct from equid herpesvirus I. Another serotype, equid herpesvirus III, was recovered from foal kidney cultures by Karpas (1966). A fourth virus has been described as an equine cytomegalovirus. Of these only herpesvirus II is known to be associated with rhinitis.

Coital exanthema is described on pp. 103 and 154. It is caused by a herpesvirus now classed as equid herpesvirus III (Thiem 1976).

Adenovirus infection

This acute and sometimes fatal disease of young horses is characterized by fever and pneumonia. McChesney et al. (1970) reported ten cases of infection in suckling Arabian foals. Clinical signs included a deep, soft productive cough, mucopurulent nasal and occular discharges and ulcers on the labial mucosa. Moist bronchial râles were heard on auscultation and abdominal respiratory movements were exaggerated by double expiratory effort. A leucopenia affecting lymphocytes and neutrophils was present in most cases.

Gross pathology included lungs that were heavy and failed to collapse, with evidence of consolidation and a yellow mucous exudation from the bronchi and bronchioles. Numerous grey/white foci, 1–2 cm in diameter, were found in the hepatic parenchyma and white, irregularly round, slightly granular foci on the subcapsular surface of both kidneys.

Characteristic intranuclear inclusions (Cowdray types A and B) were found in conjunctival epithelium. Epithelial cells of the major bronchi were hyperplastic and contained inclusions.

McChesney et al. (1970) found that the morbidity among foals was 10% and the mortality among these 100% but they recognized the possibility that some foals may have had unrecognized infection and recovered spontaneously. They recommended control of secondary infections by antibiotics and antifungal agents and by supportive agents.

It now appears that the adenovirus infection in Arabian foals is only a secondary opportunist infection in foals suffering from combined immunodeficiency disease (see p. 412).

Rhinovirus and parainfluenza virus infection

These viruses have been isolated from horses with signs of upper respiratory infections (Ditchfield 1969).

Papovavirus

Papovaviruses cause papillomatosis (milk warts) of young horses, usually on the muzzle and lips (Fig. 7.2). The disease is self-limiting and the warts regress spontaneously in two to three months. For more details see p. 455.

Equine infectious anaemia (EIA, 'swamp fever')

This infectious disease is characterized by intermittent fever, weight loss and anaemia. The condition is well known in the USA and Europe and has been reported in the UK (Rossdale et al. 1975). The condition may occur in subclinical form, where the horse shows no obvious clinical signs; in acute form, where the horse shows profound anaemia, with pyrexia, depression, circulatory collapse and hepatitis; and in chronic form, with ill-thrift and mild anaemia. Subacute and chronic forms may suddenly become acute.

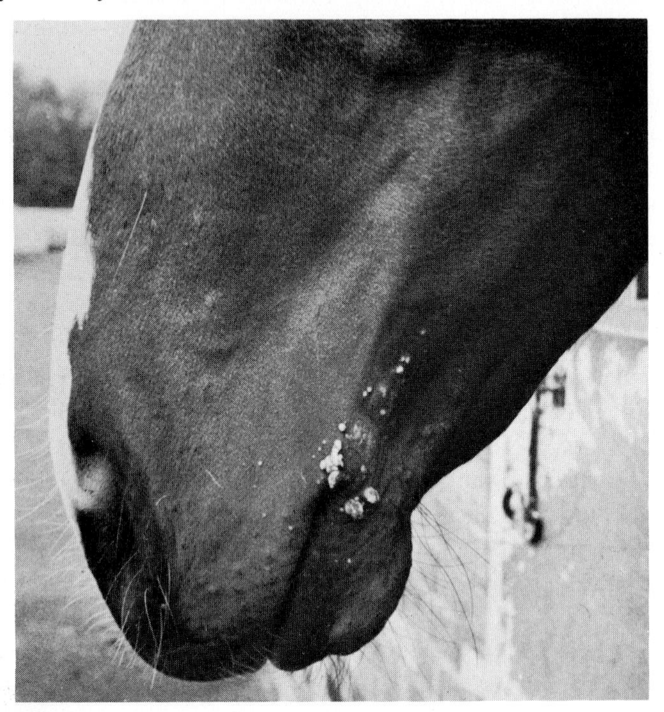

Fig. 7.2. Papillomatous warts on the muzzle of a two-year-old.

EIA is caused by an RNA virus with morphological, physical and biochemical similarities to the oncornaviruses. During the course of the disease variance of the virus, antigenically different and serologically distinguishable, appears at each febrile stage (Kono et al. 1973).

Natural transmission of the disease occurs via various blood-sucking insects, e.g. horse flies, stable flies and mosquitos. Experimental transmission from acute cases has been very easy but not from chronic cases. Accidental infection may occur via equipment such as tooth rasps, twitches, stomach tubes, curry combs, syringes, needles and any other instruments which may cause an abrasion, become contaminated with infected blood and be used on a susceptible horse. Most bodily secretions and excretions have been found to contain virus and may be relevant in disease transmission. Infected mares may or may not transmit the disease to their foals either in utero or via their milk.

The clinical signs are by no means specific but any case of profound anaemia with subcutaneous oedema should be viewed with suspicion. Sublingual haemorrhages are present in some cases (Steck 1967). Large numbers of monocytes and sideroleucocytes (leucocytes containing haemosiderin pigment) in blood films may also be a suspicious sign but not a specific one. Confirmatory diagnosis is based upon the examination of serum samples by the agar gel immunodiffusion test (AGID or Coggin's test) (Coggins et al. 1972). This test has proved to be 95% reliable in the identification of horses previously infected with EIA and detects precipitating antibodies in the sera 14–38 days after infection. Antibody has been found to persist for at least seven years. For some reason, the immunological mechanism elicited by EIA is defective, in that the horse remains viraemic for life (Gorham et al. 1977). Specific antibodies and cell-mediated immunity suppress viral activity in the intervals between disease episodes and in horses that remain subclinically infected. The immunological mechanisms do, however, play an important part in the production of the pathological signs of anaemia, glomerulonephritis, lymphadenopathy and probably hepatitis.

EIA has been a notifiable disease in the United Kingdom since June 1975 (The Ministry of Agriculture, Infectious Diseases of Horses Order (1975), S1 Number 888). Any suspected case must be notified to the Ministry of Agriculture who will investigate and have the power to place restrictions on horses and carcases and to impose control measures. All clinically suspected and AGID-positive horses should be isolated in an insect-proof area. All in-contact horses should be restricted and subjected to the AGID test. Negative cases should be re-tested after 14 days as it may take time for titres to rise and contacts should not be considered free of infection for at least 28 days after an outbreak is confirmed. A positive AGID test in a sucking foal does not necessarily confirm active infection in that foal. A positive pre-suck sample will confirm infection in utero. A foal that is not infected by a positive dam will have a negative AGID titre by six months of age (Powell 1976).

Infectious equine arteritis

This acute infectious condition is caused by an RNA virus and characterized by fever, conjunctivitis, rhinitis, oedema of the limbs, enteritis and colic. Complications include pneumonia and abortion in mares. The virus is present in the tissues and body fluids and the condition is often fatal. It is not known to occur in the UK. For a description of the condition the reader is referred to Doll et al. (1957) and Doll (1972).

Arbovirus infection

Conditions caused by arboviruses are characterized by nervous symptoms and fever. For a description of these, including Venezuelan, Far Eastern and Western equine encephalomyelitis, see Byrne (1972) and Gibbs (1976).

Reovirus infection

This RNA virus causes African horse sickness, an endemic condition in Africa and the Middle East. It is characterized by fever, pneumonia and swellings of the head, neck and dependent parts. The virus is transmitted by *Culicoides* vectors. For a description of the clinical signs and pathology the reader is referred to Maurer and McCully (1963) and Konnerup et al. (1972).

Bacteria

Streptococcal infections

Members of the genus *Streptococcus* are the most common equine bacterial pathogens. These belong to Lancefield Group C and are haemolytic. Bazeley (1940*a*, *b*, 1942*a*, *b*, 1943) and Bazeley and Battle (1940) divided Group C equine pathogenic streptococci into five types based on colonial and biochemical reactions with three sugars: lactose, trehalose and sorbitol. Type 1 they incriminated as a cause of strangles (see below) and named *Streptococcus equi.* Of the other types the most common is Bazeley's Type 2 (syn. *Str. zooepidemicus*). On blood agar it forms much smaller colonies than *Str. equi,* has a 'sparkling' jewel-like appearance and shows β-haemolysis. This organism may be isolated from suppurative processes involving joints, nasal discharges, abscesses, pneumonia, peritonitis, neoplasia and endometritis and from seminal fluid.

Although these streptococci are probably incapable of initiating infection, they are important as secondary causes of disease. Their clinical significance in any particular lesion must be assessed in relation to other factors and disease processes which may be present. For example, streptococcal bronchopneumonia may develop following primary viral infection and in these circumstances it must be treated as if it were a primary condition.

Most strains of streptococci are sensitive to penicillin, although resistant strains are probably increasing. Cloxacillin, ampicillin and neomycin might therefore be preferred.

Strangles

This is an acute infectious condition of the upper respiratory tract and adjacent lymph nodes.

Aetiology. The cause is *Streptococcus equi,* a Gram-positive coccus occurring in chains and surrounded by capsular material. On blood agar it forms a large (2 mm in diameter) mucoid, honey-coloured colony surrounded by a wide zone of haemolysis. In its most virulent form the colony has a 'matt' appearance. During the mucoid phase the organism is heavily capsulated and the capsule is associated with virulence.

Str. equi belongs to Lancefield Group C and must be identified from other strains of haemolytic streptococci, notably *Str. zooepidemics.* Besides the characteristic appearance of the colonies and the presence of a capsule, *Str. equi* fails to ferment trehalose, lactose and sorbitol, in contrast to *Str. zooepidemicus*, which ferments trehalose and lactose.

Incidence. The distribution of strangles is world-wide, although in recent years the incidence in most countries has declined. In the UK it occurs more often in ponies than Thoroughbreds. The disease is often restricted to horses under four years. The mortality rate is low but complications of purpura haemorrhagica and laryngeal hemiplegia may occur.

Pathogenesis. Str. equi is present in the nasal and abscess discharge of infected animals and contaminates pasture, feed and water mangers. Affected horses can spread infection for at least four weeks after the onset of clinical signs and the organism is relatively resistant so that premises can harbour it for several weeks. Infection, after droplets have been ingested or inhaled, initially causes a pharyngitis and rhinitis. The organism is carried to the local lymph nodes and causes abscesses. Infection may spread to the kidney, liver, spleen, brain and muscles, forming abscesses.

Clinical signs. The incubation period is four to eight days and the disease may start suddenly with anorexia and fever of 39.5–40.5°C. A serous nasal discharge, becoming purulent, develops within about 24 hours. The pharyngitis and laryngitis may cause difficult swallowing, regurgitation of food through the nostrils and a soft, moist cough. Characteristic abscesses develop in the pharyngeal and submandibular lymph nodes, causing swellings of considerable size. The affected nodes become hot, swollen and painful and may obstruct swallowing and respiration. By about the fifth day from onset the glands begin to 'sweat' and a few days later rupture to discharge a thick, creamy-yellow pus. Fever may continue until the abscesses rupture.

Occasionally abscesses may burst into the pharynx or develop on various parts of the body, such as the face, limbs and hind-quarters.

Various complications occur due to metastatic abscesses in parenchymatous organs; pneumonia, peritonitis, paralysis, nervous excitability and emaciation may develop.

Diagnosis. Nasal discharge, swellings in the head and neck region and fever are suggestive and the diagnosis may be confirmed by isolation of *Str. equi* from nasal and abscess discharges. Respiratory viral infections may cause similar clinical signs.

Treatment. Practitioners have differing views on treatment. Some claim excellent results with the early use of large quantities of penicillin (an initial dose of 5–10 megaunits of crystalline penicillin intravenously maintained thereafter with 6 million units of procaine penicillin daily). Others have found that the use of antibiotics increases the likelihood of chronic 'metastatic' spread producing 'bastard' strangles. If possible, it is better to treat the abscesses locally with hot fomentations until they burst or are ready to be lanced. Premature surgical intervention is contraindicated. After rupture, the abscess cavity should be washed out with a weak antiseptic solution.

In cases of acute dyspnoea and cyanosis due to mechanical respiratory obstruction, a tracheotomy may be necessary.

General measures include a soft palatable diet and a clean, dry and warm atmosphere, which is well ventilated. The horse should not be exercised until at least ten days after signs subside.

Control. Infected animals should be isolated immediately. Bedding should be burnt and utensils thoroughly disinfected.

A vaccine may be prepared but several antigenic strains of the organism can occur. Vaccines containing organisms obtained from a current outbreak or in endemic strains are the most reliable: four- to six-hour cultures killed by heat not exceeding 56°C are most effective. The vaccine is administered in gradually increasing doses two or three times at 10–14-day intervals.

Tetanus (lockjaw)

This is a neuromuscular disorder caused by a specific neurotoxin.

Aetiology. The cause is *Clostridum tetani,* a Gram-positive, anaerobic, sporulating and toxin-producing bacillus.

Incidence. Cases occur sporadically and the disease is endemic on certain fields or farms. Foals are particularly susceptible in the first seven weeks post-partum due to umbilical infection.

Pathogenesis. The organism is present in soil and faeces. It enters the body through a wound and develops away from air under scabs, in abscesses (e.g. in the umbilical vein of newborn foal) or in deeply penetrating wounds where it produces a neurotoxin. The toxin is thought to migrate along peripheral nerve trunks to reach the central nervous system. Here it causes an exaggerated nervous response resulting in spasms of flexor and extensor muscle groups.

Clinical signs. The usual incubation period is five to 21 days but spores may remain dormant in the tissues for months and become activated by changes due to trauma or other semipathological processes which produce conditions suitable for anaerobic development. Signs usually start as stiffness causing the horse to move reluctantly and in 'one piece' when turned (Fig. 7.3). Head and ears are extended, the tail slightly raised and the affected horse soon shows evidence of muscular spasms, when stimulated by sound, light or touch. Sweating, flaring nostrils, inability to swallow and dyspnoea may develop within 24–48 hours of onset. Painful spasms affect the muscles of mastication and make eating difficult. Saliva may drool from the mouth. The horse may become recumbent or fall over and once down is unable to get up. In recumbency the muscular spasms are accentuated and opisthotonus evident. Death occurs in about 70% of cases, due to exhaustion, circulatory failure and pneumonia.

Diagnosis. Clinical signs and the characteristic spasm of nictitating membranes when the face is tapped lightly differentiate the condition from injury to the thoracic and lumbar spine or associated structures, strychnine poisoning and myoglobinuria (azoturia).

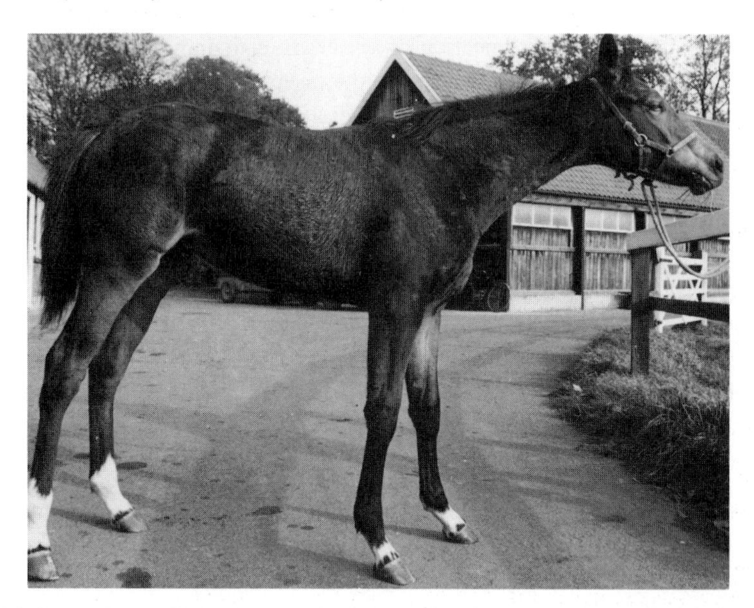

Fig. 7.3. A yearling suffering from tetanus. Note that the head is extended, the tail slightly raised, food held in the mouth and the ears directed forward.

Treatment. Antibiotics, e.g. penicillin 10 megaunits intramuscularly twice a day, and 10 000–20 000 units of tetanus antitoxin serum should be given. The serum neutralizes excess toxin but cannot affect that already attached to the nervous tissue. The skin and hooves should be searched for wounds and these should be cleansed of scabs and necrotic material. After debridement the wounds should be washed with hydrogen peroxide and, if necessary, covered with an antiseptic dressing.

Muscular spasms may be controlled by the intravenous or intramuscular injection of tranquillizers such as acetylpromazine or chlorpromazine every three hours. Mephenesin may be administered through a stomach tube in doses up to 15 g three times a day.

Water, at regular intervals, at the rate of 1 litre/10 kg body weight/day, may be administered through an oesophageal tube. The tube can be left in situ and the proximal end sutured to the skin overlying the side of the face and poll region. Glucose and skimmed cow's milk, liquid paraffin or gruel made by sifting oats soaked in water may be given, but care should be taken to avoid causing diarrhoea. Intravenous normal saline is indicated if dehydration develops.

Affected horses should be placed in a cool, darkened, quiet stable. Bed-sores should be dressed with antiseptic and emollient ointment. Therapy should continue until the spasms abate and the horse is able to get up and down without assistance. It may be necessary to continue therapy for several weeks and euthanasia is indicated if the individual fails to respond.

Muylle et al. (1975) describe the treatment of tetanus in the horse by injections of tetanus antitoxin into the subarachnoid space. Forty affected horses were immobilized by intravenous injection of a solution containing 5% glycerylguaiacol ether and 10% glucose. The area between the occipital protuberance and the atlas was shaved and thoroughly disinfected. The cisterna magna was penetrated with an 18 gauge spinal needle and about 50 ml of CSF was withdrawn with a syringe; 50 ml of tetanus antitoxin (1000 units per ml) was slowly injected into the subarachnoid space. In foals 30 ml of CSF was replaced with 30 ml of tetanus antitoxin. In addition, horses were given 3000 units of tetanus antitoxin subcutaneously and 20 000 units of long-acting penicillin per 100 kg body weight intramuscularly. Supportive treatment and sedation were also used. In all the horses that recovered, disease stabilized immediately after the injection. The results (77.5% recovery) were much better than in a previous series of horses with tetanus (50% recovery), in which tetanus antitoxin was injected intravenously, intramuscularly or in the epidural space.

Prevention. Tetanus toxoid provides substantial protection. An initial dose followed by a booster at four weeks and thereafter annually will protect horses over the age of three months. Foals under three months can be protected by immunizing their dams and administering a booster dose within a month of foaling. Alternatively, 1500 units of tetanus antitoxin, given within three days of birth and repeated three to four weeks later, will protect the newborn foal until it can receive toxoid.

Tetanus antitoxin 1500 units subcutaneously or intramuscularly gives temporary protection in non-immunized subjects for three to four weeks.

Glanders

An infectious condition of most mammalian species including man, although primarily a disease of horses (Hickman 1970), the disease has not been present in the UK since 1928 and is rare on the American continent.

Glanders is caused by a Gram-negative bacillus *Pfeifferella mallei.* Natural infection probably occurs by ingestion and once the disease is introduced into a susceptible population it spreads very rapidly. The incubation period is longer than six months.

Two clinical types occur, one in which the lungs are always affected and the other, farcy, in which skin lesions are present. However, the two types usually exist together. Lung lesions consist of rounded, firm nodules in the lung parenchyma. These have a whitish centre, dark red periphery and a central core of pus.

Nodules may also occur on the nasal mucosa and trachea and in the mandibular lymph nodes. Skin lesions consist of swelling in the subcutaneous tissue, especially the extremities and flanks. Lymphangitis and ulcerated skin are characteristic and the enlarged lymphatic glands are known as 'farcy buds'.

Diagnosis is based on finding the glanders bacilli in fresh lesions and on the mallein test.

For the intradermopalpebral test, 0.1 ml of mallein is injected into the skin of the lower eyelid and examination of the site of injection is made after 24 and 48 hours. A positive reaction is indicated by a marked oedematous swelling of the eyelid and there may be a purulent discharge from the inner canthus or conjunctival sac. The reaction which is usually accompanied by a rise of temperature may persist for several days.

In the ophthalmic test a drop is instilled into the eye at the canthus. In an infected animal the eyelids and sometimes the side of the face become swollen and there may be a certain amount of discharge from the eye; the reaction may also occur, to a lesser extent, in the non-injected eye.

Al-Kafawi et al. (1977) describe the haematological changes in three Arabian stallions suffering from the chronic form of the infection. The horses were anaemic (RBC = $4.32 \pm 1.17 \times 10^{12}$/litre, Hb = 6.83 ± 0.76 g/dl, PCV = 0.22 ± 0.02 litre/litre) and showed a total leucocytosis ($13.88 \pm 4.11 \times 10^9$/litre) and neutrophilia ($10.21 \pm 3.44 \times 10^9$/litre).

Salmonellosis

Salmonellosis is principally a disease of young foals, causing severe and often fatal enteritis. Abortion caused by *Salmonella abortivoequina* is also recorded (see p. 199). Salmonellosis in older horses is unusual but has occasionally been reported as an epizootic in veterinary hospitals (Dorn et al. 1975).

The organisms are Gram-negative bacilli which are motile and fail to ferment lactose. About 300 strains exist and identification rests on serological techniques of agglutination. In the horse, *S. typhimurium* is the most common pathogenic member of the group. It is particularly prevalent in horses up to about 12 months old. The organism, as its name suggests, is a parasite of rodents which presumably act as a reservoir of infection for horses and other animals.

The characteristic disease is an acute enteritis with blood-stained diarrhoea, fever and acute colic. In cases that recover, diarrhoea persists for five to ten days, although some individuals may suffer chronically and act as carriers. It has been suggested that symptomless carriers may occur in the horse population rather more frequently than suspected and stressful situations, e.g. housing, surgery, worming, farriery, etc., may, on occasions, stimulate the production of the acute condition (Owen 1975).

Roberts and English (1979) report that about 5–10% of the horse population in the USA is, or has been, infected, and may remain asymptomatic carriers or sporadic faecal shedders. They also report that at the Queensland Veterinary School almost 10% of hospitalized horses are carriers or intermittent excretors, although no clinical cases of salmonellosis have been seen. Ingram and Edwards (1980) report that the Royal Veterinary College, London, have also experienced deaths of horses from *Salmonella* infections following surgical procedures. During 1975–7 at post-mortem examination they cultured sites in 85 horses that had died from a variety of causes other than salmonellosis. Salmonellae were found in one or more sites in 17. The mucous membranes of the caecum and large colon were the predominant sites and there were no macroscopic lesions in the intestines. These authors suggest that 20% of the horses examined were carriers of salmonellae. Over the same period daily faecal samples were examined from 300 horses after surgical procedures; 15 excreted salmonellae in their faeces. Excretion began shortly after the operation and persisted usually for only a few days. In none was the faecal shedding of salmonellae associated with enteric or other clinical signs. These results suggested that carrier horses are mainly intermittent shedders and that the stress of surgical procedures may result in transient excretion of the organisms. It is suggested that tetracycline therapy, under these conditions, may exacerbate the problem by removing the normal intestinal bacterial antagonists of *Salmonella.* Colitis X (see p. 468) may be part of the same syndrome.

Jensen (1959) reported two outbreaks of salmonellosis on separate premises which were connected in that a mare and foal had been moved from one stud farm to the other. Faecal examination revealed that two mares were carriers but clinical signs were confined to foals, three of which died. Carriers ceased to excrete the organism after two months and the source of infection was found to be a leaking drain which had contaminated the paddock. We know of one outbreak in the Newmarket area in which a human carrier was involved.

Diagnosis is confirmed by recovery of *Salmonella* in the faeces. This is much easier in acute cases than in chronic ones or suspected carriers (Graham et al. 1920). These authors recovered salmonellae in only 22% of spontaneous clinical cases of horses with suspected enteric salmonellosis. Post-mortem examination reveals the mucosa of the large intestines to be haemorrhagic and the mesenteric lymph nodes enlarged and acutely congested. Salmonellae may be cultured from the intestinal lymph nodes.

When a case of salmonellosis is suspected or confirmed, strict isolation, disinfection and hygiene procedures must be used. In view of the risk to public health, attendants should be instructed to take care with personal hygiene. Attempts should be made to investigate the source of the infection and useful help may be obtained from local agriculture and public health authorities.

The success of treatment directed towards eliminating salmonellae from the gastrointestinal tract, lymph nodes and major organ systems has not been encouraging or consistent (Roberts & English 1979). Local and/or systemic specific antimicrobial treatment, based on in vitro antibiotic sensitivity tests, usually fails to prevent chronic shedding and in many cases has little effect on the course of the clinical disease. Clinical recovery is more likely when vigorous supportive therapy and nursing are employed, even though animals may remain faecal excretors.

For a review of equine salmonellosis see Gibbons (1980).

Brucellosis

Clinical manifestations of *Brucella abortus* infection in horses are comparatively rare but serological surveys have shown significant serum titres in 15% of horses in the UK, Ireland, the Netherlands and Australia (Denny 1972, 1973). Van der Hoeden (1964) described symptoms of intermittent fever, laziness and general weakness. He found that a high percentage of horses with fistulous withers and poll evil had significant titres and he cultured *Brucella* from the lesions. Cosgrove (1961) incriminated *Brucella abortus* in intermittent lameness characterized by inflammation of the bursae and tendon sheaths. Brucellosis has been reported as a cause of stallion infertility by Vandeplassche and Devos (1960) and of abortion by McCaughey and Kerr (1967) and Hinton et al. (1977). The latter case involved a mare who had developed a painful swelling of the right stifle joint when about eight months pregnant. She subsequently gave birth to a normal foal. During the next pregnancy, the right stifle joint again became swollen and painful and at about 8 months of pregnancy she aborted dead twins. *Brucella abortus* was isolated in pure culture from the fetal stomach and serological examinations of the mare revealed an active infection.

Denny (1972) surveyed 232 animals presented at the University of Bristol School of Veterinary Science between September 1969 and October 1970; 7.8% had serum agglutination titres of 1 in 40 (80 IU) or more and 2% were considered active cases of *Brucella* infection. The author found cattle to be the main source of infection and recognized a general form of equine brucellosis in which there was stiffness, fluctuating temperature and lethargy. Infection became local and the organism was twice cultured from joints.

Diagnosis was made on titres of greater than 1 in 40, but for a positive diagnosis Denny considered that a rising titre should be demonstrated. He advocated a repeat serum agglutination test seven to 14 days after the original test.

Dawson and Durrant (1975) and Dawson (1977) have described serological reactions to *Brucella* antigen in the horse. They conclude that the Rose Bengal plate test (RBPT), which is extensively used as a screening test for cattle, may have some value as a simple test. The RBPT, the serum-agglutination test (SAT), the complement-fixation test (CFT) and the antiglobulin (Coombs') test (AGT) were not always conclusive in any particular case and the use of all four tests, if possible, was advised. The AGT and CFT gave a higher proportion of diagnostic positive titres then the SAT. The AGT was a more sensitive indicator of exposure to infection and it is also simpler to perform than the CFT, assuming standardization of antiglobulin supplies. Titres suggestive of positive infection were SAT > 4/40; CFT > 2/4; AGT > 4/160. SAT of 2/20 to 3/40 and AGT of 1/40 to 3/160 were considered inconclusive and titres of 1/20 for SAT and 3/20 for AGT were non-significant.

Treatment may be attempted with:

1. British Ministry of Agriculture equine vaccine (Duff 1936).
2. Strain 19 vaccine (Cosgrove 1961; Millar 1961). However, this vaccine may cause severe reaction at the site of injection.
3. Broad-spectrum antibiotics, such as chloramphenicol and oxytetracycline (Daykin 1960).
4. Surgical intervention where an abscess is located.

Tuberculosis

This chronic disease affects all mammalian species, but is of diminishing incidence. Horses are comparatively resistant and pathologically the disease takes a rather different form from that in other domesticated animals and in man (Innes 1949). Caseation is rare and lesions are usually prolific, affecting the lungs, liver, spleen and bone. Tumour-like lesions appear in the liver and spleen as firm, well circumscribed, whitish masses up to several centimetres in diameter (Bostock & Owen 1975). Their cut surface has an obviously fibrous appearance but usually contains a number of tiny foci of yellowish necrosis. Similar lesions are also present in the mesenteric lymph nodes. The histological appearance is typical of a granulomatous inflammatory reaction but acid-fast organisms are usually difficult to find.

If the cervical vertebrae are affected they produce a characteristic sign of a stiff or a 'kinked' neck. Clinical signs include a persistent fever and increasing loss of weight and respiratory rate.

Diagnosis is difficult because the intradermal and subcutaneous tuberculin tests are unreliable and produce false positives and negatives.

PARASITES

Our account of parasitology is confined to aspects of particular practical significance and importance to practitioners. For a detailed description the reader should consult Lapage (1968), Soulsby (1968) and Ogborne and Duncan (1977).

Endoparasites

There is a general belief that some endoparasites are always more harmful than others; for example that *Strongylus vulgaris* is more pathogenic than *Parascaris equorum.* Although this is true in most instances, individual host tolerance and managerial factors may alter usual roles. For instance, ascarids may cause rupture of the caecum and the relatively less harmful small strongyle may ulcerate the foal's colon. The clinician must balance the circumstances of individual situations against a knowledge of the usual life cycle and pathogenicity of various equine parasites. Tables 7.3 and 7.4 set out the main endoparasites affecting horses, and the life history of the major groups is summarized in Figs 7.4 and 7.5.

TABLE 7.3 Common equine endoparasites

Genus	*Species*	*Size* (mm)	*Habitat* Adult	*Habitat* Parasitic larva
Subfamily strongylinae				
Strongylus	*equinus*	26–47	Caecum and colon	Wall of caecum and colon, liver
Strongylus	*edentatus*	23–44	Caecum and colon	Subperitoneal nodules and mesentery
Strongylus	*vulgaris*	14–24	Caecum and colon	Cranial mesenteric artery
Triodontophorus	*tenuicollis*	9–25	Right dorsal colon	
Craterostomum	*acuticaudatum*	9–11	Colon and caecum	
Oesophagondontus	*robustus*	13–22	Large intestine	
Subfamily trichoneminae				
Trichonema		4–26	Colon	Nodules in wall of large intestine
Poteriostomum		9–21	Colon	Nodules in wall of large intestine
Trichostrongylus	*axei*	4–7	Stomach	Mucosa of stomach

TABLE 7.4 Common equine endoparasites

Genus	*Species*	*Size* (mm)	*Habitat* Adult	*Habitat* Parasitic larva
Dictyocaulus	*arnfieldi*	36–60	Bronchi and air passages	Intestines, lymph, heart, lungs
Onchocerca	*cervicalis*	140	Ligamentum nuchae	Blood
Setaria	*equina*	50–150	Peritoneal cavity, scrotum, lungs	Blood
Anoplocephala	*magna*	800	Small and large intestines	Intermediate host
Anoplocephala	*perfoliata*	80	Small and large intestines	Intermediate host
Paranoplocephala	*mamillana*	6–50	Stomach and small intestine	Intermediate host
Parascaris	*equorum*	150–500	Small intestine and caecum	Liver, lungs (kidneys)

Strongyles (red worm) (Figs 7.6, 7.7, 7.8)

The direct life cycle of these parasites makes them reasonably susceptible to practical measures of control, the essence of which is to reduce the number of infective larvae on pastures grazed by susceptible stock, i.e. particularly horses under three years of age. There is evidence that both age and acquired immunity to *Strongylus vulgaris* infection develops in horses under field conditions, but as this immunity is not complete control measures are necessary throughout a horse's life (Duncan 1975).

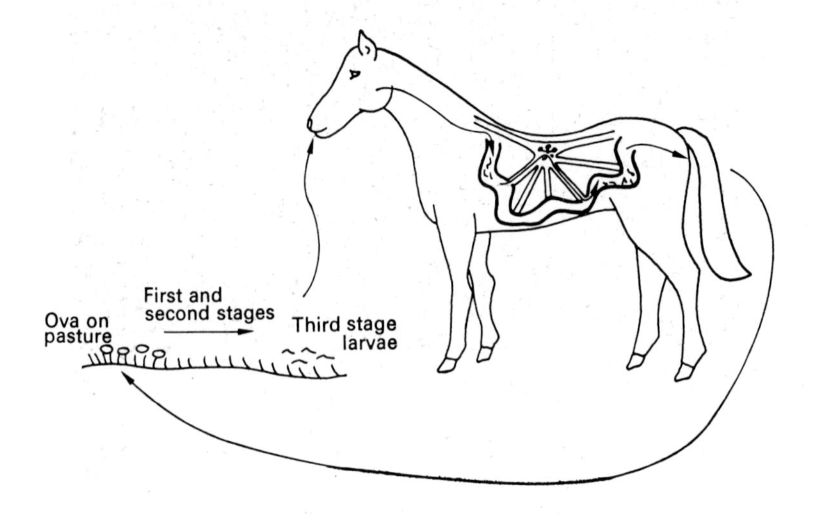

Fig. 7.4. The life cycle of *Strongylus vulgaris.* Third-stage (infective) larvae penetrate the large and small intestines. After a week they enter the submucosal arteries and migrate to the mesenteric root, where they develop for about four months and return to the intestine. After forming nodules in the intestinal wall they enter the lumen and become sexually mature in the colon about six months after entering the host. (*After Duncan 1973*)

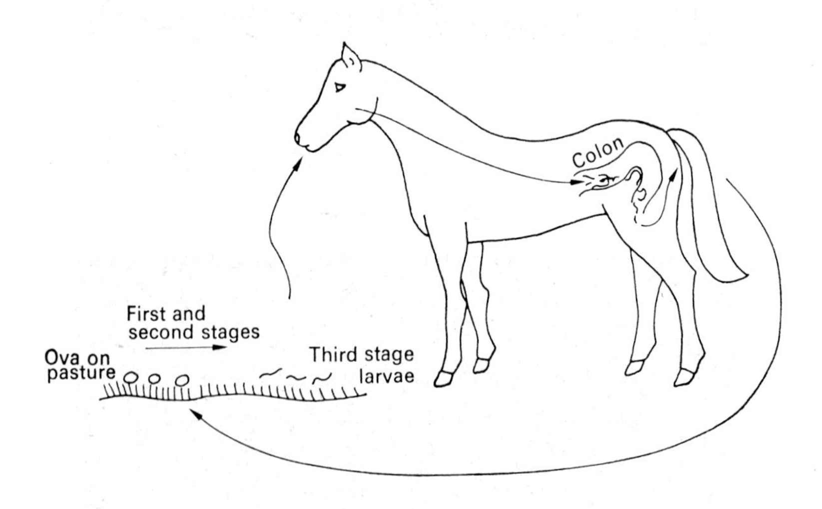

Fig. 7.5. The life cycle of *Strongylus edentatus.* Third-stage larvae moult and burrow into the colon wall forming nodules. The larvae stay in the nodules for a month or so, burrow back into the colon wall, and then break into the lumen as adult worms. Adults and ova pass out in the faeces.

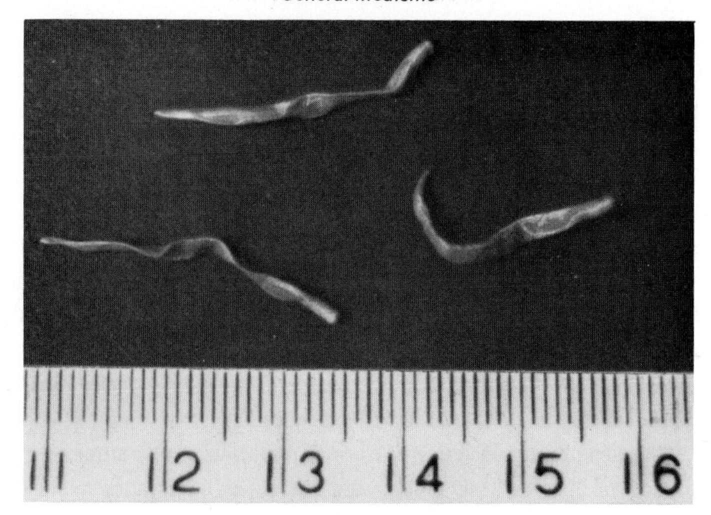

Fig. 7.6. *Strongylus edentatus.*

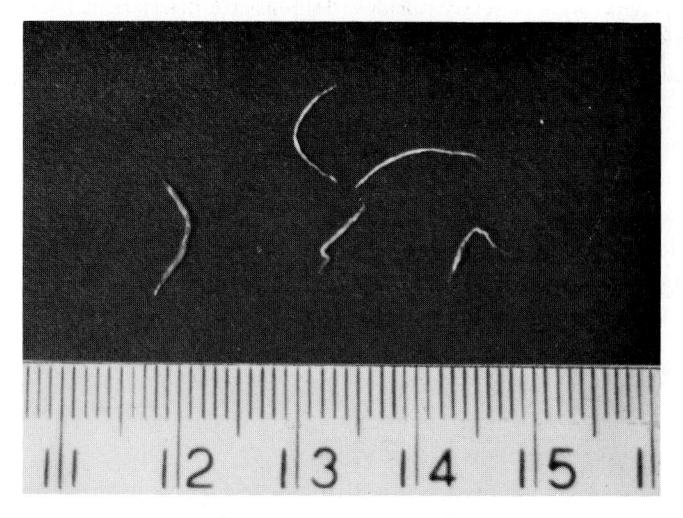

Fig. 7.7. *Strongylus vulgaris.*

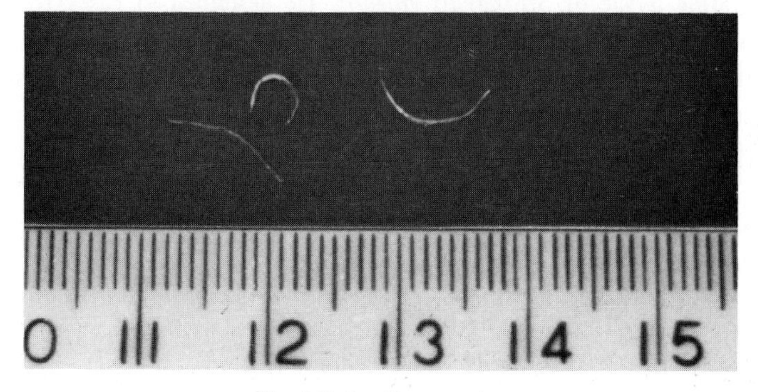

Fig. 7.8. Small strongyles.

Strongylus vulgaris is the species which causes most clinical problems (Drudge 1979). Administration of large numbers of larvae to worm-free foals produces a very acute clinical syndrome within one to three weeks of infection (Duncan 1974). Clinical signs are marked pyrexia, anorexia and severe colic, with death due to infarction of the small and large intestinal wall. This acute syndrome is not often seen under field conditions as immunological factors of continual challenge by mixed strongyle infections (Duncan 1975) and commonly practised anthelmintic programmes afford protection. The adult worms cause damage to the intestinal mucosa by their feeding habits, resulting in the formation of crater-like ulcers and damage (Duncan 1974). This damage may cause anaemia, unthriftiness and poor performance. The most serious clinical problems seen in practice are, however, caused by the migratory activities of the developing larval stages (Drudge 1972; Duncan 1974). The common lesion is an inflammation of the anterior mesenteric and ileocaecocolic arteries frequently referred to as 'verminous aneurysm'. This lesion, in fact, is usually a thrombosis and marked thickening of the arterial wall and thus may be more correctly called 'verminous arteritis' (Wright 1972; Slocombe et al. 1977). Inflammation at this site and infarction of the intestine caused by thrombosis and embolism of branches of the ileocaecocolic artery are responsible for many cases of acute and low-grade recurrent colic amongst horses.

Duncan and Pirie (1972) followed the migratory route of *S. vulgaris* larvae in nine worm-free pony foals, killed at intervals over a period of nine months. They found that infective larvae exsheath and penetrate the intestine within a few days of infection. These larvae then moult into the submucosa, penetrate small arteries and have migrated within the lumina of intestinal arteries to the anterior mesenteric site by 14 days. In the predilection site larvae develop from early to late first stage and after three to four months the first moult is completed and young adults return to the intestine through the lumina of the arteries. Nodules are formed with the subsequent release of young adults into the intestinal lumen. The migration is complete six to seven months after infection.

Greatorex (1975) has described a diarrhoeic syndrome, with ulceration of the colonic and caecal mucosae, which may be caused by thromboembolism associated with migrating larvae of *Strongylus vulgaris*. He described 91 cases, the majority of which had a history of diarrhoea of sudden or gradual onset which had been present for weeks or months. Others had a history of acute diarrhoea with associated shock. Post-mortem examination of 35 cases showed areas of necrosis and ulceration of the mucosa of the colon and caecum. There was evidence of *S. vulgaris* larval migration and thromboembolic vascular disease in the intestinal arterial system of these horses. The degree and extent of necrotic and ulcerative lesions varied according to the duration of the case.

It is unlikely that any individual can be kept completely free of strongyle infection if allowed access to pasture. It may even be harmful to rear individuals free from infection, because there is evidence that tolerance is developed after initial infection (Duncan 1975). Experimental studies showed that some immune mechanism develops in horses reared under worm-free conditions until three years of age. In another controlled experiment involving naturally infected horses, acquired resistance to infection was demonstrated, since the naturally infected cases showed no clinical abnormalities and no evidence of significant arteritis lesions following experimental infection. The control animals showed typical signs of acute infection with pyrexia, anorexia and colic and a severe arterial lesion at post-mortem

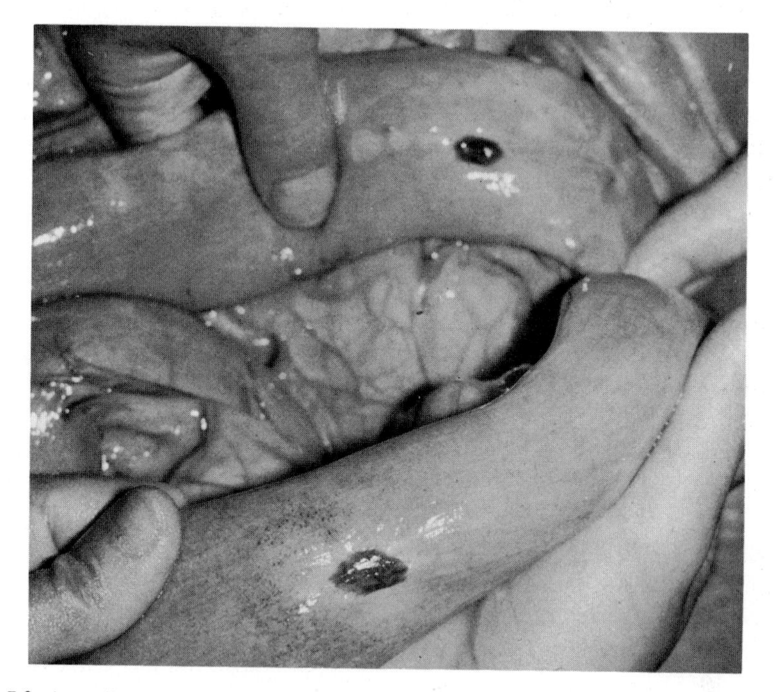

Fig. 7.9. A small intestine exteriorized at laparotomy, showing subserosal haemorrhage caused by the migration of strongyle larvae.

examination. It is clear that immunity is not complete, as there is a high field incidence of infection with both adult and immature parasites. Several possibilities exist to explain this deficit:

1. Challenge by *S. vulgaris* infection in very young foals may cause a degree of acquired immunological unresponsiveness which persists into adult life.

2. *S. vulgaris* larvae found in arterial lesions of field cases may have been inhibited in their development and thus may remain in the arteries for considerable period.

3. Heavy field infections with other strongyles may interfere with the normal operation of the immune mechanisms in the gastrointestinal mucosa, causing a degree of immunosuppression which allows the development and maturation of a proportion of *S. vulgaris* larvae in an otherwise immune animal.

Diagnosis is thus not concerned with whether or not a horse is parasitized but with whether the dynamic equilibrium of the host–parasite relationship is satisfactory. Faecal worm egg counts (see p. 528) performed on individuals are of little value as figures reflect only the egg-laying activity of the adult worms in the intestines at that particular moment. Heavily parasitized horses may have very low counts and *vice versa.* Serial examinations on all the horses on a premises or representative batches is, however, a very useful guide to the efficiency of the over-all worm control programme. In individual cases of suspected disease, clinical signs and the results of haematological and blood biochemical examinations are of greater value (see pp. 520, 521 and 525). The presence of anaemia, eosinophilia and raised beta-globulin are highly suggestive of serious arterial disease.

Treatment

Treatment must be designed in two ways: first the routine and regular treatment of all horses as an attempt to maintain a satisfactory host–parasite relationship and secondly the 'emergency' treatment of heavily parasitized animals where the host–parasite relationship is acting to the detriment of the host and clinical symptoms are present.

Routine worm control. The most important aspect of control is to avoid situations in which individuals, especially young animals, are subjected to high levels of infestation. The following measures, based on personal experience and on recommendations from various authorities, are presented as a basis for control on stud farms which are grazed by relatively large numbers of horses each year.

Regular administration of anthelmintic drugs such as thiabendazole (Round 1968), mebendazole (Walker & Knight 1972), fenbendazole (McBeath et al. 1978) and pyrantel embonate (Lyons et al. 1975) helps to reduce the adults in the large intestine and the number of eggs passed in the faeces. Phenothiazine (Poynter & Hughes 1958) was a useful drug, either monthly or in small daily doses (Gibson 1960), but is now seldom used because of its risk of liver toxity. Newly acquired horses should be treated on arrival and all horses on the premises should be treated monthly as a routine (Duncan 1976). There is evidence that *S. vulgaris* can become resistant to anthelmintic drugs (Drudge & Elam 1961; Round et al. 1974) and thus it is important that the anthelmintics used are varied between those of the thiabendazole group and pyrantel embonate. Routine examination of faecal samples on all animals on the stud farm, at least twice a year, preferably in spring and mid-summer, will check that control is effective and resistance has been avoided.

Stud farms cannot avoid the problems of parasitic disease by anthelmintic treatment programmes alone. Sensible grazing and the maintenance of 'clean' pastures are essential. Strongyle eggs develop into infective larvae only during the period March to October (Duncan 1976) and development is most rapid during summer. Infective larvae can survive the winter but in spring there is a rapid disappearance of larvae from pastures with increasing ambient temperatures. The two sources of infection for susceptible animals are thus over-wintered larvae and larvae which develop from eggs passed by other infected horses during the early grazing season. Over-wintered larvae on the pastures die out by June and thus the latter is the most important source. High levels of infective larvae may accumulate during the summer on pastures grazed by horses but regular and effective monthly dosing will reduce this contamination. There is little point in dosing foals under two months of age as the pre-patent period of the small strongyles varies between eight and ten weeks and their developmental stages have not been shown to be susceptible to most anthelmintics (Duncan 1974). When a paddock has been grazed for a number of years by infected horses, ploughing and re-seeding will reduce the pasture larvae population to a minimum. If this is not practical, the paddock should be rested until the summer months (June) by which time the over-wintered larval population will have largely disappeared. Young animals should not be allowed access to such pasture before July/August and, where possible, 'clean' paddocks should be provided for nursing mares and foals. In-foal and nursing mares should be treated before going out to grass and routinely throughout the grazing season. Manual removal of faeces from paddocks ('dropping picking') once or twice weekly and mixed grazing with cattle or sheep are very useful in reducing pasture contamination. 'Vacuum cleaner' attachments for tractors are available to aid the mechanization of 'dropping picking'.

Severely parasitized cases. Routine monthly treatment with manufacturers' recommended doses of anthelmintic drugs kills adult worms in the intestinal lumen but, in general, has little effect on the migrating larval stages. With thiabendazole and fenbendazole, markedly increased doses can be larvicidal. Drudge (1972) recommends that a single dose of 440 mg/kg thiabendazole on each of two successive days may be effective if administered early in the course of infection. Horses treated in this manner within two weeks of experimental infection responded dramatically, but after this the comparative refractoriness of late fourth- and fifth-stage larvae, present in aneurysms, presents a problem. In our experience, this dose regimen has been extremely useful but owners should be warned that untoward effects cannot be ruled out. In our experience, some treated horses may become dull and anorexic for two or three days after treatment.

We have heard of cases where treatment may have precipitated a 'larval shower' and fatal intestinal thromboembolic infarction. On general principles, one imagines that the death of large numbers of larvae in various tissue sites might lead to serious local reaction and even possibly allergic or anaphylactic manifestations.

In cases where signs of serious intestinal damage, with acute or low-grade repetitive colic, are seen, such treatment may not be successful. Many of these cases eventually require laparotomy either for exploration or as an emergency treatment. Pearson et al. (1975) analysed 140 laparotomy cases and found that 50% of the cases regarded as inoperable resulted from parasitic larval migration. The removal of a section of infarcted small intestine may on occasions be a 'surgical' success. The primary cranial mesenteric arteritis will, however, remain and most of these cases will either fail to thrive or return with another section of infarcted small intestine.

Greatorex (1975) suggests that the treatment of diarrhoea associated with ulceration of the colon and/or caecum is difficult and is only practical under hospital conditions. Treatment may take weeks or even months and temporary lapses are common.

The cost of drugs and intensive care may be considerable and uneconomic in many cases. Nevertheless, Greatorex has had some success in these difficult cases by using blood transfusions and fluid and electrolytes intravenously and orally to combat shock and circulatory collapse. Oxygen inhalation was given if there were signs of anoxia. Intravenous bicarbonate and Ringer's lactate solution were given to correct acidosis. Proprietary amino acid and lipid solutions (Aminosol and Intralipid) were given intravenously and orally to provide nutrition. To combat the thrombo-occlusive vascular lesions associated with the intestinal ulcers, anti-coagulants were given, but Greatorex obtained greater success with 6% Dextran-70 in dextrose (Macrodex). The treatment was not without untoward reactions and was given slowly and with great caution. Chalk, light kaolin, chlorodyne and powdered catechu were given orally to protect inflamed intestinal mucosae and a strained suspension of normal horse faeces to correct derangements of the intestinal bacterial flora. Stables were kept scrupulously clean and disinfected and the tail and hind-quarters were frequently washed, powdered and dried. Cases that would eat were allowed hay only at first, then supplemented gradually with oats, bran and high protein cubes. Warmed water was allowed ad lib.

Ascarids (roundworms) (Figs 7.10, 7.11)

Parascaris equorum infection is common in foals, yearlings and horses under three years of age. The rate of infection in foals is close to 100% (Clayton 1978) but clinical disease is rarely seen because of successful anthelmintic control measures and age immunity.

The life cycle is shown diagramatically in Fig. 7.10. Immature eggs are passed in the faeces and may become infective within ten days. If environmental temperature is less than 10°C the eggs may remain viable for many years because of their thick three-layered protective shell. The infective ensheathed second-stage larva hatches from the egg after ingestion by a suitable host. The larvae penetrate the intestinal wall and reach the liver within 48 hours where they remain for several days. From seven to 14 days after infection the larvae travel to the lungs, probably by way of the circulatory system. They migrate towards the larger airways and up the trachea into the mouth and are then swallowed and return to the small intestine. The migratory phase is completed within four weeks and the worms then grow for about ten weeks, increasing in length from 2 mm to about 20 cm. Preferred sites for growth and development are the duodenum and proximal jejunum, but heavy infestations may be found throughout the length of the small intestine. With large infestations, many of the worms die and are passed out in the faeces, often in a partially digested state. Under natural conditions ascarid eggs first appear in the eggs from 80 days of age onwards suggesting that infections are acquired very soon after birth. Eggs found in faeces prior to this age are probably a result of coprophagia of dam's droppings. These immature eggs pass through the foal's intestinal tract unchanged.

During their migration, ascarid larvae cause small subcapsular haemorrhages in the liver which resolve in one or two weeks. Small white rounded or irregular lesions appear beneath the capsule or within the hepatic parenchyma. These also resolve but new ones appear with repeated infection. Narrow migration tracts, surrounded by eosinophils, may be seen on microscopic examination. Lesions

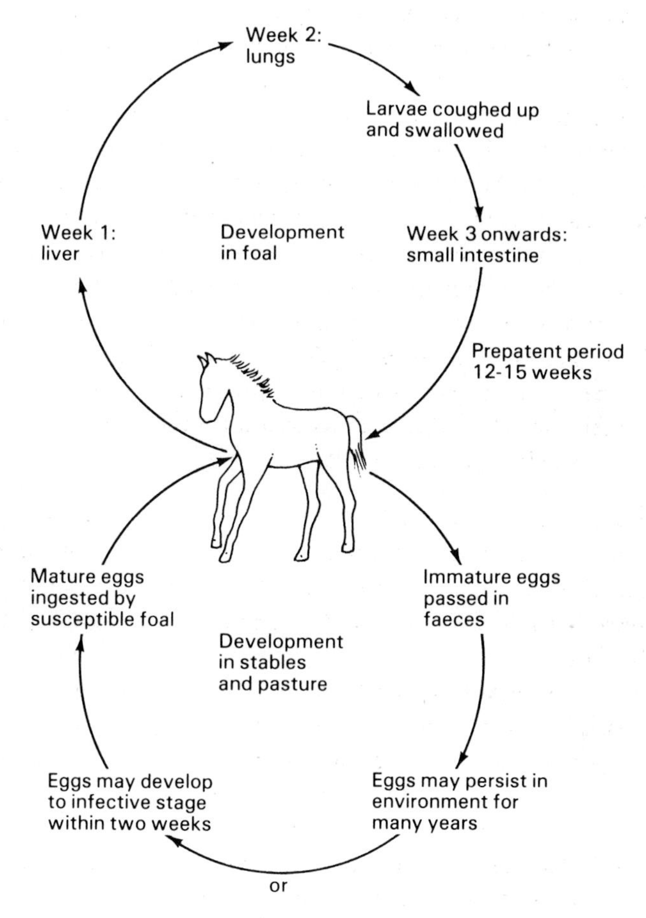

Fig. 7.10. The life cycle of *Parascaris equorum.* (*After Clayton 1978*)

eventually become replaced by fibrous tissue which is accompanied by a lymphocytic infiltration. These lesions may be seen grossly as small white spots. Penetration of the lungs causes petechial and ecchymotic haemorrhages on the surface and within the substance of the lungs. Microscopically oedema and eosinophil infiltrations and then perivascular and peribronchiolar lymphocytic accumulations may be seen. From the fourth to the sixth week after infection, subpleural lymphocytic nodules may be seen scattered over the surfaces of the lungs. They appear grey or greenish, slightly raised and may measure up to 1 cm in diameter. These nodules may be a reflection of an immunological reaction and may contain dead or dying larvae surrounded by lymphocytes and fibrous tissue.

Clinical signs include pyrexia, cough, nasal discharge, nervous disturbances, colic and unthriftiness. Occasionally, a tangled mass of adults in the small intestine has been reported, causing impaction, rupture and peritonitis.

Haematological changes are not specific but include an eosinophilia, proportional to the magnitude of the infection, and occurring 10–14 days after infection.

Diagnosis, as in the case of *Strongylus vulgaris,* is a matter of assessment of the host–parasite relationship. The number of ascarid worm eggs in an individual's

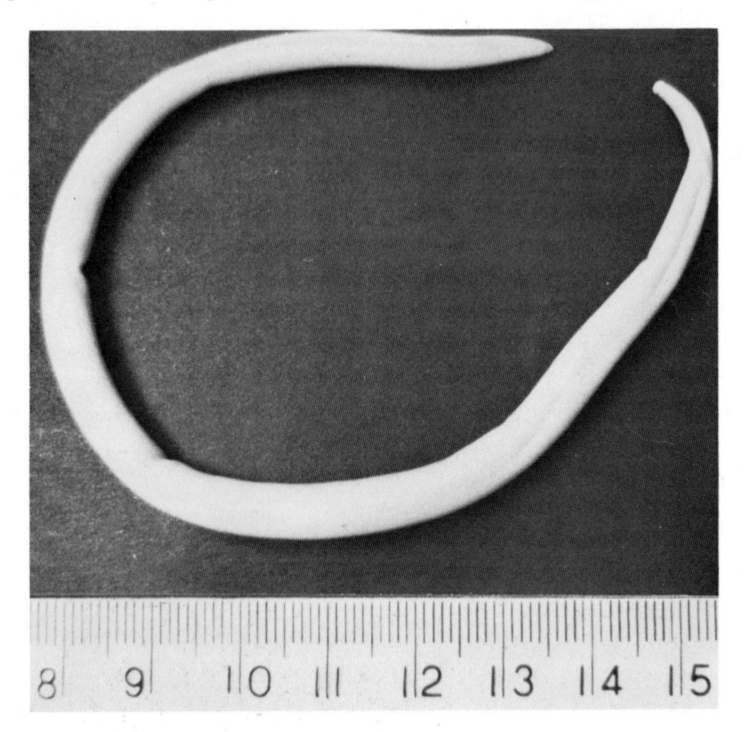

Fig. 7.11. *Parascaris equorum.*

faecal sample does not accurately reflect the state of the relationship, but the presence of large numbers plus typical clinical signs should be viewed with suspicion.

Treatment

Treatment may again be divided into routine preventive measures and the emergency treatment of heavily parasitized cases.

Routine preventive measures. Foals should be treated on a regular four-week basis from the age of one month. The intestinal stages of *Parascaris equorum* are susceptible to the action of most anthelmintics at the recommended dosage rate, but there are no data on the efficacy of these compounds against the migratory stages. Thiabendazole is not a very satisfactory anthelmintic for *Parascaris equorum* when used at the dose rate normal for *Strongylus vulgaris,* i.e. 44 mg/kg. At 88 mg/kg, however, it is highly efficient (Duncan 1976) and when treating foals, yearlings and horses up to three years of age, we have found a mixture of thiabendazole at 44 mg/kg and piperazine citrate at 100 mg/kg to be very useful. This can make an inexpensive and efficient broad-spectrum anthelmintic which can be used in rotation with pyrantel embonate, fenbendazole and mebendazole. In addition, the frequent removal of faeces, together with thorough cleansing of loose boxes and grooming of animals, will prevent the build-up of the very sticky parasite eggs in the stable. Good hygiene and cleanliness are more important than disinfection as ascarid eggs can remain viable in certain strong disinfectant solutions. Clayton (1978) recommends that foaling boxes should be rigorously cleaned and disinfected with 5% lysol or a phenol-based disinfectant in an attempt to remove this source of infection. Ideally, clean pastures should be reserved for young foals; this is seldom practical as eggs can remain viable over winter. Prior grazing with cattle or sheep helps significantly.

Heavily parasitized cases. There are few data regarding the efficacy of anthelmintic drugs against the migratory stages of *Parascaris equorum* (Clayton 1978). Treatment with an effective drug (e.g. piperazine citrate) at the recommended dose rate is advised as it is mostly the adult stages that are involved with clinical disease. In cases of intestinal impaction, perforation and peritonitis, emergency laparotomy may be indicated.

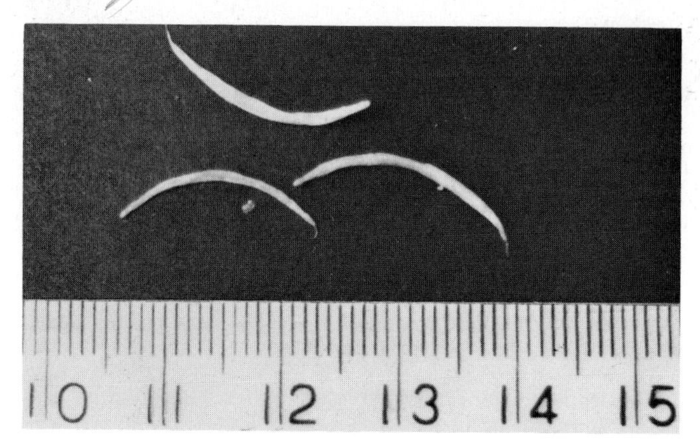

Fig. 7.12. *Oxyuris equi.*

Oxyuriasis (pin-worm) (Fig. 7.12)

Oxyuris equi infestations are not serious; they cause intense irritation of the anal region which may encourage horses to rub and bite their tails. Piperazine compounds are recommended for treatment.

Dictyocaulus (lungworm)

Dictyocaulus arnfeldi (Fig. 7.13) is more common in donkeys than in horses (Round 1976; Nicholls et al. 1978). It may, however, be common in horses who share grazing with donkeys. Round surveyed 333 donkeys from 12 stud farms in England and found that 243 had patent infection. Round's data suggest that infestations in horses may be more common than generally suspected, but the incidence of clinical disease with symptoms is very low.

Eggs are passed onto the pasture in faeces and the larvae hatch within a few hours. They survive a maximum of 14 days in direct sunlight and 24–42 days in the shade. Migration in the host is via the mesenteric lymph nodes and it is presumed that larvae reach the heart by the thoracic duct (Round 1976). Horse foals first pass larvae 12–14 weeks after grazing pasture stocked with heavily infected donkeys. Infections remain patent for six to 31 weeks in horse foals and up to eight months in naturally infected adult horses.

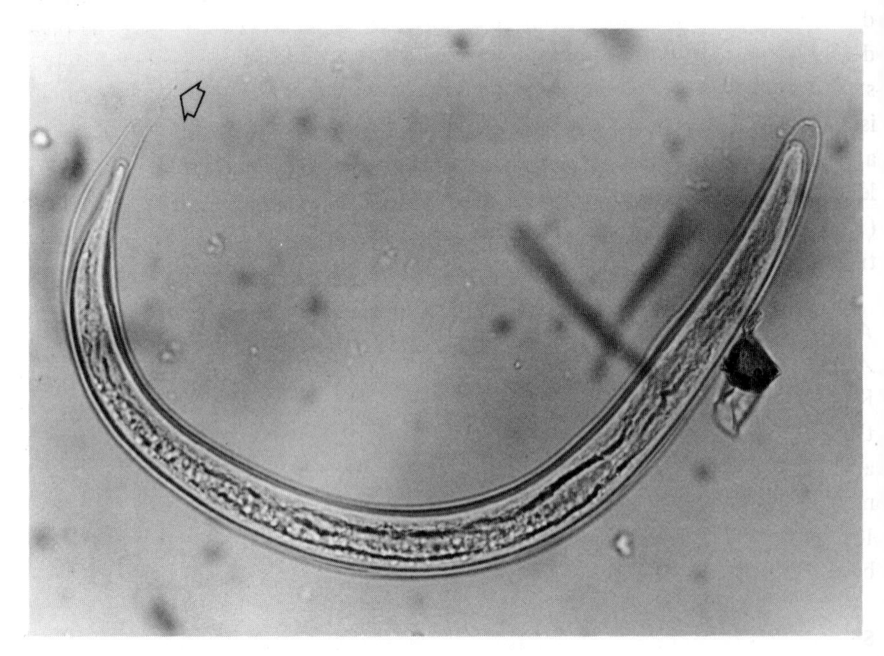

Fig. 7.13. *Dictyocaulus arnfeldi* (lungworm) larvae. The diagnostic feature is the tip of the tail (arrowed). × 400.

The response of adult horses to infection varies considerably. Some develop patent infections without clinical signs; in others, patency follows clinical disease, while some adults show neither clinical signs nor patency. Round found that, contrary to previous belief, age immunity does not occur.

There has been considerable debate as to the pathogenicity of *Dictyocaulus arnfeldi* as a 'disease-producer' in donkeys and in horses. Large numbers of lungworms may be tolerated by some horses without clinical effect but moderately severe microscopic lesions may be present in the lungs.

In experimental infections, coughing may begin as early as the twelfth day, in severe cases, or in mild cases be delayed for several weeks. The condition is generally afebrile. Coughing, increased respiratory rates and adventitious lung sounds are most intense during the third to fifth weeks with paroxysmal coughing and forced expiration. Thereafter, the signs diminish in intensity but coughing, particularly on exercise, may persist for several months and in some cases for more than a year. The animals remain alert and appetite is not usually affected.

Haematological examinations show eosinophilia from the third to the seventh week but no changes in beta-globulin levels. Confirmatory diagnosis is by the demonstration of larvae in the faeces, which is best done by overnight recovery from 50 g amounts of faeces, using the Baermann technique (see p. 529). Positive results may be interpreted with far more confidence than negative ones. Several repeated examinations may be necessary. Most cases of clinical disease in horses are seen during the pre-patent phase and larvae may not be present in the faeces (Round 1976). Most infected horses, although showing respiratory signs, do not develop patent infections. If lungworm infection is suspected on clinical and epidemiological grounds, it may be wise to treat even though larvae can not be demonstrated in the faeces. The most effective treatment appears to be the oral administration, on alternate days, of 440 ml/kg thiabendazole. Diethylcarbamazine appears to have no value in the treatment of lungworm in horses and tetramisole or levamisole are variable in effect and frequently unsatisfactory. Urch and Allen (1980) found fenbendazole, with repeated high dose rates, unsatisfactory in the treatment of lungworm infections in donkeys.

Anoplocephala (tapeworm)

Anoplocephala perfoliata is the only tapeworm found in horses in the United Kingdom (Duncan 1976). It occurs in the ileum around the ileocecal valve and in the caecum itself. Occasionally the parasites are found in the faeces (they are white and 45 cm in length) but their pathogenicity is not understood. Prophylactic treatment is not considered necessary but it has been shown that niclosamide is 98–100% efficient against *Anoplocephala perfoliata* at a dose rate of 200–300 mg/kg body weight, the lower dose rate being used for foals and yearlings.

Strongyloidosis

Strongyloides westeri infestation is common in foals under six months of age but clinical symptoms are seldom seen. Severe infestations may cause diarrhoea in two- to four-week-old foals and treatment with thiabendazole is recommended (Duncan 1976). Lyons et al. (1973) demonstrated that foals obtained their infections from larvae passed in mares' milk from five to 19 days post-partum.

Hydatidosis (Echinococcus granulosus)

Thompson and Smythe (1975) found that clinical manifestations of the disease in horses are rare but massive infestations are seen in apparently healthy aged animals at slaughter. In this situation, the disease may have public health importance and result in the condemnation of affected livers. Their epidemiological surveys suggested that within the last decade the prevelance of equine hydatidosis in Great Britain has been as high as 60%. The disease is widespread throughout the country and occurs in young as well as aged horses. From epidemiological and experimental evidence, dogs would appear to be the most likely definitive hosts of the disease, especially those with access to raw, uninspected flesh and offal. The role of the fox is uncertain. Thompson and Smythe (1975) visited 21 hunt kennels and 11 (52%) harboured *Echinococcus*-infected dogs and the worms recovered were identified as the 'horse' strain of *E. granulosus.* Infected hunting dogs cover wide areas of countryside and widespread contamination of grazing land may take place. Surveys of the incidence and significance of equine hydatidosis in Sweden and Ireland have been reported by Ronéus (1975) and Hatch (1975). Hatch suggest that the breaking of the hound/horse cycle is easily achieved by removing the liver and lungs from all carcases before they are fed to the hounds. The livers and lungs should be disposed of in such a manner that no dog has access to them. Hounds which have had access to uncooked liver and lungs should receive treatment for *Echinococcus* infection.

Fascioliasis (liver fluke)

Owen (1977) described 38 cases of *Fasciola hepatica* infection in horses with clinical signs, including loss of weight, capricious appetite, poor performance and lethargy. Some cases exhibited diarrhoea and urticaria. Some were slightly anaemic but otherwise there was no evidence of haematological or blood biochemical abnormality. Diagnosis was by the detection of eggs in faecal samples (see p. 528).

Oxyclozanide is the recommended treatment at a dose rate of 15 ml/50 kg body weight with a maximum of 100 ml. Some cases of very mild colic and transient diarrhoea following treatment were observed by Owen (1977).

This disease is undoubtedly unusual in horses but it must not be overlooked under certain conditions such as wet summer seasons and where grazing is shared with infected cattle and sheep. Nansen et al. (1975) were able to establish patent infection in only one of ten experimental horses after oral dosing with up to 800 metacercariae. They concluded that horses have a pronounced resistance to the establishment of liver fluke infection.

Ectoparasites

Lice

The biting louse (*Haematapinus asini*) and the sucking louse (*Bovicola* (*Damalinia*) *equi*) are found on horses (Fig. 7.14). Their activities irritate the skin and the horse bites, scratches and rubs the affected parts. This may cause considerable damage. With continual irritation the skin becomes scurfy and sometimes scabby. Infections are more common in winter when the lice burrow in thick hair coats. They lay eggs at the base of the hairs. The eggs hatch and the young lice crawl along the hairs where they are easily seen with the naked eye. Topical application of gammexane is the usual treatment.

Ticks

Ticks are found on horses in isolated, often wooded areas. The cattle and sheep tick (*Ixodes ricinis*) is occasionally seen on horses but does not usually cause symptoms.

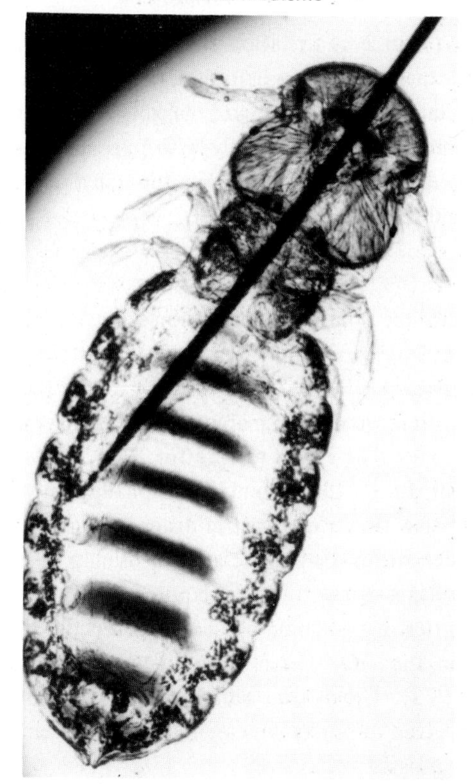

Fig. 7.14. A louse, *Damalinia equi,* attached to a horse hair.

Ticks can be removed safely after applying benzyl benzoate, ether or chloroform which releases their mouth parts, ensuring the head is not left behind. If this happens an abscess or an oedematous skin plaque may form. Equine piroplasmosis (see p. 480), an erythrocyte protozoon infection causing profound haemolytic anaemia and pyrexia, is transmitted by ticks. This condition is not seen in Great Britain.

Harvest mites

Trombicula autumnalis is a small orange mite which may infest horses in summer. It occurs in isolated geographical areas where the problem may recur year after year. The heels and coronary region are often affected by pruritus and erythema which may result in a stringhalt action or lameness behind. Some cases are more general, causing intense pruritus and eczematous lesions over the head, neck, body and legs. Diagnosis is made by examining a skin scraping and treatment with benzyl benzoate should be followed by emollient and anti-inflammatory ointments.

Myiasis

Flies are a problem on stud farms in summer. They annoy horses at pasture and may bite them, especially around the head. Any cut or wound is liable to be infested and become a source of irritation and secondary infection. Skin tumours are also likely to be attacked, causing irritation, bleeding and secondary infection. If neglected, eggs are laid in the wound and maggots hatch. Any wound should be kept clean and powdered at least once daily with pyrethrum or similar powder. If possible, surgery should not be attempted when flies are a problem unless the horse can be kept indoors and sprayed regularly.

Bot flies

Gastrophilus intestinalis are common around horses in summer and the adults are a nuisance, but cannot bite or sting. The eggs are laid at the tips of the hairs and are licked off and ingested by the horse. The larvae hatch in the stomach and attach to the stomach wall, often around the margo plicatus. Large numbers can be found in clinically normal horses. The larvae mature for 10–12 months, detach and pass out in the faeces to pupate on the ground. Occasionally there may be so many bot larvae in the stomach that they cause gastric distension, colic and even rupture of the stomach and sudden death. Bot larvae are not usually killed by normal anthelmintics and, if prophylaxis or treatment is required, it is necessary to use organophosphorus anthelmintics, e.g. dichlorvos or haloxon. For prophylaxis, one dose in late autumn, when the larvae have accumulated in the stomach, should be sufficient (Waddel 1972). Great care should be taken that organophosphorus anthelmintics are not given to horses who are ill from other causes and in particular have evidence of liver disease.

SKIN DISEASES

Parasitic skin diseases have been described above.

Ringworm

Both *Trichophyton* and *Microsporum* species cause skin lesions. These are usually on the chest, behind the elbow or on the neck or head, but can occur anywhere. Typical lesions are round, first as a raised area of skin. The hairs then break off and cause crusty lesion. Positive identification rests on the result of a skin scraping (see p. 535). Legoretta (1975) found that the normal duration of the disease varies from eight to 12 weeks. It is seldom of more than 'nuisance value' in horses on stud farms except where the disease occurs prior to export certification.

Treatment is by oral griseofulvin (Hiddleston 1970) and topical applications of fungicides, e.g. methylene-*bis*(4-chlorophenol) (Halophen). Oldenkamp (1979) described the use of the antibiotic natamycin in 83 horses affected by ringworm. The preparation was sponged on to the affected areas according to the manufacturers' recommendation. The mycological clearance rate was 97% and treatment successfully eliminated the disease within four weeks. The most common species involved in the series was *Trichophyton equinum* but the antibiotic seems similarily successful against *Microsporum equinum, Trichophyton verrucosum* and

Microsporum gypseum. After treatment the recovered animals showed no evidence of reinfection for up to six months. This preparation is also recommended for the treatment of the horse's surroundings and saddlery or harness, which can also transmit infection (Legoretta 1975).

Rain scald

When horses are turned out in wet weather, the actinomycete *Dermatophilus congolensis* may cause an exudative dermatitis especially affecting the back and hindquarters. Matting of the hair occurs with accumulations of seropurulent material. The exudate dries and hardens and on removal of an affected tuft, an inverted saucer-shaped crust is seen, filled with orange-yellow purulent material (Thomsett 1979).

Diagnosis is confirmed by the demonstration of *D. congolensis* in smears of exudate or crushed scab. Treatment is by housing the horses so that their skin dries. Severely infected cases may need systemic antibiotic treatment with penicillin and streptomycin. Thomsett (1975) suggests treatment by the application to the affected areas of a solution of 1% potash alum in water or an equal mixture of powdered potash alum with chalk. We have found an equal mixture of sulphanilamide powder and liquid paraffin to be very useful in the treatment of cases of rain scald. This mixture is also useful as an antibacterial 'water-proofing' agent where complete housing is not possible.

Cracked heels/mud fever

This is a common problem in brood mares turned out in wet and muddy conditions during the early part of the breeding season. In some cases, infection by *Dermatophilus congolensis* may be involved (Thomsett 1979) but in others, constant wetting and 'chapping' of the skin allows bacterial infection, especially *Staphylococcus aureus,* to gain entry. The heel areas show exudative dermatitis with scab formation. Oedema of the legs may occur and some cases may be extremely sore and lame.

Treatment is by housing affected animals so that the legs may dry. Severely affected cases may need antibiotic treatment with penicillin and streptomycin and tetanus antitoxin should always be administered, if the horse is not vaccinated. We have found an equal mixture of sulphanilamide powder and liquid paraffin to be a very useful local treatment and this may be used as an antibacterial 'water-proofing' agent where complete housing is not possible.

Papilloma

Papillomatosis is seen in horses up to two years of age, frequently around the muzzle and nostrils. The condition is viral in origin and is self-limiting. Treatment is seldom necessary but in serious cases an autogenous vaccine, made by suspending fresh wart material in 0.1% formalin, may be used (Bostock & Owen 1975). This vaccine may be injected subcutaneously 5–10 ml at a single dose on each of four occasions at one-week intervals.

Equine sarcoid

Sarcoids (Jackson 1936) occur on the legs, head, shoulders and abdomen, usually in mature horses up to middle age (Thomsett 1979). The lesions arise as small dermal nodules covered by thin smooth epidermis. These enlarge and become ulcerated and the whole lesion may be several centimetres in diameter. The tumour may occur at sites of previous wounds (Ragland et al. 1970; Lane 1977). It has also been suggested following transmission studies that viral infection may be involved (Voss 1969). Thomsett (1979) reports that the condition occasionally appears in stables in epidemic form.

Diagnosis is by histological examination of biopsy specimens (see p. 540). There has been considerable disagreement on the histopathological definition of the lesion (Baker & Leyland 1975; Bostock & Owen 1975). Lane (1977) described the sarcoid as a fibroblastic tumour with variable epithelial participation, which behaves in a unique manner. Histologically it has the appearance of a fibrosarcoma but does not metastasize and is not therefore typically malignant.

The clinical significance of the tumours depends on their site and size. They are most troublesome when they occur around the genitalia in stallions or on the inner aspect of the thighs and close to the mammary glands in mares. Surgical removal often exacerbates the condition and the growths recur, rapidly forming a soft granulating mass which bleeds easily. If surgery is attempted an area of surrounding skin should be removed. Lane (1977) described the treatment of 50 horses by cryosurgery; 33 were cleared of neoplasia and the majority of the others were rendered suitable for work. Wyn-Jones (1979) reported the treatment of three periocular sarcoids using radio-active gold-198 grains. He suggested that the technique was very useful, especially when the tumours are close to important structures. Radioactive implant material may, however, be contraindicated when growths occur close to the testes. Whatever method of treatment is used, there is no doubt that the earlier treatment is started, the better the results are likely to be.

Sweet itch

This allergic skin disease may affect ponies on stud farms between the months of April and October (Mellor & McCaig 1975). These authors found that affected ponies were hypersensitized to the bites of *Culicoides* and reacted annually when re-challenged. Insects crawl down the mane and tail to the skin where they initiate the allergic response. The ponies itch, rubbing the mane and the base of the tail where an exudative dermatitis forms.

Diagnosis rests with the type of animal, the seasonal nature of the disease and the body areas affected.

Affected horses should not be grazed over marshy ground or other wet areas where midges are found (Thomsett 1979). Ponies should be stabled at times when the midges are most active, i.e. dusk, and the stable should be as insect-proof as possible and fitted with fly killers. Systemic treatment with corticosteroid preparations and antihistamines may control the problem and local treatment with soothing antiseptic creams or benzyl benzoate emulsion may help. Baker and Quinn (1978) suggests that midge repellants such as dimethylphthallate may be useful.

Warble flies

Hypoderma bovis is a parasite of cattle but can be a great nuisance to horses, causing them to rear and bolt. The adults land on the horse's legs and, with a specially adapted ovipositor, lay eggs on the basal part of the hairs. Usually only horses under three years old are affected by the larvae, which hatch and penetrate the skin to wander in the hypodermal space, travelling up the legs and flanks. Eventually after several months they reach the skin on the back or withers and form a capsule where they mature. Clinically they look like a small boil with a central opening. If tack does not press on the area the warble may not be a problem. The larvae should never be squeezed as this will release enough antigen to cause a hypersensitive reaction and a large, unsightly, oedematous skin plaque. This may become secondarily infected. A better way to cope with the problem is to wait until the larva is ready to emerge, or poultice the area, then remove the larvae surgically. Oral or local parasiticides are not effective once this stage has been reached.

Mange

Mange can be caused by three types of mite: *Sarcoptes scabei* and *Psoroptes communis* are notifiable in Great Britain. *Sarcoptes scabei* is sometimes seen in horses, but is more common in ponies, especially those kept in suboptimal conditions. The female burrows in the skin causing intense pruritus. Eggs are laid in the tunnel she makes and the larvae hatch in three to seven days. The activity of the parasite causes raised erythematous areas which exude and dry. These scabs irritate, often causing the horse to rub or bite itself so that large areas of skin are abraded, exude and/or bleed. Body condition quickly deteriorates and the horse becomes emaciated. Gammexane and local wound treatment should be applied.

Psoroptes communis does not burrow in the skin, so irritation is not as intense. Hair falls out over the back and withers and self-mutilation occurs. Treatment is as for sarcoptic mange. The mites are occasionally found in horses' ears, sometimes causing head-shaking. They should be treated with ear drops (Otoryl).

Mange caused by *Chorioptes equi* is not notifiable and is now rare. The mites cause irritation below the hock or knee and the affected horses, usually of a heavy breed with 'feathered' legs, stamp and kick. Gammexane and local wound treatment should be applied.

Demodectic mange

Demodex mite infestations have been reported in horses (Thomsett 1979). We have seen it only twice and in these cases six-month-old foals out of the same mare were involved in successive years. The foals showed irritation and skin thickening around the eyes and the base of the ears. Characteristic mites were demonstrated in skin scrapings. Treatment with rotenone was followed by complete recovery in both cases.

DIGESTIVE SYSTEM

Dysphagia

Difficulty in swallowing may be caused by injury to the pharynx and associated structures, the presence of a foreign body in the pharynx or oesophagus (choke), enlargement of the pharyngeal lymph nodes (as in strangles), pharyngeal oedema (sometimes seen in acute allergic states) or paralysis of the muscles associated with swallowing (as in grass sickness or mouldy corn poisoning (Bridges 1972).

Varying amounts of food and saliva are discharged from the nasal passages. The discharge is coloured green if the affected horse has recently been eating grass.

Choke

Oesophageal obstruction may be caused by a bolus of dry food or a foreign body such as a lump of wood. Signs include distress, refusal to eat or drink, a profuse nasal discharge, repeated arching of the neck and retching.

Treatment of simple choke, where the lodged material is not excessive or where there are no complicating factors such as ulcerated or ruptured oesophagus, consists of administering a tranquillizer, e.g. acetylpromazine. The condition then usually clears spontaneously within about two hours.

Colic

Aetiology

The term 'colic' is used to describe a number of conditions, the chief symptom of which is abdominal pain (Greatorex 1972). The syndrome has been divided into 'true' colic, i.e. involving the stomach and or intestines, and 'false' colic, i.e. involving other abdominal organs or structures.

False colic

False colic may involve a number of systems:

Urinary system. These conditions are unusual in the horse but cystitis, urinary calculi and nephritis may cause signs of abdominal pain (see p. 486).

Genital system. Rupture of the vagina, cervix and uterus in the mare, haemorrhage into the broad ligament of the uterus after foaling, foaling itself and the contractions of the uterus during expulsion of the placental membranes, involution, abortion and hypermotility of the fetus in late gestation may all cause signs of abdominal pain (see Chapters 3 and 4). In the stallion, orchitis and rotation or strangulation of the testes may cause signs of abdominal pain (see p. 154).

Liver. Acute hepatitis may cause abdominal pain (see p. 471).

Abdominal tumours. Mesotheliomas may produce marked ascites and acute colic (Ricketts & Peace 1976). Lipomas may become pedunculated and may obstruct the intestine either by encirclement or by local pressure and stenosis.

Peritonitis. Peritonitis, either diffuse or localized, usually causes severe abdominal pain. This frequently occurs as a secondary sequel to a 'true' colic (see below) or following rupture of a mesenteric lymph node abscess with *Streptococcus equi* or *Corynebacterium equi* infection. Horses appear to have a low threshold of pain associated with inflammation of, or stretching of, the peritoneum (Greatorex 1972).

Set-fast/azoturia/myoglobinuria. Some acute cases present clinical signs suggesting abdominal pain. The history of recent strenuous exercise, especially following a period of rest, and the laboratory estimation of serum AST and CK levels should allow an accurate diagnosis (see p. 489).

True colic

True colic may be caused by:

Distention of the stomach. Gas or fluid may distend the stomach after a sudden change of food or the ingestion of unsuitable food. Sudden fermentation of the intestinal contents may cause a build-up of gas. Distension of the stomach by fluid is seen in cases of small intestinal obstruction, e.g. volvulus or intussusception (see below) and in acute grass sickness (see p. 469). In severe cases, rupture of the stomach may occur, and on occasions, when the condition is peracute, the horse may be found dead, with a ruptured stomach, before signs of abdominal pain have been noticed. It has been suggested that rupture or perforation of the stomach may be associated with very heavy infestations with *Gastrophilus intestinalis* (bot) larvae.

Enteritis. Abdominal pain is often associated with diarrhoea, especially in the early stages. Sometimes, abdominal pain, pyrexia and hypermotility of the intestines precede observable diarrhoea (see p. 470).

Distension of the small intestine. Fluid and/or gas may cause distension after diarrhoea or in cases of excessive fermentation of intestinal contents after sudden nutritional changes or the ingestion of unsuitable feed. Massive small intestinal fluid accumulations are seen in cases of small intestinal obstruction, e.g. volvulus and intussusception (see below) and in acute grass sickness.

Volvulus ('twist') of the small intestine. This may occur spontaneously in young or old horses and results in intestinal torsion or 'knot' formation with embarrassment to the blood supply to the section of intestine involved. Infarction then follows with signs of severe abdominal pain and cardiovascular shock. Rooney (1970) suggests that such cases may be caused by parasitic larval damage, which then acts as a focus for torsion or 'knot' formation as peristaltic waves are impeded.

Intussusception of the small intestines. This condition usually occurs in foals and yearlings. Pearson et al. (1975) described nine cases of intussusception, involving ileum into caecum, caecum into colon, invagination of the caecal apex and jejunum into jejunum. Four cases were attributed to intestinal hypermotility or atony caused by verminous arteritis and in one case it occurred at the site of a primary intestinal neoplasm. In one case, invagination of the caecal apex might have resulted from the use of parasympathomimetic drugs. Intussusception results in infarction of the intestine, signs of acute abdominal pain and cardiovascular shock.

Peri-intestinal adhesions. Intraperitoneal adhesions have a variety of causes such as parasitic larval damage, local abscess formation, peritonitis and previous abdominal surgery. Adhesions involving a section of the small intestine may result in stenosis or may form a 'focus' for torsion, volvulus or strangulation (see above).

Small intestinal herniation and strangulation. Pearson et al. (1975) reported 12 cases of intestinal strangulation involving mesenteric tear, epiploic foramen, umbilical hernia, ruptured prepubic tendon, suprapreputial rupture, ruptured diaphragm, haemorrhagic ovary, mesocolonic lipoma, adventitious mesenteric band and retracted spermatic cord. Depending on the site and degree of embarrassment to the intestinal blood vessels, the severity of the abdominal pain may vary. Where strangulation is complete, infarction of the intestinal segment occurs with acute abdominal pain and cardiovascular shock.

Infarction of small intestines. Obstruction of the blood supply to a section of small intestine may occur following small intestinal volvulus, intussusception, strangulation or peri-intestinal adhesion formation (see above). Infarction may also occur after torsion of the root of the mesentery (Pearson et al. 1975) and where end-arterial thromboembolism has followed parasitic intestinal arteritis (Wright 1972). This is a characteristic feature of experimental and natural infection with *Strongylus vulgaris* (see p. 442). The condition causes acute abdominal pain and cardiovascular shock.

Small intestinal ileus. This may occur as a sequel to small intestinal volvulus, intussusception, strangulation or infarction or in some cases of colonic inpaction. It may be a problem following intestinal surgery (Boles 1975). Ileus may occur as a specific intestinal neurological 'paralysis' in cases of grass sickness (see p. 469).

Distension of the large intestine and caecum. Gas and/or fluid distension may occur with enteritis, with lower large intestinal displacement, torsion or impaction and following abnormal fermentation reactions of the large intestinal contents. The latter may follow sudden nutritional changes or the ingestion of unsuitable food material. The severity of the abdominal pain shown by large intestinal distensions is usually not as great as with small intestinal distensions.

Displacement and torsion of the large intestine. For reasons not understood, some sections of the large intestine, especially the pelvic and sternal flexures and the caecum, may become displaced inside the abdominal cavity or undergo torsion about their axes. This may result in a functional blockage of the large intestine with first low-grade pain, usually associated with impaction. The severity of pain may increase as gaseous distension of the proximal large intestine occurs and may become severe, with cardiovascular shock, if obstruction of the colonic blood supply with infarction occurs.

Impaction of the large intestine and caecum. One of the most common causes of 'colic' seen in equine practice is an impaction of the large intestine, palpable at the pelvic flexure. At stud farms it invariably involves mares stabled because of weather conditions and/or foal illness and therefore not receiving exercise. Some cases may be associated with a period of inadequate water supply caused by managerial oversight. Page and Amstutz (1972) described an impaction at the ileocaecal junction consisting primarily of ground corn cobs. Blue (1979) described 30 cases of obstruction of the large intestine by enterolith formation. These cases were in horses older than four years and most obstructions were found near the beginning of the small colon. They were formed by mineral deposition in concentric layers about a central nidus of ingested material and were spherical or tetrahedral in shape. These concretions were found to consist primarily of ammonium magnesium phosphate. Impaction of the caecum may occur, especially among horses grazing on light sandy soil (Greatorex 1972). The severity of the abdominal pain is usually low-grade unless associated with displacements or torsions.

Pericolonic adhesions. These may occur in a similar manner to, and sometimes associated with, peri-intestinal adhesions (see above).

Colitis. An acute, sporadic, oedematous and haemorrhagic colitis (colitis X) is sometimes seen in mares at stud (see p. 468). Variable clinical signs are seen from sudden death, to acute abdominal pain with circulatory collapse to low-grade abdominal pain which later becomes more severe. Some cases are associated with diarrhoea. Low-grade abdominal pain may be associated with chronic diarrhoea caused by a granulomatous enteritis involving both large and sometimes small intestines (Merritt et al. 1976). These authors describe nine cases, between one and 11 years of age, in which persistent weight loss was a feature. Four cases had chronic diarrhoea. A parallel is drawn between granulomatous enteritis in horses and Crohn's disease in man which may be associated with some form of heritable immunological defect. Other possible causes are tuberculosis, chronic fungal infections, cytomegalovirus and enteric anaerobic bacterial infection (Merritt et al. 1976).

Rectal damage. Damage to the rectum may follow accidental anal penetration by the stallion, accidents during rectal examinations (see p. 512) and, rarely, human criminal interference. If the damage is retroperitoneal, the signs of abdominal pain may be low-grade but if penetration into the peritoneal cavity has occurred, acute peritonitis, severe acute abdominal pain and cardiovascular shock occur.

Neoplasia. Lymphosarcoma of the intestine is probably the most commonly seen abdominal neoplasm, but carcinoma of the stomach, carcinoma of the intestine, granulosa cell tumours of the ovary, cortical and medullary tumours of the adrenal gland, serosal lipomas, carcinoma of the pancreas, bile duct carcinoma and hepatic cell carcinoma have been reported (Cotchin 1977). Roberts and Pinsent (1975) described three horses suffering from alimentary lymphosarcoma, predominantly affecting the small intestine and the associated lymph nodes. Malabsorption, followed by progressive weight loss, with or without abdominal pain and diarrhoea, were the clinical features.

Clinical signs

Cardinal signs of colic are inappetence, unusual attitudes (prolonged recumbency, looking round at the flanks, crouching, lying on the back) and restlessness (pacing the box, pawing the ground and rolling). Anxious expression, grunting, increased skin temperature, profuse or patchy sweating are other signs, but are not confined to cases of colic.

Pulse rate may be normal or increased, the quality varying from strong and full to weak and small. Heart rate may be irregular and murmurs develop (possibly after tranquillizing and other drugs).

The temperature varies from subnormal to fever, depending on the severity of the case. Mucous membranes may be normal, injected, purple or brick-red.

Borborygmi may be increased or abolished and quality of sound (from high-pitched, tympanitic, to fluid) may be distinguished generally or locally.

Faeces may be normal, hard, soft, diarrhoeic, blood-stained, black, brown or green. The odour may vary from normal to foetid or necrotic and the faeces may be covered with a catarrhal slime (resembling white worms). The quantity of faeces passed in 24 hours (normally 10–20 kg for an adult) varies. Faecal matter may be present in the rectum but in acute obstruction there may be a complete absence. At the start of signs, ingesta posterior to the lesion may be passed giving a deceptive impression of normality. Ingesta anterior to the lesion may not be voided until hours or days later.

Diagnosis

The diagnosis of colic is relatively simple because of the characteristic clinical signs. It is the diagnosis of the primary abnormality causing the clinical signs that is sometimes very difficult. Firstly one must try to distinguish 'true' from 'f colics (see above). In cases that may be 'set-fast', a rapid estimation of serum A and CK levels is invaluable. In pregnant mares, genital causes such as uterine tors and signs of impending abortion or birth must be eliminated, if possible. With true colic it is then essential to establish the specific lesion as a basis for therapy. In particular the clinician must decide, as early as possible, whether medical treatment alone is indicated or if surgical exploration of the abdomen will be necessary (Stashak 1979). If the latter is the case, the sooner it is performed, the greater the chances of success.

Recommended lines of investigation are:

1. The *history* of the affected animal and its age and sex are an important starting point. Foals, yearlings and mares at grass are unlikely to suffer from large intestinal impaction whereas mares are unlikely to suffer from small intestinal intussusception. Mares with a history of current low-grade abdominal pain and inadequate past worm control may well be suffering from the effects of parasitic larval migration.

2. The animal's *behaviour* should be noted for a subjective assessment of pain. Lethargy, lying about, looking round at the flanks and occasionally pawing the ground are taken as signs of dull pain. Profuse sweating, rolling, frequently changing position and vigorously pawing the ground are signs of acute pain.

3. *Skin temperature* is a subjective sign varying with climatic conditions and the individual. The presence and degree of sweating help to differentiate between severe and less severe conditions. A cold clammy state is a bad sign and suggests a state of shock and/or rupture of the alimentary canal.

4. In general, *abdominal pain* causes a non-specific rise in rectal temperature. Cases of peritonitis or salmonellosis may have a marked pyrexia. In many cases of colic, rectal temperature has little accuracy because of rectal atony and ballooning, especially after repeated rectal examinations.

5. *Pulse* rate and quality are important diagnostic parameters. A strong full pulse carries a good prognosis and a weak thready pulse a poor one.

6. *Abdominal sounds* are a useful guide to diagnosis and prognosis. Absence of borborygmi is usually associated with acute conditions and a grave prognosis. Normal or increased sounds indicate a favourable prognosis. Abdominal signs do, however, change throughout the course of several conditions. In intestinal volvulus or intussusception, hypermotility may occur prior to ileus.

7. Passage of a *stomach tube* may be very useful. Cases of distension of the stomach and small intestine may show acute pain when the stomach tube reaches the gastric cardia. When the tube does pass into the stomach, there may be a rush of foul-smelling gas, in the case of acute small intestinal obstruction or fermentation of abnormal intestinal contents, or of fluid, in the case of acute small intestinal obstruction or grass sickness. When medicines are passed down the stomach tube, in these cases, there is usually an increase in abdominal pain.

8. *Rectal palpation* is an essential diagnostic procedure (Greatorex 1968). A large intestinal impaction may be readily palpated and the absence of faeces in the rectum may denote a higher obstruction. Soft, sloppy, foul-smelling faeces may indicate abnormal fermentation of the intestinal contents. Care should, however, be taken to differentiate between faeces that are present initially and those that appear subsequently. A series of rectal examinations should be performed during the course of the illness. A dry mucosal surface and rectal wall that clings to the operator's arm indicate severe conditions, such as volvulus, infarction or acute peritonitis. Ballooning of the rectum may be present in diarrhoea and spasmodic colic. A dry sticky rectum with sparse, dry, sticky faeces sometimes covered in 'slime' may occur in grass sickness. Structures felt through the rectal wall must be interpreted with care. Faecal impactions may be reliably diagnosed, but tense band-like structures may give a false impression of twisted mesenteries and soft masses may be mistaken for adhesions.

9. *Serial laboratory examinations* of packed cell volume and white cell count are very valuable. In cases of large intestinal impaction, despite the sometimes increasing severity of the pain, packed cell volume remains usually below 0.55 litre/litre. A rising PCV of 0.6 litre/litre and above indicates a severe circulatory disturbance and usually acute obstruction such as volvulus or infarction. Serial estimations are essential and, for example, an increase from 0.30 to 0.35 litre/litre in foals or from 0.40 to 0.50 litre/litre in adults is significant when it occurs over three or four hours. Nelson et al. (1968) studied clinical and biochemical changes caused by infarction of the colon. They found a decreased total blood leucocyte count, decreased aortic blood pressure and increased peritoneal fluid with a reddish turbidity and bacteria content. They also found a decrease in serum proteins and electrolytes and an increasing acidosis. Moore et al. (1976) evaluated blood lactate levels in 36 horses with signs of abdominal pain. There was a correlation between increasing blood lactate levels and decreasing percentage survival. The authors suggest that blood lactate determinations may be used as a prognostic rather than diagnostic aid.

10. *Paracentesis abdominis* (see p. 536) is a simple, safe technique which may yield very useful information (Table 7.5). In general, a total nucleated cell count of 10×10^9/litre should be a cause for concern and may be very useful in making the final decision that abdominal surgery is indicated. Moore et al. (1977) studied lactate acid concentrations in peritoneal fluid of 15 clinically healthy horses and five horses with acute abdominal disease. The normal range was 0.027–0.134 g/litre. Simultaneous blood and peritoneal blood samples from healthy horses revealed consistently lower concentrations in the peritoneal fluid than in the blood. Peritoneal fluid levels were consistently greater than blood levels in diseased horses. These had highly significant increases in both blood and peritoneal fluid concentrations when compared with healthy horses.

11. The *response to pain-relieving drugs* provides a useful guide to diagnosis and prognosis. In general, intestinal impactions and 'spasmodic' colic associated

TABLE 7.5 The interpretation of the gross appearance of the peritoneal fluid in relation to abdominal disease

Peritoneal fluid	*Differential diagnosis*
Pale yellow, clear or slightly opalescent, normal cell count	Normal Impaction or tympany Diarrhoea Early intussusception Fibrotic abdominal abscess Aneurysm Well encapsulated tumour
Yellow, turbid, increased cell count	Peritonitis Ruptured rectum Lymphosarcoma Acute abdominal abscess Aneurysm
Amber yellow, slight turbidity, red blood cells, increased cell count	Normal, with blood-staining Early infarction Intussusception Volvulus Strangulation Incarceration Strongyle larva migration
Amber, turbid, red blood cells, increased cell count	Infarction Late intussusception Incarceration Volvulus Strangulation Pancreatic carcinoma
Blood	Blood vessel tap Splenic tap Hepatic or splenic carcinoma Diffuse carcinomatosis
Brown, granular	Intestinal tap Intestinal rupture

After Bach and Ricketts (1974).

with abnormal fermentation reactions respond readily to visceral analgesic, but acute obstructions, such as volvulus, intussusception and infarction, do not. In general, the more anterior the lesion the more severe the pain. If fluid is put into the stomach and there is an anterior lesion, signs will be exacerbated. Posterior lesions of fatal proportions (e.g. adhesions of the small colon) may cause a slowly developing condition, the intensity of signs increasing over several days until death results from rupture of the colon and peritonitis.

A summary of diagnostic criteria is shown in Table 7.6.

Treatment

A great number of different drugs and remedies are used to treat colic. Here we are concerned with general principles rather than detail. In all cases the control of pain is essential. Hyocine-*N*-butylbromide is a useful starting point and most cases that

TABLE 7.6 Various types of colic

Type of colic	*Temperature*		*Pulse rate*	*Pulse quality*	*Abdominal sounds*	*Rectal palpation*	*Packed cell volume* (litre/litre)	*Paracentesis abdominis*	*Response to treatment*	*Special features*
	Skin	Rectal								
Simple impaction	Warm	Normal or sub-normal	Normal	Full	Periodically increased; intervals of quiet; tympanitic sounds	Large faecal mass	0.35–0.45	Normal	Slow but pain can be con-trolled	Dull pain
Simple spasmodic	Sweating	Normal or slightly elevated	Normal or increased	Normal	Greatly increased	Clinging rectal wall Wet faeces in rectum	0.35–0.45	Normal	Pain relatively easily controlled	Some cases in violent pain but of short duration
Infarction, adhesions, volvulus	Profuse or patchy sweating	Normal or raised	Rapid and increasing	Strong becoming weak and thready	Initially present then ceasing or inter-mittent	Tense bands or a small tender mass. Absence of faeces in rectum	Usually rises steadily to above 0.60	Rising cell count	Pain not controlled by drugs except for short period	Acute signs and un-remitting pain continuing > 3 hours

will not need surgical interference will respond readily. In cases of severe acute pain pethidine may be more useful and again the response is often a good prognostic sign. Boles (1975) reports that phenylbutazone appears to have some visceral analgesic properties in addition to its usual action as a controller of musculoskeletal pain. It has been argued that both pethidine and hyocine-*N*-butylbromide may reduce intestinal motility, which may be contraindicated in cases of ileus and intestinal impaction. The clinician is, however, in a 'cleft stick', in that pain must be relieved.

Simple impactions may be treated with 2 litres or more of liquid paraffin via a stomach tube. Dioctyl sodium sulphosuccinate is also a very useful 'faecal softner' but is not always commercially available. In cases of obvious large intestinal impaction, additional oral treatment with danthron at a dose rate of 9 g with sodium chloride and water usually speeds recovery. Attendants should be warned that some cases of large intestinal impaction, especially where danthron is used, may appear to get worse before they get better. Purgatives are contraindicated in all cases other than simple large intestinal impaction consisting of dry food material.

Spasmodic, tympanitic and diarrhoeic colic cases may be given 2 g chloramphenicol through a stomach tube daily for two or three days.

If diagnostic procedures suggest that surgical interference may be indicated, then the sooner it is performed the better. Pearson et al. (1975) describe the indications for laparotomy in 140 horses and found an overall recovery rate of only 28%. They point out that 48 of the 82 animals with 'colic' had lesions which were considered to be inoperable and they might concede that, as a referral institution, they would tend to see a higher volume of 'poor prognosis' cases than might be seen by veterinary surgeons in practice. Huscamp (1977) described some problems associated with intestinal surgery in the horse and emphasized the need for a highly organized, experienced, fast and atraumatic approach. Ideally, clinicians should be prepared to embark upon exploratory laparotomy with the confidence that there would be no serious adverse effects in those cases that, in retrospect, did not require it. Such a situation cannot be arrived at easily. The confidence of veterinary surgeons and horse owners in surgical exploration is marred by the fact that surgery is often only resorted to in severe and 'hopeless' cases after all else has failed. This is a situation that needs to be remedied.

To achieve the best results with abdominal surgery the following are required:

1. An experienced surgical team with assistance and laboratory 'back-up' as well as a properly organized 'theatre' (Huscamp 1977).

2. Facilities for extensive preoperative diagnostic studies.

3. Experienced anaesthetic facilities to which the horse is subjected for the minimum possible time. Apart from the problems of anaesthetizing a horse with some degree of cardiovascular shock, there are special cardiopulmonary problems associated with the recumbent horse (Gillespie et al. 1969; Weaver 1970; McDonell et al. 1979).

4. An experienced approach to the preoperative and postoperative assessment of metabolic function with particular reference to fluid and electrolyte therapy and the postoperative restoration of intestinal function (Donawick & Alexander 1970; Lucke 1972; Nelson & Meagher 1972; Boles 1975; Waterman 1977; Kohn 1979).

Regarding surgical technique, details sometimes vary between experienced surgical teams, but most conclude that the midline approach, with the horse in dorsal recumbency, gives the best approach to the abdominal contents and the best results. Readers wishing to pursue this in greater detail are referred to Messervy (1970), Pearson and Gibbs (1970), Donawick et al. (1971), Pearson et al. (1971, 1975), Huscamp (1977) and Weaver and Adams (1979).

Colitis X

Rooney and Bryans (1963) and Bryans (1963) described a sporadic peracute fatal disease of horses characterized by severe diarrhoea and toxaemia. The signs include a profuse, watery or blood-stained diarrhoea, depression, sweating and abdominal pain. Some cases were found dead before evidence of diarrhoea had been noticed. The cause was unknown and thus the disease was called colitis X.

Experimental studies suggested that the clinical and pathological manifestations might have been related to endotoxaemia. It was found that endotoxins, prepared from several strains of *E. coli,* caused an identical disease syndrome when injected intravenously (Carroll et al. 1965).

If the duration of the disease is long enough, severe dehydration occurs, denoted by a rise in packed cell volume to greater than 0.55 litre/litre. There may be a total leucopenia with the white blood cell count dropping to less than 3×10^9/litre. Horses of all ages are susceptible and death occurs after three to four hours with or without treatment. Most spectacular lesions are found in the caecum and colon. These are a dull reddish-blue cyanotic colour, easily seen from the serosal surface. There is a large quantity of fluid, foaming, evil-smelling ingesta. The mucosa is intensely hyperaemic with fine petechiae apparent in a dull, plum-red background. Frequently there is oedema or haemorrhage, or both, of varying degress in the submucosa; rarely there is free blood in the colon contents.

Treatment consists of giving large quantities (20–40 litres) of normal saline, Hartmann's solution, sodium bicarbonate and 5% dextrose. Antibiotics and corticosteroids are also used but the treatment of this disease is rarely, if ever, effective.

As the disease has become better understood, it would appear that it may be a local 'allergic' or 'anaphylatic' reaction, involving endotoxic shock and cardiovascular collapse (Rooney et al. 1966; Vaughan 1973). A variety of 'stress' factors may be involved as trigger mechanisms, including foaling, colic, viral rhinitis, myocarditis, local pneumonia, chronic pleuritis, chronic metritis, purulent cholangiolitis, long-distance transport, especially if draughts of cold water are given afterwards, anthelmintic treatment, fasting, surgical procedures and work, e.g. racing, especially if early in a period of convalescence from influenza (Vaughan 1973).

The use of intravenous tetracycline has also been incriminated (Andersson et al. 1971; Cook 1973), especially in cases which may be *Salmonella* carriers (Owen 1975) (see p. 435). On stud farms we have seen the condition most frequently in mares approximately two to three weeks after foaling and occasionally a similar period after weaning. Sometimes cases are seen in which there appears to be no obvious 'stress' factor.

Grass sickness

This condition of unknown aetiology causes degenerative lesions in the nerves of the sympathetic ganglia, producing intestinal 'paralysis' which results in various degrees of abdominal pain (Greig 1928; Obel 1955). Acute, subacute and chronic cases occur and signs include difficult swallowing, absence of peristaltic sounds, rock hard impaction of the large intestine, sweating, fine muscular tremors affecting the fore-legs and flanks and a rise in packed cell volume to more than 0.55 litre/litre. Acute cases die in one to five days, subacute in two to three weeks and chronic cases may survive for months, but usually suffer emaciation. Cases do not respond to treatment and giving fluid through an oesophageal tube usually exacerbates the signs of colic. Syphoning off stomach fluid and administering physiological fluids intravenously may give some relief. Peracute and acute cases develop massive anterior intestinal fluid effusions which may be regurgitated down the nostrils or, if a stomach tube is passed, down the tube under pressure.

The epidemiology of the condition has been studied extensively (Gilmour & Jolly 1974). This is a disease which affects horses out at grass. Those between the ages of four and eight years are particularly at risk and especially those that have been turned out after having been previously stabled in training. The highest incidence is during April, May and June.

The disease is basically one of intestinal paralysis and characteristic degenerative lesions are seen in the neurones of the stellate, coeliacomesenteric and thoracic sympathetic chain ganglia as well as in nuclei in the spinal cord and brain stem (Mahaffey 1959). Gilmour (1973*a, b*) confirmed these findings but warned that post-mortem diagnosis of the disease by histological examination of the sympathetic ganglia is not always as straightforward as it may seem unless the ganglia are removed very rapidly after death. He concluded that in the pathogenesis of grass sickness, gut paralysis follows autonomic neurone degeneration.

The cause of the disease remains unknown but it appears to be mediated, via the nerve supply to the intestines, by a neurotoxin (Thompson 1979, personal communication). This toxin has been chemically isolated from the serum of affected horses and when injected into healthy horses has produced the disease. Its origin is not known.

There is no known specific treatment at present. Symptomatic treatment, replacement of fluid and electrolytes and feeding by stomach tube are usually attempted. Rarely, chronic cases do survive but the end product is usually unsatisfactory from the onwer's point of view.

Logical preventive measures at the stud farm are:

1. Move all horses away from the 'offending' paddock. Epidemics involving a series of horses may be seen.
2. House all 'at risk' horses at night and feed hay and concentrates to reduce the grass intake and give the intestines more roughage.
3. Crop the 'offending' paddock with cattle or sheep.
4. Never graze paddocks with a confirmed history of disease during April, May and June.

Diarrhoea

Diarrhoea in adult horses is fortunately not seen commonly in horses at stud. Foal diarrhoea is much more common and has been discussed previously (see p. 402). Merritt et al. (1975) suggest that the most common causes of acute diarrhoea are acute salmonellosis (see p. 435), colitis X (see p. 468), acute peritonitis, e.g. following contaminated abdominal surgery, manual rupture of the rectum, ruptured intra-abdominal abscess, intestinal leakage or rupture secondary to strongyle larval induced ischaemia, and *Corynebacterium equi* infection. The latter is usually seen in foals and yearlings (see p. 401). These authors define chronic diarrhoea as that which has persisted for at least one month and which has proved refractory to the usual symptomatic treatment. They report the most common causes of chronic diarrhoea to be strongyle larva migration (see p. 442), granulomatous enteritis (see p. 461), chronic liver disease (see below), *Corynebacterium equi* infection in foals and yearlings (see p. 401), salmonellosis (see p. 435) and intestinal neoplasia, e.g. lymphosarcoma and gastric carcinoma (see p. 462). Cases may be differentially diagnosed on historical, clinical and clinicopathological grounds (see Table 7.7).

Treatment must be designed to remove the aetiological agent responsible, if possible, restore normal metabolism, replace fluids and electrolytes and treat symptoms. The first two of these are the most important as, if they are successful, the symptoms will usually look after themselves; if not, intestinal absorbents and spasmolytics may have little effect. As well as a loss of fluid (Carlson 1979) and electrolytes, the loss of albumin through the intestines (protein-losing enteropathy) (Menten et al. 1978) is sometimes a serious part of acute or chronic diarrhoea and may lead to intravascular haemodynamic collapse. Diagnosis may be made by serum protein estimations (see p. 523) and attempts at replacement must be made by the use of intravenous plasma expanders and increasing the total protein oral intake. A total serum albumin level of under 15 g/litre tends to be a poor prognostic sign.

Liver disease

Liver disease may be more common in the horse than is recognized because the amazing capacity of the liver for compensation and regeneration leaves many cases subclinical until they are very advanced. Signs include jaundice, wasting, unthriftiness, staring coat, disturbed intestinal function and neurological signs (head-pressing, circling, incoordination and irritability).

Jaundice is recognized chiefly by a yellowing of the visible mucous membranes. Various degrees of 'yellowing' or 'dirtiness' of the membranes may be present without lesions and may complicate a clinical diagnosis. For example, inanition invariably causes a degree of jaundice.

Primary obstructive jaundice is quite rare but may be associated with parasitic invasion of the bile duct by, for example, *Fasciola hepatica, Gastrophilus intestinalis* or ascarid larvae. Space-occupying hepatic lesions, such as abscesses, calculi or neoplasms, may cause mechanical obstruction of the bile duct. Chronic *Senecio* (ragwort) poisoning causes periportal fibrosis which may obstruct the bile canaliculi and result in an obstructive jaundice.

Haemolytic jaundice is caused by massive destruction of erythrocytes as in equine infectious anaemia (see p. 428), piroplasmosis (see p. 480) or phenothiazine poisoning. Haemolytic disease of the newborn foal is described in the section on newborn foals (see p. 345).

Damage to liver cells impairs their functions, among which is to process bile pigment. Hepatocellular jaundice may be caused by various metallic or chemical poisons (arsenic, lead, copper, phosphorus, nitrate and carbon tetrachloride); by bacterial toxins; by plant poisoning with *Senecio* (ragwort), *Equisetum* (horse tails), locoweed and alsike clover; and by infectious conditions such as those caused by EHV-I arteritis virus, β-haemolytic streptococci, *Leptospira,* and contagious pleuropneumonia organisms.

Cirrhosis of the liver follows poisoning by plants of *Crotolaria, Atalya, Senecio* and *Amsinckia* species. Cirrhosis is characterized by hepatic and neurological signs and may be present in a chronic or acute form.

An often fatal disease of horses, characterized by an acute hepatic insufficiency with neurological signs, caused by extensive hepatic necrosis, is known as Theiler's disease (Hjerpe 1964; Panchera 1972). It is found in horses vaccinated or given serum against African horse sickness. It became known as 'serum sickness' and has subsequently been reported to occur after antiserum prophylaxis against encephalomyelitis or influenza and, in sporadic cases, after the use of pregnant mare serum and tetanus antitoxin. The cause is not known but is thought in many cases to be a virus. Signs are of jaundice and sweating without pyrexia. There was also depression and anorexia. Neurological signs include restlessness, excitement, mania, head-pressing, circling and blindly walking into objects. Individuals may become positively dangerous for handlers. Clinicopathological changes include leucocytosis, neutrophilia, hypoglycaemia, bilirubinaemia, haemoglobinaemia, haemoglobinuria, albuminuria, bilirubinuria, and a marked rise in serum AST and SDH levels. The histological lesions consist of extensive liver necrosis with mononuclear cell infiltrations.

TABLE 7.7A Differential diagnosis of acute diarrhoea

Acute salmonellosis
1. History of recent abdominal surgery or rectal examination
2. High fever
3. Profuse watery stool – frank blood present?
4. Initial degenerative then regenerative left shift
5. Hyponatraemia with mild hypokalaemia
6. Hypoalbuminaemia
7. Mild metabolic acidosis
8. Culture *Salmonella* organism from stool

Haemorrhagic oedematous colon (colitis X)
1. History of recent stress
   – Virus infection plus continued training
   – Massive antibiotic (tetracycline?) therapy
2. Marked tachycardia (80–100 beats per minute)
3. Cold extremities
4. Copious explosive water diarrhoea
5. Hyperaemic mucous membranes/slow capillary refill
6. Hypothermia
7. Marked hypovolaemia
8. Very high PCV (0.6–0.7 litre/litre)
9. Severe metabolic acidosis

Acute peritonitis
1. History of recent abdominal surgery or rectal examination
2. Abdominal pain
3. Stool watery but not profuse
4. Fever?
5. Rectal examination
   – Tear
   – Mass
   – Adhesions
   – Ingesta on serosal surfaces
6. Any subcutaneous abscesses?
7. Peritoneal fluid, WBC count 10 000, mainly neutrophils

Corynebacterium equi
1. Farm history
2. Young animals
3. Stool watery but not profuse
4. Bronchopneumonia?
5. Leucocytosis with moderate shift
6. Gram stain stool – Gram-positive pleomorphic rods
7. Culture *Corynebacterium* from stool

After Merritt et al. (1975).

TABLE 7.7B Differential diagnosis of chronic diarrhoea

Strongyle larval migrans
1. History of recurrent colic
2. Anterior mesenteric arteritis and/or aneurysm
3. Abdominocentesis
   - Increased number of eosinophils
   - Increased phagocytic activity
4. Faeces usually cow-like consistency
5. Dermatosis
   - Patchy alopecia
   - Severe scaling
   - General thinness of hair
   - Acute endothelial proliferation in dermis
6. Abnormal D(+)xylose absorption
7. Eosinophilia
8. Increased serum beta globulin
9. Normal ^{51}Cr loss in faeces

Granulomatous enteritis
1. Thin-to-emaciated body condition
2. Rectal examination
   - Roughened friable rectal mucosa
   - Thick-walled intestines
   - Prominent enlarged mesenteric lymph nodes
3. Abdominocentesis
   - Decreased phagocytic activity
4. Faeces very watery consistency
5. Marked hypoalbuminaemia
6. Acid-fast organisms in faeces or rectal biopsy
7. Excessive ^{51}Cr loss in faeces

Chronic liver disease
1. Thin body condition
2. Faeces soft or watery, not profuse
3. Hypoalbuminaemia
4. Increased serum beta globulin
5. Decreased bromosulphaphthalein clearance
6. Increased prothrombin time

Corynebacterium equi infection
1. Farm history/young animals
2. Progressive weight loss
3. Significantly increased amounts of watery faeces
4. Rectal examination (if possible)
   - Enlarged soft mesenteric lymph nodes
5. Demonstration of organisms in faeces
   - Gram stain
   - Culture

Salmonellosis
1. Farm/stable history
2. Onset characterized by severe acute illness
   - Fever
   - WBC changes
   - Blood in faeces
3. Rectal examination painful
4. Neutrophilia – left shift
5. Mild hypoalbuminaemia
6. Culture organism in faeces

After Merritt et al. (1975).

Differentiation of hepatic pathology is based on clinical signs and blood biochemistry. In haemolytic jaundice, total and indirect (unconjugated) bilirubin is increased whereas other liver function tests are normal. The packed cell volume falls to less than 0.3 litre/litre and ghost cells may be seen on erythrocyte examination.

In hepatocellular jaundice, total and direct (conjugated) bilirubin are increased. SAP is sometimes reduced and AST, SDH, LDH and α-GT are increased. Bromsulphalein (BSP) clearance (see p. 526) is delayed when damage is sufficient to impair gross hepatic function.

In biliary obstruction, the total direct (conjugated) bilirubin is increased and SAP is greatly increased whereas other liver function tests, except α-GT, may be normal. α-GT is a useful indicator of chronic liver damage. Liver biopsy (see p. 543) is useful to confirm liver pathology.

Acute hepatitis and advanced chronic hepatic damage, especially where biliary obstruction occurs, is usually easy to define on clinicopathological grounds. Cases of subclinical liver disease, not associated with biliary obstruction, are very difficult to confirm as there is no acute hepatocellular damage to increase the levels of AAT, SDH, and LDH, and SAP is normal.

In the absence of abnormality of the more specific liver enzymes, we find the interpretation of abnormal bilirubin levels very difficult. In cases with adequate hepatic compensation, BSP clearance tests are usually within the normal range.

The treatment of liver disease is frequently unrewarding in that it is only supportive. Therapy in cases of hepatic necrosis is aimed at allowing time for regeneration to occur. Supportive therapy includes intravenous fluids, glucose orally or intravenously, oral methionine and vitamin B1 and antibiotics administered parenterally if infection is present.

Diabetes mellitus

Reported cases of diabetes mellitus in the horse have been reviewed by Baker and Richie (1974). Most have been associated with pituitary neoplasia but two reports incriminated pancreatic degeneration. Baker and Richie described disease in a 21-year-old pony mare which was showing polydipsia, polyuria and loss of bodily condition. The animal became emaciated and at one stage a plasma glucose estimation revealed a level of 22.9 mmol/litre (normal range = 3.4–5.9 mmol/litre). The urine had a specific gravity of 1.029, a pH of 7, protein 300 g/litre and more than 0.1 mmol/litre glucose. The glucose tolerance test was abnormal, with prolonged elevation, and there was no response to insulin. A post-mortem examination revealed a tumour of the pars intermedia of the pituitary gland, adrenocortical hyperplasia and depletion of the beta cells of the pancreatic islets.

Pancreatic disease

Pancreatic disease is rarely seen in the horse but a case of acute necrotizing pancreatitis has been reported by Baker (1978).

CARDIOVASCULAR SYSTEM

The clinician is not called upon to diagnose or treat cardiovascular disease as frequently in stud farm as in stable practice. The main aspects are prognosis for insurance of stallions and, to a lesser extent, mares and the diagnosis of lesions which are causing clinical signs.

The assessment of cardiovascular status to recommend underwriters to insure a horse or a client to buy one are common tasks in stud farm medicine, but the same limits of interpretation apply as in other branches of equine medicine. Investigation is restricted to auscultation and electrocardiography. Measuring blood pressure or radiography of the heart are, for various reasons, seldom practised. At best, a clinical

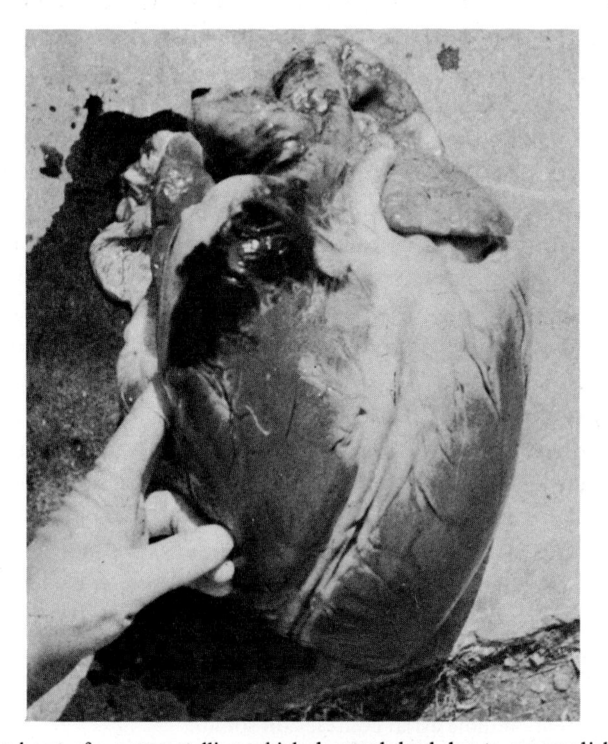

Fig. 7.15. The heart of a young stallion which dropped dead due to myocardial haemorrhage. Tracing from a small rupture of the aorta close to one of the semilunar valves.

appraisal is a matter of an accurate recording of findings followed by their subjective interpretation. Stallions may continue to cover mares for years despite a Grade III mitral systolic murmur or evidence of atrial fibrillation. But a young stallion with no detectable 'abnormalities' on auscultation or electrocardiography may die suddenly from myocardial haemorrhage or aortic rupture (Fig. 7.15).

Chronic cardiac disease in stud farm horses is usually confined to atrial fibrillation or vegetative lesions on the heart valves. Systemic signs of heart disease are often not apparent in these cases although intermittent fever, wasting and lassitude may be present. Conversely, heart murmurs and jugular pulse may be absent even in cases where, at post-mortem, gross lesions are present on the valves, which makes diagnosis hazardous. However, careful examination on several occasions will usually reveal some signs if such lesions are clinically significant.

The diagnosis of equine cardiovascular disease is a unique challenge to veterinarians because of the difficulties, and the aura which surrounds the subject in lay minds. A knowledge of available information is therefore essential and readers are recommended to a review by Detweiler and Patterson (1972) in which 295 references are cited.

The treatment of atrial fibrillation in three racehorses has been described by Rose and Davis (1977). They were treated with 10 g quinidine sulphate, every two hours, until auscultation of the heart demonstrated that 'cardioversion' had occurred. The total dose varied between 20 and 30 g. All three cases showed normal sinus rhythm at six months and went on to win races. Detweiler and Patterson (1972) suggest that a 5 g test dose is given before larger doses are started. The side effects of quinidine sulphate include urticarial weals, gastrointestinal disturbances (inappetence, colic, diarrhoea), erythema and oedema of the nasal mucosa (with respiratory embarrassment), vascular collapse, laminitis, congestive heart failure and sudden death. Treatment may be continued in the presence of mild urticaria and/or gastrointestinal disturbances. Any of the untoward sequelae indicate the necessity to stop treatment.

The diagnosis of atrial fibrillation is based on the following (Detweiler & Patterson 1972):

1. Absolutely irregular ventricular rhythm.
2. Elevated heart rate (between 50 and 90/minute), although bradycardia, normal rate and rates exceeding 100/minute sometimes are found.
3. 'Pulse deficit', i.e. pulse rates less than the audible heart beat rate.
4. Absence of the second heart sound when, following a short diastolic period, the ventricles fail to fill sufficiently with blood to permit opening of the semilunar valves.
5. Variation in the strength of the peripheral pulse.
6. Variation in the intensity of heart sounds and murmurs.
7. Absence of an audible atrial contraction sound.

An electrocardigraphic examination completes the diagnosis by the absence of P-waves and the presence of rapid atrial oscillations (fibrillation or F-waves).

RESPIRATORY SYSTEM

Conditions of the respiratory system are usually infectious and they are referred to earlier in this chapter or in discussing pulmonary diseases of the newborn or older foal.

Here we shall confine ourselves to a summary of non-infectious diseases which originate in the respiratory tract or lungs.

Epistaxis

Nose bleeds may follow accident, ulceration of the guttural pouch or nasal mucosa, pulmonary disease (Robinson 1979), or neoplasia, e.g. ethmoid haematoma (Cook & Littlewort 1974). These authors described it in 16 horses varying in age from four to 20 years who all showed signs of slight unilateral epistaxis. The diagnosis is made endoscopically by the observation of a trickle of blood seen escaping either from the nasomaxillary duct, at the caudal end of the middle meatus, or from the ethmoidal meati. In others, the great ethmoturbinate bone shows a greenish yellow discoloration. In advanced cases, the haematoma itself becomes visible in the ethmoid region, sometimes obscuring normal anatomical land-marks. An abnormal radiopacity may sometimes be seen in the paranasal sinuses and even in the nasal cavity and nasopharynx. Cook and Littlewort described surgical resection of the haematoma and the effected ethmoid labyrinth in 13 cases but the lesion recurred in five. Histologically the capsule of the haematoma is composed of respiratory epithelium and fibrous tissue and the stroma contains blood, macrophages, multinucleate giant cells and some fibrous tissue. The disease is not yet fully understood.

Guttural pouch disease

The features of guttural pouch disease have been reviewed by McAllister (1977). The paired pouches are ventral diverticula of the eustachian tubes, situated beneath the base of the cranium and the atlas and apposing each other medially. The pouches are dorsal to the nasopharynx and bounded laterally by the vertical rami of the mandible and parotid salivary glands. Each pouch is divided into a medial and lateral compartment by the hyoid bones. The cranial nerves VII, IX, X, XI and XII, the cranial sympathetic trunk and the internal and external carotid arteries are involved with the pouches. Each pouch communicates with the nasopharynx through the nasopharngeal orifice of the eustachian tube.

Tympany of the guttural pouch sometimes occurs in foals and may be diagnosed by marked distention of the guttural pouches with air. The cause of this condition is probably a maldevelopment or malfunction of the mucosal flap on the inner aspect of the nasopharyngeal orifice. Treatment is by surgical fenestration of the medial septum of the two pouches (Cook 1966, 1974).

Guttural pouch empyema may follow upper respiratory infections or, more usually, are associated with guttural pouch mycosis (Cook 1968). This condition usually presents as a foul-smelling, greenish, unilateral chronic nasal discharge which may be intermittently blood-tinged. Repeated epistaxis or a single fatal haemorrhage may occur. Diagnosis is by endoscopy (see p. 512) and treatment is by drainage and local irrigation of the guttural pouch using a suitable antibiotic and antifungal agent. Drainage may be by surgical intervention through Viborg's triangle (Baker 1972) or via the nasopharynx using an indwelling mare uterine cather (see p. 72) or through a fibreoptic endoscope (Cook 1974; Mansman & Wheat 1972).

In cases where serious epistaxis has occurred, or is likely, surgical ligation of the internal carotid artery is recommended (Owen 1974).

Chronic obstructive pulmonary disease (pulmonary emphysema, 'heaves')

McPherson and Lawson (1974) discussed the difficulty of defining 'heaves' as a clinical or pathological entity. McPherson et al. (1978*a, b*) used the definition chronic obstructive pulmonary disease (COPD) and showed that affected horses had all or some of the following features: poor work performance, a history of previous febrile illness, chronic cough, dyspnoea, double expiratory effort, increased breathing sounds, wheezing and crepitant breathing sounds and prolonged coughing. Affected horses improved when contact with hay and straw was reduced.

McPherson et al. (1979) found that COPD was most commonly detected in show-jumping and hacking horses between the ages of six and ten years. The incidence of the disease did, however, increase with age. Ponies were more frequently affected than Thoroughbred horses but there is no doubt that 'broken-winded' Thoroughbred brood mares and stallions are seen. These authors suggest that the high incidence in ponies is related to the more frequent exposure to poor-quality fodder and bedding. Exposure to moulds and poor ventilation increase the incidence of the disease. Sex, body weight and season of onset of coughing had no influence on the recurrence of the disease. An allergic aetiology has long been suspected (Alexander 1959; Mahaffey 1962; Cook & Rossdale 1963; Gillespie & Tyler 1969 Eyre 1972) and parallels have been drawn to the condition of asthma in human (Cook 1976; Gerber 1973). Mansmann et al. (1975) reported on a study of two horses that were exposed to chickens. They demonstrated an allergic, hypersensitivity-type reaction, leading to 'heaves' which was believed to be similar to the Arthus-like hypersensitivity pneumonitides reported in man.

Macpherson et al. (1979) identified the fungi *Micropolysporum faeni* and *Aspergillus fumigatus* as common causes of respiratory hypersensitivity in horses affected with COPD. Rye grass pollen and Actinomycetes produced respiratory allergy in a few horses. Not infrequently, individual horses were found to have respiratory hypersensitivity to two or more antigens. These authors used an intradermal test with an antigen extract suitable for diagnostic use. Lawson et al. (1979) found that serum precipitins to *M. faeni* and *A. fumigatus* occurred more frequently in case of COPD than in unaffected horses. Many animals without detectable precipitin responded clinically to inhalation challenge with these antigens. Matthews (1979 investigated the possible role of serum antiproteases in the onset of COPD, in an analogous manner to the hereditary dysproteinaemia of α_1 antitrypsin in man There was no evidence of a genetically determined variation in the protease-binding proteins, but an increased frequency of the electrophoretically slower Pr antitrypsin alleles was present in COPD cases. The significance of this observation could not be critically assessed.

Mansman and Mansman (1969) and Gerber (1973) found eosinophils and inflammatory cells in the nasal secretions of horses with chronic allergic pulmonary disease.

Gerber (1973) described the histopathological lesions seen in affected horses. There was moderate chronic bronchiolitis in all cases and in most there was a mononuclear cell infiltration of the peribronchiolar tissue. The bronchiolitis appeared to be purulent in some cases but as a rule it was bacteriologically sterile. In fewer than a third of all cases, eosinophil leucocytic infiltration was demonstrable. The interstitial tissues occasionally showed infiltration with eosinophil leucocytes. There was hyperplasia of bronchiolar mucous glands, hyperplasia of smooth muscle and vasculitis in some cases. In cases which were destroyed for reasons of advanced COPD, panlobular bullous emphysema was seen. The emphysema sometimes spread into the interstitial tissues and in one-third of the cases a focal hyperplasia of the respiratory epithelium was observed.

The condition is undoubtedly progressive in that continual exposure to the allergens results in advanced pulmonary histopathological changes and 'broken wind' occurs.

Treatment is aimed at trying to reduce challenge by the allergens and at suppressing the allergic response mechanisms. Recommended treatment is usually to turn affected horses out to grass at all times. This may not always be possible, or desirable, as is the case with brood mares with young foals. In these cases all one can do is to try to reduce environmental dust and moulds. A large, clean, well ventilated stable should be used and peat moss should be used for bedding. Complete pelleted rations should be fed and any hay given should be of the very best quality and thoroughly soaked before use. Injections of corticosteroids, with systemic antibiotic cover, are useful and antihistamines are sometimes given.

BLOOD AND BLOOD-FORMING ORGANS

Primary problems are rare in the horse. Haematological changes are usually secondary to other systemic problems and are a useful aid to diagnosis in systemic disease (see p. 519). Anaemias are seldom primary but secondary to trauma, strongylosis, poor nutrition or chronic infections. Some viral diseases, especially equine infectious anaemia, cause a profound anaemia. Haemolytic anaemias may occur with some plant poisoning, phenothiazine administration and in haemolytic disease of the newborn foal.

Equine infectious anaemia

This infectious condition is a serious problem in North America and some parts of Europe but few cases have been reported in Great Britain. This disease has been discussed previously (see p. 428).

Piroplasmosis

Piroplasmosis is a protozoal disease caused by *Babesia equi* and *Babesia caballi* which is seen in some parts of America and the European continent (Ristic 1975). It manifests as a profound haemolytic anaemia with haemoglobinuria and the clinical signs are very similar to those of EIA. Various species of ticks are capable of transmitting the disease. Diagnosis is by the identification of the protozoa in blood smears from capillary vessels, for example the pinna of the ear, and the serological detection of babesial antibodies. The drugs of choice for treatment of *Babesia caballi* infections are:

1. Phenamidine isethionate at a dose rate of 0.03 ml of a 40% solution per kg body weight subcutaneously. Occasionally there may be a local reaction at the site of injection.

2. Quinuronium sulphate at a dose rate of 0.6–1 mg/kg body weight subcutaneously. Signs of intolerance may occur 10–15 minutes after injection, consisting of restlessness, muscular spasms and salivation. Toxic symptoms may be controlled by the administration of adrenaline or atropine.

Barnett (1974) has discussed the anomaly associated with the complement-fixation test against *B. caballi* and *B. equi* antigens. Although he believes that the UK is 'free' of the disease, he reports that 7% of tests carried out by the US Department of Agriculture on horses for export from the United Kingdom to the USA reacted positively to one or both of the equine babesial species. He suggests that an infection rate of this order would indicate that endemic disease is present in the UK, that the test is detecting non-specific antibodies or that the UK re-exports a very large number of horses originating from other infected countries. The Ministry of Agriculture favours the latter view and Barnett suggests that the UK must protect itself by testing all horses coming from the USA. Barnett was not able to trace the origin of the horses involved and on epidemiological grounds he was sceptical of the validity of a complement-fixation test as an indicator of infection. He suggests that all past positive reactors to the complement-fixation test, especially those that are undisputedly indigenous and have never been outside the British Isles and Ireland, should be tested for infection by inoculating their blood into splenectomized horses. Piroplasmosis is a notifiable disease in Great Britain.

Trypanosomiasis

Trypanosomiasis is another protozoal disease affecting the erythrocytes and causing anaemia and is not seen in the United Kingdom. Ristic (1975) has reviewed the disease in horses. Nagana (*Trypanosoma brucei*) is confined to the African continent and is transmitted by the tsetse fly. Symptoms include anaemia, intermittent fever and oedema. In the early state of the disease, trypanosomes can be found in the peripheral blood. As the disease progresses, the organism is more readily detected in the fluid obtained by puncturing lymph glands. Surra (*Trypanosoma evansi*) has been reported from the Far East, the Middle East, South and Central America and through importations, from Australia and the United States. The disease is transmitted by the horse fly (*Tabanus*). Clinical signs are similar to those of nagana. Mal del caderas (*Trypanosoma equinum*) is seen in South America and is transmitted by biting flies and vampire bats. Clinical symptoms are similar to surra and nagana. Murrina (*Trypanosoma hippicum*) occurs in Panama and parts of Central and South America. The disease is transmitted by biting flies and vampire bats and symptoms are similar to those previously described. Dourine (*Trypanosoma equiperdum*) occurs in Asia (USSR), Africa, Mediterranean countries, the Republic of South Africa, southern and eastern Europe, South America and Mexico. The disease is notifiable in the United Kingdom. It is a venereal disease, transmitted by coitus, and is seldom seen in the blood. This disease has been described previously (see p. 156).

Ehrlichiosis

Ehrlichiosis is an infectious disease manifested by fever, anorexia, stiffness and oedema of the legs and thrombocytopenia (Ristic 1975). *Ehrlichia equi*, a Rickettsia-like organism, is found in the cytoplasm of neutrophils and eosinophils and is easily detectable at the time of acute infection. The disease is restricted to the west coast of the United States and the mode of transmission is unknown.

Autoimmune haemolytic anaemia

Autoimmune haemolytic anaemia is rare in the horse but has been discussed by Collins (1975). It is a manifestation of an immunological dyscrasia which results in the production of antibodies operative against the body's own erythrocytes or erythrocytic precursors. Autoantibodies have been incriminated in the pathogenesis of acute haemolytic anaemia observed both during the terminal stages of abdominal lymphomatosis and following purpura haemorrhagica. Idiopathic autoimmune haemolytic anaemia has also been described. Cases may show dullness, ventral abdominal oedema, marked jaundice and sometimes pyrexia. The most striking clinicopathological feature is the rapid autoagglutination of erythrocytes following blood sampling. Positive agglutination may also occur with anti-horse globulin.

Haemophilia

Haemophilia is rarely seen in young foals and has been described previously (see p. 411). Haemophilia-like syndromes may occur after a haemorrhagic episode and loss of platelets, causing a vicious circle of further haemorrhage. This can be corrected by a platelet transfusion with packed erythrocytes.

Disseminated intravascular coagulopathy

Disseminated intravascular coagulopathy (DIC) is a syndrome recognized in man and dog following systemic infections and some neoplastic lesions (Archer 1977).

A similar condition has been seen in horses (Lewis 1972, personal communication) and responds to heparinization.

Purpura haemorrhagica

Purpura haemorrhagica may be a complication of other infectious disease, e.g. strangles, influenza and various suppurative conditions (Greatorex 1969). The condition usually appears either while the acute symptoms are subsiding or at the commencement of the convalescent period. Clinical signs are extensive oedema of the head and limbs and the wide-spread development of petechial haemorrhages. Urticarial lesions may also be present over various parts of the body surface. The aetiology of the condition is obscure but, because of its common association with streptococcal infections of the upper respiratory tract, the suggestion has been made that it is an allergic reaction to streptococcal protein. Cases have, however, been encountered without a prior history of streptococcal infection. As the disease progresses, respiratory distress may become acute. Oedematous limbs may become acutely painful and pit easily on pressure. The oedematous swellings on the limbs may terminate abruptly at the level of the stifle or elbow joints but occasionally the oedema merges into the surrounding unaffected tissues.

An anaemia of varying severity occurs (PCV less than 0.30 litre/litre) and prothrombin times are above the upper limit of the normal range. There is leucocytosis with a 'shift to the left' and an eosinopenia is usually present. In a majority of cases there is associated hypocalcaemia (1.25–1.5 mmol/litre).

Treatment consists of early administration of 2–3 litres of blood intravenously without waiting for the thrombocyte and prothrombin estimations, followed by 1000 ml of calcium borogluconate intravenously and 200–250 mg vitamin K intramuscularly. Antihistamine preparations may be administered if there is no sign of improvement within 12 hours of the initial treatment. Systemic antibiotic cover is given. Thiamine and corticosteroid preparations have been advocated but Greatorex is of the opinion that they do not influence the course of the condition. Cold applications to the affected limbs are useful and short spells of walking exercise should be given immediately the patient is capable. Rugs, harness etc. should be removed, as this may increase the risk of sloughing of the oedematous parts.

If cases are recognized and treated early, the prognosis may be favourable, but as the condition progresses and there are signs of respiratory distress, diarrhoea, sudden rises in temperature and recumbency, the prognosis becomes grave.

Myeloma

Multiple myeloma has been described in a horse by Cornelius et al. (1959). This is a plasma cell lesion causing lameness and weakness progressing to paralysis. A profound anaemia occurs due to space-occupying lesions in the bone marrow.

Lymphosarcoma

Lymphosarcoma is the most common tumour of the haemopoietic system of the horse (Vaughan 1969). It is also the most common abdominal tumour of the horse and has been previously described (see p. 462). Roberts (1977) described progressive leukaemic changes and a persistant anaemia in a seven-year-old gelding which showed signs of lowered performance and unthriftiness and later developed dependant oedema and became listless. The total leucocyte count, initially within the normal range although reflecting an absolute lymphocytosis, increased four-fold in six days, from excessive lymphoid production involving predominately the more immature cell types (lymphoblasts, prolymphocytes and large lymphocytes). The severity of the condition was confirmed by bone marrow biopsy. We have had the opportunity to examine a blood sample from a leukaemic horse where the total white cell count was in the region of 100×10^9/litre.

Lymphangitis

This disease is also known as Monday morning disease, big leg and ulcerative, sporadic or epizootic lymphangitis. The terminology surrounding inflammatory conditions of the lymphatic system is confused because of the different synonyms that have been used to describe a variety of entities in which lymphangitis is a sign.

There are multiple causes. Overloaded lymphatics and circulatory disturbances are responsible for simple, uncomplicated attacks of lymphangitis in which oedematous swelling is the cardinal sign. Infective lymphangitis, in which heat, swelling and pain are present, may be caused by *Str. pyogenes, Staph. aureus, E. coli, Corynebacterium pseudotuberculosis* and *Histoplasma farcinnosum.* In most cases lymphadenitis is also present.

Hot, painful swellings associated with the lymphatics occur in the legs, especially hind-legs, on the abdomen, in front of the mammary glands in advanced gestation and in tracts from subcutaneous abscesses and *Hypoderma* larvae on the flank, back or shoulder. In the legs the condition starts as a local swelling, often confined to one side in the fetlock or pastern region. The swelling soon spreads up the leg, to include the cannon, hock and thigh in the hind-limb and the knee and fore-arm in the fore-limb. The swelling is oedematous and pits on pressure. A ridge is formed at its upper limits, which in the hind-limb is usually level with the stifle (Fig. 7.17). The condition is usually confined to one limb and often starts from a depigmented marking on the pastern.

In peracute cases, the limb increases to two or three times its normal diameter within 24 hours. The affected individual is disinclined to move and when forced to do so uses the leg in short, painful strides. Anorexia and 'constipation' are usually present and there may be rapid loss of weight. Sweating and distress may occur if the horse is made to move.

After 24–72 hours serum exudes onto the skin and rolls down the leg. Small bullae develop and burst at various points along the lymphatic system leaving scabs

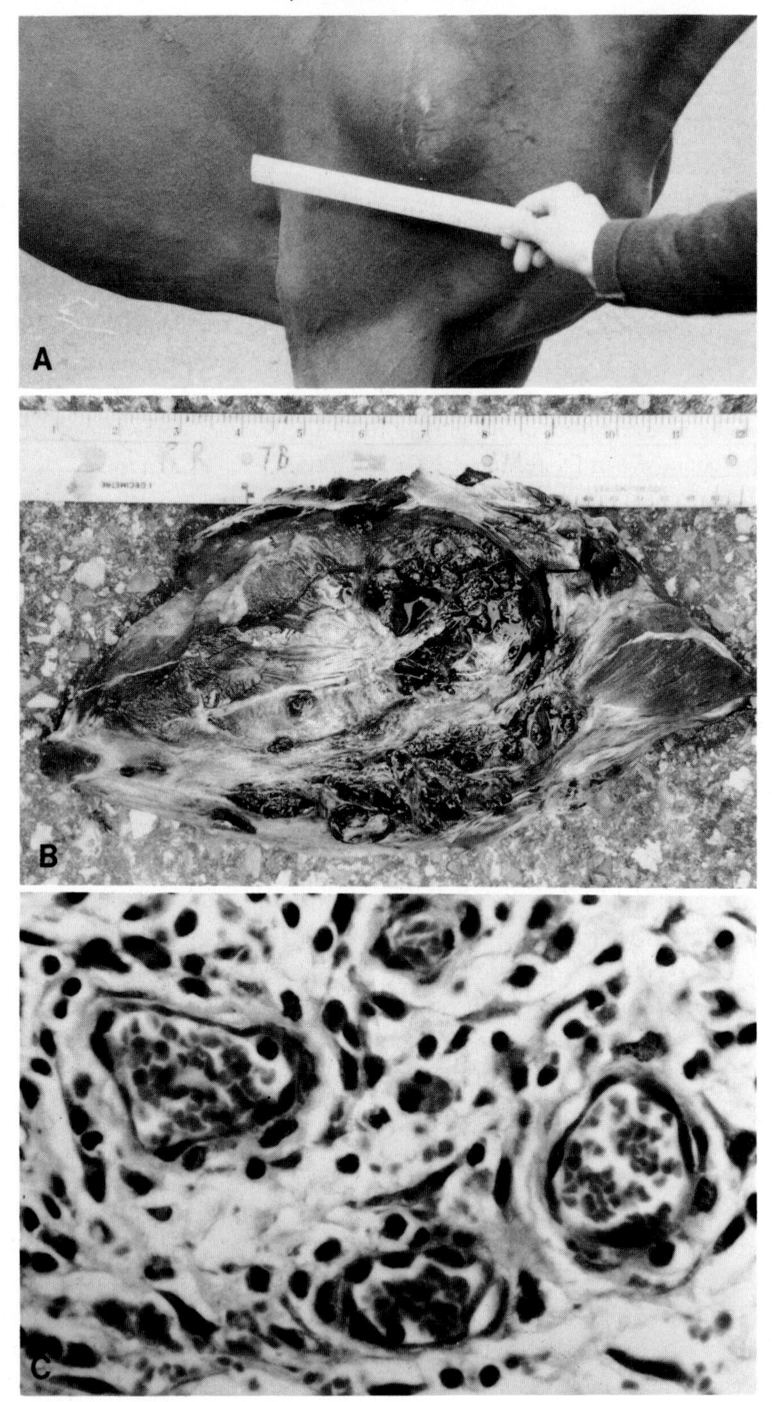

Fig. 7.16. A, Haemangio-endothelioma of the right shoulder in a yearling Thoroughbred filly, which had regrown following previous attempts at surgical excision. B, Gross structure at post-mortem. C, Poorly circumscribed invasive lesion with oval hyperchromatic cells lining irregular sinusoidal spaces containing some erythrocytes. H & E × 450.

of serum and matted hair. These eruptions usually coincide with a weakening of signs.

Repeated occurrences are probable and the leg may become permanently thickened by chronic subcutaneous inflammatory tissue.

Wounds, small abrasions and pustular areas should be liberally treated with ointment containing a broad-spectrum antibiotic, e.g. terramycin, and a corticosteroid. Scabs should be gently removed. If they are thick and persistent they may

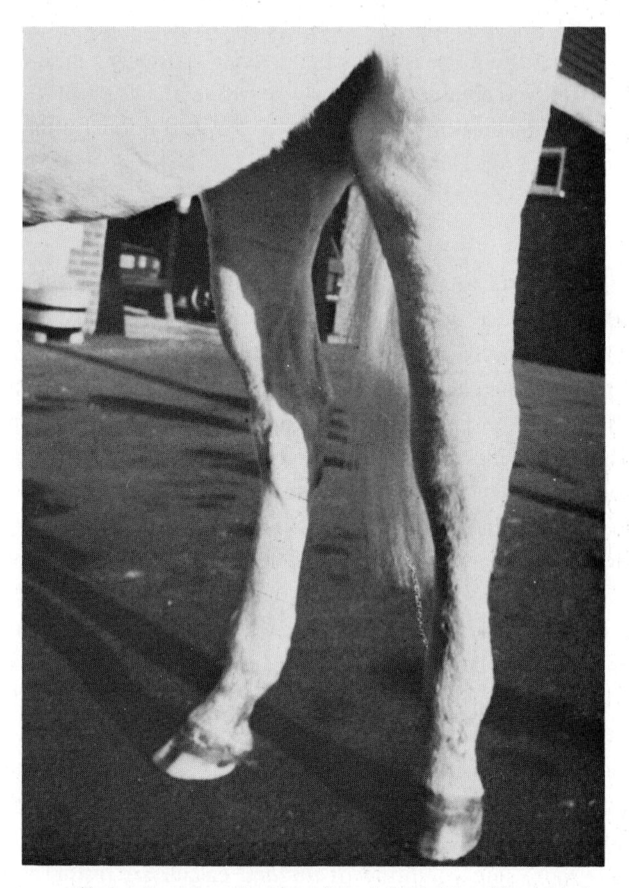

Fig. 7.17. A mare suffering from lymphangitis of the left hind-leg. Note the characteristic ridge inside the stifle. For details see text.

be first softened with cetrimide ointment. Parenteral antibiotics (terramycin or penicillin) or sulphonamides should be administered for two to three days until the acute phase has subsided. Corticosteroids and diuretics may be used to reduce swelling and phenylbutazone to relieve pain. Naproxen, if used early enough, is sometimes useful in reducing swelling. Saline and liquid paraffin should be administered through a stomach tube, depending on faecal consistency. Gentle exercise should be encouraged and affected horses made to move about the paddock or led in hand. In the acute phase straw bedding should be reduced to a minimum or be replaced by peat or wood shavings. The horse should, if possible, be turned onto a paddock or large yard. When appetite returns the protein content of the diet should be reduced and the quantity of concentrates limited. Susceptible horses with access to spring grass should not receive concentrates.

URINARY SYSTEM

Urinary and renal abnormalities are comparatively rare in the horse. The horseman's complaint that this horse is 'thick in his water' is usually a misconception.

Diagnosis of urinary conditions is made on urine analysis (see p. 529), raised blood urea and serum creatinine levels (see p. 527), abnormal urinary creatinine clearance ratios (see p. 527) and rectal palpation.

Calculi

Urinary calculi consist of accumulations of mineral substances in the urinary tract. These form in the bladder, urethra and, rarely kidneys. Those most commonly seen are composed of calcium carbonate. Their surfaces are rough and they are coloured yellow-brown. Phosphate calculi are smooth and white. Carbonate calculi are more common in horses fed on pasture or high-roughage diets whereas phosphate calculi occur in horses fed on high-phosphate rations. The most common site of calculi is in the bladder where they form by precipitation and not, as sometimes happens in other species, in the kidneys. A particulate nucleus is thought to be necessary for the formation of such masses and a low-water, high-mineral diet may predispose to their formation.

The presence of calculi causes signs of vague abdominal discomfort and excessive straining to pass urine. The calculus may work as a 'ball' in a valve and obstruct the passage of urine. When this occurs incontinence is often seen and voiding of urine during exercise. Complications include cystitis accompanied by fever, inappetance and blood-stained urine. Urine analysis reveals large amounts of mineral crystals and palpation of the calculi on rectal examination completes the diagnosis. Treatment is by surgical removal.

Signs of the more rare condition of *urethral* calculi are restlessness, colic and frequent attempts at urination. Such calculi may be detected on passing a catheter and they may sometimes be dislodged in this way. There is usually an associated urethritis with blood and debris in the urine. Smooth muscle relaxants, e.g. proquamazine fumerate, may be useful in aiding their expulsion from the urethra. Urethral calculi seldom cause problems in mares but in colts and geldings urethrotomy may be necessary to remove the calculus.

Renal calculi are very rare. One was reported by Jackson (1972) in a 10-year-old gelding found in routine inspection at an abattoir. This was primarily composed of calcium carbonate. No history was available for the gelding as to whether it had shown symptoms or been under veterinary treatment.

Cystitis

Cystitis is usually seen as a secondary phenomenon. Signs are frequent urination, colic and the presence of blood and purulent material in the urine. Organisms cultured are streptococci, staphylococci, coliforms, corynebacteria and klebsiellae. Treatment is by the administration of antibiotics to which the particular organisms is sensitive. A primary cystitis has been reported in America with horses grazing Sudan grass.

Nephrosis

Nephrosis is rarely seen but is characterized by histological degeneration of tubular or glomerular tissue. Tubular degeneration has been reported as a post-mortem finding in cases of chemical poisoning with mercury, arsenic, copper, carbon tetrachloride, sodium nitrate, phenothiazine, tetrochloroethylene and chlorinated hydrocarbon insecticides. Bile pigment, bacterial toxins, haemoglobinuria and myoglobinuria also produce lesions.

Glomerular nephrosis with the production of anti-glomerular basement membrane (GBM) antibody has been reported by Banks and Henson (1972). One case showed clinical signs of renal failure and died. The authors suggest that carcinomas may in some cases produce antigens which result in the formation of anti-GBM.

Nephritis

Nephritis is rare in horses and is most commonly seen as *Actinobacillus* infection in newborn foals (see p. 308). Purulent foci may also occur in the kidneys of foals with strangles or in other chronic streptococcal infections. Buntain et al. (1979) described a case of chronic nephritis in a 17-year-old pony. Clinical symptoms were weight loss over a six-month period despite dental attention, anthelmintic treatment and supplementary feeding. Serial blood samples revealed high blood urea and creatinine and occasional slight elevations in SAP and AST. The circulating albumin levels and the albumin/globulin ratio were low to low-normal throughout. Serum electrophoresis confirmed a low albumin peak. Analysis of urine samples showed a consistantly low-normal specific gravity and a high level of protein. Hyaline casts were seen on one occasion. The horse's condition deteriorated and the pony was destroyed. At post-mortem examination the kidneys were reduced in size. The capsules were stripped with difficulty to reveal pale, irregular surfaces and there was diffuse thinning of the cortices. Microscopic examinations of the kidneys disclosed a variety of glomerular changes. Many were completely hyalinized while others were partially destroyed. The latter showed varying degrees of mesangial cell proliferation with exudation of fibrin and adhesions between the capillary loops and Bowman's membrane. Glomeruli in the outer cortex were hypertrophied but otherwise relatively normal. In the vicinity of affected glomeruli there was extensive tubular atrophy with interstitial fibrosis and small aggregations of lymphocytes and plasma cells. The surviving functional tubules were dilated and many contained hyaline casts.

We have had the opportunity of investigating an almost identical case to the one just described. The clinical, clinicopathological and pathological findings were almost identical but in addition urine creatinine clearance ratios (see p. 527) were performed. These showed significant elevation in urinary clearance of sodium, potassium, chloride and phosphate, indicating gross renal incompetence. The glomerular damage accounted for the protein-losing nephropathy. As with the case of Buntain et al. the aetiological factors associated with this case were obscure.

Bladder paralysis

Paralysis of the bladder may be a sequel to equid herpesvirus I (rhinopneumonitis) infection, neuritis of the cauda equina and incontinence following a difficult parturition.

NERVOUS SYSTEM

The subject of nervous diseases is extensive yet in equine stud farms most conditions are related to accidents which result in trauma of the cranial nerves and cause paralysis of the facial or limb muscles. Blindness, due to cranial haemorrhage involving the optic nerves, is also a common sequela of cranial injury.

Wobbler disease and cerebellar hypoplasia have been described in Chapter 6. *Setaria* spp. (cerebrospinal nematodiasis) are a cause of equine incoordination in the Far East (Shoho 1954) and aberrant *Hypoderma* or strongyle larvae may occasionally enter the cranium and cause nervous signs. Abscesses of the brain and hydatid cysts (Miller & Poynter 1956) are sometimes found; meningitis and encephalitis are rare except in young foals and in specific arbovirus infections.

Segmental myelitis has been recorded by Rooney et al. (1970) who described focal lesions in grey and white matter and destructive, inflammatory lesions in the spinal cord. Clinical signs vary with the site of the lesions but cases often cross legs when pushed sideways and drag the feet when backed. Incoordination may become marked until recumbency occurs. Treatment is not successful.

Neuritis of the cauda equina is an inflammatory lesion of the caudal part of the spinal cord and sometimes the cranial nerves, causing anaesthesia of the perineum, paralysis of the tail and bladder and degrees of posterior incoordination. The trigeminal is the most often affected of the cranial nerves (Rooney 1971; Greenwood et al. 1973).

Incoordination associated with equid herpesvirus I infection has been described before (see p. 425).

Encephalitis caused by louping-ill virus has been described by Timoney et al. (1976) in a group of free-range horses in Ireland. Three of the four horses displayed signs of CNS disturbance and two died after illness ranging from two to 12 days duration. Cases showed muscular tremors, incoordination and a tendency to knuckle over in front. In one case, the condition progressed to recumbency and the mare exhibited hyperexcitability, incoordination and opisthotonus. In two cases that died, a variable degree of viral polioencephalomyelitis was observed. A virus, antigenically indistinguishable from a reference strain of louping-ill virus, was isolated from the brain and cervical cord of one mare. Serum samples obtained from three of the horses contained haemagglutination-inhibition, complement-fixation, precipitating and neutralizing antibodies to louping-ill virus, with a rise in antibody titre being demonstrated in two cases. Timoney (1976) described a serological survey of horses in Ireland and demonstrated a positive serum neutralizing antibody reaction to louping-ill virus in 10.6% of cases. Many of the positive cases were cross-bred horses destined for slaughter and the incidence in Thoroughbred mares was only 0.7%. Timoney suggested that the considerable differences in the environmental background of the two types of horses accounted for the different infection rates. The disease is spread by the tick *Ixodes ricinis* which is more prevalent in Ireland than in Britain. Timoney studied the susceptibility of the horse to louping-ill virus and indicated that, although the horse could act as a reservoir of the virus, the infection had little if any clinical significance.

MUSCULOSKELETAL SYSTEM

The subject of lameness does not fall within the scope of this book and readers are referred to Adams (1974) and Rooney (1972).

Set-fast

However, we must mention set-fast (myoglobinuria) because it is frequently encountered when heavily pregnant mares or those that have foaled are turned onto the paddock for the first time following confinement to a loosebox. The aetiology and pathogenesis of the condition are still obscure although a number of hypothese (Carlstrom 1950; Rowland 1964; McLean 1967) suggest lactic acid release in abnormal physiological situations, hormonal disturbances and vitamin A and E deficiencies.

Signs include stiffness, sweating, distress and in some cases the passing of red or black urine due to the presence of myoglobin and haemoglobin. Some cases may need differentiation from a 'true' colic (see p. 495). Muscles over the rump or loin are hard and painful.

Diagnosis is made on the clinical signs and history of recent strenuous exercise, especially following a period of rest. Serum CK levels may rise to 250 IU/litre and greater. In severe cases, CK levels are as high as several thousand units and these cases may become recumbent and their prognosis is poor.

Very mild cases may need only tranquillization and rest. In more severe cases, salicylates and phenylbutazone may be used. Corticosteroids and intravenous sodium bicarbonate may reduce the effects of progressive muscle damage and may therefore hasten recovery. Following an initial period of rest, slow regular exercise should begin after the acute phase has subsided.

In mares that seem particularly prone to this problem, it may sometimes be prevented by the administration of 28 g sodium salicylate orally, daily, prior to exercise after a period of enforced rest. Some degree of prevention may also be obtained by initially turning the mare out in a small paddock or, if exercise is restricted because of foal disease, letting the mare exercise for a short while, daily, on her own. Vitamin E and selenium therapy appears useful in some cases.

Laminitis

Laminitis is associated with a transient inflammation of the sensitive laminae of the hoof followed by their congestion (Colles & Jeffcott 1977). The disease may occur in one or all four feet and may be acute, subacute or chronic. Ponies are

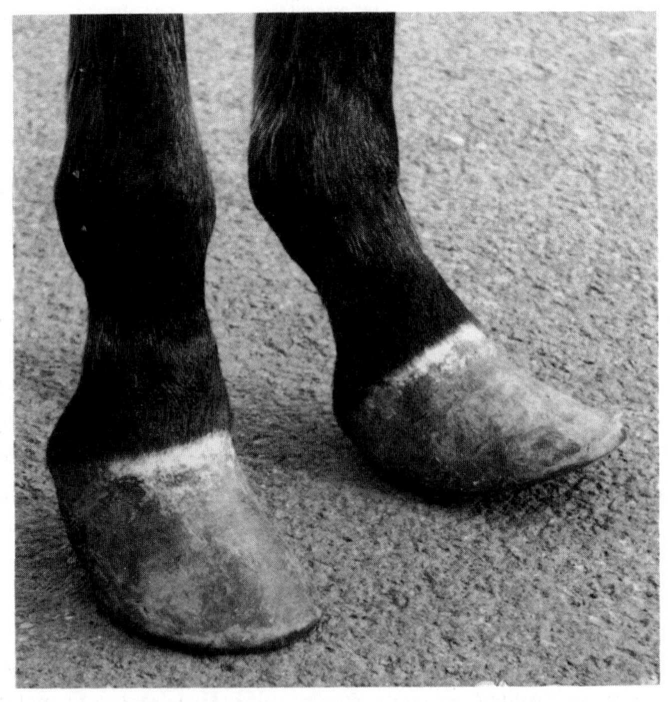

Fig. 7.18. Chronic laminitis in a pony mare. Inadequate hoof trimming has led to marked overgrowth at the toes and a 'chinese slipper' effect.

affected more frequently than Thoroughbreds and those that are fat, overweight and unfit appear prone to the disease. There is a higher incidence of the acute and subacute forms of the disease in April and May with the flush of new grass, and in August and September.

Acute cases are depressed and anorexic and show a great reluctance to stand. There is always marked resistance to exercise and the horse has a characteristic stance with the fore-legs forward and hind-legs drawn under the body, in order to take weight on the heels. If forced to walk, affected cases show a slow, crouching, short-striding gait, with each foot lifted and replaced as quickly as possible. There is usually heat in the region of the coronary band and a bounding pulse in the digital arteries. Pain may cause muscular tremors. Rotation of the pedal bone may occur during or after the acute stage if early treatment is not successful. In cases where a blood-stained exudate seeps from the coronary band, the prognosis is considered hopeless.

Subacute cases show similar signs to those described above but to a lesser degree. Acute and subacute forms may tend to recur and develop into the chronic form.

TABLE 7.8 Some precipitating factors in equine laminitis

Excess carbohydrate intake ('grain overload')
Post-parturient metritis septicaemia
Toxaemia – associated with enteritis, colitis X (exhaustion shock) and endotoxic shock
Management and type – concussion in unfit horses or susceptible animal (e.g. fat pony)
Unilateral leg lameness putting excess strain on contralateral limb
High level corticosteroid administration
Fatty liver syndrome

Other suggested factors:
- Hypothyroidism
- Allergic-type reaction to certain medication (e.g. anthelmintics, oestrogens and androgens)
- High oestrogen content of pasture

After Colles and Jeffcott (1977).

Chronic laminitis is characterized by changes in the shape of the hoof with bands of irregular horn growth (laminitic rings), close at the toe and diverging at the heel. The hoof itself becomes contracted (narrow and elongated) with a wall almost vertical at the heel and horizontal at the toe. In neglected cases, the toe may turn upwards ('chinese slipper'). The sole becomes thickened and flattened and somewhat convex in outline. When standing, the horse shifts weight from one foot to the other and, when moving, the gait is abnormal and similar to that described above. Radiographic examination reveals rotation and sometimes osteoporosis of the pedal bone. In severe cases, the tip of the pedal bone may penetrate the sole, just in front of the point of the frog.

The full details of the pathogenesis of laminitis are still incompletely understood but many precipitating factors have been incriminated (Table 7.8). Raised blood pressure (hypertension) appears to be involved and a disturbance in blood circulation to the foot probably causes the pain. Laminitic rings and pedal bone rotation may be caused by chronic hypoxia and a lack of sulphur-containing amino acids to the corium of the hoof, slowing or stopping keratinization.

Treatment must be started as early as possible if permanent damage is to be avoided. Where there is a history of alimentary involvement or if the cause is unknown, the administration of liquid paraffin and purgatives by stomach tube is indicated. The diet should be restricted to hay and water. Antibiotic cover is indicated in horses where the precipitating factor may be an infectious agent or when secondary infection is suspected. To encourage the circulation in the foot, local anaesthetic blocks of the posterior digial nerves should be performed. This relieves pain and allows the horse to stand and walk normally. Acetylpromazine will reduce blood pressure and suppress the animal's response to pain. Corticosteroids may be valuable initially, but appear to be contraindicated after the first day, as they may produce proteolysis and encourage pedal bone rotation. Phenylbutazone is useful for long-term analgesia. The value of antihistamine treatment is uncertain.

Improving the blood circulation to the foot by walking on soft ground is extremely useful but is contraindicated if there may be rotation of the pedal bone. Support to the sole of the foot may be given by standing the horse on sand or packing the sole with tar and tow or hoof repair material. Hot-water bathing is probably more beneficial than cold, as warmth tends to dilate the arterioles and ease the spasm and hypertension.

To help keratinization, methionine may be administered at a dose rate of 10 g daily for four days followed by a 5 g daily for a further 10 days. In cases where fatty liver and hypothyroidism are suspected, appropriate treatment should be given.

With chronic laminitis, careful attention to the feet and the prevention of further acute or subacute attacks (i.e. by restriction of diet and controlled exercise etc.) is indicated. Secondary infection should be eliminated by debridement of infected sinuses and any rotting horn should be carefully pared away. The toes should be shortened and the heels lowered regularly and frequently to try to restore the conformation of the hoof in relation to the pedal bone. In cases of marked rotation, radical hoof surgery may be indicated but in general the prognosis in these cases is poor.

Laminitis is occasionally seen in brood mares at stud. Steps to prevent its occurrence should be taken following traumatic parturition, retention of the placenta and uterine prolapse. The condition may be seen in stallions, as they get older, especially where management has allowed them to become excessively fat due to excess food and/or inadequate exercise.

References and further reading

Adams O.R. (1974) *Lameness in Horses*, 3rd ed. Philadalphia: Lea & Febiger

Alexander, A.F. (1959) Chronic alveolar emphysema in the horse. *Am. Rev. resp. Dis.*, **80**, 141.

Al-Kafawi, A.A., Al-Ani, F.K., Al-Bassam, L.S. & Youkob, A.T. (1977) Haematological changes in Arabian horses infected with glanders. *Vet. Rec.*, **101**, 427.

Andersson, G., Ekman, L., Mansson, Z., Persson, S. Rubarth, S. & Tufvesson, G. (1971) Lethal complications following administration of oxytetracycline in the horse. *Nord. VetMed.*, **23**, 9.

Andrewes, C., Pereira, H.G. & Wildy, N.P.L. (1978) *Viruses of Vertebrates*, 4th ed. London: Baillière Tindall.

Archer, R.K. (1977) The nature of blood and its disorders. In *Comparative Clinical Haematology*, ed. R.K. Archer & L.B. Jeffcott, p. 11. Oxford: Blackwell Scientific.

Bach, L.G. & Ricketts, S.W. (1974) Paracentesis abdominis as an aid to the diagnosis of abdominal disease in the horse. *Equine vet. J.*, **6**, 116.

Baker, C.J. (1972) Surgery of the head and neck. In *Equine Medicine and Surgery*, ed. E.J. Catcott & J.F. Smithcors, 2nd ed., p. 752 Wheaton, I11.: American Veterinary Publications.

Baker, J.R. & Leyland, A. (1975) Histological survey of tumours of the horse with particular reference to those of the skin. *Vet. Rec.*, **96**, 419.

Baker, K.P. & Quinn, P.J. (1978) A report of the clinical aspects and histopathology of sweet itch. *Equine vet. J.*, **10**, 243.

Baker, R.H. (1978) Acute necrotizing pancreatitis in a horse. *J. Am. vet. med. Ass.*, **172**, 268.

Baker, R.R. & Ritchie, H.E. (1974) Diabetes mellitus in the horse: a case report and review of the literature. *Equine vet. J.*, **6**, 7.

Barnett, S.F. (1974) Babesiasis of horses in Britain. *Vet. Rec.*, **95**, 346.

Banks, K.L. & Henson, J.B. (1972) Immunological mediated glomerulitis of horses. II. Antiglomerular basement membrane antibody and other mechanisms in spontaneous disease. *Lab. Invest.*, **26**, 708.

Bazeley, P.L. (1940*a*) Sulphanilamide treatment of streptococcal infections in horses. *Aust. vet. J.*, **16**, 187.

Bazeley, P.L. (1940*b*) Studies with equine Streptococci. 2. Experimental immunity to *Str. equi. Aust. vet. J.*, **16**, 243.

Baseley, P.L. (1942*a*) Studies with equine Streptococci. 3. Vaccination against strangles. *Aust. vet. J.*, **18**, 141.

Bazeley, P.L. (1942*b*) Studies with equine Streptococci. 4. Cross-immunity to *Streptococcus equi. Aust. vet. J.*, **18**, 189.

Bazeley, P.L. (1943) Studies with equine Streptococci. 5. Some relations between virulence of *Streptococcus equi* and immune response in the host. *Aust. vet. J.*, **19**, 62.

Bazeley, P.L. & Battle, J. (1940) Studies with equine Streptococci. 1. A survey of betahaemolytic Streptococci in equine infections. *Aust. vet. J.*, **16**, 140.

Beveridge, W.I.B., Mahaffey, I.W. & Rose, M.A. (1965) Influenza in horses. *Vet. Rec.*, **77**, 57.

Blood, D.C., Henderson, J.A.& Radostits, O.M. (1979) *Veterinary Medicine*, 5th ed. London: Baillière Tindall.

Blue, M.G. (1979) Enteroliths in horses: a retrospective survey of 30 cases. *Equine vet. J.*, **11**, 76.

Böhm, H.O. (1964) Uber die Isolierung und Charkterisierung eines Picornavirus vom Pferd. *Zentbl. VetMed.*, **11**, 240.

Boles, C. (1975) Postoperative management of equine abdominal patients. *J. S. Afr. vet. med. Ass.*, **46**, 123.

Bostock, D.E. & Owen, L.N. (1975) *Neoplasia in the Cat, Dog and Horse.* London: Wolfe Medical Publications.

Breese, S.S. & McCollum, W.H. (1969) Electron microscopic characterization of equine arteritis virus. *Proc. 2nd int. Conf. equine infect. Dis.*, 133.

Bridges, C.H. (1972) Mycotoxicosis. In *Equine Medicine and Surgery*, ed. E.J. Catcott & J.F. Smithcors, 2nd ed., p. 134. Wheaton, I11.: American Veterinary Publishers.

Bruner, D.W. & Gillespie, J.H. (1966) *Hagan's Infectious Diseases of Domestic Animals*, 5th ed., p. 331. New York: Comstock.

Bryans, J.T. (1963) The colitis syndrome. *Proc. 9th ann. Conv. Am. Ass. equine Practnrs*, 25.

Bryans, J.T., Doll, E.R. & Wilson, J.C. (1966) Immunising for equine influenza. *J. Am. vet. med. Ass.*, **148**, 413.

Bryans, J.T., Doll, E.R., Wilson, J.C. & Zent, W.W. (1967) Epizootiologic features of disease caused by Myxovirus influenza A equine. *Am. J. vet. Res.*, **28**, 9.

Bryans, J.T., Swerczek, T.W., Darlington, R.W. & Crowe, M.W. (1977) Neonatal foal disease associated with perinatal infection by Equine Herpesvirus I. *J. equine Med. Surg.*, **1**, 20.

Buntain, B., Greig, W.A. & Thompson, H. (1979) Chronic nephritis in a pony. *Vet. Rec.*, **104**, 307.

Burrows, R. & Goodridge, D. (1975) Experimental studies on equine herpesvirus type 1 infections. *J. Reprod. Fert.*, Suppl. **23**, 611.

Byrne, R.J. (1972) The Arbovirus encephalitides. In *Equine Medicine and Surgery*, ed. E.J. Catcott & J.F. Smithcors, 2nd ed. Wheaton, Ill.: American Veterinary Publications.

Carlson, G.P. (1979) Fluid therapy in horses with acute diarrhoea. *Vet. Clins N. Am. lge Anim. Pract.*, **1** (2), 313.

Carlstrom, B. (1950) Deficiency diseases in domestic animals. *Vet. Rec.*, **62**, 351.

Carroll, E.J., Schalm, O.W. & Wheat, J.D. (1965) Endotoxemia in a horse. *J. Am. vet. med. Ass.*, **146**, 1300.
Catcott, E.J. & Smithcors, J.F. (1972) *Equine Medicine and Surgery*, 2nd ed. Wheaton, I11.: American Veterinary Publications.
Charlton, K.M., Mitchell, D., Girard, A. & Comer, A.H. (1976) Meningoencephalitis in horses associated with equine herpesvirus 1 infection. *Vet. Path.*, **13**, 59.
Clayton, H.M. (1978) Ascariasis in foals. *Vet. Rec.*, **102**, 553.
Coggins, L., Norcross, N.L. & Nusbaum, S.R. (1972) Diagnosis of equine infectious anaemia by immunodiffusion test. *Am. J. vet. Res.*, **33**, 11.
Colles, C.M. & Jeffcott, L.B. (1977) Laminitis in the horse. *Vet. Rec.*, **100**, 262.
Collins, J.D. (1975) Autoimmune haemolytic anaemia in the horse. *Proc. 1st int. Symp. equine Haemat.*, 342.
Cook, W.R. (1966) Observations on the etiology of epistaxis and cranial nerve paralysis in the horse. *Vet. Rec.*, 78, 396.
Cook, W.R. (1968) The clinical features of gutteral pouch mycosis in the horse. *Vet. Rec.*, **83**, 336.
Cook, W.R. (1973) Diarrhoea in the horse associated with stress and tetracycline therapy. *Vet. Rec.*, **93**, 15.
Cook, W.R. (1974) Some observations on diseases of the ear, nose and throat in the horse and endoscopy using a flexible fiberoptic endoscope. *Vet. Rec.*, **94**, 533.
Cook, W.R. (1976) Chronic bronchitis and alveolar emphysema in the horse. *Vet. Rec.*, **99**, 448.
Cook, W.R. & Littlewort, M.C.G. (1974) Progressive haematoma of the ethmoid region in the horse. *Equine vet. J.*, **6**, 101.
Cook, W.R. & Rossdale, P.D. (1963) The syndrome of 'broken wind' in the horse. *Proc. R. Soc. Med.*, **56**, 972.
Cornelius, C.E., Goodbary, R.F. & Kennedy, P.C. (1959) Plasma cell myelomatosis in a horse. *Cornell Vet.*, **49**, 478.
Cosgrove, J.S.M. (1961) Symposium on equine practice. 2. Clinical aspects of equine brucellosis. *Vet. Rec.*, **73**, 377.
Cotchin, E. (1977) A general survey of tumours in the horse. *Equine vet. J.*, **9**, 16.
Cruickshank, R. (1965) *Medical Microbiology*, 11th ed. Edinburgh and London: Livingstone.
Daubney, R. & Mahlau, E.A. (1957) Near-Eastern equine encephalomyelitis. *Nature, Lond.*, **179**, 584.
Dawson, F.L.M. (1977) Further serological reactions to *Brucella* antigen in the horse. *Equine vet. J.*, **9**, 158.
Dawson, F.L.M. & Durrant, D.S. (1975) Some serological reactions to *Brucella* antigens in the horse. *Equine vet. J.*, **7**, 137.
Daykin, P.W. (1960) *Veterinary Applied Pharmacology and Therapeutics*, pp. 493 and 519. London. Baillière, Tindall & Cassell.
Denny, H.R. (1972) Brucellosis in the horse. *Vet. Rec.*, **90**, 86.
Denny, H.R. (1973) A review of brucellosis in the horse. *Equine vet. J.*, **5**, 121.
Detweiler, D.K. & Patterson, D.F. (1972) The cardiovascular system. In *Equine Medicine and Surgery*, ed. E.J. Cattcott & J.F. Smithcors, 2nd ed., p. 277. Wheaton, I11.: American Veterinary Publications.
Dickson, R.J., Hartley, W.J., Hutchins, D.R., Lepherd, E.E., Feilon, C., Jones, R.E., Love, D.N., Sabine, M. & Wells, A.L. (1978) Perinatal foal mortality associated with a herpesvirus. *Aust. vet. J.*, **54**, 103.
Dimock, W.W. & Edwards, P.R. (1933) Is there a filterable virus of abortion in mares? *Bull. Ky agric. Exp. Stn*, Suppl. 333, 297.
Dimock, W.W., Edwards, P.R. & Bruner, D.W. (1942) Equine virus abortion. *Bull. Ky agric. Exp. Stn*, 426.
Dinter, Z. & Klingeborn, B. (1976) Serological studies of an outbreak of paresis due to equid herpesvirus 1 (EHV-1). *Vet. Rec.*, **99**, 10.
Ditchfield, W.J.B. (1969) Rhinoviruses and parainfluenza viruses of horses. *J. Am. vet. Med. Ass.*, **155**, 384.
Ditchfield, J. & MacPherson, L.W. (1965) The properties and classification of two new Rhinoviruses recovered from horses in Toronto, Canada. *Cornell Vet.*, **55**, 181.
Ditchfield, J., MacPherson, L.W. & Zbitnew, A. (1965) Upper respiratory disease in Thoroughbred horses: studies of its viral etiology in the Toronto area, 1960–1963. *Can. J. comp. Med. vet. Sci.*, **29**, 18.
Ditchfield, J., Zbitnew, A. & MacPherson, L.W. (1963) Association of Myxovirus parainfluenza 3 (RE55) with upper respiratory infection of horses. *Can. vet. J.*, **4**, 175.

Doll, E.R. (1952) Seasonal incidence and fetal age in equine virus abortion. *Cornell Vet.*, **42**, 505.

Doll, E.R. (1972) Viral arteritis. In *Equine Medicine and Surgery*, ed. E.J. Catcott & J.F. Smithcors., 2nd ed., p. 22. Wheaton, Ill.: American Veterinary Publications.

Doll, E.R., Bryans, J.T., McCollum, W.H. & Crowe, M.E.W. (1957) Isolation of a filterable agent causing arteritis of horses and abortion by mares. Its differentiation from the equine abortion (influenza) virus. *Cornell Vet.*, **47**, 4.

Donawick, W.J. & Alexander, J.T. (1970) Laboratory and clinical determinations in the management of the horse with intestinal obstruction. *Proc. 16th ann. Conv. Am. Ass. equine Practnrs*, 343.

Donawick, W.J., Christie, B.A. & Stewart, J.V. (1971) Resection of diseased ileum in the horse. *J. Am. vet. med. Ass.*, **159**, 1146.

Dorn, C.R., Coffman, J.R., Schmidt, D.A., Garner, H.E., Addison, J.B. & McCune, E.L. (1975) Neutropenia and salmonellosis in hospitalized horses. *J. Am. vet. med. Ass.*, **166**, 65.

Drudge, J.H. (1972) Metazoal disease. In *Equine Medicine and Surgery*, ed. E.J. Catcott & J.F. Smithcors, 2nd ed., p. 157. Wheaton, Ill.: American Veterinary Publications.

Drudge, J.H. (1979) Clinical aspects of *Strongulus vulgaris* infection in the horse: emphasis on diagnosis, chemotherapy and prophylaxis. *Vet. Clins N. Am. lge Anim. Pract.*, **1** (2), 251.

Drudge, J.H. & Elam, G. (1961) Preliminary observations of the resistance of horse strongyles to phenothiazine. *J. Parasit.*, **47**, 38.

Duff, H.M. (1936) Fistulous withers and poll-evil due to *Brucella abortus*. *Vet. Rec.*, **48**, 175.

Duncan, J.L. (1973) The life cycle, pathogenesis and epidemiology of *S. vulgaris* in the horse. *Equine vet. J.*, **5**, 20.

Duncan, J.L. (1974) *Strongylus vulgaris* infection in the horse. *Vet. Rec.*, **95**, 34.

Duncan, J.L. (1975) Immunity to *Strongylus vulgaris* in the horse. *Equine vet. J.*, **7**, 192.

Duncan, J.L. (1976) The anthelmintic treatment of horses. *Vet. Rec.*, **98**, 233.

Duncan, J.L. & Pirie, H.M. (1972) The life cycle of *Strongylus vulgaris* in the horse. *Res. vet. Sci.*, **13**, 374.

Eyre, P. (1972) Equine pulmonary emphysema. A bronchopulmonary mould allergy. *Vet. Rec.*, **91**, 134.

Gerber, H. (1966) The clinical differentiation of some equine viral diseases. *Proc. Br. equine vet. Ass. Conf.*, 3.

Gerber, H. (1969) Clinical features, sequelae and epidemiology of equine influenza. *Proc. 2nd int. Conf. equine infect. Dis.*, 63.

Gerber, H. (1973) Chronic pulmonary disease in the horse. *Equine vet. J.*, **5**, 26.

Gibbons, D.F. (1980) Equine salmonellosis. A review. *Vet. Rec.*, **106**, 356.

Gibbs, E.P.J. (1976) Equine viral encephalitis. *Equine vet. J.*, **8**, 66.

Gibson, T.E. (1960) Some experience with small daily doses of phenothiazines as a means of control of Strongylid worms in the horse. *Vet. Rec.*, **72**, 37.

Gillespie, J.R. & Tyler, W.S. (1969) Chronic alveolar emphysema in the horse. *Adv. vet. Sci. comp. Med.*, **13**, 59.

Gillespie, J.R., Tyler, W.S. & Hall, L.W. (1969) Cardiopulmonary dysfunction in anaesthetized laterally recumbent horses. *Aust. J. vet. Res.*, **39**, 61.

Gilmour, J.S. (1973*a*) Experimental reproduction of the neurological lesions associated with grass sickness. *Vet. Rec.*, **92**, 565.

Gilmour, J.S. (1973*b*) Grass sickness: the paths of research. *Equine vet. J.*, **5**, 102.

Gilmour, J.S. & Jolly, G.M. (1976) Some aspects of the epidemiology of equine grass sickness. *Vet. Rec.*, **95**, 77.

Gorham, J.R., McGuire, T.C., Henson, J.B. & Crawford, T.B. (1977) Review of the pathogenesis of equine infectious anaemia. *J. equine Med. Surg.*, **1**, 71.

Graham, R., Reynolds, F.H.K. & Hull, J.F. (1920) Bacteriological studies of peracute disease of horses and mules. *J. Am. vet. med. Ass.*, **56**, 378, 489, 586.

Greatorex, J.C. (1968) Rectal examination as an aid to diagnosis of some medical conditions in the horse. *Equine vet. J.*, **1**, 26.

Greatorex, J.C. (1969) Urticaria, blue nose and purpura haemorrhagica in horses. *Equine vet. J.*, **1**, 157.

Greatorex, J.C. (1972) The clinical diagnosis of colic in the horse. *Equine vet. J.*, **4**, 182.

Greatorex, J.C. (1975) Diarrhoea in horses associated with ulceration of the colon and caecum resulting from *S. vulgaris* larval migration. *Vet. Rec.*, **97**, 221.

Greenwood, A.G., Barker, J. & McLeish, I. (1973) Neuritis of the cauda equina in a horse. *Equine vet. J.*, **5**, 111.

Greenwood, R.E.S. (1979) Equine rhinopneumonitis outbreak at Newmarket, *Vet. Rec.*, **104**, 534.

Greenwood, R.E.S. & Simson, A.R.B. (1980) Clinical studies of an outbreak of a paralytic syndrome affecting mares and foals in a Thoroughbred stud farm. *Equine vet. J.*, **12**, 113.

Greig, J.R. (1928) Acute 'grass disease': an interpretation of the clinical symptoms. *Vet. Rec.*, **8**, 31.

Hatch, C. (1975) Observations on the epidemiology of equine hydatidosis in Ireland. *Irish vet. J.*, **29**, 155.

Heller, L., Espmark, A. & Viriden, P. (1956) Immunological relationship between infectious cough in horses and human influenza A. *Arch. ges. Virusforsch.*, **7**, 120.

Hickman, J. (1970) Glanders: A contribution to epidemiology. *Equine vet. J.*, **2**, 153.

Hiddleston, W.A. (1970) The use of griseofulvin mycelium in equine animals. *Vet. Rec.*, **87**, 119.

Hinton, M., Marker, G.L. & Morgan, T.L.A. (1977) Abortion in a mare associated with *Br. abortus* infection and torsion. *Vet. Rec.*, **101**, 526.

Hjerpe, C.A. (1964) Serum hepatitis in the horse. *J. Am. vet. med. Ass.*, **144**, 734.

Hsiung, G.D., Fischman, H.R., Fong, C.K.Y. & Green, R.H. (1969) Characterization of a cytomegalo-like virus isolated from spontaneously degenerated equine kidney cell culture. *Proc. Soc. exp. Biol. Med.*, **130**, 80.

Huck, R.A. (1964) The classification of viruses. *Vet. Bull.*, **34**, 239.

Huscamp, B. (1977) Some problems associated with intestinal surgery in the horse. *Equine vet. J.*, **9**, 111.

Ingram, P.L. & Edwards, C.B. (1980) Salmonella infections in horses. *Trans. R. Soc. trop. Med. Hyg.*, **74**, 113.

Innes, J.R.M. (1949) Tuberculosis in the horse. *Br. vet. J.*, **105**, 373.

Jackson, C. (1936) The incidence and pathology of tumours of domesticated animals in South Africa. *Onderstepoort J. vet. Sci. Anim. Ind.*, **6**, 1.

Jackson, O.F. (1972) Renal calculi in a horse. *Vet. Rec.*, **91**, 7.

Jackson, T. & Kendrick, J.W. (1971) Paralysis of horses associated with Equine Herpesvirus I Infection. *J. Am. vet. med. Ass.*, **158**, 1351.

Jackson, T.A., Osborn, B.I., Crosby, O.R. & Kendrick, J.W. (1977) Equine herpesvirus 1 infection of horses: studies on the experimentally induced neurological disease. *Am. J. vet. Res.*, **38**, 709.

Jensen, P.T. (1959) *Salmonella typhimurium* in foals and mares. *Medlemsbl. danske Dyrlaegeforen.*, **42**, 1.

Karpas, A. (1966) Characterization of a new herpes-like virus isolated from foal kidney. *Annls Inst. Pasteur, Paris,* **110**, 688.

Kemeny, L. & Pearson, J.E. (1970) Isolation of herpesvirus from equine leukocytes: comparison with rhinopneumonitis virus. *Can. J. comp. Med.*, **34**, 59.

Kohn, C.W. (1979) Preoperative management of the equine patient with an abdominal crisis. *Vet. Clins N. Am. lge Anim. Pract.*, **1** (2), 289.

Konnerup, N., Gluckstein, F.P. & McCully, R.M. (1972) African horse-sickness. In *Equine Medicine and Surgery*, ed. Catcott, E.J. & Smithcors, J.F., 2nd ed., p. 64. Wheaton, Ill.: American Veterinary Publications.

Kono, Y. & Kobayashi, K. (1964) Cytopathogenic equine orphan (CEO) virus in horse kidney cell culture. I. Isolation and properties. *Natn. Inst. Anim. Hlth Q. Tokyo,* **4**, 10.

Kono, Y., Kobayashi, K. & Fukinaga, Y. (1973) Antigenic drift of equine infectious anaemia virus in chronically infected horses. *Arch. ges. Virusforsch.*, **41**, 1.

Lane, J.G. (1977) The treatment of equine sarcoid by cryosurgery. *Equine vet. J.*, **9**, 127.

Lapage, G. (1968) *Veterinary Parasitology*, 2nd ed. Edinburgh and London: Oliver & Boyd.

Lawson, G.H.K., McPherson, E.A., Murphy, J.R., Nicholson, J.M., Wooding, P., Breeze, R.C. & Pirie, H.M. (1979) The presence of precipitating antibodies in the sera of horses with chronic obstructive pulmonary disease. (COPD). *Equine vet. J.*, **11**, 172.

Legoretta, G.G.L. (1975) Dermatological Studies in the Horse with Special Reference to Ringworm in the Thoroughbred Horse. MSc Thesis, University of Cambridge.

Little, P.B., Thorsen, J. & Moran, K. (1974) Virus involvement in equine paresis. *Vet. Rec.*, **95**, 575.

Lucke, J.N. (1972) Fluid and electrolyte balance relating to intestinal surgery. *Equine vet. J.*, **2**, 56.
Lyons, E.T., Drudge, J.H. & Tollins, S.C. (1973) On the life cycle of *Strongyloides westeri* in the equine. *J. Parasit.*, **59**, 780.
Lyons, E.T., Drudge, J.H. & Tollins, S.C. (1975) Field tests of three salts of pyrantel against internal parasites of the horse. *Am. J. vet. Res.*, **36**, 161.
McAllister, E.S. (1977) Guttural pouch disease. *Proc. 23rd ann. Conv. Am. Ass. equine Practnrs*, 251.
McBeath, D.G., Best, J.M.J., Preston, N.K. & Duncan, J.L. (1978) Studies on the faecal egg count output of horses after treatment with fenbendazole. *Equine vet. J.*, **10**, 5.
McCaughey, W.J. & Kerr, W.R. (1967) Abortion due to brucellosis in a Thoroughbred mare. *Vet. Rec.*, **80**, 186.
McChesney, A.E., England, J.J., Adcock, J.L., Stackhouse, L.L. & Chow, T.L. (1970) Adenovirus infection in suckling Arabian foals. *Path. vet.*, **7**, 547.
McDonell, W.N., Hall, L.W. & Jeffcott, L.B. (1979) Radiographic evidence of impaired pulmonary function in laterally recumbent anaesthetized horses. *Equine vet. J.*, **11**, 24.
McIntyre, R.W. (1949) Virus papular dermatitis of the horse. *Am. J. vet. Res.*, **10**, 229.
McLean, J.G. (1967) 'Tying-up' syndrome in horses. II. Biochemical aspects. *Vict. Vet. Proc.*, **26**, 35.
McPherson, E.A. & Lawson, G.H.K. (1974) Some aspects of chronic pulmonary disease of horses and methods used in their investigation. *Equine vet. J.*, **6**, 1.
McPherson, E.A., Lawson, G.H.K., Murphy, J.R., Nicholson, J.M., Fraser, J.A., Breeze, R.G. & Pirie, H.M. (1978*a*) Chronic obstructive pulmonary disease (COPD): identification of affected horses. *Equine vet. J.*, **10**, 47.
McPherson, E.A., Lawson, G.H.K., Murphy, J.R., Nicholson, J.H., Breeze, R.G. & Pirie, H.M. (1978*b*) Chronic obstructive pulmonary disease (COPD): factors affecting the incidence. *Equine vet. J.*, **11**, 167.
McPherson, E.A., Lawson, G.H.K., Murphy, J.R., Nicholson, J.M., Breeze, R.G. & Pirie, H.M. (1979) Chronic obstructive pulmonary disease (COPD) in horses: Aetiological studies: responses to intradermal and inhalational antigenic challenge. *Equine vet. J.*, **11**, 159.
Mahaffey, L.W. (1959) Ganglionic lesions in grass sickness of horses. *Vet. Rec.*, **71**, 170.
Mahaffey, L.W. (1962) Respiratory conditions in horses. *Vet. Rec.*, **74**, 1295.
Mahaffey, L.W. (1966) Influenza in the young foal. Clinical aspects and histopathology. *Proc. 1st int. Conf. equine infect. Dis.*, 68.
Mansman, R.A. & Mansman, J.A. (1969) Cytology of equine nasal secretions. *J. Am. vet. med. Ass.*, **154**, 1037.
Mansman, R.A. Osburn, B.I., Wheat, J.D. & Frich, O. (1975) Chicken hypersensitivity pneumonitis in horses. *J. Am. vet med. Ass.*, **166**, 673.
Mansman, R.A. & Wheat, J.D. (1972) The diagnosis and treatment of equine upper respiratory diseases. *Proc. 18th ann. Conv. Am. Ass. equine Practnrs*, 375.
Matthews, A.G., (1979) Identification and characterisation of the major antiproteases in equine sera and an investigation of their role in the onset of chronic obstructive pulmonary disease (OPD). *Equine vet. J.*, **11**, 177.
Maurer, F.D. & McCully, R.M. (1963) African horse sickness, with emphasis on pathology. *Am. J. vet. Res.*, **24**, 235.
Mayr, A.J., Pette, J. & Pape, J. (1966) The 1965 epidemic of coughing in horses (Hoppengarten cough) in the German Federal Republic (in German). *Tierarztl. Umsch.*, **6**, 281, 285, 289.
Mellor, P.S. & McCaig, J. (1974) The probable cause of 'sweet itch' in England. *Vet. Rec.*, **95**, 411.
Menten, D.J., Butcher, D.G., Thomson, G.W. & Lumsden, J.H. (1978) Chronic enteritis associated with malabsorption and protein-losing enteropathy in the horse. *J. Am. vet. med. Ass.*, **172**, 326.
Merritt, A.M., Bolton, J.R. & Cimprich, R. (1975) Differential diagnosis of diarrhoea in horses over 6 months of age. *J. S. Afr. vet. med. Ass.*, **46**, 73.
Merritt, A.M., Cimprich, R.E. & Beech, J. (1976) Granulomatous enteritis in horses. *J. Am. vet. med. Ass.*, **169**, 603.
Messervy, A. (1970) Surgical approach to abdominal surgery. *Equine vet. J.*, **2**, 52.
Millar, R. (1961) Disease of the ligamentum nuchae associated with *Brucella abortus* infection in the horse and its treatment with Strain 19 vaccine. *Br. vet. J.*, **117**, 167.

Miller, W.C. & Poynter, D. (1956) Hydatid cysts in a Thoroughbred mare. *Vet. Rec.*, **68**, 51.

Moore, J.N., Travers, D.S., Turner, M.F., White, F.J., Huesgen, J.G. & Buttera, T.S. (1977) Lactic acid concentrations in peritoneal fluid of normal and diseased horses. *Res. vet. Sci.*, **23**, 117

Moorse, J.N., Owen, R. ap R. & Lumsden, J.H. (1976) Clinical evaluation of blood lactate levels in equine colic. *Equine vet. J.*, 8, 49.

Moyer, W. & Rooney, J.R. (1972) An epidemic central nervous system disease in horses. *Proc 18th ann. Conv. Am. Ass. equine Practnrs*, 307.

Mumford, J.A. & Edington, N. (1980) EHV-I and equine paresis. *Vet. Rec.*, **106**, 277.

Muylle, E., Oyaert, W., Ooms, L. & Decraemore, H. (1975) Treatment of tetanus in the horse by injections of tetanus antitoxin into the subarachnoid space. *J. Am. vet. med. Ass.*, **167**, 47.

Nansen, P., Anderson, S. & Hesselholt, M. (1975) Experimental infection of the horse with *Fasciola hepatica. Exp. Parasit.*, **37**, 15.

Nelson, A.W., Collier, J.R. & Griner, L.A. (1968) Acute surgical colonic infarction in the horse. *Am. J. vet. Res.*, **29**, 315.

Nelson, A.W. & Meagher, D.M. (1972) Septic shock. *Proc. 18th ann. Conv. Am. Ass. equine Practnrs,* Appendix IV, 531.

Nicholls, J.M., Duncan, J.L. & Greig, W. (1978) Lungworm (*Dictyocaulus arnfeldi*) infection in the horse. *Vet. Rec.*, **102**, 216.

Obel, A.L. (1955) Studies on grass disease. The morphological picture with special reference to the vegetative nervous system. *J. comp. Path.*, **65**, 334.

Oldenkamp, E.P. (1979) Treatment of ringworm in horses with natamycin. *Equine vet. J.*, **11**, 36.

Ogborne, C.P. & Duncan, J.F. (1977) *Strongylus vulgaris* in the horse: its biology and veterinary importance. Miscellaneous Publication No. 4. Farnham Royal: Commonwealth Institute of Helminthology.

Owen, J.M. (1977) Liver fluke infection in horses and ponies. *Equine vet. J.*, **9**, 29.

Owen, R. ap R. (1974) Epistaxis prevented by ligation of the internal carotid artery in the guttural pouch. *Equine vet. J.*, **6**, 143.

Owen, R. ap R. (1975) Post-stress diarrhoea in the horse. *Vet. Rec.*, **96**, 267.

Ozawa, Y. (1968) Studies on the properties of African horse sickness virus. *Jap. J. med. Sci. Biol.*, **21**, 27.

Page, E.H. & Amstutz, H.E. (1972) Colitis X (haemorrhagic colitis, acute colitis, colitis syndrome). In *Equine Medicine and Surgery*, ed. E.J. Catcott & J.F. Smithcors, 2nd ed., p. 269. Wheaton, I11.: American Veterinary Publications.

Panchera, R.J. (1972) Serum disease (Theiler's disease, staggers, secondary disease, liver necrosis-encephalosis, acute yellow atrophy, postvaccinal hepatitis. In *Equine Medicine and Surgery,* ed. Catcott, E.J. & Smithcors, J.F., 2nd ed., p. 275. Wheaton, I11.: American Veterinary Publications.

Pascoe, R.R., Spradbrow, P.B. & Bagust, T.J. (1969) An equine genital infection resembling coital exanthema associated with a virus. *Aust. vet. J.*, **45**, 166.

Pearson, H. & Gibbs, C. (1970) Review of sixty equine laparotomies. *Equine vet. J.*, **2**, 60.

Pearson, H., Messervy, A. & Pinsent, P.J. (1971) Surgical treatment of abdominal disorders in the horse. *J. Am. vet. med. Ass.*, **159**, 1344.

Pearson, H., Pinsent, P.J.N., Denny, H.R. & Waterman, A. (1975) The indications for equine laparatomy: an analysis of 140 cases. *Equine vet. J.*, **7**, 131.

Plummer, G. (1962) An equine respiratory virus with enterovirus properties. *Nature, Lond.*, **195**, 519.

Plummer, G. & Waterson, A.P. (1963) Equine herpesviruses. *Virology*, **19**, 412.

Porterfield, J.S., Hill., D.H. & Morris, A.D. (1958) Isolation of a virus from the brain of a horse with 'staggers' in Nigeria. *Br. vet. J.*, **114**, 425.

Powell, D.G. (1975) Equine infectious respiratory disease. *Vet. Rec.*, **96**, 30.

Powell, D.G. (1976) Equine infectious anaemia. *Vet. Rec.*, **99**, 7.

Powell, D.G. & Felmingham, D. (1977) Equine influenza. *Vet. Rec.*, **101**, 191.

Poynter, D. & Hughes, D.L. (1958) Phenothiazine and piperazine: an efficient anthelmintic mixture for horses. *Vet. Rec.*, **70**, 1183.

Ragland, W.L., Keown, G.H. & Spencer, G.R. (1970) Equine sarcoid. *Equine vet. J.*, **2**, 2.

Ricketts, S.W. & Peace, C.K. (1976) A case of peritoneal mesothelioma in a Thoroughbred mare. *Equine vet. J.*, 8, 78.

Ristic, M. (1975) Equine ehrlichosis with emphasis on biology and immune response to the agent. *Proc. 1st int. Symp. equine Haemat.*, 386.

Roberts, M.C. (1977) A case of primary lymphoid leukaemia in a horse. *Equine vet. J.*, **9**, 216.

Roberts, M.C. & English, P.B. (1979) Antimicrobial chemotherapy in the horse. The application of antimicrobial therapy. *J. equine Med. Surg.*, **3**, 308.

Roberts, M.C. & Pinsent, P.J.N. (1975) Malabsorption in the horse associated with alimentary lymphosarcoma. *Equine vet. J.*, **7**, 166.

Robinson, N.E. (1979) Functional abnormalities caused by upper airway obstruction and heaves: their relationship to the etiology of epistaxis. *Vet. Clins N. Am. lge Anim. Pract.*, **1** (1), 17.

Ronéus, O. (1975) Presence and longevity of hydatid cysts of *Echinococcus granulosus* in imported horses in Sweden. *Nord. VetMed.*, **27**, 49.

Rooney, J.R. (1969) Quoted by Manahan, F.F. (1970) Diarrhoea in horses with particular reference to a chronic diarrhoea syndrome. *Aust. vet. J.*, **46**, 231.

Rooney, J.R. (1970) *Autopsy of the Horse: Techniques and Interpretation.* Baltimore: Williams & Wilkins.

Rooney, J.R. (1971) *Clinical Neurology of the Horse.* Pennsylvania: KNA Press.

Rooney, J.R. (1972) The musculoskeletal system. In *Equine Medicine and Surgery,* ed E.J. Catcott & J.F. Smithcors, 2nd ed., p. 489. Wheaton, I11.: American Veterinary Publications.

Rooney, J.R. & Bryans, J.P. (1963) Colitis X of horses. *J. Am. vet. med. Ass.*, **142**, 510.

Rooney, J.R., Bryans, J.T., Prickett, M.E. & Zent, W.W. (1966) Exhaustion shock in the horse. *Cornell Vet.*, **56**, 220.

Rooney, J.R., Prickett, M.E., Delaney, F.M. & Crowe, M.W. (1970) Focal myelitis-encephalitis in horses. *Cornell Vet.*, **40**, 494.

Rose, R.J. & Davis, P.E. (1977) Treatment of atrial fibrillation in three racehorses. *Equine vet. J.*, **9**, 68.

Rose, M.D., Vopes, R., Rossdale, P.D. & Beveridge, W.I.B. (1974) Virus infections of horses at Newmarket. *Vet. Rec.*, **95**, 484.

Rossdale, P.D., Hunt, M.D.N., Peace, C.K., Hopes, R. & Ricketts, S.W. (1975) A case of equine infectious anaemia in Newmarket. *Vet. Rec.*, **97**, 207.

Round, M.C. (1968) Experiences with thiabendazole as an anthelmintic for horses. *Br. vet. J.*, **124**, 248.

Round, M.C. (1976) Lungworm infection (*D. arnfeldi*) of horses and donkeys. *Vet. Rec.*, **99**, 393.

Round, M.C., Simpson, D.J., Haseldon, C.S., Glendinning, E.S.A. & Baskerville, R.E. (1974) Horse strongyles' tolerance to anthelmintics. *Vet. Rec.*, **95**, 517.

Rowland, L.P., Fahn, S., Hirsberg, E. & Harter, D.H. (1964) Myoglobinuria. *Archs Neurol., Chicago,* **10**, 537.

Saxegaard, F. (1966) Isolation and identification of equine rhinopneumonitis virus (equine abortion virus) from cases of abortion and paralysis. *Nord. VetMed.*, **18**, 504.

Scott, G.R. (1971) Guide lines for the control of equine viral infections. *Equine vet. J.*, **3**, 1.

Shoho, C. (1954) Prophylaxis and therapy in epizootic cerebrospinal nematodiasis of animals by diethylcarbamyl-methylpiperazine dihydrogen citrate. Report of a second field trial. *Vet. Med.*, **49**, 459.

Slocombe, J.O.D., Owen, R. ap R., Pennock, P.W., McCrow, B.M. & Rendano, V.T. (1977) Arterographic presentation of the early development of vascular lesions in ponies infected with *Strongylus vulgaris. Proc. 23rd ann. Conv. Am. Ass. equine Practnrs,* 305.

Soulsby, E.J.L. (1968) *Helminths, Arthopods and Protozoa of Domestic Animals,* 6th ed. London: Baillière, Tindall & Cassell.

Stashak, T. (1978) Clinical evaluation of the equine colic patient. *Vet. Clins N. Am. lge Anim. Pract.*, **1** (2), 275.

Stannard, A.A. (1972) The skin. In *Equine Medicine and Surgery,* ed. E.J. Catcott & J.F. Smithcors, 2nd ed., p. 381. Wheaton, I11.: American Veterinary Publications.

Steck, W. (1967) The epidemiology of equine infectious anaemia. *Vet. Rec.*, **81**, 205.

Theiler, A. (1918) Acute liver atrophy and parenchymatous hepatitis in horses. *5th & 6th Rep. Dir. vet. Res. S. Afr.*, 7.

Thiem, P. (1976) Association of EHV-II infection with keratitis and research on the occurence of equine coital exanthema, EHV-III of horses, in Germany. *Proc. 4th int. Conf. equine infect. Dis.*, 33.

Thomas, R.E. & Jones, L.P. (1960) Lungworm infection in the burro. *Vet. Med.*, **55**, 38.
Thomason, G.R., Mumford, J.A., Campbell, J., Griffiths, L. & Clapham, P. (1976) Serological detection of equid herpesvirus 1 infections of the respiratory tract. *Equine vet. J.*, **8**, 58.
Thomsett, L.R. (1979) Skin diseases of the horse. *In Practice*, **1**, 15.
Thomson, R.C.A. & Smyth, J.D. (1975) Equine hydatidosis: a review of the current status in Great Britain and the results of an epidemiological survey. *Vet. Parasit.*, **1**, 107.
Thorsen, J. & Little, P.B. (1975) Isolation of equine herpesvirus 1 from a horse with acute paralytic disease. *Can. J. comp. Med.*, **39**, 358.
Timoney, P.J. (1976) Louping ill: a serological survey of horses in Ireland. *Vet. Rec.*, **98**, 303.
Timoney, P.J., Donnelly, W.J.C., Clements, L.O. & Fenlon, M. (1976) Encephalitis caused by louping ill virus in a group of horses in Ireland. *Equine vet. J.*, **8**, 113.
Urach, D.L. & Allen, W.R. (1980) Studies on fenbendazole for treating lung and intestinal parasites in horses and donkeys. *Equine vet. J.*, **12**, 74.
Vandeplassche, M. & Devos, A. (1960) Excretion of brucella in the semen of stallions. *Vlaams diergeneesk. Tijdschr.*, **29**, 199.
Van der Hoeden, J. (1964) *Zoonoses*, p. 108. Amsterdam: Elsevier.
Vaughan, J.T. (1973) The acute colitis syndrome: colitis X. *Vet. Clins N. Am.*, **3**, 301.
Vaughan, S.M. (1969) A case of equine lymphosarcoma. *Vet. Rec.*, **84**, 474.
Voss, J.L. (1969) Transmission of equine sarcoid. *Am. J. vet. Res.*, **30**, 183.
Waddell, X.X. (1972) The pathogenicity of *Gasterophilus intestinalis* larvae in the stomach of the horse. *Aust. vet. J.*, **48**, 332.
Walker, D. & Knight, D. (1972) The anthelmintic action of mebendazole: a full trial in horses. *Vet. Rec.*, **90**, 58.
Waterman, A. (1977) A review of the diagnosis and treatment of fluid and electrolyte disorders in the horse. *Equine vet. J.*, **9**, 43.
Weaver, B.M.Q. (1970) Role of the anaesthetist. *Equine vet. J.*, **2**, 53.
Weaver, A.D. & Adams, C.M. (1979) A specialist German practice. *Vet. Rec.*, **105**, 147.
Wright, A.I. (1972) Verminous arteritis as a cause of colic in the horse. *Equine vet. J.*, **4**, 169.
Wyn-Jones, G. (1979) Treatment of periocular tumours of horses using radioactive gold 198 grains. *Equine vet. J.*, **11**, 3.
Zwick, W. & Witte, J. (1929) Weitere Beitrage zur Erforschung der Bornaschen Krankheit des Pferdes. *Arch. wiss. prakt. Tierheilk.*, **59**, 511.

Clinical and Further Examinations

8

At college the student is taught clinical examinations. When he enters practice he modifies these to meet particular circumstances, such as differences of species, clientele and location. In short, he develops the art, not at the expense of the science, but largely as a means of economic survival. Clinical experience entitles him to take short cuts to diagnosis, often by employing an intuitive rather than an objective approach. Equine practitioners are fortunate because the value of their 'patients' demands individual attention; most cases allow considerable scope for advanced techniques of diagnosis and therapy.

In this chapter we are concerned primarily with differences in approach dictated by species variation and with highlighting those areas where established procedures are not popularly used in equine practice, but which the reader might like to consider to enlarge his or her experience.

Before embarking on a description of special examinations and procedures we will take the opportunity to comment on equine clinical examinations.

In the general approach, consistency is important and habit a definite aid to clinical examintion. By adopting a fairly rigid programme towards investigation the clinician is less liable to forget a critical part in any particular case. The order adopted does not matter so much, provided it is roughly the same each time.

The age of the animal under investigation should be considered first. Certain conditions are more prevalent in various age groups, e.g. joint-ill in foals, epiphysitis in yearlings, pulmonary emphysema and myoglobinuria in older horses. The status of a mare should also be considered, i.e. pregnant, barren or recently covered by the stallion.

A detailed history is usually available because of the individual attention provided. Attendants are usually reliable, although the stableman is apt to colour his account from previous experience. One of the arts a practitioner must learn is to judge the accuracy of an account of the case's history.

Keeping case notes and records is valuable but time-consuming and not always practical. However, it should be the aim of every practitioner as it forms the basis of objectivity. There are many systems of quick recording, such as a diagrammatic representation of heart sounds and murmurs (Littlewort 1962).

Management obviously plays a large part in many conditions encountered in stud farm practice. A painstaking investigation of managerial factors, such as nutrition, pasture management, stabling and other environmental factors, may be particularly rewarding in understanding each case.

A physical examination of a horse should be conducted in a manner similar to that adopted for other species. Temperature, respiratory rate, heart rate, pulse quality, quantity and quality of faeces passed and appetite should be noted. The chest and abdomen should be auscultated on both sides and visible mucous membranes examined.

Change in behaviour may be pathognomonic for disease and particular conditions. Normal behavioural patterns conform to narrow limits. Dullness (reduced activity), uneasiness (increased activity) and other signs which indicate pain, fever or interference with normal activity, e.g. choke, provide a basis for most other examinations.

The clinician should take note of the way horses are handled. For example it is customary to approach them from the left side. Particular care should be taken therefore when an approach on the right side is necessary during an examination. Individual idiosyncrasies must be acknowledged and the advice of attendants heeded. Restraint in the form of a twitch on the nose or neck skin may be more appropriate to one individual than another.

Horses as well as owners can distinguish the competent from the timid approach. Sudden movements, intolerance or undue roughness should be avoided. When handling a fractious horse we have often found it helpful to grasp a fold of skin on the neck. This not only quietens the horse but enables the handler to keep close and move with it; this is usually safer than to be a foot or two away. Wherever there is a doubt as to the safety of clinician or attendants a tranquillizer must be used. The days of heroics or when a veterinarian had to be a horseman are receding into the past. In equine practice common sense allied to scientific training is as useful now as it has always been in other branches of veterinary practice.

HYGIENE AT GYNAECOLOGICAL EXAMINATION

It is important that adequate facilities are available to allow veterinary examinations to be performed in a clean and hygienic manner. Assistants, and all other personnel who may handle the genital organs of horses at any time, should be directed to wear disposable plastic gloves. Adequate facilities for the washing of hands and boots should be provided at areas where these procedures are to occur. Ideally, there should be, at a central convenient area, a specialized veterinary examination facility. This should include areas for the maintenance of clean overalls and boots, gynaecological examination equipment and a sterilizer to provide an

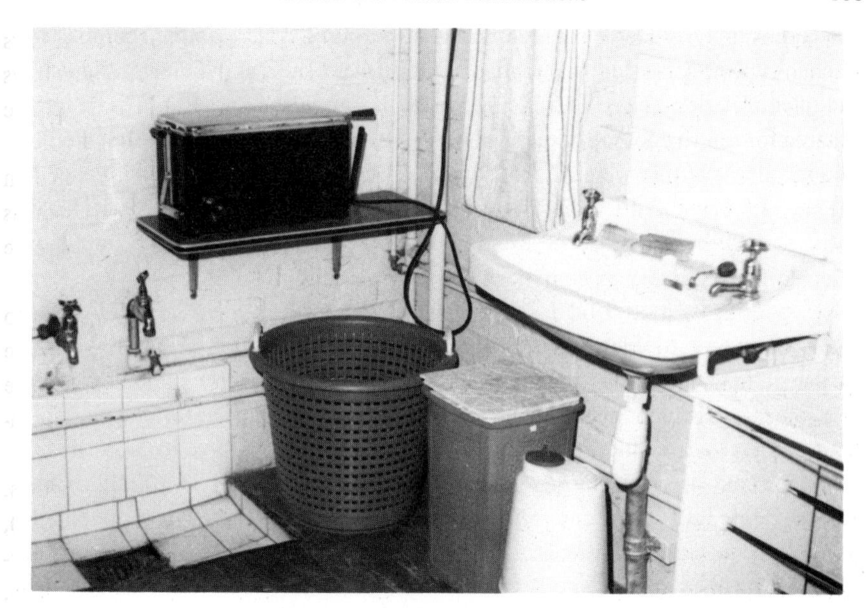

Fig. 8.1. An example of the facilities provided on a stud farm for washing hands and boots and sterilizing instruments. Distilled water should be used in the sterilizer to prevent calcareous deposits forming on the instruments. Before sterilization the specula should be scrubbed to remove grease and washed in disinfectant solution.

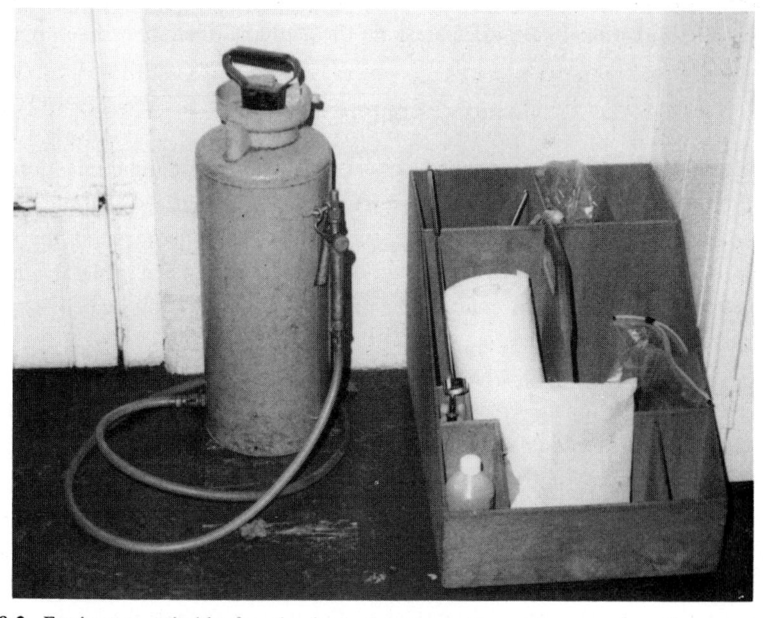

Fig. 8.2. Equipment suitable for the hygienic examination of mares when the examiner is travelling from box to box. Warm water is provided under pressure in a portable spray washer with a flexible and adjustable hand-held nozzle. The wooden box contains disposable plastic gloves, lubricant, disposable paper towels, sterilized specula, swab extension rods and speculum light unit.

adequate supply of sterile specula. For these purposes, a clean room, equipped with kitchen-type units, including cupboards and drawers, sinks and drainer, boot washer and plentiful hot and cold running water, is suitable (Fig. 8.1). The sterilizer, suitable for the vaginoscope described on p. 512, is a medical boiling water sterilizer of adequate length in which distilled water is used. Tap water should not be used or specula will become discolored, brittle and covered with calcarious deposit. Ideally, there should be an adjacent examining area containing stocks or loose boxes reserved for veterinary examinations only. For reasons including tradition and man-power shortages, most stud farms in the UK still prefer the veterinarian to travel from loose box to loose box without a central examination area. This requires sufficient help, transport facilities and boxes for the necessary equipment. Under this system, it is recommended that portable spray equipment (Fig. 8.2) should be used rather than disinfectant buckets carried from loose box to loose box. *K. aerogenes* and probably *P. aerugenosa* can remain viable in 1 in 200 dilutions of chlorhexidine gluconate and cetrimide antiseptic (Ricketts 1976, unpublished). Thus, such solutions, carried in buckets from mare to mare during veterinary examinations, could become a potential source of spread of venereal disease. A variety of portable sprayers is available and some are being marketed for this specialized purpose. The one chosen should be sturdy enough to withstand the amount of use required and must be capable of delivering a good plentiful wetting spray. In view of the shortcomings and possible dangers of chemical disinfectants, it may be preferable to use a spray of warm clean water with no disinfectants, for the washing of the perineal areas of mares and the genitalia of stallions (see pp. 80 and 136).

HYPODERMIC INJECTION

If is often said that horses are more likely to react to hypodermic injections than are other species. This is probably false, having its origins in the attitude of horse owners who tend to be resentful when untoward reactions occur at the site of injections. The principles governing hypodermic injections in general apply to the horse and here we are concerned only with special points which may help students and young graduates.

1. Opinions differ as to whether the site of injection should be cleansed with spirit or the hair clipped. From an aesthetic point of view it is preferable to use spirit, and for intravenous injections it has a definite practical value in exposing the vein.

2. Intramuscular injections should be made direct into a muscle mass, such as that of the hind-quarters (Fig. 8.3), neck or brisket, in order of preference. Reaction is most likely in the pectoral muscles. If the neck is used it is advisable to avoid injecting into the ligamentum nuchae. In very young foals the triceps muscles may be used, and some clinicians also prefer these muscles in older animals.

3. Within limits the choice of needle is a matter for personal preference. We prefer a gauge 19 or 21 for intramuscular or subcutaneous injection and a gauge

16 or 19 for intravenous ones. In adults a length of 3 cm is preferred, inserted to the hilt; in foals it should be about 2 cm.

4. The operator should avoid moving the needle once it is inserted into muscle and if there is haemorrhage, a fresh site should be selected. Bleeding appears to predispose to reaction, especially when vaccines or oily solutions are administered.

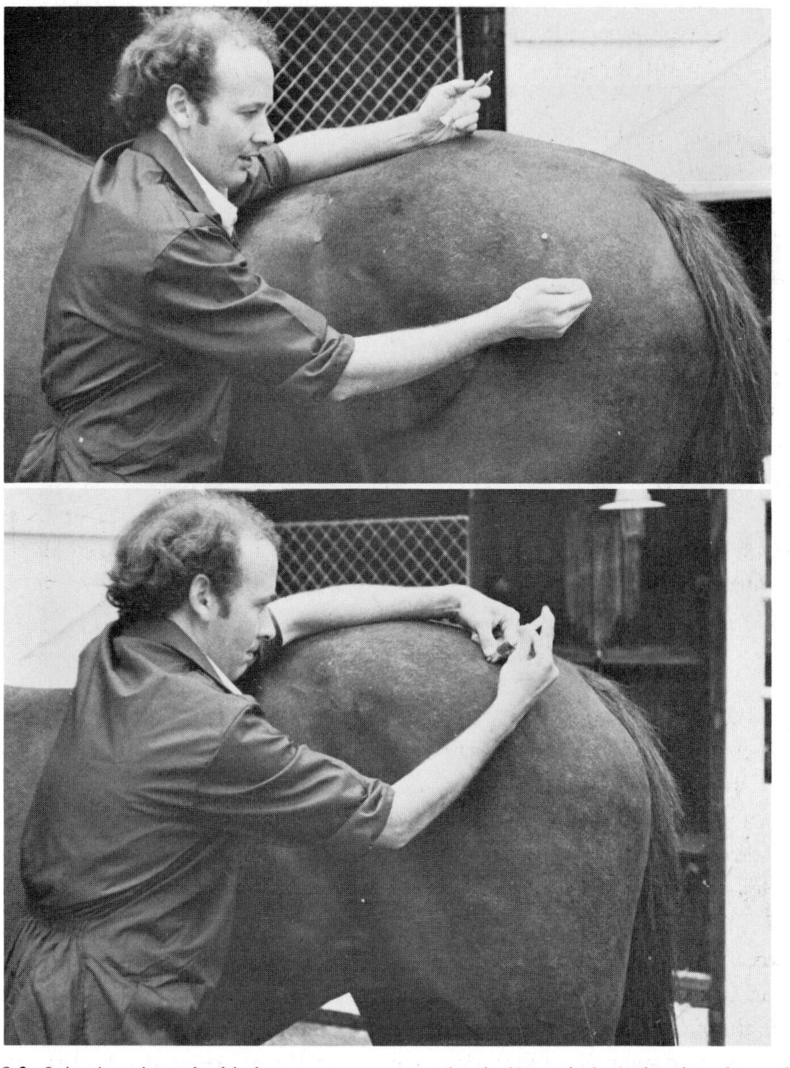

Fig. 8.3. Injections into the hind-quarters can conveniently be made into the gluteal muscles, as demonstrated. Note the position of the operator who has inserted the needle before attaching the syringe.

A convenient method of restraining fractious animals is to grasp a fold of neck skin with the left hand using the right to insert a needle attached to a syringe making the injection in the same movement (Fig. 8.4). For all other intramuscular injections the needle should be inserted before the syringe is attached. Intravenous injections are made relatively easily into the large jugular vein. Adequate restraint should be applied so that the horse remains still and positioned with adequate light on the injection site. A thumb should be pressed into the lower aspect of the jugular furrow, which visibly 'raises' the vein. A disconnected hypodermic needle is then placed into the vein, either by one quick direct motion or by slow gentle pressure through the tissues. Horses respond differently to these methods and one can only judge each case on its merits at the time. Ideally, the needle should be

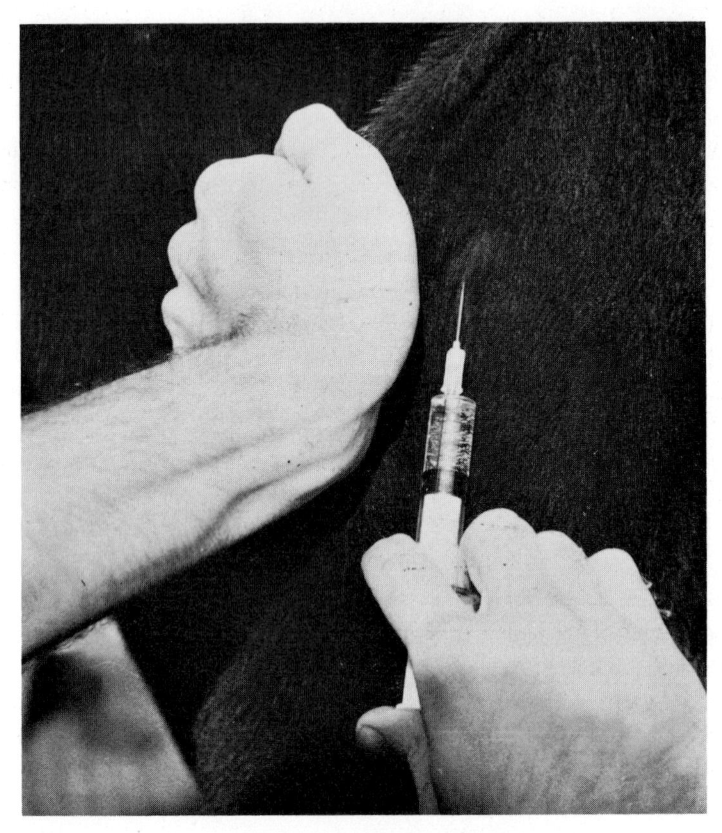

Fig. 8.4. A fractious horse can be restrained by grasping a fold of neck skin with one hand and injecting with the other.

placed in the vein in the direction of the heart. Venous blood should flow freely from the needle before the syringe is attached and its contents slowly injected, occasionally stopping to withdraw blood to check that the needle is still correctly placed. Despite careful technique, untoward reactions sometimes follow intravenous injections (Gabel 1977). These are:

1. Perivascular injection of irritant drugs, e.g. barbiturates, sulphonamides, tetracyclines, phenylbutazone. This can result in a severe local reaction with phlebitis and sloughing of local tissues. If sloughing of the vein occurs, threatening fatal haemorrhage, the vein should be ligated above the slough. If perivascular injection

or leakage is detected, large volumes of normal saline should be injected into the area to dilute the drug. Local anaesthetic (e.g. xylocaine), injected locally, is useful to neutralize alkaline drugs such as phenylbutazone and barbiturates. Local hot and cold physical therapy also helps.

2. Rapid injection of irritant solutions, e.g. phenylbutazone, may cause a severe phlebitis resulting in complete occlusion of the vein.

3. Intracarotid arterial injection may result in almost immediate convulsions and death. Prevention of injury, during convulsions, is important in those horses that do not die. The use of a large-bore needle, directed towards the heart, enables one to be confident that an accidental carotid puncture has not been made, before a drug is injected.

Indwelling catheters are sometimes useful where irritants solutions are used (e.g. induction of anaesthesia with barbiturates) or where repeated or long-term injections are used (Bishop & Boles 1972). Catheters must be carefully and correctly placed and their use is not without risk (Gabel 1977; Meagher 1977*a*). These risks are:

1. Local infection. The placing of an intravenous catheter should be performed as a surgical procedure.

2. 'Lost' catheters. Great care should be taken to avoid piercing the wall of the catheter with the introducing needle.

3. Emboli. Catheters should be occluded and should contain either saline or heparin solution to prevent internal clotting.

PASSING A STOMACH TUBE

Administering drugs or fluid through a tube inserted into the oesophagus (Adams 1977) is important in equine therapeutics and is a considerable improvement on older methods such as 'balling'. The tube may be plastic or rubber and its external diameter should be about 3 cm for adults of large breeds, 2 cm for ponies and 1 cm for young foals. The distal end should be blunt and the proximal end enlarged to receive a funnel stem or pump nozzle.

The tube should be lubricated with oil or water and introduced into the left or right nostril with an attendant restraining the horse on the opposite side to the operator (Fig. 8.5). It may be necessary to depress the tube with the forefinger of the passing hand so that it slips into the ventral meatus beyond the turbinate bones. With the distal end in the pharynx it may be necessary to flex the horse's head to ensure that the tube is swallowed.

As the tube enters the oesophagus the increased resistance felt by the operator indicates that the tube is not in the trachea. The trachea may be shaken, laterally, and if the tube is inside it will be heard and felt to rattle. The horse often, but not always, coughs when the tube enters the trachea. With the tube in the oesophagus, the operator may blow and observe the wave of air passing down. This procedure also demonstrates that the tube has not become buckled, when it must be withdrawn and reinserted.

The tube should be passed to the entrance of the chest and it is helpful to have a mark on the tube coinciding with the level of the nostril when the tube is in situ. Confirmation of the tube's presence in the oesophagus may be obtained by blowing further boluses of air which may be seen or felt passing in each direction

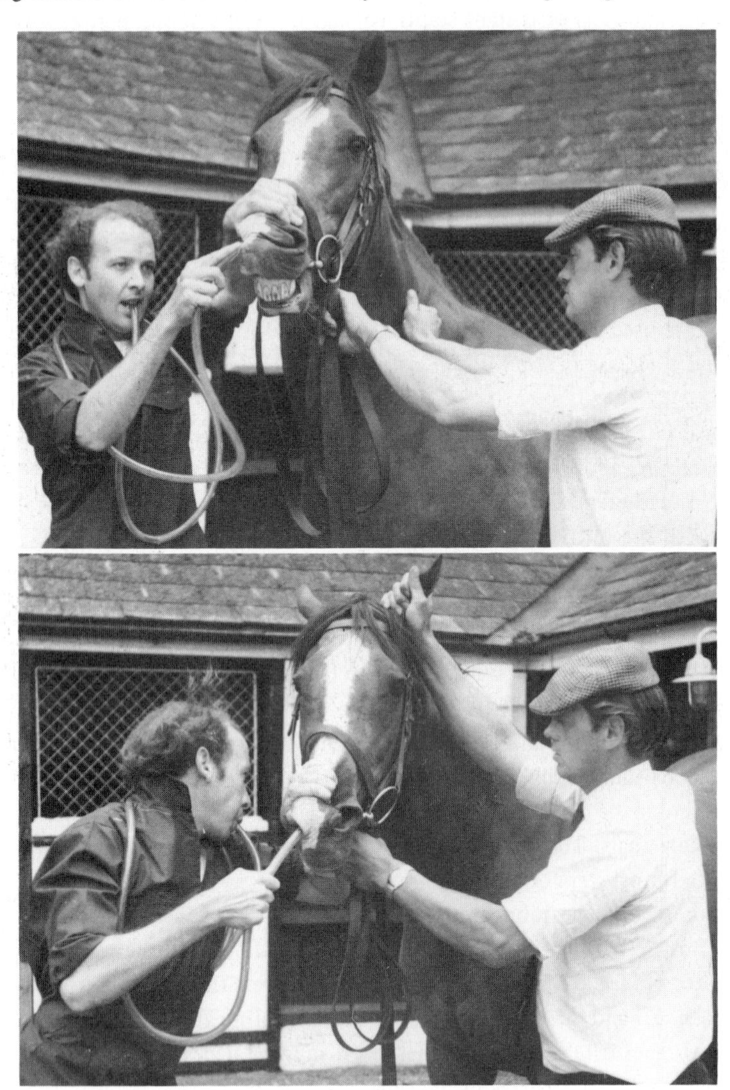

Fig. 8.5. Passing a stomach tube from the right side. Note the positions of the veterinarian and handler.

along the left side of the neck. (Fig. 8.6). The end of the tube can also be seen or felt as it passes down the neck; stomach sounds of fluid can be heard at the proximal end of the tube.

On withdrawal, the proximal end should be sealed to prevent escape of fluid in the pharynx and nasal passages. The tube should be withdrawn slowly as the distal end leaves the oesophagus to avoid abrupt contact with the turbinate bones which may cause haemorrhage. Bleeding may also occur on insertion if the tube scrapes the nasal or pharyngeal mucosa or if it is driven against the turbinate bones.

If the tube is difficult to pass, it is usually due to the distal end entering the pharynx in a position from which it is not easily swallowed. In this case the head should be flexed and/or the tube passed through the opposite nostril.

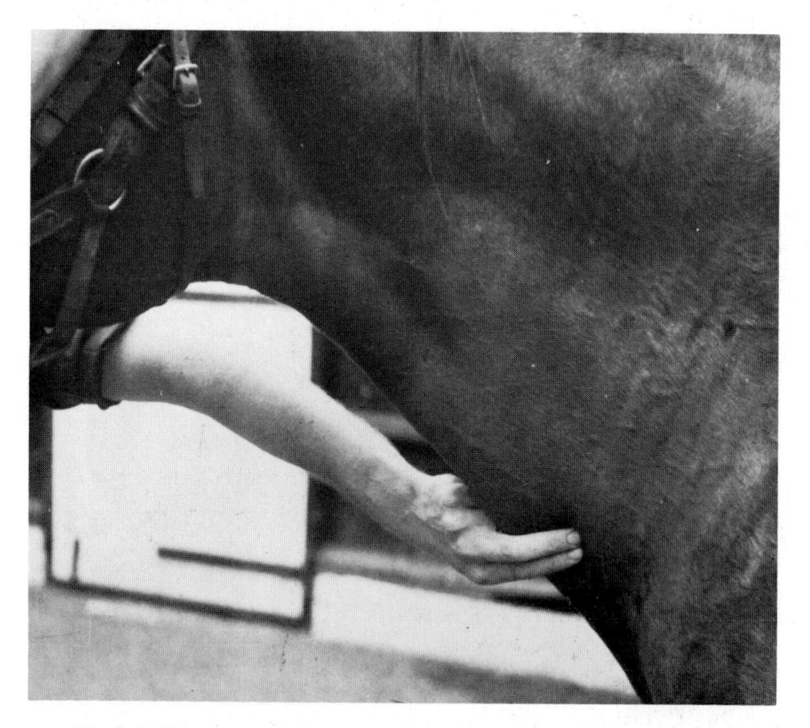

Fig. 8.6. The operator feeling for the end of the tube or for a bolus of air.

It may be necessary to pass the tube when a newborn foal is recumbent. The same principles apply except that the foal should be placed so that its head lies on the operator's lap.

RECTAL EXAMINATION

This is performed in the following cases:

1. In conditions affecting the abdominal organs, as in colic and wasting diseases, i.e. to palpate the alimentary tract and its mesenteries, the bladder, kidneys, liver and spleen.

2. In acute lameness of a hind-limb, to palpate parts of the pelvis and sublumbar muscles.

3. In gynaecological examinations to palpate the ovaries, uterus and cervix of the mare and the accessory sex glands and pelvic part of the urethra in the stallion.

The procedure adopted varies between veterinarians and according to circumstances. The standard methods are (*a*) in stocks and (*b*) with the horse alongside a partition or backed against bales of straw. The horse should be bridled and placed with the hind-quarters at an opening or doorway (Fig. 8.7). An attendant should stand at the head end, another at the flank, both on the opposite side to the veterinarian, and take the tail across the hind-quarters or vertically over the back. For reasons of hygiene and venereal disease control, attendants holding tails should

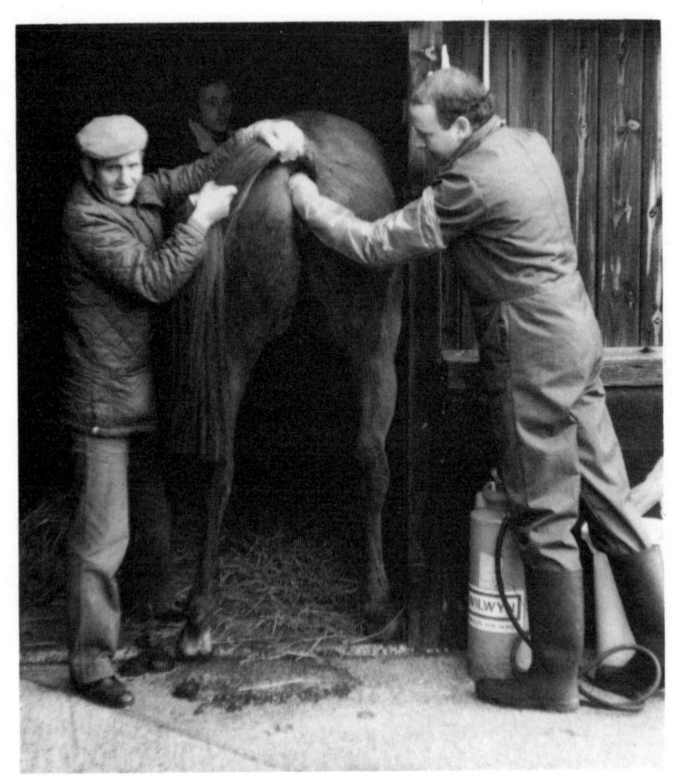

Fig. 8.7. Rectal examination. Note the position of the operator with the doorpost between him and the mare's hind-legs.

wear a separate pair of disposable gloves for each mare. Additional restraint may be applied in the form of a twitch and/or by grasping a fold of skin in the neck. If a fore-leg is raised, care should be taken as the horse may plunge and fall over. A twitch should not be applied to mares immediately after foaling because of the risk that this will precipitate haemorrhage. If necessary a tranquillizer should be given half an hour before examination.

There is no particular advantage in a left or right approach; most veterinarians seem to favour use of the left arm and therefore approach from the right side. The following points are listed for safety:

1. The reaction of the mare when the attendant takes the tail should be closely watched, especially as he places his hand on the base of the tail. The operator

should then wash the perineum and anal region while standing with the end of the partition between the mare's hind-legs and his own body. If the mare shows signs of kicking or resentment a decision must then be made whether or not to apply further restraint.

2. The operator should wear long plastic disposable gloves. Gloves are worn to protect the rectal mucosa from being scraped by the fingernails, to protect the operator's arm from allergic and infective conditions and to prevent the possible spread of contagious disease between horses.

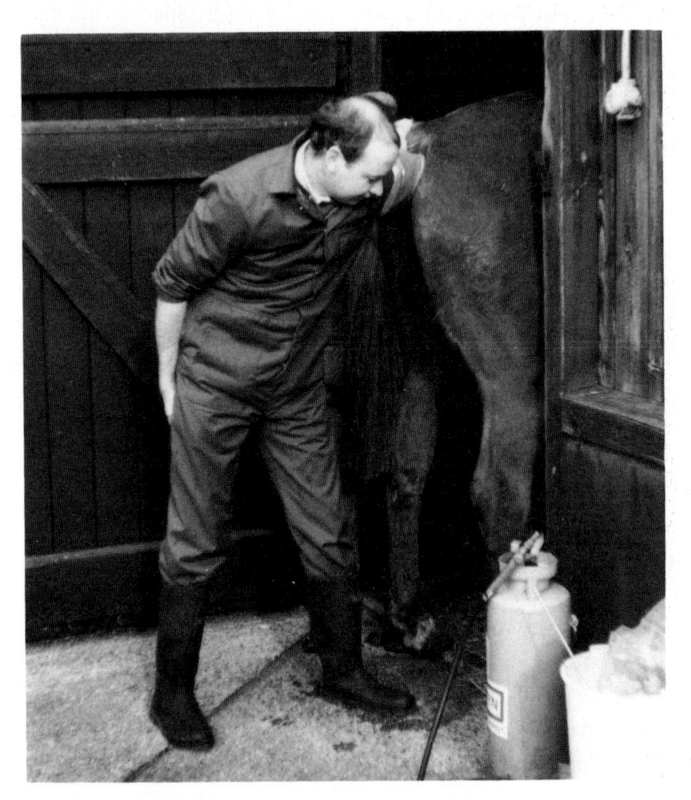

Fig. 8.8. When the arm is fully inserted the operator is still to one side but cannot avoid standing to some extent behind the mare.

3. The gloved arm should be well covered with obstetrical lubricant and the index finger placed into the anus. With the operator still standing well to one side (Fig. 8.7) the hand is then passed into the rectum and the faeces removed.

4. At this point the operator must stand closer to the horse to pass the full arm's length into the rectum (Fig. 8.8). It is safer to stand close to the hocks and sideways, rather than at a distance.

If the examination is in the centre of a box, as in a suspected fracture, the same approach applies but in the initial stages the operator should stand alongside the horse, level with the flanks, before taking a position behind.

Care must be taken when performing rectal examinations (Witherspoon 1977; Proctor 1977; Meagher 1977*b*; Vaughan 1977) as a ruptured rectum usually results in acute peritonitis and, unless the tear is retroperitoneal, often death. When inserted through the anus, the fingers should be coned and when inside the rectum the fingers should be together and the hand and arm should be relaxed. Faeces should be removed carefully and slowly, without any attempts to evacuate the rectum with one sweep. 'Poking' with the fingers is hazardous and should be used with extreme caution only by experienced operators. If a peristaltic wave reaches the hand, the arm should be withdrawn with the wave. Special care must be taken with older and debilitated horses (Meagher 1977*b*), who may have weaker or thinner rectal walls, and those that strain on the arm. This is particularly found in mares enjoying the 'spring flush' of grass. Sometimes the use of a twitch or the man at the head pulling out the horse's tongue reduces straining. Surgery for repair of a ruptured rectum should be contemplated only if the tear is cranial to the pelvis and an early diagnosis is made (Vaughan 1977).

The palpable contents of the abdomen of the horse are described by Greatorex (1968). Palpation of viscera is an art gained by experience, in conjunction with a good knowledge of anatomy. The position of sections of large and small colon, liver, spleen, ovaries, uterus, bladder, etc., must be accurately determined before rectal examinations are of value in routine diagnosis.

ENDOSCOPIC EXAMINATIONS

Vaginoscopy

The cervix may be observed through a speculum. Several patterns are available but for reasons of practicality and disease control, a separate plastic tubular speculum for each mare, with a distal light source, is preferred (Fig. 8.9). The perineum should be cleaned of faeces, washed and dried before examination (Fig. 8.10). During routine gynaecological examinations, vaginal examinations should be made before rectal examinations, if possible, as rectal examinations heavily contaminate the vulval lips with faecal material and sticky lubricant. The visible changes in position, shape, tone and colour during the oestrous cycle and in the presence of disease have been described in Chapter 1.

Endoscopy of pharynx and larynx

This procedure has been described by Cook (1970*a, b*) and Johnson (1971) for the rigid endoscope and by Cook (1974) and Johnson et al. (1977*a*) for the flexible fibreoptic endoscope. Rigid endoscopes are less expensive and portable; flexible ones are more versatile, as they allow small biopsies to be taken. The horse is tranquillized and restrained with a twitch. The endoscope is passed up the ventral meatus. When it is in the pharynx, the larynx may be viewed for the diagnosis of laryngeal hemiplegia (Johnson et al. 1977*b*), soft palate paresis, epiglottic

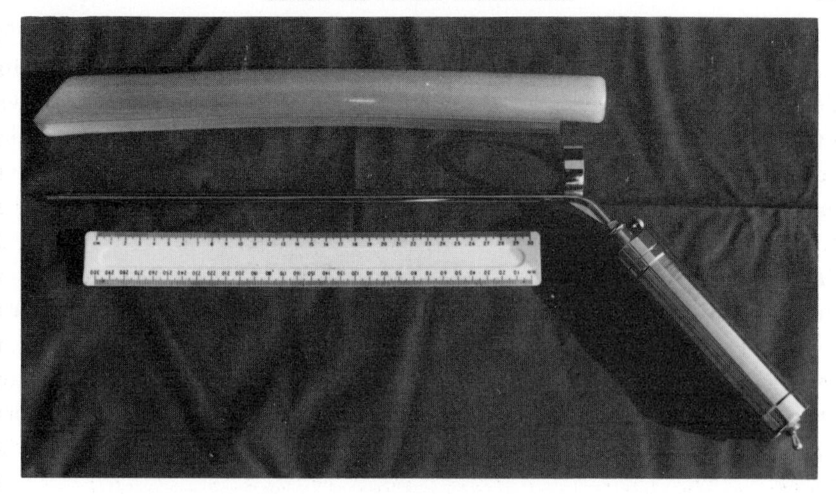

Fig. 8.9. A speculum set consisting of a distal light source with batteries in the handle and a detachable plastic sterilizable (boiling water) speculum. A separate sterilized speculum is used for each mare.

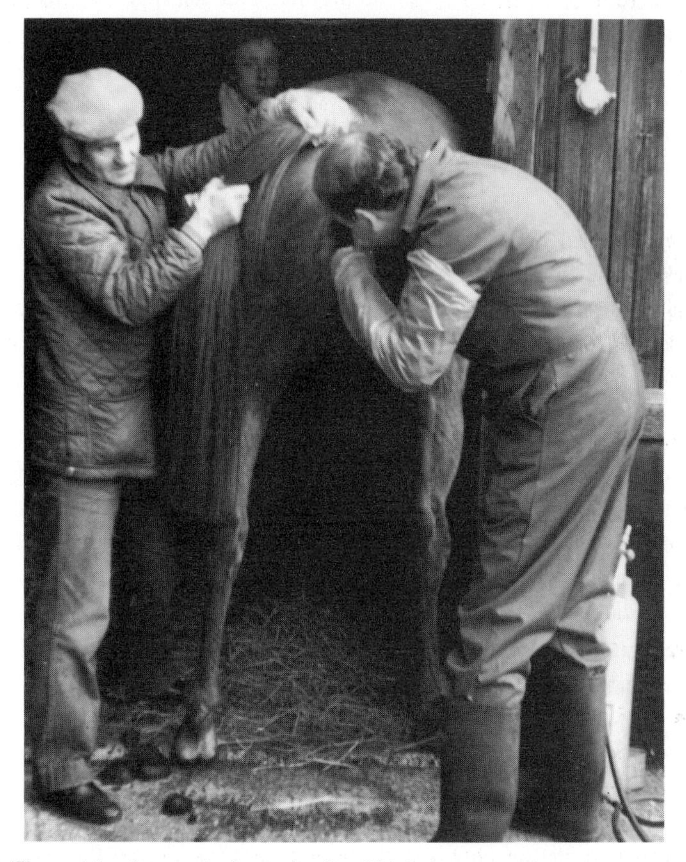

Fig. 8.10. The position for a vaginal examination. If it is necessary to stand behind the mare the operator should be close to her hocks rather than at a distance.

entrapment and follicular pharyngitis (Boles 1975). The guttural pouch may be entered either with the rigid endoscope (using a 60° pro-grade angled bulb) or with the flexible endoscope (using a blunt-ended nylon rod or the biopsy attachment through the 3 mm channel as a guide). Guttural pouch disease has been reviewed by McAllister (1977), who describes empyema, tympany, mycosis and chronic guttural pouch disease as a possible cause of chronic pharyngeal lymphoid hyperplasia.

Laparoscopy

This has been described by Heinze et al. (1972). It is necessary for the peritoneal cavity to be insufflated with oxygen for the abdominal viscera to be seen. A rigid or flexible endoscope may be passed through a trochar inserted into a skin incision made in the sublumbar fossa. This may be useful as more information on ovarian disease, abdominal neoplasia and intestinal disorders becomes available.

Cystoscopy

A rigid endoscope may be used in the mare and a flexible one in the stallion or gelding to pass into the bladder via the urethra. This can help diagnose cystitis or calculus formation.

Endoscopy of the uterus

To view the uterus a semi-flexible endoscope or a flexible one may be passed through the cervix. Insufflation with air or oxygen is necessary to see the endometrium. The flexible endoscope allows small biopsies to be taken, but these are considered too small for accurate interpretation (see Fig. 8.26). The procedure has been described by Brandt and Manning (1969) and Mather et al. (1979). The technique may be useful in demonstrating the extent of lymphatic cyst development.

NERVE BLOCKS

Lameness in stud farm animals is common. In many cases the cause is readily apparent, but not always. Local anaesthetic injected over specific nerves will remove sensation to the parts supplied by these nerves. If the horse goes sound after this, it indicates the seat of lameness. A good anatomical knowledge of the limbs is necessary to make the best use of the technique. Full details of techniques are available in Adams (1974) and Hall (1971). The most useful nerve blocks are:

1. *Post-digital.* This removes sensation from the posterior aspect of the foot and is used to diagnose such conditions as navicular disease, corns, thrush and pedal ostitis.

2. *Low volar.* This removes sensation from the entire foot, the majority of the pastern and posterior part of the fetlock and sesamoid bones. If the horse goes sound with a low volar block, but not with a posterior digital block, conditions such as pyramidal disease, ring bone, side bone and fractures of the pastern should be suspected.

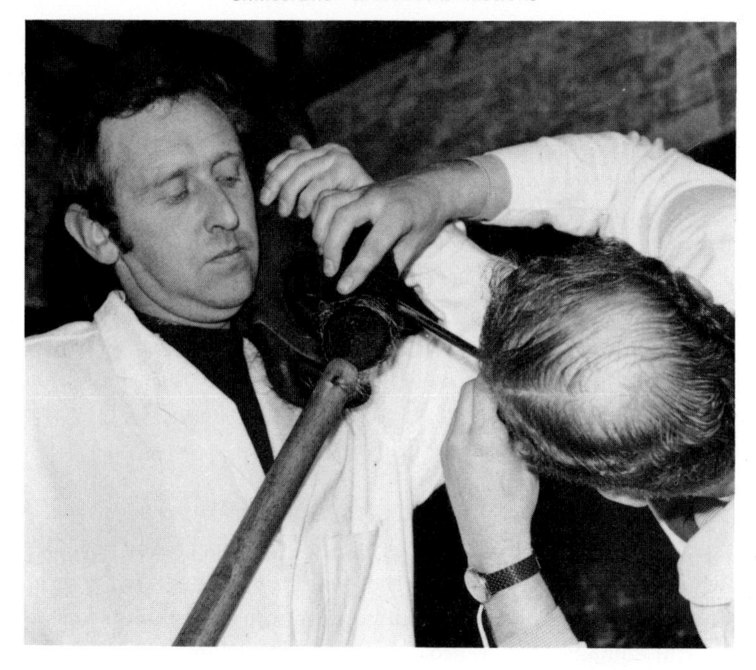

Fig. 8.11. A laryngoscopic examination with a rigid endoscope. Note the position of the twitch and the man holding the head, with the instrument in the left nasal passage.

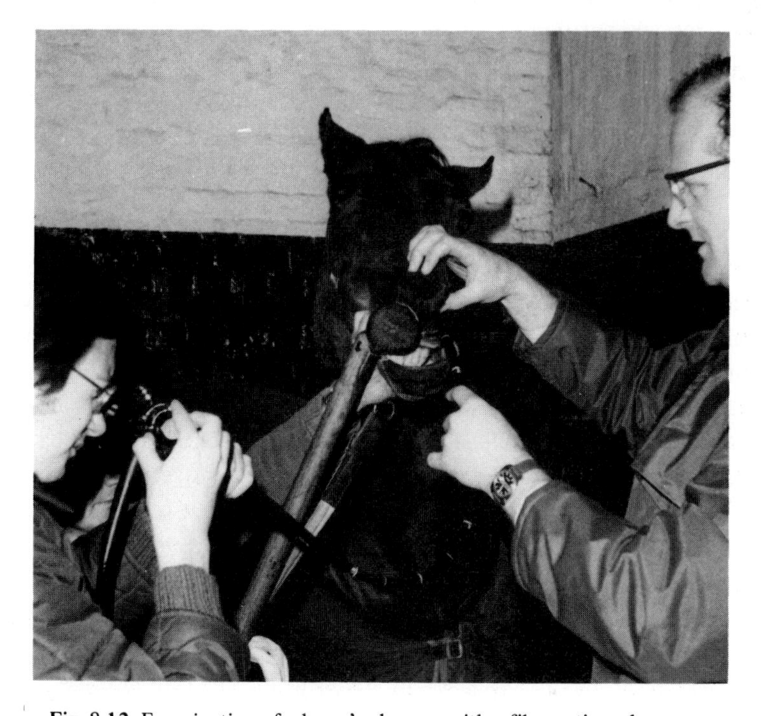

Fig. 8.12. Examination of a horse's pharynx with a fibreoptic endoscope.

3. *High volar.* This removes sensation from the foot, pastern, fetlock and distal cannon area. A diagnosis of splint bone problems, bucked shins or tendon problems is made if a horse is sound after high volar, but not after digital or low volar, block.

4. *Median, ulnar* and *musculocutaneous.* These blocks remove sensation from the carpus downwards.

5. *Tibial* and *peroneal.* These blocks remove sensation from the hock downwards.

Local anaesthetic may also be injected into joints to diagnose specific joint lameness (Tufvesson 1963). Joints which can be injected or blocked are the radiocarpal and intercarpal, the metacarpophalangeal, the tibiotarsal and the femoropatellar. It is also possible to block the trochanteric bursa of the hip, the navicular bursa in the heel, the P1/P2 and P2/P3 joints of the pastern. The intertarsal joints are very difficult to block adequately (Tufvesson 1963).

RADIOGRAPHY

Radiography is essential to diagnose many cases of lameness. Any possible osseous or joint lesion indicates radiography. The procedure is often used after a clinical examination and a nerve block. A small portable machine is useful for limbs, but more powerful equipment is needed for the thorax, abdomen and/or hips, except sometimes in young foals.

Common indications for radiography are foals with suspected fractured proximal sesamoid bones (Ellis 1978), joint-ill or arthritis (see Chapter 6). In epiphysitis in yearlings, the combination of an abnormal epiphysis on radiography plus clinical signs of a hot, painful enlarged epiphysis indicates confinement and treatment. It is impossible to contemplate surgery of fracture cases without adequate radiographs. Douglas and Williamson (1980) describe techniques of radiographic examination and the use of equipment.

DIAGNOSTIC PHYSIOTHERAPY

In some cases of lameness the seat of lameness is still not apparent after usual clinical examination, nerve blocks and radiography. In these cases faradic stimulation (rhythmic muscular contractions) to investigate muscle groups is advised. The technique has been reported by Strong (1946) and Hopes (1970). A rhythmic electrical current is passed (via an exploratory electrode held in the hand) through specific muscle bodies to a fixed electrode strapped to the horse's back. This current causes the muscles to contract and if they are damaged the horse reacts to the pain at low amplitude current. It is essential to rule out fracture or periosteal damage before using this technique. After the diagnosis of muscular damage, the same equipment can be used for physiotherapy to restore the muscle to normal use.

CLINICAL PATHOLOGY

Clinicopathological aids to diagnosis are useful to the clinician in disease, preventive medicine, the application and monitoring of treatment and the fulfilment

TABLE 8.1 Equine haematological parameters* in use at the authors' practice laboratory

Test	*Units*	*Birth to 36 hours*	*3 weeks*	*Yearlings*	*Horses in training*	*Mares at stud*
Red blood count	× 10^{12}/litre	9.9 (7.8–11.9)	10.7 (8.8–12.6)	10.8 (8.7–12.9)	9.4 (6.5–12.3	11.5 (9.0–14.0)
Packed cell volume	litre/litre	0.38 (0.31–0.45)	0.36 (0.30–0.42)	0.40 (0.33–0.47)	0.41 (0.33–0.49)	0.41 (0.35–0.47)
Haemoglobin	g/dl	13.1 (11.6–14.6)	12.0 (10.0–14.0)	12.9 (10.9–14.9)	13.7 (11.2–16.2)	14.0 (11.1–16.9)
Mean corpuscular volume	fl	36.6 (31.7–41.5)	36.0 (29.7–42.3)	35.5 (28.3–42.7)	42.7 (36.2–49.3)	36.0 (31.0–41.0)
Mean corpuscular haemoglobin concentration	g/dl	33.8 (31.0–36.6)	34.2 (30.0–38.4)	33.6 (30.0–37.2)	33.3 (29.9–36.7)	34.0 (32.0–36.0)
Mean corpuscular haemoglobin	pg	12.8 (10.5–15.1)	12.3 (10.1–14.5)	11.8 (8.6–15.0)	13.9 (11.3–16.5)	12.1 (10.0–14.2)
White blood count	× 10^9/litre	7.9 (3.7–12.1)	7.3 (5.9–8.7)	10.3 (6.1–14.5)	7.5 (3.7–11.3)	7.1 (4.1–10.1)
Segmented neutrophils	%	75 (59–61)	60 (43–79	48 (34–62	55 (39–71	52 (36–68)
	× 10^9/litre	5.9 (1.7–10.1)	4.3 (1.1–7.5)	5.0 (2.2–7.8)	4.0 (1.6–6.4)	3.6 (1.4–5.8)
Lymphocytes	%	24 (10–30)	38 (22–54)	48 (34–62)	43 (27–59)	45 (39–61)
	× 10^9/litre	1.7 (0.5–2.9)	2.8 (0.8–4.8)	4.9 (2.7–7.1)	2.9 (0.7–5.1)	3.0 (1.4–4.7)
Monocytes	%	1 (0–3)	1 (0–3)	1 (0–3)	2 (0–4)	1 (0–3)
	× 10^9/litre	0.05 (0–0.2)	0.07 (0–0.3)	0.06 (0–0.2)	0.1 (0–0.3)	0.07 (0–0.2)
Eosinophils	%	1 (0–3)	1 (0–3)	3 (0–9)	1 (0–3)	3 (0–5)
	× 10^9/litre	0.01 (0–0.08)	0.03 (0–0.2)	0.3 (0–1.0)	0.08 (0–0.4)	0.2 (0–0.5)

*Mean (±2 SD).

TABLE 8.2 Equine biochemical parameters* in use at the authors' practice laboratory

Test	*Units*	*Birth to 36 hours*	*3 weeks*	*Yearlings*	*Horses in training*	*Mares at stud*
Total serum proteins	g/litre	45 (31–59)	45 (41–49)	58 (48–68)	57 (47–67)	58 (46–70)
Albumin	g/litre	25 (17–33)	25 (19–31)	27 (21–33)	34 (27–40)	27 (17–37)
Globulin	g/litre	20 (8–32)	22 (12–32)	31 (19–43)	25 (17–34)	31 (21–41)
Bromsulphalein clearance	sec	–	–	168 (138–198)	168 (138–198)	168 (138–198)
Sorbitol dehydrogenase	IU/litre	0.7 (<2.0)	0.65 (<2.0)	0.4 (<1.0)	0.4 (<1.0)	0.4 (<1.0)
Lactic dehydrogenase (LDH)	IU/litre	670 (400–940)	540 (260–820)	243 (76–409)	243 (76–409)	243 (76–409)
Gamma glutamyl transferase	IU/litre	12.8 (8.6–17.0)	15.7 (9.1–22.3)	18.1 (<41.2)	18.1 (41.2)	18.1 (41.2)
Aspartate aminotransferase (AST)	IU/litre	70 (<130)	117 (<220)	140 (<230)	160 (<250)	140 (<230)
Creatine kinase (CK)	IU/litre	57 (<107)	53 (<135)	43 (<80)	68 (<100)	43 (<105)
Serum alkaline phosphatase	IU/litre	472 (<778)	172 (<280)	118 (<196)	86 (<145)	71 (<131)
Total bilirubin	mmol/litre	54.9 (15.6–94.2)	37.8 (21.7–53.9)	34.1 (22.4–45.8)	25.9 (13.0–38.8)	25.9 (13.0–38.8)
Direct bilirubin	mmol/litre	19.7 (5.6–33.8)	11.7 (5.3–18.1)	11.5 (4.9–18.1)	9.5 (4.2–14.8)	9.5 (4.2–14.8)
Calcium	mmol/litre	3.2 (2.7–3.6)	3.2 (2.5–4.0)	3.4 (2.7–4.0)	3.4 (2.6–3.9)	3.4 (2.9–3.9)
Phosphate	mmol/litre	2.5 (1.2–3.8)	2.5 (1.6–3.4)	1.8 (1.4–2.3)	1.3 (1.1–1.5)	1.1 (0.5–1.6)
Urea	mmol/litre	6.0 (4.3–9.3)	6.0 (4.5–7.5)	6.0 (3.5–8.0)	5.4 (3.7–7.3)	6.0 (3.5–8.0)
Creatinine	mmol/litre	175.3 (98.3–252.3)	157.0 (89–225)	141.4 (106.1–168.0)	125.0 (87–163)	141.4 (10.6–168.0)
Glucose	mmol/litre	3.1 (1.1–5.1)	4.2 (2.2–6.2)	4.7 (3.4–5.9)	4.7 (3.4–5.9)	4.7 (3.4–5.9)
Sodium	mmol/litre	136 (126–146)	137.5 (130–144)	138.5 (133.7–143.3)	138.5 (133.7–143.3)	138.5 (133.7–143.3)
Potassium	mmol	4.8 (3.7–5.4)	4.5 (3.6–5.4)	4.3 (3.3–5.3)	4.3 (3.3–5.3)	4.3 (3.3–5.3)
Magnesium	mmol/litre	0.83 (0.57–1.09)	0.81 (0.66–0.96)	0.78 (0.62–0.86)	0.78 (0.62–0.86)	0.78 (0.62–0.86)

* Mean (± 2 SD).

of regulations governing export of horses. If used correctly, they are invaluable, but if samples are incorrectly taken, handled, examined or interpreted, they may be counter-productive. Haematological and serum biochemical references parameters for Thoroughbred horses of varying ages, as seen in our practice laboratory, are

TABLE 8.3 Conversion factors – old and SI units

Test	*Old units*	*SI units*	*Multiplication factor*	
			Old to SI	SI to old
RBC	$\times 10^6/mm^3$	10^{12}/litre	10^6	10^{-6}
PCV	%	litre/litre	0.01	100
Hb	g/100 ml	g/dl	No change	No change
MCV	μm^3	fl	No change	No change
MCHC	%	g/dl	No change	No change
MCH	pg	pg	No change	No change
WBC	$\times 10^3/mm^3$	10^9/litre	10^6	10^{-6}
TSP	g/100 ml	g/litre	10.0	0.1
Albumin	g/100 ml	g/litre	10.0	0.1
Globulin	g/100 ml	g/litre	10.0	0.1
BSP Clearance	min	sec	60	0.0167
SDH	mU/ml	IU/litre	No change	No change
LDH	mU/ml	IU/litre	No change	No change
Gamma GT	mU/ml	IU/litre	No change	No change
AST (SGOT)	mU/ml	IU/litre	No change	No change
CPK	mU/ml	IU/litre	No change	No change
SAP	mU/ml	IU/litre	No change	No change
Bilirubin	mg/100 ml	μmol/litre	17.1	0.0585
Calcium	mg/100 ml	mmol/litre	0.250	4.008
Phosphate	mg/100 ml	mmol/litre	0.323	3.10
Urea*	mg/100 ml	mmol/litre	0.166	6.01
Creatinine	mg/100 ml	μmol/litre	88.4	0.0113
Glucose	mg/100 ml	mmol/litre	0.0555	18.02
Sodium	mEq/litre	mmol/litre	No change	No change
Potassium	mEq/litre	mmol/litre	No change	No change
Magnesium	mg/100 ml	mmol/litre	0.411	2.43
Chloride	mEq/litre	mmol/litre	No change	No change

*To convert BUN to urea multiply by 2.14.

shown in Tables 8.1 and 8.2. The modern use of SI (Système International) units aids the comparison of such data, but to help those not familiar with this system, Table 8.3 has been produced.

Haematology

The examination of peripheral blood samples for evidence of systemic disease is one of the most useful tests in equine medicine. Interested readers are referred to two excellent reviews on this subject by Archer and Jeffcott (1977) and the American Association of Equine Practitioners (1975). Samples should be taken into sequestrated (dipotassium EDTA) containers and, if possible, from a quiet resting animal. Excitement raises the packed cell volume, haemoglobin content and erythrocyte count due to the mobilization of large erythrocyte reserves, principally in the spleen. This phenomenon also occurs in acute pain or shock.

Packed cell volume (haematocrit)

The packed cell volume is a very simple, quick and practical guide to red cell numbers and to fluid balance. High values, in the absence of excitement at the time of collection, suggest haemoconcentration, whereas low values suggest anaemia (Table 8.4), blood loss or over-hydration. The 'supernatant' plasma may be yellow, red/orange or milky/white, suggesting jaundice, intravascular haemolysis (provided the sample is relatively fresh and well handled) or hyperlipaemia. The 'buffy'

TABLE 8.4 Causes of anaemia in the horse

Direct blood loss	Haemorrhage from trauma and surgery
	Epistaxis
	Defective coagulation
	Haemophilia
	Warfarin poisoning
	Primary idiopathic thrombocytopenic purpura
Haemolysis	Haemolytic disease of newborn
	Infections
	Equine infectious anaemia (EIA)
	Babesiosis
	Ehrlichiosis
	Trypanosomiasis
	Leptospirosis
	Poisons and toxic chemicals
	Lead
	Phenothiazine
	Onion poisoning
	Autoimmune haemolytic anaemia
	Idiopathic haemolytic anaemia
Dyserythropoiesis	Primary
	Nutritional – iron and folate deficiency
	Idiopathic hypoplastic anaemia
	Secondary
	Parasitic infestation
	Chronic inflammatory disease and debility
	Purpura haemorrhagica
	Malignant neoplasia
	Aplastic anaemia

From Jeffcott (1977).

coat may be very thick and obvious, suggesting a high white cell count. Stud farm animals, being relatively unfit, usually have lower packed cell volumes than do fit horses in training. The packed cell volume is useful in monitoring cardiovascular shock and following the progress of colic cases; it drops in the early stages of intestinal impaction but may rise as the condition develops (De Groot 1971); it rises in intestinal infarction (Nelson 1964; Nelson et al. 1968); it provides a rough guide to the quantity of fluids needed to correct cardiovascular shock (Carlson 1979). Assuming there is no continuing fluid loss, 1 litre of fluid reduces the packed cell volume by approximately 1%. The packed cell volume forms a useful screen for haemolytic diseases and for haemoconcentration due to diarrhoea or convulsions.

Haemoglobin content and erythrocyte count

High values (in the absence of excitement at the time of collection) are found in cases of dehydration and low ones in anaemia. Haemoglobin values, like the packed cell volume, are usually lower in stud farm animals than in Thoroughbreds in training. Anaemias associated with parasitism are common in stud farm animals. The erythrocyte count (in the absence of excitement at the time of collection) is used to indicate blood loss, anaemia or haemoconcentration and in the assessment of 'fitness' in racehorses. It is of questionable value unless electronic particle counting techniques can be used. Manual erythrocyte counts are subject to large technical errors and in this situation it is best to rely on the measurement of packed cell volume and haemoglobin. This applies also to mean corpuscular volume (MCV), mean corpuscular haemoglobin (MCH) and mean corpuscular haemoglobin concentration (MCHC) as these are all computed from the erythrocyte count.

The most commonly seen anaemias in stud farm animals are normocyctic/macrocytic and are invariably of parasitic, traumatic or haemolytic origin. Microcytic anaemia is usually associated with chronic infection or debilitating disease. A classification of equine anaemias is shown in Table 8.4.

Leucocytes

The leucocyte count is a useful diagnostic aid in many diseases, but particularly in the presence of infection (Table 8.5). Bacterial infections (acute or chronic) usually result in a leucocytosis (high white cell count). The exception to this rule is in newborn septicaemic foals and in acute peritonitis and other overwhelming infections where a leucopenia (low white cell count) may be found. Viral infections usually result initially in a leucopenia, rising to normal and then a leucocytosis, as secondary bacterial infection and/or recovery occurs.

A differential count gives added useful information (Table 8.5). Students are always told that differential percentages are of little value and that absolute figures must be used. While this is basically true, experience with clinical interpretation has suggested that 'relative' neutrophilias or lymphocytoses may be a useful guide at some stages of bacterial or viral infections, even though 'absolute' figures are well within the 'normal' limits. 'Normal' limits are not always as straightforward to use as they may seem (Blackmore 1975) and the traditional two standard deviations from a mean may be too wide for certain individuals.

Lymphocytosis is often encountered without apparent clinical signs, probably due to upper respiratory tract viral infections frequently present in young horses. Monocytosis is associated with a chronic infection or a convalescent phase of a viral infection and eosinophilia with states of histamine release in allergy or during the migratory phase of parasitic larvae. Archer (1954) and Round (1968) have demonstrated a rise in eosinophil count that occurs in the autumn during strongyle larvae migration. This phenomenon must be recognized in interpreting routine blood samples in preventive medicine. In acute bacterial infections a polymorphonuclear leucocytosis is usual and severity can be estimated by the number of

TABLE 8.5 Alterations of the leucocyte count in the horse

	Total leucocytes	*Neutrophils*		*Lymphocytes*	*Monocytes*	*Eosinophils*
		Juvenile	Segmented			
increase ↑	Infection Inflammation Severe parasitism	Acute bacterial infection	Infection Inflammation 'Fitness'	Acute viral infection Adrenocortical insufficiency Convalescence after infection	Chronic infection EIA EHV I	Virus infection Parasitism Allergy
decrease ↓	Acute viral infection Acute salmonellosis Peritonitis Neonatal septicaemia Neonatal immune 'incompetence'		Viral infection Hypersensitivity Peritonitis Acute salmonellosis	Immunological incompetence CID		

juvenile forms. The acute phase is indicated by more than 5% band forms (shift to the left). During a viral infection, a neutropenia or lymphocytosis may occur depending on the stage of sampling.

Nitroblue tetrazolium (NBT). Benjamin et al. (1975) have described the use of this cytochemical staining test with heparinized or sequestrated equine blood samples. Neutrophils, when involved in phagocytosis, have an increased cell membrane permeability which allows the entry of the blue/black NBT dye. The presence of more than 10% stained neutrophils suggests that active phagocytosis of bacteria is occurring and that this may be a useful additional diagnostic aid to the total and differential leucocyte count. In 'negative' cases (less than 10% stained neutrophils), in vitro 'stimulation' of the neutrophils with a proprietary bacterial extract may differentiate between a 'true' negative and a case of bacteraemia with a basic defect in the phagocytic system. Benjamin et al. (1975) found this to be particularly useful as a prognostic aid in neonatal foal septicaemias. They also found the test useful in the differentiation of bacterial and viral respiratory infections.

Biochemistry

Most routine blood biochemical tests are performed on serum samples. Samples should be obtained by jugular venepuncture into a plain sterile tube. Shaking is not necessary and may be undesirable. The blood should be allowed to clot by leaving it to stand at room temperature. When the clot contracts, serum is left above the red cells and fibrin and may be withdrawn by a pipette for examination.

Kaneko and Cornelius (1970) provide a useful general account of equine biochemistry. The reader is also referred to the work on serum enzyme determination by Gerber (1969), Gerber et al. (1975), Coffmann et al. (1977) and Jeffcott (1977).

Serum proteins

Low total serum protein values may suggest gross nutritional or metabolic deficiency. This chiefly involves the albumin fraction and values are characteristically low in starvation or cachexia, liver disease and protein-losing enteropathy or nephropathy. If serum albumin levels fall below 15 g/litre in an adult horse, there is a danger of intravascular haemodynamic collapse which, if not corrected, is usually fatal. Foals, yearlings and sometimes two-year-olds in training have a very significant drain on their protein reserves for growth and adequate supplementation is sometimes necessary.

The total serum proteins of newborn foals are very low but rise rapidly after adequate colostral ingestion. This, to some extent, involves albumin but is mostly due to the absorption of colostral gammaglobulins during the immediate postpartum period (see p. 294). Low globulin levels in newborn foals, at approximately 36 hours of age, may indicate inadequate colostral ingestion or absorption and subnormal immune status. Such foals are considered to be at risk of infectious challenge. High total serum protein values, usually involving the globulin fractions,

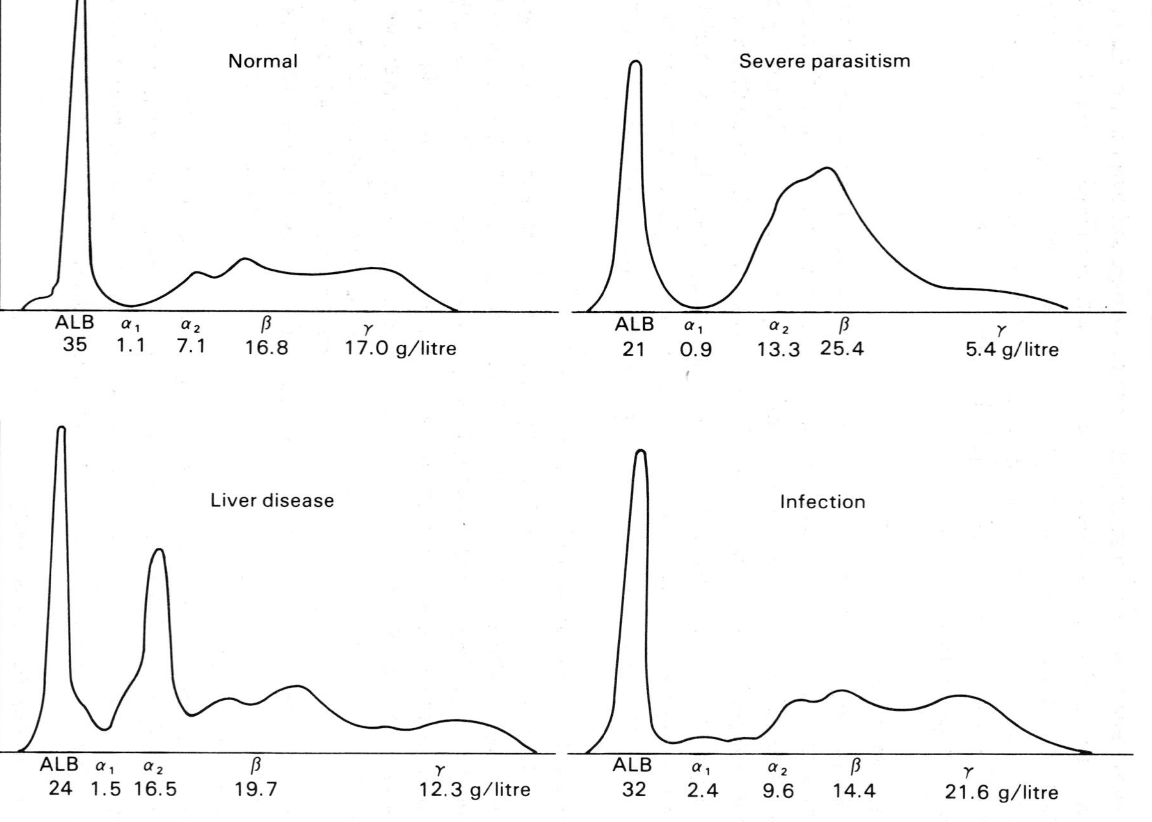

Fig. 8.13. Electrophoretic patterns of serum proteins traced from the records of actual cases.

are most commonly seen in infections, parasitic damage and liver disease. Protein electrophoresis (Fig. 8.13) is useful in cases of raised total globulin to differentiate rises in gamma fraction (>14 g/litre) (usually infection), beta fraction (>21 g/litre) (usually parasitism, specifically strongylosis, see p. 444) and alpha$_1$ (>4 g/litre) and alpha$_2$ (>13 g/litre) fractions (alpha$_2$-globulin rises may be seen in the presence of tissue damage; Erickson 1975).

Plasma fibrinogen

Plasma fibrinogen levels may be determined by subtracting the results of total protein estimations on a plasma sample and a serum sample collected at the same time. Alternatively, total protein estimations may be performed after heating a plasma sample in a water bath at 58°C for three minutes. Normal adult plasma fibrinogen levels are 2.58 ± 0.072 g/litre (Schalm 1975; Jeffcott 1977) and there is no obvious age or breed variation. High levels are seen in inflammatory, neoplastic and traumatic disease and levels over 10 g/litre are usually a poor prognostic sign.

Aspartate aminotransferase (AST) (formerly AAT or SGOT)

This intracellular enzyme is released by acute hepatic or muscular pathology. Cardinet et al. (1963), Cornelius et al. (1963), Mullen (1969), Blackmore and Elton (1975), Anderson (1975) and Mullen et al. (1979) have described how AST levels are higher for horses in training than in less active horses. Their results also show that AST activity rises at the beginning of training, then decreases as training progresses. This presumably indicates less muscular damage as the horse becomes more 'fit'. The authors also demonstrated marked rises in AST levels in horses with clinical signs of 'tying up' or myoglobinuria. Their results suggest that these horses had significantly high levels before the exercise and this may help anticipate the clinical actuality.

Gerber (1969) suggests that AST is a non-specific but sensitive indicator of acute hepatocellular damage. However, the muscular effects described above may tend to mask or dominate these effects. Levels seen in uncomplicated acute hepatitis (see p. 471) are not as high as those in acute muscular damage.

Serum alkaline phosphatase (SAP)

This enzyme is involved in the mineralization of bone and excreted by the liver. High levels in adult horses suggest a liver abnormality with biliary obstruction, e.g. chronic ragwort poisoning, or an abnormality in the bone mineralization process. 'Intestinal' phosphatase (Blackmore & Palmer 1977), i.e. that component originating from the intestines and differentiated from other phosphatases by analysis at a pH of 9.5 and inhibition with 15 mM/litre phenylalanine, may be elevated in cases of intestinal damage, e.g. enteritis. Total serum alkaline phosphatase levels decrease with age, presumably due to decreasing bone mineralization. Levels greater than 150 IU in adult horses suggest an obstructive jaundice or an abnormality in the mineralization process. Abnormal values are sometimes seen in yearlings with epiphysitis, sometimes associated with an imbalance of serum calcium and phosphorus.

Bromosulphalein (BSP) clearance

BSP clearance is useful to assess gross hepatic insufficiency. The dye is warmed in a water bath and 1 g is injected into one jugular vein of the resting horse. A stopwatch is started at that moment and blood samples are taken from the opposite vein at two, four, eight and 16 minutes. The results are expressed graphically and the dye should normally be cleared from the blood by the liver at a half-time rate of less than 200 seconds.

Bilirubin

Jaundice may be defined and classified by the level of conjugated and unconjugated bilirubin in the serum. Unconjugated bilirubin is increased in haemolytic jaundice and conjugated bilirubin in hepatocellular and obstructive jaundice. The horse, however, has an unusual biliary excretion system (Tennant et al. 1975) and levels vary considerably, making the interpretation of some elevations difficult. Levels rise in horses which do not eat for even a few days and in some mares out at grass in late summer (Jeffcott 1977).

Blood glucose

Normal whole blood levels are less than plasma levels because the erythrocyte cell membranes are impermeable to glucose molecules. Diet and time of day will affect blood glucose values. Diabetes mellitus classically results in a hyperglycaemia but diabetes is rare in horses. Hypoglycaemia may occur in a newborn foal but is usually symptomless (Rossdale 1966). The foal is normally able to maintain blood glucose levels, even when starved, in contrast to human infants and piglets.

Serum creatine kinase (CK, formerly CPK)

This intracellular enzyme is involved in muscular activity. Serum levels, measured in conjunction with AST, differentiate liver from muscular pathology. Exercise, of even mild degree, especially in unfit horses, may cause moderate rises in CK and thus values should not be considered to be significantly elevated unless higher than 150 IU/litre. High AST and CK values suggest a muscular problem and a high AST with a normal CK suggest a hepatocellular problem or a recovering muscular problem. Raised CK and AST levels are associated with myoglobinuria (setfast, azoturia, the tying-up syndrome). After the acute attack, the CK levels return to normal in a matter of days whereas AST levels may take several weeks.

Electrophoretic separation of CK isoenzymes has been described (Nealon & Henderson 1975) and may be useful to differentiate CK of brain (CK_1), heart (CK_2) and skeletal muscle (CK_3) origin.

Blood urea

High levels may be seen in renal malfunction. A dietary history is important when considering results as a high-protein diet, e.g. horses in training, produces a rise in blood urea.

Serum creatinine

This product of muscle metabolism is excreted by the kidneys and high levels may be seen in renal disease.

Serum calcium and inorganic phosphate

Calcium levels remain relatively stable but inorganic phosphate declines with age. There are seasonal changes and variations associated with nutrition. Abnormalities in the calcium/inorganic phosphate status may be associated with epiphysitis and bone disease in young horses. The homeostatic mechanisms responsible for controlling these mineral levels are so efficient that many cases of actual disease have normal serum levels (Traver et al. 1976). Urinary clearance ratios for phosphate in relation to creatinine may be a more accurate assessment (see below).

Serum electrolytes

Metabolic disturbances may change values and measurements are useful in evaluating therapy in horses suffering from shock and intestinal conditions such as acute colic and diarrhoea. Low serum potassium occurs in cases of chronic diarrhoea and should be corrected by feeding extra potassium. Urinary clearance ratios for these electrolytes in relation to creatinine is a useful additional assessment (see below).

Urinary, mineral and electrolyte clearance ratios

A practical method of estimating the percentage urinary clearance of inorganic phosphate, sodium, potassium and chloride in relation to creatinine has been described by Traver et al. (1976). It involves collecting a single urine sample (without the use of a diuretic) and serum sample and calculating the clearance ratio from the following equation:

$$\text{Percentage clearance ratio (X)} = \frac{[X]_u}{[X]_s} \times \frac{[\text{Creatinine}]_s}{[\text{Creatinine}]_u} \times 100$$

where X $= PO_4^-, Na^+, K^+, Cl^-$

$[X]_u$ = concentration of X in urine

$[X]_s$ = concentration of X in serum

Normal clearance ratios for adult horses are: Na^+ 0.02–1%; K^+ 15–65%; $PO4^-$ 0–0.5% and Cl^- 0.04–1.6%. High percentage phosphate clearance suggests hyperparathyroidism (primary or secondary). Low dietary calcium may cause hyperparathyroidism which may cause epiphysitis in growing stock or chronic non-specific lameness in adults. These conditions may be corrected by supplementing calcium in the diet. High percentage sodium, potassium and chloride clearances suggest renal tubular malfunction.

Blood pH and gas analysis

Arterial and venous pH, $P\text{CO}_2$ and $P\text{O}_2$ are used to determine the balance between respiratory and metabolic buffer systems in cases undergoing intensive care after surgery and those suffering shock or diarrhoea. Values in normal subjects and pathological states have been reported in foals (Rossdale 1968; Rossdale & Mullen 1970) and in older horses (Gillespie et al. 1964).

In diarrhoea the rapid loss of intestinal bicarbonate normally retained results in metabolic acidosis. In respiratory distress, pneumonia, lung consolidation and emphysema a respiratory acidosis is often present.

PARASITOLOGY

Parasitism in general and strongylosis in particular is the most important cause of disease in stud farm animals. Under intensive systems of management it is a constant and practically insoluble problem; at best it is restricted by regular prophylactic treatment. The faecal worm egg count has, traditionally, been the method of investigating parasitism but its limits have been discussed on p. 443.

Every horse on the stud farm from weaning onwards should be sampled on a regular basis. In this way the efficacy of an anthelmintic programme can be assessed. Individuals with a high worm count may even be a clue to an unconnected systemic problem.

Faecal samples for worm egg counts should be collected when fresh into a clean pot or plastic bag and sealed. Clear and adequate labelling is essential when large numbers of samples are involved. Samples should be stored in a cool dark place until the examination, which should be as soon as possible. If left for any length of time, especially in the warm, the eggs will hatch and make the test even more inaccurate. The egg count is expressed as eggs per gram of faeces (epg) and the method recommended by the late Leo Mahaffey is:

1. Weigh 3 g of faeces and emulsify in 42 ml of water until they are thoroughly broken up. It is helpful to use an electric mixer for three minutes.

2. Centrifuge 15 ml of the emulsion at 1500 rpm for five minutes. Discard the supernatant fluid and shake deposit free from the sides of the tube.

3. Fill the tube to within 1 cm of the top with saturated NaCl and mix by inverting two or three times, taking care to avoid bubbles.

4. Completely fill the tube to a slight convex meniscus with saturated NaCl, avoiding bubbles.

5. Place a 18 × 18 mm coverslip over the fluid and press gently onto the lip of the centrifuge tube, which should then be spun for one minute at 1000 rpm.

6. Carefully reduce the speed of the centrifuge and remove the coverslip with a sudden vertical movement and transfer it to a slide. Eggs that are present in the liquid adhere to the coverslip.

7. Count the eggs in the total area under a 16 mm objective and multiply by 5/4. The result is expressed as epg.

If the specimen has more than 400 epg, proceed to stage 1 as above and then:

1. Measure 15 ml of a representative sample of fluid into a smaller container, shaking continuously.

2. Place 0.15 ml of the fluid onto a slide and cover with 12 × 12 mm coverslip, then examine the whole area under a 16 mm objective.

3. Multiply the total eggs seen by 100 to obtain the total epg.

Various worm egg count levels have been quoted as criteria of significance but the presence of any eggs is significant as far as control and treatment are concerned.

A complete laboratory 'screen' for strongylosis is a worm cell count, an eosinophil count, a measurement of packed cell volume, mean cell volume, haemoglobin and serum beta-globulin levels.

The identification of *Dictyocaulus arnfeldi* (lungworm) larvae is best accomplished by the examination of 50 g amounts of faeces, removed manually from the rectum (Round 1976), after leaving overnight in a Baermann funnel (Fig. 8.14). The larvae descend to the bottom of the funnel and are drawn off in the first 1–2 ml of fluid. *D. arnfeldi* larvae characteristically have a 'tipped' tail (see Fig. 7.13) which distinguishes them from other nematode larvae.

A method for the examination of faecal samples for *Fasciola hepatica* eggs has been described by Owen (1977). The method is as follows:

1. 30–40 g of faeces are washed through a 100 mesh sieve, 20 cm in diameter, with a forced jet of tap water, and the filtrate is collected on a 200 mesh sieve.

2. The residue which contains any fluke eggs is washed off the 200 mesh sieve into a 250 ml beaker.

3. After the contents have been allowed to settle for 2–3 minutes the supernatant is poured off.

4. The beaker is again refilled, the debris allowed to settle and the water decanted off again. This is repeated until the fluid contents of the beaker are clear, when a final decantation is made leaving about 10–15 ml of water and the non-floating debris.

5. This is agitated, poured on to an 8 cm Petri dish and examined for fluke eggs under the low power of a microscope. Scanning of the Petri dish is made easier if it is marked with parallel lines. The presence of one egg in the faeces of a suspect animal is sufficient to advise treatment (see p. 452).

URINE ANALYSIS

Inflammation of the urinary tract is diagnosed by the presence of leucocytes and sometimes casts and necrotic debris in a urine sample. Pathogenic bacteria may be isolated from such cases but growths can only be interpreted, with confidence, in samples taken by catheter in an aseptic manner. Equine urine usually contains carbonate and oxalate crystals but abnormally high numbers may indicate calculus formation. The normal specific gravity of equine urine is 1.025–1.060. The pH varies with the diet; the higher the carbohydrate ration the more acid the urine.

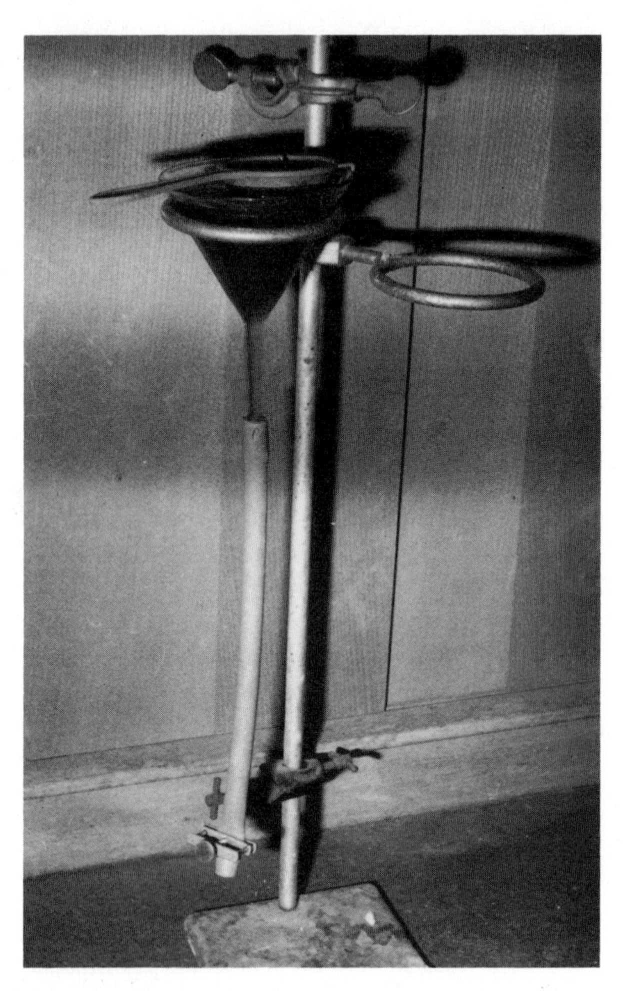

Fig. 8.14. Baermann funnel system for the examination of fresh faecal samples for *D. arnfeldi* (lungworm) larvae.

Horses at grass or on a high roughage diet have an alkaline urine. Horse urine is normally mucoid and contains no sugar or protein. The presence of blood, myoglobin, protein, glucose or ketones may indicate a metabolic condition, muscle damage, blood abnormality or pathological condition of the kidney or bladder.

BACTERIOLOGY

The culture, identification and antibiotic sensitivity testing of infectious agents is a valuable aid to diagnosis, prognosis and therapy. Material to be cultured is usually collected with a sterile swab which is then placed in a sterile container or into suitable medium for transport to the laboratory. The results of bacteriological examination depend on correct swabbing, transport and culturing techniques. Cases that have received antibiotic therapy may give spurious results.

Swabs are usually plated out onto blood agar and incubated aerobically for cultural characteristics and initial identification. McConkey's agar is used to differentiate Enterobacteriacae by their ability to ferment lactose. For *Haemophilus equigenitalis,* swabs received in Amies charcoal transport medium are plated onto a chocolated blood agar, and incubated under micro-aerophilic conditions (Platt et al. 1977). In addition to the 'selective' agar containing streptomycin, useful for the strain of the organism seen in the United Kingdom at the present time, streptomycin-free agar is also used to identify streptomycin-sensitive strains which have been seen in other countries (Swerczek 1978). Enrichment media are used for certain organisms that do not grow well on blood agar, for example DCA media for *Salmonella* species.

Further identification of organisms may be by Gram stain, catalase, coagulase and oxidase tests, biochemical 'sugar' tests, slide agglutination tests with prepared antisera, e.g. salmonellae, fluorescent antibody tests, phage typing for *E. coli* and capsule typing for *Klebsiella aerogenes.* Definitive *Klebsiella* capsule typing is a specialized technique but differentiation of some of the more commonly isolated strains is sometimes possible on the basis of colonial characteristics and urease, citrate and ornithine biochemical reactions (Atherton 1975). As a very crude 'rule of thumb', urease production usually suggests a potentially pathogenic strain, e.g. K1 or K5, whereas negative urease production suggests a less significant strain, e.g. K7 or *Enterobacter aerogenes* type 68.

Cervicouterine swabs

This routine procedure in stud farm practice is performed early in oestrus to protect the stallion from transmissible pathogenic organisms, such as *Klebsiella aerogenes, Pseudomonas aeruginosa* and *Haemophilus equigenitalis.* It has also been used as an indirect indication of the presence of acute cervicitis or endometritis, when organisms such as *Streptococcus zooepidemicus* (beta-haemolytic streptococci), *E. coli* (haemolytic) or *Staphylococcus aureus* (coagulase-positive) are grown. The accuracy of the technique for this purpose has been increased by the additional technique of cervical cytology (see p. 537).

Several different methods (Allen & Newcombe 1979) are used to collect material from the cervix and uterus for bacteriological and cytological examination. Instrumentation and technique vary according to personal preference but certain principles must be observed for the best results. Swabs should be taken only when the mare is in oestrus and the cervix is relaxed and moist. At that time there is a greater of recovering pathogenic organisms (David et al. 1978) and a greater chance of obtaining a true endometrial swab. Unless the mare is in oestrus there is little correlation between cervical bacteriological findings and the endometrial flora (Brandt 1970). We prefer the use of the tubular speculum (Fig. 8.15) with a distal light source for the following reasons:

1. A separate sterile speculum may be used for each mare, thus eliminating the risk of mechanical transfer of potential venereal-disease-producing organisms.
2. The distal light source, built in, leaves one hand free for taking swabs etc.

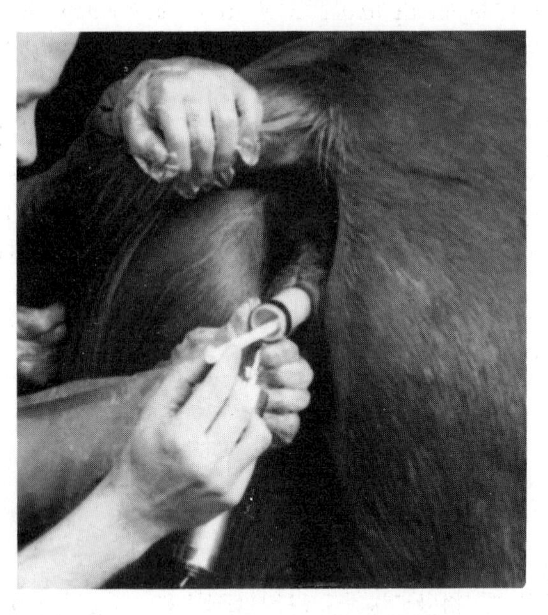

Fig. 8.15. A detachable tubular speculum with a distal light source is used with a swab extended by a sterilizing rod.

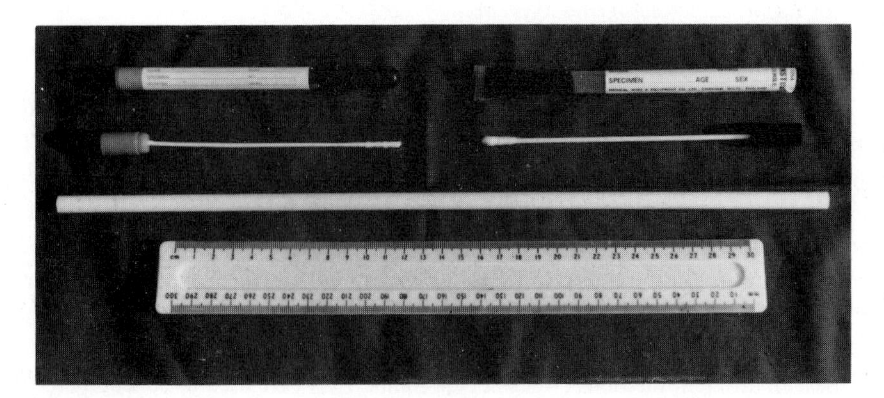

Fig. 8.16. Swabs suitable for bacteriological examination of mares. Narrow tipped swabs (*left*) with containers of Ames charcoal transport medium suitable for swabbing clitoral sinuses. Larger tipped swabs (*right*) with container of Ames charcoal transport medium suitable for swabbing cervix, urethral opening and clitoral fossae. A plastic disposable sterilized tipped extension rod is shown underneath.

3. The small-diameter speculum distorts the vulva and vagina less than the traditional duck-billed speculum.

Prior to the insertion of the speculum, the perineum of the mare must be thoroughly cleansed and examinations should be performed in as clean an atmosphere as possible, since air is drawn into the vagina, through the speculum, and contamination will occur.

The swabs used must be reliably sterilized and guarded swabs are preferred. Unfortunately, no satisfactory practical and economic guarded swab is at present commercially available, incorporating transport medium suitable for the isolation of *Haemophilus equigenitalis*. Most clinicians now use unguarded short swabs lengthened by attachment to sterile aluminium or plastic rods (Fig. 8.16).

Swabs are passed into the os of the cervix, as far forward as is possible, ideally into the uterine lumen. The swab is then gently rotated against the wall of the endometrium, to pick up material and then withdrawn and placed immediately into suitable transport medium. If a sterile tubular speculum is used and swabbing technique is careful, the speculum may be considered to be a 'guard'. There is no doubt, however, that the isolation of aerobic 'contaminants' has increased since this method has been used and the concomitant use of cervical smear cytology is, in our opinion, essential to aid interpretation.

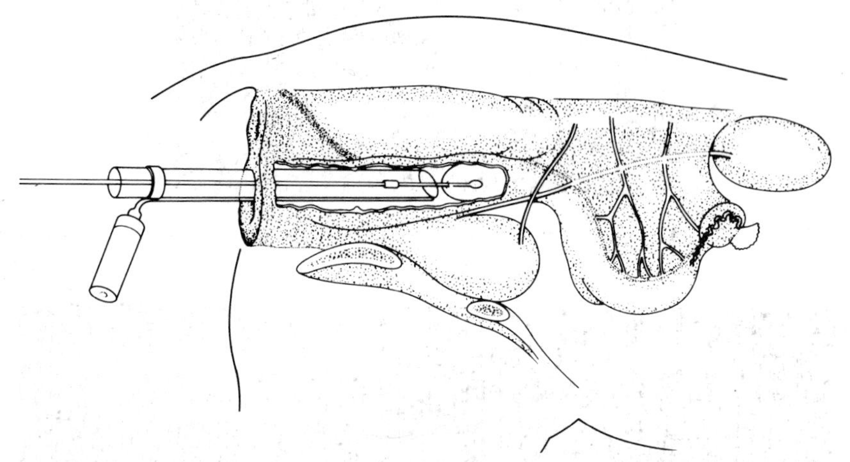

Fig. 8.17. The use of a cervicouterine swab. The swab (attached to a sterile extender) is passed through a sterile speculum, through the oestrous cervix and into the body of the uterus.

Similar short unguarded swabs, with suitable transport medium, may be used for the collection of urethral and clitoral fossa swabs. With a gloved hand, the vulval lips are parted and the swab is placed in the area of the urethral opening. By this means, the swab is naturally 'moistened' before being placed in the everted clitoral fossa. To obtain material from the clitoral sinuses, the body of the clitoris may be gently squeezed, sometimes producing small 'peas' of smegma. Caution must be used during this procedure as some mares object violently. A smaller tipped swab may be used to obtain material from inside the clitoral sinuses (see Fig. 1.4).

Nasal swabs

A sterile flexible polythene tubular swab is best for this procedure. The tube is passed up the nostril into the nasopharynx and the swab is extruded and withdrawn. The nasopharynx usually has a mixed flora of organisms but growth of *Str. equi* is diagnostic of strangles.

Rectal swabs

For this a short stick swab is adequate. A mixed bacterial growth is usually obtained and the problem is to identify significant organisms. *Salmonella* spp. should be further identified and interpreted in regard to clinical signs but specific pathogenic serotypes of *E. coli* have not been determined for the horse (Davies 1978). A profuse growth of haemolytic *E. coli* is often seen in diarrhoea cases and is probably significant in some. Fungal growths may also be diagnostic of mycotic diarrhoea, usually occurring after prolonged antibiotic therapy.

Abscess and sinus tract swabs

For this a short stick swab is used. It is important to clean off the skin and surface area to be swabbed and to obtain a deep sample of material.

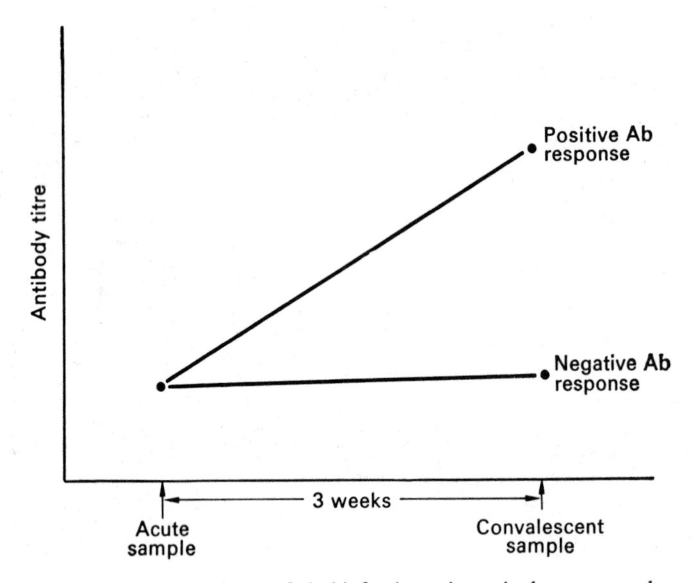

Fig. 8.18. Indirect evidence of viral infection using paired serum samples.

VIROLOGY

Samples for virus isolation are usually obtained from swabs (as above), by washing, or biopsy tissue material. Care is necessary to obtain a representative sample which is then put into specialized transport medium. The virus is grown in tissue or other culture systems and is recognized by characteristic cytopathic effects (CPE).

Indirect evidence of virus infection may be obtained by paired serum samples collected in the acute phase of the condition and in the convalescent phase two to three weeks later. The sera are tested against specific antisera and a rising antibody titre is indirect evidence of infection by the specific antigen (Fig. 8.18).

MYCOLOGY

Samples for fungal culture are obtained from swabs or tissue material such as scabs or skin scrapings. Wet smears, cultured organisms and tissue sections may be stained with cotton blue, Grocott, PAS or Feulgan's method. These stain the fungal hyphae. Fungi are cultured on specific Saboraud's medium for at least three weeks.

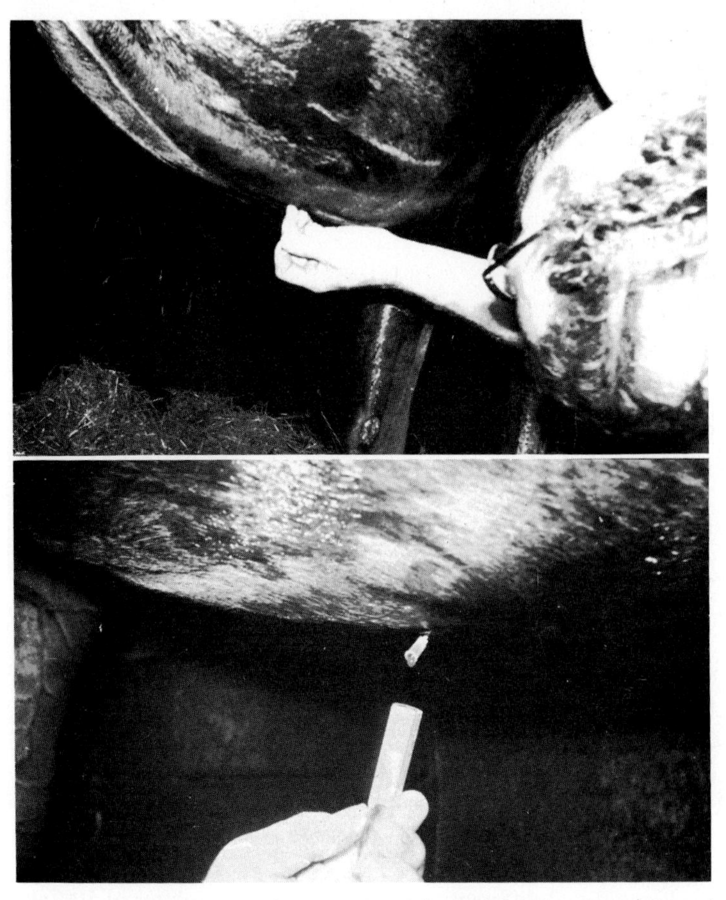

Fig. 8.19. The site of paracentesis abdominis. The abdominal fluid is collected through a small-bore needle into a sterile bottle. For full details see text.

Hair samples are examined for ringworm by clearing the hairs in warm 10% potassium hydroxide and examining them under the microscope. Ringworm (*Trichrophyton* and *Microsporon* spp.) can be seen as small, refractile chain-like arthrospores in the substance of the hairs. Where initial results are negative, samples are left overnight in blue/black ink and then re-examined in the morning. The species can be identified by culture on Saboraud's medium and the vegetative forms differentiated.

CYTOLOGY

The examination of body fluids often reveals valuable information of pathological processes. Immediate fixation of the cells in the fluid is necessary to prevent them degenerating. Two samples must be obtained, one in dipotassium EDTA (sequestrene)

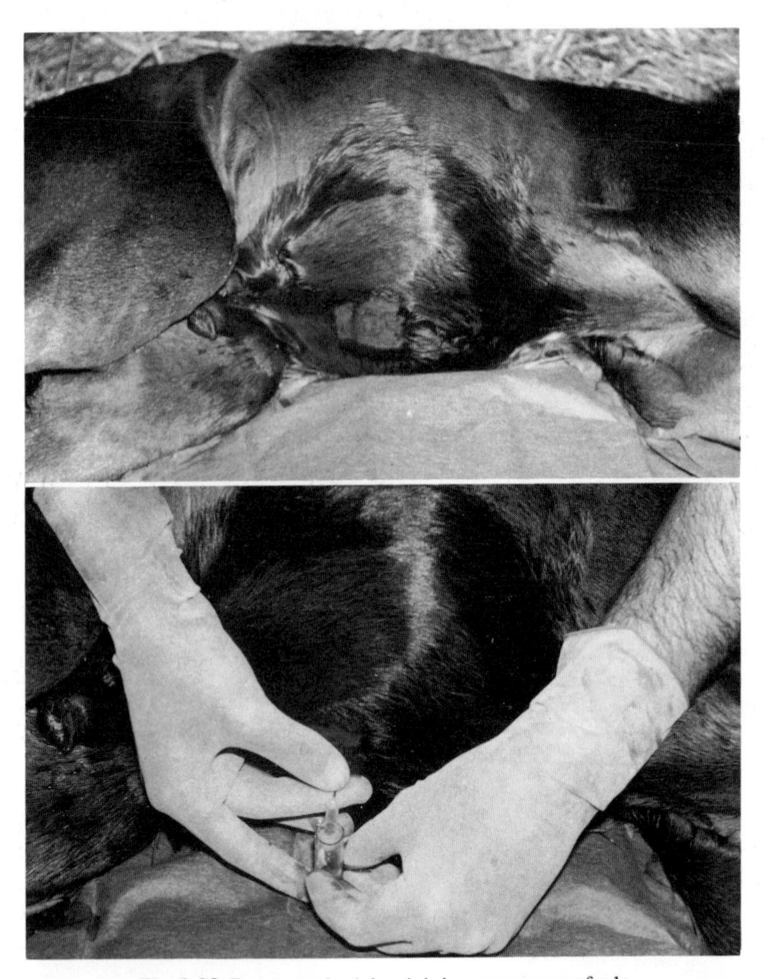

Fig. 8.20. Paracentesis abdominis in a very young foal.

for total cell count and differential and one in an equal volume of 50% alcohol for specific cytological studies. Wright's or Giemsa's stains are adequate for cytological examination, although more sophisticated stains are useful, e.g. a rapid trichrome stain (Pollack 1944; Sano 1949). If fluid samples are not available then a wet swab may be examined but this technique is not a quantitative one.

Paracentesis abdominis

The examination of peritoneal fluid in cases of chronic and acute abdominal disease in the horse has been described by Maksic (1964), Coffman (1973), Bach and

Ricketts (1974), McGrath (1975) and Nelson (1979). The abdomen 10 cm either side of the midline from sternum to umbilicus may be clipped and prepared as for surgery. A 19 gauge 4 cm needle is passed through the skin in the midline, at the lowest point of the abdomen, with the horse standing (Fig. 8.19). The needle is then carefully advanced; entry into the peritoneal cavity is indicated by a slight pain reaction and

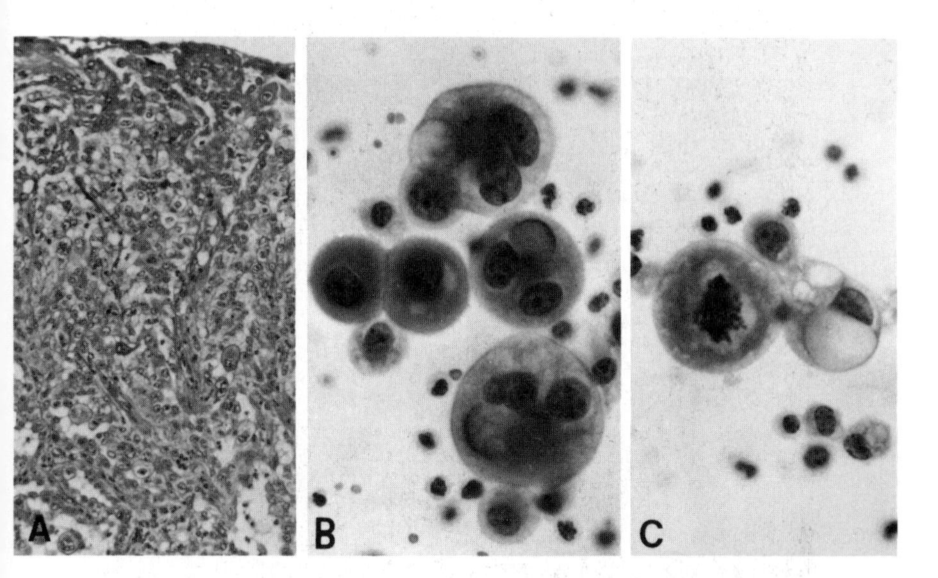

Fig. 8.21. Peritoneal mesothelioma. A, Greater omentum from a 12-year-old Thoroughbred mare with signs of acute colic and ascites. A densely cellular structure composed of branching twisting areas of connective tissue covered by eosinophilic cells of varying shapes and sizes. H & E × 100. B, C, Peritoneal fluid sample showing grossly enlarged multinucleate cells with vacuolated cytoplasm (B) and a mitotic figure (C). Trichrome × 300.

the passage of fluid through the needle. A total white cell count of more than 9×10^9/litre with a predominantly polymorphonuclear leucocyte differential may indicate intestinal pathology and warrant an exploratory laparotomy. The technique is used in the young foal with the subject restrained in lateral recumbency (Fig. 8.20). Intra-abdominal neoplasia may be encountered. Lymphosarcoma is the most common intra-abdominal tumour (Roberts & Pinsent 1975) and may sometimes be diagnosed by abdominal paracentesis (Bach & Ricketts 1974). A case of peritoneal mesothelioma (Fig. 8.21) has been reported in a brood mare with acute colic and ascites (Ricketts & Peace 1976).

Cervicouterine cytology

Smears are taken from the endometrium of the mare, via a tubular speculum, as described above for swabs, through the relaxed oestrous cervix. A simple short swab on a sterile extension is used and transport medium is not required. The wet swab is rolled, as soon as possible after it has been taken, on to gelatine-coated slides, fixed in 95% ethanol for at least two hours or by the use of Spraycyte aerosol and then stained as described above (Fig. 8.22). The technique and interpretation of this invaluable diagnostic aid has been described by Wingfield-Digby (1978), who has found that polymorphonuclear leucocytes are not present in smears taken and examined by this method from oestrous mares with healthy endometria. One exception is seen in some maiden mares during their first oestrous

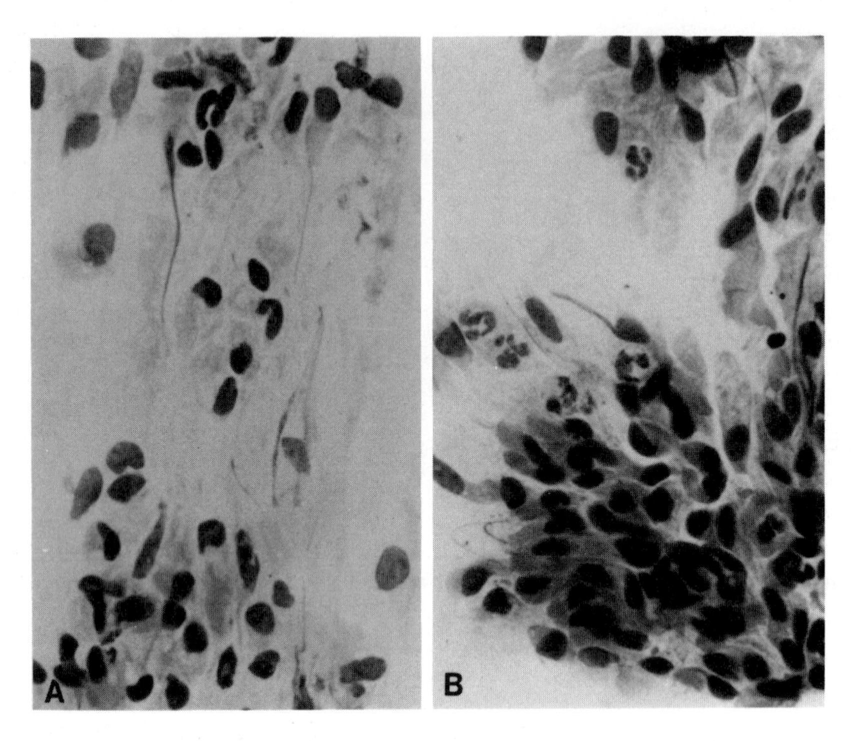

Fig. 8.22. Endometrial smears. A, Normal epithelial cells. B, Acute endometritis showing polymorphonuclear leucocytes among epithelial cells. Trichrome × 400.

period following winter anoestrus (Wingfield-Digby, unpublished). This technique has the great advantage of giving rapid results. The presence of polymorphonuclear leucocytes in a cervicouterine smear denotes the presence of an acute endometritis which may mean that an infection of the uterus is present. Such mares will not be covered until the swab results are satisfactory for the absence of potential veneral-disease-producing organisms and treatment has been successful, as shown by follow-up smears. The presence or absence of polymorphonuclear leucocytes in a smear allows the clinician to decide more accurately upon the significance of aerobic bacterial cultures with opportunist organisms (see p. 70). Chronic endometritis may show the presence of mononuclear leucocytes in endometrial smears (Knudsen 1964).

Milk

In suspected cases of mastitis, milk samples are stained with methylene blue or Gram stain for the presence of polymorphonuclear leucocytes, macrophages, debris and bacteria.

Trans-tracheal aspiration

By this technique a deep tracheal washing may be obtained for bacteriological and cytological examination. This is a useful diagnostic aid in pneumonia and chronic pulmonary emphysema (Mansmann et al. 1971; von Schatzmann et al. 1972; Beech 1975, 1979). The trachea is palpated in the midline of the neck between the sterno-cephalicus muscles midway down. An area at this point is clipped and prepared as for surgery. A local anaesthetic bleb is put under the skin and a 2 cm incision made over the midline. The subcutaneous tissue is parted and the muscles are divided. The trachea is identified and a large-bore needle pushed into the lumen of the trachea between two rings. A 45 cm long flexible polythene tube is passed down the needle into the trachea. The needle is withdrawn to prevent severance of the tube on movement. The tube is advanced down the trachea to the bifurcation of the bronchi, at which point the horse usually coughs; 20–50 ml of sterile saline are then injected down the tube and immediately aspirated, at the same time as the tube is withdrawn slowly. This technique collects washings from the walls of the trachea. Washings may be collected via a fibreoptic endoscope passed through the larynx and down the trachea.

Large numbers of polymorphonuclear leucocytes and pathogenic bacteria are diagnostic of a pneumonic process. Antibiotic sensitivity tests are performed on bacterial growths and this indicates optimal therapeutic measures.

Arthrocentesis

The cytology of synovial fluid is a useful guide to differentiation of arthritis and arthropathy (Van Pelt 1974). The joint to be tapped must be accurately defined anatomically. The skin over the joint is clipped and prepared as for surgery. A 19 gauge 4 cm needle is pushed through the skin into the joint and synovial fluid usually escapes (Fig. 8.23). This should be collected into calcium EDTA (sequestrene). The presence of polymorphonuclear leucocytes indicates an infective arthritis.

Occipital puncture

Examination of cerebrospinal fluid is a useful guide to diagnosing meningitis. Cerebrospinal taps should be performed with the animal heavily sedated or, preferably, under general anaesthesia, in lateral recumbency. It is important to place the nose of the animal so that it lies in a horizontal line with the long axis of the spine. This ensures correct identification of the site of the tap. The area over the atlanto-occipital junction is clipped and scrubbed as for surgery. A drape is not used as it obscures the essential landmarks. The correct site should be accurately delineated before proceeding with the tap and should be in the midline halfway between an imaginary line drawn between the occipital protuberances and the widest part of the atlantal protuberances. In large animals a 20 gauge needle should be used with a stylette. After piercing the skin the needle should be advanced very slowly and the stylette withdrawn to see if fluid is forthcoming; if not the stylette should be replaced before advancing the needle further. The fluid should be allowed to drip from the needle by gravity only and not aspirated as this may distort the results of cytology.

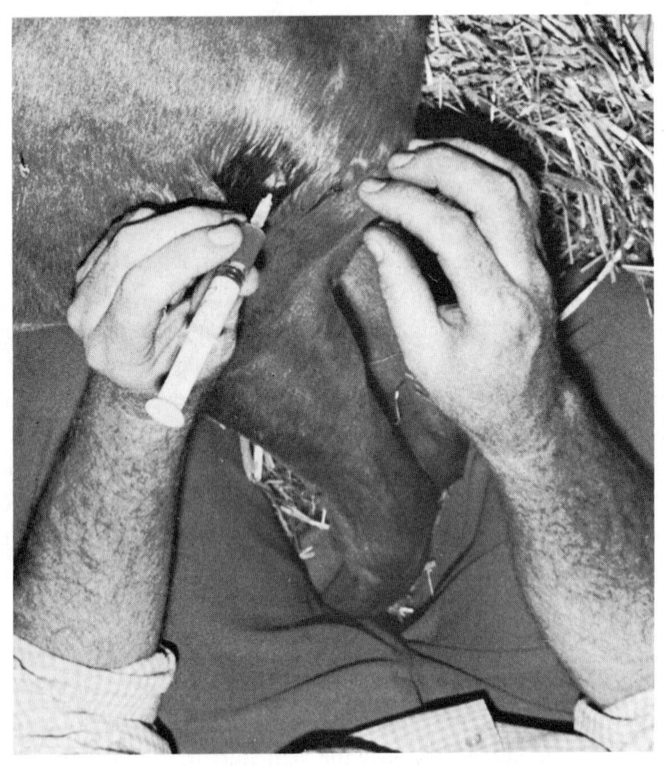

Fig. 8.23. The site of entry into the shoulder joint of a foal with infective arthritis.

Significant numbers of leucocytes are evidence of pathology. Normally the cell count is very low. The differential count helps to identify the type of pathology involved. Levels of protein greater than 100 mg/dl are found in maladjustment syndromes, especially in foals suffering from convulsions (see Tables 5.15 and 5.16).

HISTOLOGY

The histological differentiation of equine pathology is of great value in post-mortem or biopsy techniques. In each case 1 cm^2 samples should be fixed in 10% formol saline immediately after removal and before transport to the laboratory.

Histological examination is important in any post-mortem, particularly in cases of abortion or neonatal death. Liver cells should be examined for the presence of eosinophilic intranuclear inclusion bodies which signify equid herpesvirus I (rhinopneumonitis) infection (see p. 200).

Uterine biopsy has become a routine diagnostic and prognostic procedure for infertile mares, and liver, lung, skin and testicular biopsy are also more widely used.

Uterine biopsy

A suitable instrument is essential (Fig. 8.24); an alligator-jawed biopsy forceps, 55–60 cm in length with basket jaws approximately 2 × 1 cm in size, is preferred (Greenhof & Kenney 1975, Ricketts 1975*a*, *b*, 1978).

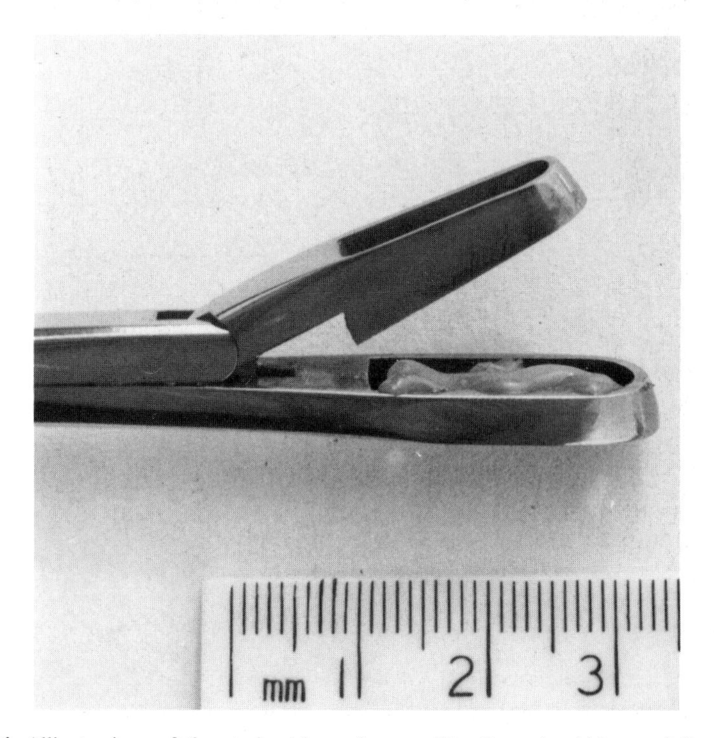

Fig. 8.24. Alligator jaws of the uterine biopsy forceps. The tissue should be carefully removed with fine forceps or a hypodermic needle and placed immediately in Bouin's fluid.

The mare should be restrained as for a rectal examination. The tail should be bandaged and held to one side. Faeces should be removed from the rectum and the perineum thoroughly washed. A clean disposable and lubricated glove should be worn. Biopsy forceps are inserted into the vagina, guarded by the fingers. The cervix is palpated and the index finger inserted into the uterus through the cervix. The biopsy forceps is then advanced through the cervix into the uterus along the index finger. Holding the forceps in place, the arm is removed from the vagina and placed in the rectum. The uterus is palpated with the forceps inside. The forceps is further advanced and guided gently into the horn or wherever the biopsy is to be taken. The jaws of the punch are opened and a piece of endometrium pushed into its jaws through pressure from the rectum. The jaws are shut and the punch is drawn back until the endometrium can be felt trapped. A sharp pull will then complete the biopsy and the forceps is withdrawn. The biopsy material is carefully removed and placed in Bouin's solution for fixation before histological processing. It is found that Bouin's is preferable to formol saline because it produces a harder

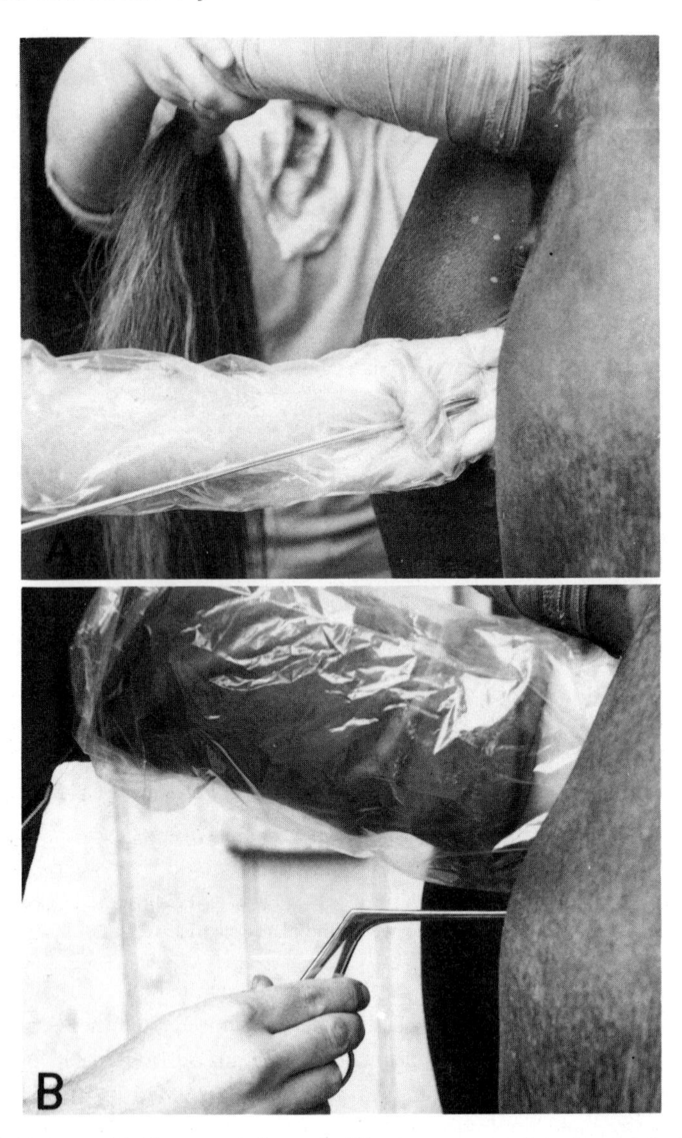

Fig. 8.25. Endometrial biopsy technique. A, The instrument is introduced into the vagina guarded in a gloved hand. B, Once the instrument is in the uterus the arm is withdrawn and placed in the rectum where the instrument may be palpated and biopsy performed at the required site.

tissue for processing, causes less tissue shrinkage and inhances the haematoxylin and eosin stain. Tissues should not be left in solution for longer than three days or deterioration will occur and if there is to be any delay it is preferable to transfer the specimen into 70% ethanol after 24 hours fixation. Fresh tissues are suitable for frozen sections using a cryostat and histochemical staining techniques may be used (Ricketts 1978).

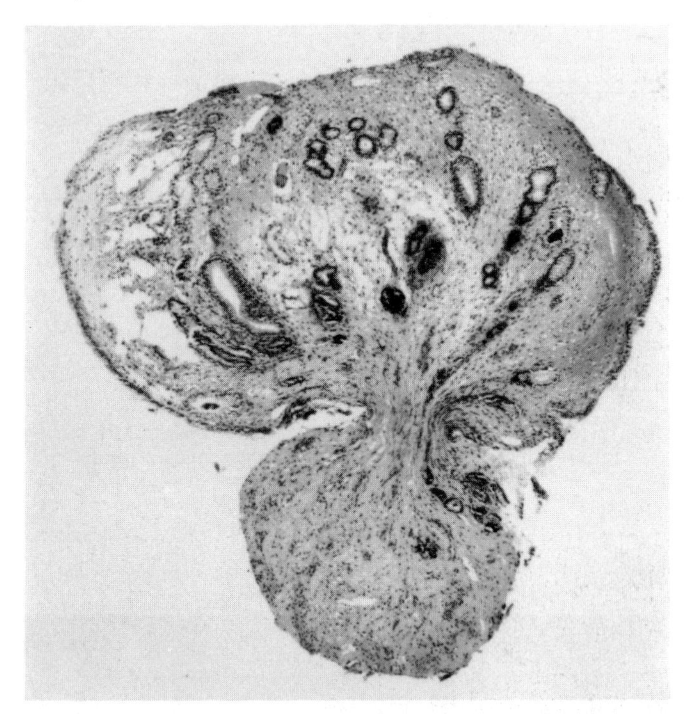

Fig. 8.26. Endometrial biopsy specimen taken with a fibreoptic endoscope. The tissue specimen is too small and badly affected by artefactual damage to interpret adequately. Compare with Figs 1.12 and 1.43, taken with the recommended instrument. H & E × 50.

In the absence of palpable uterine abnormality, Bergman and Kenney (1975) and Ricketts (1978) found that a single mid-horn biopsy specimen was diagnostically representative of the whole endometrium. In cases where the endometrium is not palpably homogeneous, more than one biopsy specimen should be taken. Biopsy specimens may be taken at any time during the oestrus cycle but for the standard end-of-season barren mare examination, a mid-dioestrous sample is recommended.

Liver biopsy

The technique of liver biopsy using a trocar and cannula (Fig. 8.27) recommended by Mullen (1976) is as follows. An area 5–10 cm square is clipped and shaved on the right flank as shown in Fig. 8.28. The site is prepared as for aseptic surgery. Local anaesthetic is infiltrated between the fourteenth and fifteenth rib and projected down through the intercostal muscles into the parietal pleura. At this point

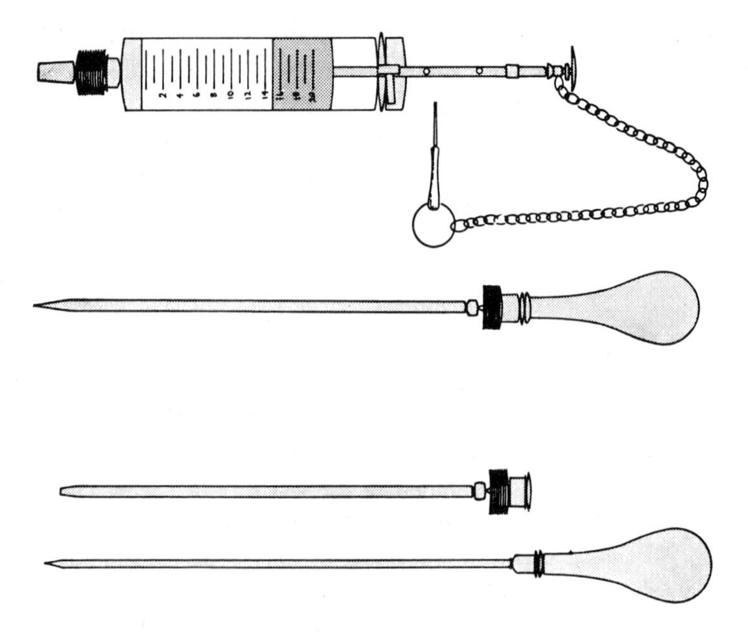

Fig. 8.27. Liver biopsy instruments. From top to bottom: syringe with screw connection, trocar with cannula inserted and trocar and cannula separate.

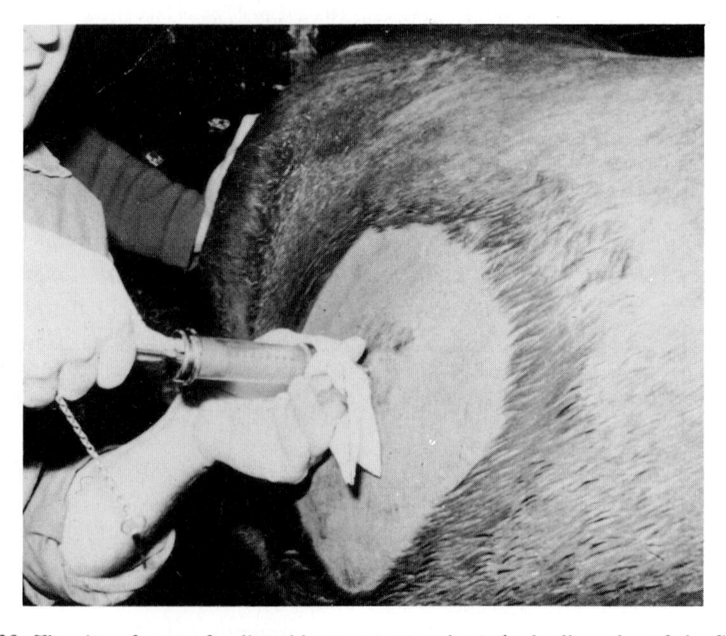

Fig. 8.28. The site of entry for liver biopsy puncture is at the leading edge of the fifteenth rib at the point of intersection of a line from the point of the hip to the shoulder joint.

the operator should ensure full anaesthetic dispersal to anaesthetize the pleura, before proceeding through the thoracic cavity to the diaphragm. 5–10 ml of 2% lignocaine are usually sufficient. After allowing time for the anaesthesia to take effect, a small incision is made through the skin along the leading edge of the fifteenth rib, at a point of intersection of an imaginary line between the point of the hip and shoulder joint on the right side. Trocar and cannula are then inserted through the incision and pushed by pressure from the palm of the operator's hand through the intercostal musculature. Rotation of the cannula will help this passage. Quite a strong force is required but care must be taken to control the instrument as resistance is released when the pleura is punctured. Once the pleura is penetrated the presence of the diaphragm is appreciated from the doughy response when the cannula is pressed against it. Further penetration brings the trocar through the diaphragm and this position may be confirmed by observing the regular movement of the trocar caused by the membrane in respiratory movement. A solid mass may then be appreciated by the sensation transmitted through the trocar. Generally at this point the trocar has been inserted no more than 7 cm from the original skin incision. The trocar is now withdrawn and a 20 ml syringe attached to the exposed end of the cannula. It is important to ensure an air-tight seal to the syringe and cannula. The cannula is now plunged a further 6 cm into the liver. It is rotated to the left and right through 180° and the plunger of the syringe withdrawn to create a negative pressure to hold the liver core in position. The cannula is now withdrawn slowly with the negative pressure maintained. The liver samples and hepatic blood are usually flushed up into the syringe in the process of withdrawal. Mullen considers that a large rush of blood into the syringe is welcome as it confirms that the liver has been penetrated.

The skin incision is closed in a surgical manner and tetanus antitoxin given. The contents of the cannula and syringe are separated and their contents expelled onto a gauze swab and the core of liver transferred to 10% formol saline.

Liver biopsy may also be performed, using similar sites and landmarks, with a Truecut biopsy instrument.

ENDOCRINOLOGY

The assay of specific hormones is a specialized technique, but readily available and easily interpreted 'hormonal profiles' would be useful to diagnose abnormality in stud animals. Too often 'hormonal imbalance' is incriminated in low libido stallions or infertile mares without factual evidence.

At present the progesterone assay (radio-immunoassay) represents an adjunct to the 19–21-day manual pregnancy diagnosis. Mares with plasma levels less than 4 ng/ml are unlikely to be pregnant. But high levels do not indicate pregnancy, only an active corpus luteum. The assay can be used to diagnose a persistent corpus luteum and forms the basis of prostaglandin therapy.

Gonadotrophin assays are a basis for therapy with pituitary releasing factors in cases of ovarian inactivity; oestrogen and progesterone assays may be useful with uterine biopsies, to compare with endometrical histochemical staining (see Table 1.2) in cases of cyclic irregularity and suspected hormonal abnormalities.

BLOOD AND URINE PREGNANCY TESTS

These have been described in Chapter 3, pp. 211–213.

CROSS-MATCHING BLOOD

Before donor blood can be transferred to a recipient, the donor's plasma and recipient's cells must be proved compatible. In the case of an exchange transfusion, both erythrocytes and plasma must be compatible. If they are not, antibodies in the donor's plasma react with antigen in the recipient's erythrocytes and cause haemolysis and embolism.

Equine erythrocytes are prone to rouleau formation which may simulate agglutination, so great care must be taken in interpreting crude slide agglutination reaction.

Blood samples from the donor and recipient are collected in EDTA and plain tubes. The plasma is removed after centrifugation and the erythrocytes suspended in normal saline at 1 : 10 dilution. Two or three drops of donor serum are then put on a white tile and a drop of recipient cells added. The mixture is carefully stirred with a glass rod or match-stick. A positive reaction is indicated by clumping, which may occur within about five minutes. The blood of positive reactors is further diluted with normal saline to differentiate agglutination from rouleau formation. In the latter case the red cell clumps will break up when diluted, which does not occur with true agglutination. False reactions may occur because the antibodies associated with haemolytic disease in the foal are usually incomplete and do not, by themselves, result in erythrocyte agglutination or lysis.

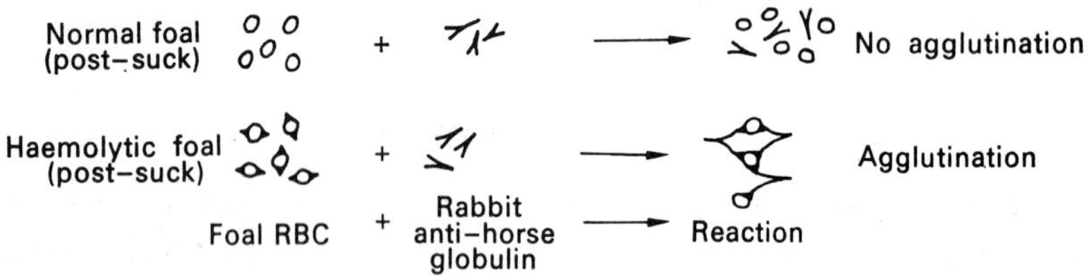

Normal foal (post-suck) + → No agglutination

Haemolytic foal (post-suck) + → Agglutination

Foal RBC + Rabbit anti-horse globulin → Reaction

Fig. 8.29. Anti-horse globulin (Coombs's) test for the diagnosis of isoimmune haemolytic disease in a foal after sucking.

A more satisfactory test of incompatibility of horse blood is the anti-horse globulin or Coombs's test. This is especially useful when testing for an isoimmune situation in a newborn foal (see Chapter 5). Foal cells are washed with normal saline to remove plasma. They are placed in rabbit anti-horse globulin. If the foal is isoimmune its red cells are coated with an 'incomplete' antibody (i.e. horse globulin) and the cells will clump (Fig. 8.29).

In cases where an isoimmune situation is suspected then an indirect form of this test may be used on the foal at birth, before it sucks. The foal should be muzzled until it has been diagnosed as negative. The foal's cells are incubated in the mare's colostrum or serum and then washed. If the foal is potentially isoimmune the mare's 'incomplete' antibodies will coat, but not agglutinate or lyse, the cells. The anti-horse globulin test is then repeated as above (Fig. 8.30).

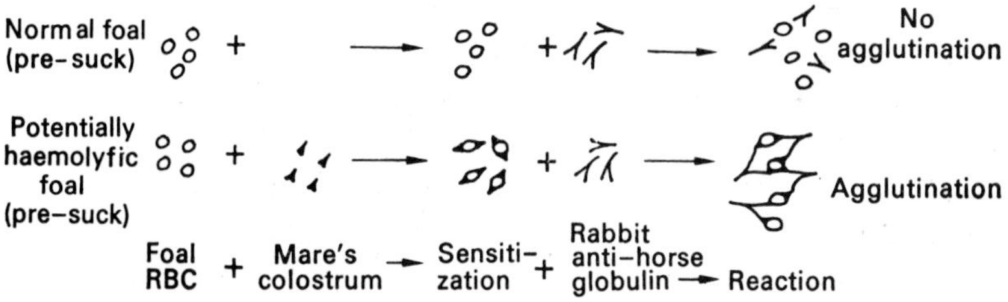

Normal foal (pre-suck) — No agglutination
Potentially haemolytic foal (pre-suck) — Agglutination
Foal RBC + Mare's colostrum → Sensitization + Rabbit anti-horse globulin → Reaction

Fig. 8.30. Indirect globulin (Coombs's) test for the diagnosis of potential isioimmune haemolytic disease in a foal after sucking.

It is helpful to be able to predict an isoimmune foal by detecting rising antibody titres in the mare in late pregnancy. This is sometimes attempted by collecting blood samples from the mare two months, one month, two weeks and one week before the expected foaling. The serum is cross-matched against a bank of washed red cells from eight to 12 different sources by the plate agglutination test. This method is not ideal as the antibodies tend to be incomplete. It also presupposes that the red cell antigen present in the foal is present in one of the bank red cells. Further, the isoimmune plasma is not covered with only one red cell antigen, but a number, and thus this method of screening is likely to be inaccurate. A Coombs's (anti-horse globulin) test may be used with serum from the mare during later pregnancy. This is a more reliable method.

BLOOD TRANSFUSIONS

Transfusions are indicated in cases of haemorrhage or intravascular haemolysis. They are not lightly undertaken in the adult horse as large volumes of blood (10–20 litres) are required. The newborn foal's blood volume is about 5 litres and transfusions are therefore more practical.

Following a compatible cross-match, blood is collected from the jugular vein of a donor horse through a large-bore needle into 500 ml bottles containing anticoagulant. The warm blood is then administered intravenously by gravity. In cases of severe haemorrhage clotting occurs when blood volume and pressure fall. Therefore a blood transfusion should be given only if death is likely from hypovolaemia.

Techniques for transfusion of foals suffering from haemolytic disease are described in Chapter 5.

References and further reading

Adams, O.R. (1974) *Lameness in Horses*, 3rd ed. Philadelphia: Lea & Febiger.

Adams, O.R. (1977) The technique of stomach tube passage and the use of this method for administering medication to the horse. *Proc. 23rd ann. Conv. Am. Ass equine Practners*, 39.

Allen, W.E. & Newcombe, J.R. (1979) Aspects of genital infection and swabbing techniques in the mare. *Vet. Rec.*, **104**, 228.

American Association of Equine Practitioners (1975) *Proceedings of the First International Symposium on Equine Haematology*, ed. H. Kitchen & J.D. Krehbiel. Golden, Colorado.

Anderson, M.G. (1975) The influence of exercise on serum enzyme levels in the horse. *Equine vet. J.*, 7, 160.

Archer, R.K. (1954) Studies upon the blood picture of equidae. Ph. D. thesis, University of Cambridge.

Archer, R.K. & Jeffcott, L.B. (1977) *Comparative Clinical Haematology*. Oxford: Blackwell Scientific.

Atherton, J.G. (1975) The identification of equine genital strains of *Klebsiella* and *Enterobacter* species. *Equine vet. J.*, 7, 207.

Bach, L. & Ricketts, S.W. (1974) Paracentesis as an aid to the diagnosis of abdominal disease in the horse. *Equine vet. J.*, **16**, 116.

Beech, J. (1975) Cytology of tracheobronchial aspiration in horses. *Vet. Path.*, **12**, 157.

Beech, J. (1979) Evaluation of the horse with pulmonary disease. *Vet. Clins N. Am. lge Anim. Pract.*, **1** (1), 73.

Benjamin, M., Kelly, A.B. & Stamp, C. (1975) The application of the nitroblue tetrazolium test (NBT) to clinical conditions in horses. *Proc. 1st. int. Symp. equine Haemat.*, 497.

Bergmann, R.V. & Kenney, R.M. (1975) Representativeness of uterine biopsy in the mare. *Proc. 21st ann. Conv. Am. Ass. equine Practners*, 355.

Bishop, R. & Boles, C.L. (1972) An indwelling venous catheter for horses. *Vet. Med. small Anim. Clin.*, 67, 415.

Blackmore, D.J. (1975) A new concept of 'normal' in haematology. *Proc. 1st int. Symp. equine Haemat.*, 276.

Blackmore, D.J. & Elton, D. (1975) Enzyme activity in the serum of Thoroughbred horses in the United Kingdom. *Equine vet. J.*, 7, 34.

Blackmore, D.J. & Palmer, A. (1977) Phenylalanine-inhibited *p*-nitrophenyl phosphatase activity in the serum as an indication of intestinal cellular disruption in the horse. *Res. vet. Sci.*, **23**, 146.

Boles, C.L. (1975) Epiglottic entrapment and follicular pharyngitis: diagnosis and treatment. *Proc. 21st ann. Conv. Am. Ass. equine Practnrs*, 29.

Brandt, C.W. (1970) The significance and interpretation of uterine biopsy in the mare. *Proc. 16th ann. Conv. Am. Ass. equine Practnrs*, 279.

Brandt, G.W. & Manning, J.P. (1969) Improved uterine biopsy technics for diagnosing infertility in the mare. *Vet. Med.*, **64**, 977.

Cardinet, G.H., Fowler, M.E. & Tyler, W.S. (1963) The effects of training, exercise and tying up on serum transaminase activities in the horse. *Am. J. vet. Res.*, **24**, 980.

Carlson, G.P. (1979) Fluid therapy in horses with acute diarrhoea. *Vet. Clins N. Am. lge Anim. Pract.*, **1** (2), 313.

Coffmann, J.R. (1973) Technic and interpretation of abdominal paracentesis. *Mod. vet. Pract.*, **54**, 79.

Coffmann, J.R., Towers, D.S., Johnson, J.H., Gower, H.E., Trischler, L.G. & Moore, J.N. (1977) Practical clinical chemistry. *Proc. 23rd ann. Conv. Am. Ass. equine Practnrs*, 161.

Cook, W.R. (1970*a*) Procedure and technique for endoscopy of the equine respiratory tract and eustachian tube diverticulum. *Equine vet. J.*, **2**, 137.

Cook, W.R. (1970*b*) Instrument specifications for endoscopy of the equine upper respiratory tract and eustachian tube diverticulum. *Vet. Rec.*, 87, 429.

Cook, W.R. (1974) Some observations on diseases of the ear, nose and throat in the horse and endoscopy using a flexible fibreoptic endoscope. *Vet. Rec.*, **94**, 533.

Cornelius, C.E., Burnham, L.G. & Hill, H.E. (1963) Serum transaminase activities of Thoroughbred horses in training. *J. Am. vet. med. Ass.*, **142**, 639.

David, J.S.E., Frank, C. & Powell, D.G. (1978) Problems of isolating CEM antigen. *Vet. Rec.*, **102**, 386.

Davies, M.E. (1978) Some studies on equine strains of *Escherichia coli*. *Equine vet. J.*, **10**, 115.

Douglas, S.W. & Williamson, H.D. (1980) *Principles of Veterinary Radiography*, 3rd ed. London: Baillière Tindall.

Ellis, D.R. (1978) Fractures of the proximal sesamoid bones in Thoroughbred foals. *Equine vet. J.*, **11**, 48.
Erickson, E.D., (1975) Alpha globulins of equine serum. *Proc. 1st int. Symp. equine Haemat.*, 152.
Gabel, A.A. (1977) Intravenous injections – complications and their prevention. *Proc. 23rd ann. Conv. Am. Ass. equine Practnrs*, 29.
Gerber, H. (1969) Serum enzyme determination in equine medicine. *Equine vet. J.*, **1**, 129.
Gerber, H., Tschudi, P. & Satub, R. (1975) 'Normal' values for different breeds of horses. *Proc. 1st int. Symp. equine Haemat.*, 266.
Gillespie, J.R., Tyler, W.S. & Eberly, V.E. (1964) Blood pH, O_2 and CO_2 tensions in exercised control and emphysematous horses. *Am. J. Physiol.*, **207**, 1967.
Greatorex, J.C. (1968) Rectal exploration as an aid to the diagnosis of some medical conditions in the horse. *Equine vet. J.*, **1**, 26.
Greenhof, G.R. & Kenney, R.M. (1975) Evaluation of the reproductive status of non-pregnant mares. *J. Am. vet. med. Ass.*, **167**, 449.
De Groot, A. (1971) The significance of low packed cell volume in relation to the early diagnosis of intestinal obstruction in the horse, based on field observation. *Proc. 17th ann. Conv. Am. Ass. equine Practnrs*, 309.
Hall, L.W. (1971) *Wright's Veterinary Anaesthesia and Analgesia*, 7th ed. London: Baillière Tindall.
Heinze, H., Klug, E. & Lepel., J.D. (1972) Optische Darstellung der inneren. Geschlechtsorgane bei Equidem zur Diagnostik und Therapie. *Dt. tierarztl. Wschr.*, 79, 49.
Hopes, R. (1970) Physiotherapy in the horse. *Physiotherapy, Lond.*, 56.
Jeffcott, L.B. (1977) Clinical haematology of the horse. In *Comparative Clinical Haematology*, ed. R.K. Archer & L.B. Jeffcott. Oxford: Blackwell Scientific.
Johnson, J.H. (1971) Endoscopy of the pharynx, larynx and gutteral pouch in the horse. *Vet. Med.*, **66**, 47.
Johnson, J.N., Moore, J.N., Goffmann, J.R., Gower, H.E., Tritschler, L.G. & Traver, D.S. (1977*a*) Selection and care of endoscopic equipment. *Proc. 23rd. ann. Conv. Am. Ass. equine Practnrs*, 239.
Johnson, J.H., Moore, J.N., Gower, H.E., Goffmann, J.R., Tritschler, L.G. & Traver, D.S. (1977*b*) Clinical characterization of the larynx in laryngeal hemiplegia. *Proc. 23rd. ann. Conv. Am. Ass. equine Practnrs*, 259.
Kaneko, J.J. & Cornelius, C.E. (1970) *Clinical Biochemistry of Domestic Animals*, 2nd ed. New York and London: Academic.
Knudsen, O. (1964) Endometrial cytology as a diagnostic aid in mares. *Cornell Vet.*, **54**, 415.
Littlewort, M.C.G. (1962) The clinical auscultation of the equine heart. *Vet. Rec.*, **74**, 1247.
McAllister, E.S. (1977) Gutteral pouch disease. *Proc. 23rd ann. Conv. Am. Ass. equine Practnrs*, 251.
McGrath, J.P. (1975) Exfoliative cytology of equine peritoneal fluid – an adjunct to haematological examination. *Proc. 1st int. Symp. equine Haemat.*, 408.
Maksic, D. (1964) Abdominal paracentesis and its use in diagnosis in the horse. *Proc. 10th ann. Conv. Am. Ass. equine Practnrs*, 319.
Mansmann, R.A., Wheat, J.D. & Jang, S.S. (1971) Diagnostic usefulness of transtracheal aspiration in the horse. *Proc. 17th ann. Conv. Am. Ass. equine Practnrs* 143.
Mather, E.C., Refsal, K.R., Gustafson, B.K., Sequin, B.E. & Whitmore, H.L. (1979) The use of fibre-optic techniques in clinical diagnosis and visual assessment of experimental intrauterine therapy in mares. *J. Reprod. Fert.*, Suppl. **27**, 293.
Meagher, D.M. (1977*a*) in discussion of paper by Gabel (1977).
Meagher, D.M. (1977*b*) in discussion of Witherspoon (1977).
Mullen, P.A. (1969) Serum constituents. *Equine vet. J.*, **1**, 190.
Mullen, P.A. (1976) The diagnosis of liver dysfunction in farm animals and horses. *Vet. Rec.*, **99**, 330.
Mullen, P.A., Hopes, R. & Sewell, J. (1979) The biochemistry, haematology, nutrition and racing performance of two-year-old Thoroughbreds through their training and racing season. *Vet. Rec.*, **104**, 90.
Nealon, D.A. & Henderson, A.R. (1975) Lability of human creatine kinase isoenzymes at 37°C: a complication of electrophoretic separation. *J. clin. Path.*, **28**, 834.
Nelson, A.W. (1964) Intestinal infarction. *Proc. 10th ann. Conv. Am. Ass. equine Practnrs*, 35.
Nelson, A.W. (1979) Analysis of equine peritoneal fluid. *Vet. Clins N. Am. lge Anim. Pract.*, **1** (2), 267.

Nelson, A.W., Collier, J.R. & Griner, L.A. (1968) Acute surgical colonic infarction in the horse. *Am. J. vet. Res.*, **29**, 315.

Platt, H., Atheton, J.G., Simpson, D.J., Taugher, C.E.D., Rosenthal, R.O. Brown, D.F.J. & Wreghitt, T.G. (1977) Genital infection in mares. *Vet. Rec.*, **101**, 20.

Pollack, O.J. (1944) A rapid trichrome stain. *Archs Path.*, **37**, 294.

Proctor, D.L. (1977) in discussion of paper by Witherspoon (1977).

Ricketts, S.W. (1975*a*) Endometrial biopsy as a guide to diagnosis of endometrial pathology in the mare. *J. Reprod. Fert.*, Suppl. **23**, 341.

Ricketts, S.W. (1975*b*) The technique and clinical application of endometrial biopsy in the mare. *Equine vet. J.*, 7, 102.

Ricketts, S.W. (1978) Histological and histopathological studies of the endometrium of the mare. Fellowship thesis, Royal College of Veterinary Surgeons.

Ricketts, S.W. & Peace, C.K. (1976) A case of peritoneal mesothelioma in a Thoroughbred mare. *Equine vet. J.*, 8, 78.

Roberts, M.C. & Pinsent, P.J.N. (1975) Malabsorption in the horse associated with alimentary lymphosarcoma. *Equine vet. J.*, 7, 166.

Rossdale, P.D. (1966) A clinical and laboratory assessment of the health status of the new-born Thoroughbred foal. Fellowship thesis, Royal College of Veterinary Surgeons.

Rossdale, P.D. (1968) Blood gas tensions and pH values in the normal Thoroughbred at birth and in the following 42 hrs. *Biol. Neonat.*, **13**, 18.

Rossdale, P.D. & Mullen, P.A. (1970) Alterations to whole blood pH, pCO_2 and plasma bicarbonate index values during a metabolic acidosis occasioned by neonatal diarrhoea in Thoroughbred foals. *Br. vet. J.*, **126**, 82.

Round, M.C. (1968) The course of naturally acquired helminth infections of horses given regular anthelmintic treatment. *Res. vet. Sci.*, **9**, 583.

Round, M.C. (1976) Lungworm infection (*Dictyocaulus arnfeldi*) of horses and donkeys. *Vet. Rec.*, **99**, 393.

Sano. E.M. (1949) Trichrome stain for tissue section, culture and smear. *Am. J. clin. Path.*, **19**, 898.

Schalm, O.W. (1975) Significance of plasma fibrinogen concentrations in clinical disorders in the horse. *Proc. 1st. int. Symp. equine Haemat.*, 159.

Von Schatzmann, U., Straub, R. & Gerber, H. (1972) Bronchialsekretaspiration beim Pferd. *Schweiz. Arch. Tierheilk.*, **114**, 395.

Strong, C.L. (1946) *Common-sense Therapy for Horses' Injuries.* London: Faber & Faber.

Swerczek, T.W. (1978) Contagious equine metritis in the USA. *Vet. Rec.*, **102**, 512.

Tennant, B., Baldwin, B.H., Silverman, S.L. & Makowski, X.X. (1975) Clinical significance of hyperbilirubinaemia in the horse. *Proc. 1st int. Symp. equine Haemat.*, 246.

Traver, D.S., Goddmann, J.R., Moore, J.N., Salem, C.A., Gower, H.E., Johnson, J.H. & Tritschler, L.G. (1976) Urine clearance ratios as a diagnostic aid in equine metabolic medicine. *Proc. 22nd ann. Conv. Am. Ass. equine Practnrs*, 177.

Tufvesson, G. (1963) *Local Anaesthesia in Veterinary Medicine.* Sodertalje, Sweden: Astra.

Van Pelt, R.W. (1974) Interpretation of synovial fluid findings in the horse. *J. Am. vet. med. Ass.*, **165**, 91.

Vaughan, J.T. (1977) in discussion of paper by Witherspoon (1977).

Wingfield-Digby, N.J. (1978) The technique and clinical application of endometrial cytology in mares. *Equine vet. J.*, **10**, 167.

Witherspoon, D.M. (1977) Exploration of the abdominal cavity by digital manipulation. *Proc. 23rd ann. Conv. Am. Ass. equine Practnrs*, 15.

Index

Abdominal pain, 458
Abortion, 56, 63, 83, 183, 195–206, 425
  aetiology, 196–7
  bacterial, 199
  clinical signs, 198–9
  diagnosis, 199
  epidemiology, 203–5
  incidence, 197–8
  infective, 196
  mycotic, 200
  non-infective, 196
  pathogenesis, 198
  pathology, 199
  preventive measures, 205–6
  treatment and control, 203–5
  viral, 200–2
Abscess swabs, 535
Acidaemia, 194, 316, 319, 409
Acidosis, 296
ACTH, 6
Actinobacillus equuli, 308, 396
Actinobacillus infection, 487
Adaptive period, 277–357
Adenocarcinoma, ovarian, 66
Adenomas, pituitary, 62
Adenovirus infection, 412, 427
Adrenal cortex hormones, 225, 296–8
Adrenocorticotrophic hormones (ACTH), 6
African horse sickness, 430, 471
Afterbirth, *see* Placenta
Agar gel immunodiffusion test (AGID), 429
Albumin/globulin (A/G) ratio, 381
Alimentary disturbance, 404
Allantoic fluid, 178, 231, 234, 243
Amnion, 180, 200, 242, 247, 375
Amnionitis, 194
Amniotic fluid, 180–1, 194, 286
Ampullitis, 67
Anaemia
  autoimmune haemolytic, 481
  equine infectious, 309, 428–9
Androgenic hormones, 127
Anoestrus, 15, 25, 32–5
Anoplocephala perfoliata, 451
Anthelmintics, 405
Antibiotics, 71, 74, 81, 93, 107, 249, 311, 398, 405
Anti-horse globulin test (AGT), 437, 546
Antihistamines, 482
Arbovirus infection, 429, 488
Arrhythmia, 292
Arteritis virus infection, 204, 429
Arthritis, infective, 396–9
Arthrocentesis, 539
Artificial insemination, 33, 41, 55, 59, 80, 81
  minimal contamination techniques, 73–4
Artificial light, 11, 13, 14, 32–3, 51, 148
Artificial vagina, 141, 151

Ascarids, 446–9
Aspartate aminotransferase (AST), 525
Aspergillus fumigatus, 478
Asphyxia, fetal, 315, 327–33
Ataxia of foals, 410
Atelectasis, 288, 290
Atresia, follicular, 3
Atrial fibrillation, 476
Autoimmune haemolytic anaemia, 481

Babesia caballi, 480
Babesia equi, 480
Bacillus piliformis, 407
Bacterial abortion, 199
Bacterial infections, 157–8, 430–8
Bacteriology, 70, 530–5
Behaviour disturbances in foal, 314–37
Behavioural signs, 18, 28–31
Beta-carotene, 35
Bilirubin, 474, 526
Biochemical standards in foal, 381–2
Biochemical tests, blood, 523
Biochemistry, 523–5
Biopsy
  endometrial (uterine), 41, 60, 63, 68, 84, 90, 95, 106, 198, 541–3
  liver, 543–5
Birth, 220–74
  abnormal conditions, 260–71
  afterbirth, retention, 249–50
  anatomy, 233–9
  'breaking water', 242
  Caesarean section, 271–4
  delivery, 231–3
  dystocia, 260–5
  effects on fetus, 251
  endocrinology, 220–5
  environmental factors, 250
  first-stage, 237–41
Birth (*continued*)
  hormonal changes, 222, 231
  induction, 225–31
  initiation, 220–5
  management of foaling mare, 251–60
  maternal behaviour, 239–51
  position, presentation and postu[re], 235–9, 261, 264
  second-stage, 231, 239, 241–7
  third-stage, 247
Birth canal, 233
Bladder
  paralysis, 488
  patent, 342–5
  rupture, 342–5
Blastocyst, 166, 183, 184
Blood
  biochemical tests, 523
  cross-matching, 546
  diseases, 479–86
  haematological status of foal, 378–9
  pH, 356, 404, 405, 528
Blood flow
  umbilical, 192
  uterine, 192
Blood gases, 356, 528
Blood glucose, 296, 356, 526
Blood lactic acid, 356
Blood lactate levels, 296
Blood sampling, 519, 546
Blood tests, 211–2
Blood transfusions, 547
  cross-matching, 546
Blood urea, 527
Bone growth, 385
Bordetella bronchiseptica, 400
Bot flies, 454
Bovicola (Damalinia) equi, 451
Bradycardia, 290
'Breaking water', 242
Breathing, *see* Respiratory
Breeding performance, 198
Breeding records, 105
Breeding season, 32, 34, 226
'Breeding soundness' in stallion, 14[6]

Breeding statistics, 109
Bromosulphalein (BSP) clearance, 526
Brucella abortus, 437
Brucellosis, 437–8
Buccal mucous membranes, 293

Caecum, rupture, 269
Caesarean section, 271–4
Calculi, urinary, 486
Campylobacter spp., 403
Candida spp., 403
Carbohydrate metabolism, 296
Cardiac, *see* Heart
Cardiac failure in NMS, 325
Cardiovascular system, 475–9
'Caslick index', 11
Caslick operation, 253
Catheters, 71, 72, 507
Cerebral haemorrhage, 314, 325
Cerebral lesions, 326
Cerebrospinal fluid, examination, 539
Cervicitis, 99
Cervix, 7, 8, 11, 25, 35, 99, 228, 233–5
  abnormal, 99
  bacteriology, 52
  cytology, 69, 537–8
  examination, 209, 512
  manipulation, 41
  state of, 51–2
  swabs, 69, 70, 79, 531–3
Choke, 458
Chorionic girdle, 183
Chorioptes equi, 457
Chromosome abnormality causing infertility, 60–1
Chronic obstructive pulmonary disease (COPD), 478
Circulation of foal, 315
Clearance ratios, urinary, 527–8
Clinical and further examinations, 501–47
Clinicopathological aids, 516–9
Clitoris, 8, 29
Clostridum tetani, 432
Coccidiosis, 403
Coggin's test, 429
Coital exanthema, 59, 103, 156
Colic, 335, 352, 404, 458–68
  aetiology, 458–62
  clinical signs, 462
  diagnosis, 462–5
  false, 458–9
  treatment, 465–8
  true, 459–62
Colitis X, 461, 468–9
Colon, rupture, 269
Colostrum, 227, 294, 368, 398
Combined immunodeficiency disease (CID), 412–3
Complement-fixation test (CFT), 437, 480
Conception, 1, 59
  probability, 55
Convulsions, *see* Neonatal maladjustment syndrome
Coombs's test, 437, 546
Coprophagia, 364
Corpus luteum (CL), 3, 12, 17, 18, 33, 38, 39, 62, 63, 107
Corticosteroids, 225, 231, 398, 426
Cortisol, 225, 296, 298
Corynebacterium equi, 397, 470
  infection, 401–2
Corynebacterium ovis, 371
Corynebacterium pseudotuberculosis, 483
Cracked heels, 455
Cryptosporidiosis, 412
Culicoides, 456
Cystitis, 487
Cystoscopy, 514
Cysts, 50, 63–4, 97, 102
Cytochemical staining test, 523
Cytology, 535
  cervix (endometrial), 69, 537–8
  synovial fluid, 539
Cytomegalovirus, 308

Daylight, extended (photoperiod), 11, 13, 14, 32–3, 51, 148
Death, fetal, 56, 105, 189, 198
Dehydration, 404, 405
Dehydroepiandrosterone sulphate (DHAS), 187
Delivery, *see* Birth
Demodex mite infestations, 458
Dermatitis, 455
Dermatophilus congolensis, 455
Desmotomy, superior check ligament, 393
Developmental abnormalities in the foal, 338–45
Diabetes mellitus, 474
Diagnostic physiotherapy, 516
Diarrhoea, 402–5, 470
  aetiology, 402–4
  clinical signs, 404–5
  treatment, 405
Dictyocaulus arnfeldi, 449–51, 529
Diet, 324, 371, 387
  artificial, 375–8
  supplements, 35
Diethylstilboestrol (DES), 191
Digestive system, 458–74
Diseases, notifiable in Great Britain, 429, 457, 481
Dioestrus, 11, 17, 25, 26, 29–31, 36, 38
  prolonged, 25, 35–9
Disseminated intravascular coagulopathy (DIC), 481
DNA viruses, 421–2
Dourine, 156, 481
Drugs, teratogenic, influence on fetus, 253
Dysmaturity, 333–5
Dysphagia, 458
Dysplasia of growth plate, 387
Dystocia, 199, 260–5

Echinococcus granulosus, 451
Ectoparasites, 451–4
Ehrlichia equi, 481
Ehrlichiosis, 481
Eimeira (globidium) leuckarti, 403
Ejaculation, 124, 129, 135, 136, 137, 142, 148
Electrocardiography, 195, 292
Electrocautery, 411
Electron microscopical studies, 25
Embryology, 165–181
Embryotomy, 271–4
Emphysema, pulmonary, 478
Encephalitis, 488
Endocrine glands, 13
Endocrinology, 545
  birth, 220–5
  gestation, 184–91
  mare, 11–18
  stallion, 123–8
Endometrium, 19, 23, 25
  atrophy, 89–91
  biopsy, 41, 60, 63, 68, 84, 90, 95, 106, 198, 541–3
  cups, 183
  curettage, 88–9, 97
  fibrosis, 197
  hyperplasia, 92–5
  hypoplasia, 91–2
  involution, 94
  neoplasia, 98–9
  'wear and tear' syndrome, 86, 87, 95, 105, 205
Endometritis, 39, 67, 205
  acute, 53, 68–75
  chronic, 84–9
Endoparasites, 438–51
Endoscopy, 477
  larynx, 512–4
  pharynx, 512–4
  uterus, 514
Entropion, 339
Epididymis, 154–5
Epiphyseal injuries in foal, 390–2
Epiphysitis, 386–7
Episiotomy, 133, 252
Epistaxis, 477
Epithelium, 23

Equid herpes virus I infection, 59, 198, 203–4, 308, 400, 425–7
Equine coital exanthema, 59, 103, 156
Equine infectious anaemia, 428–9
Equine influenza, 59
Erythrocyte count, 300, 521
Erythrocytes, 346, 347, 378, 480, 546
Escherichia coli, 308, 396, 403, 483
Exanthema, coital, 59, 103, 156
Eye, 294

Fallopian tubes, 7
  abnormal, 66–8
  function, 67–8
  patency test, 67–8
Faradic stimulation, 516
Fasciola hepatica, 452, 471
Fascioliasis, 452
Feeding, *see* Diet
Femur, fracture, 269
Fertility, 54–5, 146–7
Fertilization, 166
Fetal gonads, 169–174, 187
Fetal sac, 210
Fetlocks, knuckling over, 388–42, 489
Fetus
  death, 56, 105, 189, 198
  effect of parturition, 251
  environment and metabolism, 191–5
  growth, 168–9, 194, 206
  health, 206
  heart rate, 195
  loss of, 63, 94
  maturity, 228
  plasma glucose levels, 192
  resorption, 190
  stress, 194–5
Fibrosis, endometrial, 197
Fibrosis, stromal, 85, 86, 87, 93
Fistula, rectovaginal, 270
Flies, 454, 481
Fluprostenol, 41, 42, 64
Foal
  adaptive period, 277–357
  affinity for mare, 281
  behavioural disturbances, 314–37
  biochemical standards, 381–2
  birth-weight, 177
  breathing, onset of, 289
  cardiac status, 290–3
  circulatory status, 290–3
  developmental abnormalities, 338–45
  diet, 324
  disease in, 305–49, 386–416
  growth, 382–6
  haematological status, 300–5
  haematological standards, 378–9
  health, 361–6
  immune status, 294–5
  immunological conditions, 345–9
  infective conditions, 308–14
  isoimmune, 546–7
  metabolic assessment, 298–300
  metabolic status, 295
  neonatal conditions, 305–49
    differential diagnosis, 349–56
  non-infective conditions, 314–49
  normal newborn, 277–305
  older, 361–416
  orphan, 372–8
  perinatal mortality, 356–7
  play behaviour, 364–6
  pulmonary disturbances, 315
  pulmonary ventilation, 286–9
  shaker, 409
  standing for the first time, 281
  suck reflex, 309, 316, 323, 352
  sucking behaviour, 281, 362–4
  supplementary feeding, 371, 378
  twins, 357
Foal heat, 27–8
Foaling, *see* Birth
Foaling unit box, 251–2

Follicles, 2, 3, 17, 18, 19, 27, 34, 38, 48–50, 62, 63
Follicle-stimulating hormones (FSH), 5, 12–16, 33–4, 124, 186
Follicular atresia, 62
Follicular fluid, 17, 18
Fostering, 372–5
Fracture
  epiphyseal, 390–2
  proximal sesamoid bones, 393–5

Ganglionectomy, cervical, 15, 33
Gastrophilus intestinalis, 454, 471
Genital tract, 7–11, 80
  bacteriology, 52–3
  infection, 75–8
Gestation, 165–214
  embryology, 165–181
  endocrinology, 184–91
  fetal environment and metabolism, 191–5
  length, 213, 221, 333
  management of in-foal mare, 206
  ovarian development, 172–4
  pregnancy diagnosis, 206–13
  prenatal mammary development, 213–4
  stress, 211, 306
  uterine changes, 181–4
Glanders, 434–5
α-Globulin, 381
β-Globulin, 381
γ-Globulin, 381
Glucose, blood, 296, 356, 526
Glucose tolerance test, 474
Goitre, 406
Gonadotrophin-releasing hormones (GnRH), 11, 15–17, 33, 34, 40–1, 64
Gonad-stimulating (gonadotrophic) hormones, 5
Gonads, fetal, 169–174, 187
Granulosa cell tumours, 65, 66
Grass sickness, 469–70
Growth and growth rate in foal, 38
Guttural pouch
  disease, 477, 514
  tympany, 411
Gynaecological examination, 47
  hygiene at, 502

Haematapinus asini, 451
Haematocrit, *see* Packed cell volume
Haematological standards of foal, 378–9
Haematological status of foal, 300–5
Haematology, 519
Haematoma, 266–7
Haemoglobin content of blood, 300, 379, 521
Haemolytic disease, 345–9
Haemophilia, 411–2, 481
Haemophilus equigenitalis, 53, 59
  infection, 75–8
Haemorrhage
  after birth, 265–7
  cerebral, 314, 325
Harvest mites, 453
Heart disease, 475
  in NMS, 319
Heart murmur, 292
Heart rate, 290–2, 352
  fetal, 195
Heaves, 478
Hepatitis, 407
Hernia, umbilical, 413–6
Herpesvirus, *see* Equid herpesvirus
Hippomane, 178–80
Histology, 540–5
Histoplasma farcinnosum, 483
Homeostasis in NMS, 324
Hormones, 5–6, 17, 33–42, 124–8, 183, 185–91, 213, 221–6, 231

Hormones (*continued*)
  adrenal cortex, 225, 296–8
  adrenocorticotrophic hormones (ACTH), 6
  androgenic, 127
  assay, 545
  blood levels, 107
  controlling birth, 222, 231
  cortisol, 225, 296, 298
  follicle-stimulating (FSH), 5, 12–16, 33–34, 124, 186
  gonadotrophin-releasing (GnRH), 11, 15–17, 33, 34, 40–1, 64
  gonad-stimulating (gonado-trophic), 5
  human chorionic gonadotrophin (HCG), 39–40. 41
  'imbalance', 107
  interstitial-cell-stimulating (ICSH), 124
  luteinizing (LH), 5, 12–17, 34, 39–41, 124
  oestradiol, 40, 41
  oestrogens, 5, 13, 18, 41, 186, 222
  oxytocin, 5, 6, 223, 225
  pregnant mares' serum gonado-trophin (PMSG), 16, 33, 38, 168, 183, 185, 186, 189, 212
  progestagen, 16, 17, 35, 39
  progesterone, 3, 5, 12, 13, 33–7, 41, 63, 185, 186, 189, 190, 205, 223
  prolactin, 5, 16, 189
  prostaglandin, (PG), 13, 18, 35–9, 41, 42, 63, 185, 188, 189, 222, 223, 225
  stilboestrol, 41
  testosterone, 124, 127, 128
  thyroid, 305
  thyroid-stimulating (TSH), 6
  vasopressin, 5, 6
Human chorionic gonadotrophin (HCG), 39–40, 41, 191, 205
Hydatidosis, 451
Hygiene at gynaecological examinations, 502
Hymen, 7, 8, 102
Hyperflexion of joint, 338–42, 392–3
Hyperplasia, endometrial, 92–5
Hyperthyroidism, 406
Hypocalcaemia, 267
Hypoderma bovis, 457, 488
Hypodermic injection, 504–7
Hypoglycaemia, 296
Hypoplasia
  cerebellar, 410
  endometrial, 91–2
Hypothermia in NMS, 324
Hypothyroidism, 406
Hypoxia, 194
Hysteroscopy, 97, 107

Idiogenic infertility, 59–60
Immaturity, 333–5
Immune status of foal, 294–5
Immunoglobulin, 413
Immunological conditions in foal, 345–9
Infections, 421–38
  bacterial, 430–8
  uterine, 69, 73, 199
  virus, 421–30
Infectious equine arteritis, 429
Infective arthritis, 396–9
Infertility
  mare
    aetiology, 56–103
    definition, 55–6
    diagnosis, 105–8
    pathogenesis, 105
    prognosis, 108–111
    statistics, 59–60, 147
    treatment, 108
  stallion, 146–58
Influenza, 424–5

Infundibulitis, 67
Injections, 504–7
Insemination, artificial, 33, 41, 55, 59, 80, 81
minimal contamination techniques, 73–4
Intersex state, 60
Interstitial-cell-stimulating hormones (ICSH), 124
Intestine, small, 460
obstruction by foreign body, 406
Intrauterine and cervical manipulation, 41
Intrauterine infusion, 35, 39, 71–3, 93, 95
Isoimmune foal, 546–7
Isthmitis, 67
Ixodes ricinis, 453

Jaundice, 347, 471, 526
Joint, hyperflexion, 392–3
Joint-ill, 396–9

Klebsiella aerogenes, 53, 59, 78–80, 504
Klebsiella pneumoniae, 308
Knuckling-over, 338–42, 489

Lactation, 368–71
Lactobacillus acidophilus, 405
Lameness, 395, 397, 514, 516
Laminitis, 490–2
Laparoscopy, 108, 514
Laparotomy, 66, 407
Larynx, endoscopy, 512–4
Lavage, saline, 398
Lead poisoning, 399
Leucocytes, 300–5, 398, 483, 521–3
Libido estimation, 140
Lice, 451–2
Limbs
angular deformities, 387–90
hyperflexion, 338–342
Listeriosis, 412
Liver
biopsy, 543–5
disease, 470–4
Liver fluke, 452
Lockjaw, 432
Louping-ill virus, 489
Luminal (lymphatic) cysts of endometrium, 97
Lungs of foal, 286–9, 290
Lungworm, 449–51
Luteal phase, 39, 41
Luteinizing hormones (LH), 5, 12–17, 34, 39–41, 124
Luteolysis, 18, 35, 36, 39, 41
Lymphangitis, 483
Lymphopenia, 412
Lymphosarcoma, 483

Mal del caderas, 481
Maladjustment syndrome, *see* Neonatal maladjustment syndrome
Mammary development, prenatal, 213–4, 227–8
Mange, 457
demodectic, 458
Mare
barren, 55, 56, 59
behaviour during birth, 239–51
breeding management, 60
foal carrying ability, classificatio 108
foaling, management, 251–60
infertility/subfertility, 53–111, definition, 55–6
in-foal, management, 206
maiden, 91
physical abnormality, 61
preparation for mating, 130–3
problem, 160

Mare (*continued*)
  reproductive anatomy, 1–11
  sexual functions, management, 42–53
'Marsenac approach', 272
Mastitis, 371, 539
Masturbation, 136
Mating, 128–36
  minimal contamination techniques, 73, 83, 89, 111
    artificial insemination, 73–4
    natural cover, 74
  prolonged delay, 150
  synchronized, 41–2
Meclofenamic acid, 191
Meconium
  evacuation, 285–6
  retention, 335–7, 343
Meningitis, 308, 488, 539
Metabolic assessment of foal, 298–300
Metabolic status of foal, 295
Metritis, post-parturient, 268
Micropolyspora faeni, 478
Microsporum equinum, 454
Microsporum gypseum, 455
Midges, 456
Milk
  mares', 368
  secretion, 213, 228
  substitutes, 375–8
  see also Weaning
Minimal contamination techniques, 73, 83, 89, 111
  artificial insemination, 73–4
  natural cover, 74
Mites, 453, 457
Monday morning disease, 483
Monocytosis, 426
Mortality, perinatal, 356–7
Mud fever, 455
Murrina, 481
Musculoskeletal system, 489–92
  disorders, 386–99
Muscular dystrophy, nutritional (NMD), 393
Mycology, 535
Mycoplasma, 396
Mycotic infection, 403
Myelitis, segmental, 488
Myeloma, multiple, 482
Myiasis, 453–4
Myoglobinuria, 459, 489–90
Myometrium, 231
Myxovirus infection, 424

Nasal swabs, 426, 533
Natural cover, 70, 74, 94
  minimal contamination techniques, 73–4
Navel-ill, 396–9
Neonatal conditions, 305–49
  classification, 307
  differential diagnosis, 349–56
  Group I, 308–14
  Group II, 314–37
  Group III, 337–45
  Group IV, 345–49
Neonatal maladjustment syndrome (NMS), 314–33
  aetiology and incidence, 314
  behaviour, 320–3
  cardiac dysfunction, 319
  cardiac failure, 325
  cerebral oedema, 314
  cerebral haemorrhage, 314, 325
  clinical signs, 316
  convulsions, 316, 320–3
  course of condition, 319
  diagnosis, 319
  feeding, 323
  homeostasis, 324
  hypothermia, 324
  pathogenesis, 314
  pathology, 325
  pulmonary function, 318
  treatment, 319
Neoplasia, 462
  endometrial, 98–9
Nephritis, 487
Nephrosis, 487
Nerve blocks, 514–6

Nervous system, 488–9
Nitroblue tetrazolium (NBT) test, 523
Non-infective conditions in foal, 314–49
Notifiable diseases in Great Britain, 429, 457, 481
Nutrition, 15, 61
  disturbances, 402
  and growth, 384
  supplementary, 35
Nutritional muscular dystrophy (NMD), 393

Obesity, 61
Occipital puncture, 539
Oedema, cerebral, 314
Oestradiol, 40, 41
Oestrogens, 5, 13, 18, 41, 186, 222
Oral lactose tolerance test (OLTT), 403
Orchitis, 154
Osteochondrosis, 395–6
Oestrous cycle, 11–42
  control, 31–2
  cyclical activity, initiation, 13–15
  definition, 11
  endocrinology, 11–18
  environmental factors, 11
  irregularities, 60, 61
  physiology and behaviour correlation, 31
  variations, 25–7
Ovarian adenocarcinoma, 66
Ovarian teratomas, 66
Oviducts, 7
Ovariectomy, 18, 186–8, 190
Ovaries, 1–5, 7, 18–25, 185
  abnormal, 62–6
  development during gestation, 172–4
  palpation, 47–9, 51
Ovulation, 3, 18, 19, 26, 31–33, 38, 39–41, 48–9
Ovum, 166
Oxytocin, 5, 6, 223, 225
Oxyuriasis, 449
Oxyuris equi, 449

Packed cell volume, 300, 355, 379 464, 520
Pain, abdominal, 458
Palpation
  ovaries, 47–9, 51
  uterus, 47, 50–51, 97
  viscera, 512
Pancreatic disease, 474
Papillomatosis, 455
Papovavirus, 427
Paracentesis abdominis, 343, 464, 536–7
Parainfluenza virus infection, 427
Parascaris equorum, 438, 446–9
Parasites, 438–54
Parturition, *see* Birth
Pelvic girdle, 11, 235
Pelvic ligaments, 228
Pelvis, fracture, 269
Penis, 70, 103, 122, 153–4
Perinatal mortality, 356–7
Perineum, 8, 11, 52
  lacerations, 101, 102, 269–71
Peritoneal fluid, 536
Peritonitis, 459
Pfeifferella mallei, 434
pH, blood, 356, 404, 405, 528
Pharynx, endoscopy, 512–4
Photoperiod, increased, 11, 13, 14, 32–33, 51, 148
Physiotherapy, diagnostic, 516
Pin-worm, 449
Piroplasmosis, 480
Pituitary adenomas, 62
Pituitary gland, 5–6, 17, 61–2
Placenta, 174–8, 188, 191, 194, 199, 200, 241
  retention, 249–50
Placentitis, 194, 199
Plant poisoning, 471
Plasma fibrinogen levels, 525
Plate agglutination test, 547
Pneumocystis carinii, 412, 413

Pneumonia, 399, 400, 413
Pneumovagina, 11, 99–100
Poisoning
lead, 399
plant, 471
zinc, 399
Polioencephalomyelitis, 489
Polyarthritis, 396
Post-mortem techniques, 540
Post-parturient metritis, 268
Pregnancy
diagnosis, 187, 195, 206–13
maintenance, 188–91
manual examination, 207–11
methods of detection, 207–13
ultrasonic detection, 195, 213
Pregnant mares' serum gonadotrophin (PMSG), 16, 33, 38, 168, 183, 185, 186, 189, 212
Pregnant mares' urine, 31, 41
Prematurity, 195, 333–5
Prepuce, 123, 153–4
Progestagen, 16, 17, 35, 39
Progesterone, 3, 5, 12, 13, 33–7, 41, 63, 185, 186, 189, 190, 205, 223
Prolactin, 5, 16, 189
Prostaglandin, (PG), 13, 18, 35–9, 41, 42, 63, 185, 188, 189, 222, 223, 225
Prostate gland, 122, 139
Proteins, 35, 294
Proteinuria, 294
Pseudomonas aeruginosa, 53, 59, 80–1, 504
Psoroptes communis, 457
Pulmonary disturbances of the foal, 315
Pulmonary emphysema, 478
Pulmonary function in NMS, 318
Pulmonary ventilation of foal, 286–9
Pulse
arterial, 293
jugular, 293
Purpura haemorrhagica, 482
Pyometra, 81–3

Radiography, 516
Radio-immunoassay, 186
Rain scald, 455
Rectum
examinations, 206, 207, 509–12
palpation, 47–51, 62, 63, 97, 464
swabs, 404, 535
Rectal temperature, 293, 352
Rectovaginal fistula, 270
Redworm, 439
Reflexes, development, 280
Releasing and inhibiting factors, 6
Reovirus infection, 430
Respiratory distress, 318, 332
Respiratory rate, 355
Respiratory rhythm, 290
Respiratory system, 476–9
Respiratory tract infections, 399–401
Respirometer, 290
Resuscitation, 332
Rhinovirus infection, 427
Ringworm, 454–5
RNA virus, 423, 428, 429
Rose Bengal plate test (RBPT), 437
Rotavirus infection, 403, 406
Roundworms, 446–9
Rupture
bladder, 342–5
caecum, 269
colon, 269
uterine, 269

Salmonella spp., 403
Salmonella abortivoequina, 199, 203
Salmonella abortus, 435
Salmonella enteritides, 406

Salmonella typhimurium, 308, 396, 405, 406, 435
Salmonellosis, 59, 405–6, 435–7
Salpingitis, 67
Sarcoid, 456
Sarcoptes scabei, 457
Scrotum, 120, 139, 154
Segmental myelitis, 488
Semen, 137–46
  collection, 73, 140–2, 144, 151
  evaluation and prediction of fertility, 138–46
  examination, 142–5
  freezing, 159
  gel fraction, 142
  longevity, 143
  motility estimates, 142–3
  storage, 159
  see also Spermatozoa
Seminal vesicles, 122, 138, 139
Seminal vesiculitis, 155
Sensory awareness, 280
Septicaemia, 199, 308, 311
Serum-agglutination test (SAT), 437
Serum alkaline phosphatase (SAP), 382, 525
Serum calcium, 382, 527
Serum creatine kinase (CK), 526
Serum creatinine, 527
Serum electrolytes, 527
Serum glutamic oxalo-acetic transaminase (SGOT), *see* Aspartate aminotransferase (AST)
Serum inorganic phosphate, 527
Serum phosphorus levels, 382
Serum potassium, 527
Serum proteins, 356, 381, 523–5
'Serum sickness', 471
Setaria spp., 488
Set-fast, 489–90
Shaker foal, 409
Sinus tract swabs, 535
Skin, diseases of, 454–8
Sleepy foal disease, 308
Small intestine, 460
  obstruction by foreign body, 40
Speculum, vaginal, 512, 531–2
Spermatozoa, 129, 137–8
  concentration, 143
  daily production, 137, 139
  live/dead ratio, 144
  morphology, 145
  number per ejaculate, 145
  see also Semen
Stallion, 120–161
  abnormal behaviour, 149–51
  'breeding soundness', 146
  conditioned sexual reflexes, 130
  ejaculatory disorders, 150–1
  endocrinology, 123–8
  fertility prediction, 146
  fertility statistics, 147
  fertility testing, 138
  handler relationship, 149
  health and sexual history record 138
  infertility, 146–58
  loss of libido, 148
  maiden, 149
  managerial influences on sexual behaviour, 129, 147–14
  'mare shyness', 151
  mounting behaviour, 129, 133–
  nutritional factors affecting sexu performance, 148
  preparation for mating, 130–6
  preparation for stud, 130
  prolonged delay in mounting, 15
  reproductive anatomy, 120–3
  reproductive behaviour, 128–36
  selection, 120
  sexual maturity, 137
Staphylococcus aureus, 308, 396, 455, 483
Statistics of infertility, 59–60, 147
Steatitis, generalized, 409
Still-birth, 333
Stilboestrol, 41
Stomach tube, 463, 507–9
Strangles, 59, 430–2

reptococcal infections, 430
reptococcus equi, 430
reptococcus pyogenes, 483
reptococcus zooepidemicus, 308, 371, 396, 430
ress in gestation, 211, 306
romal fibrosis, 85, 86, 87, 93
rongyloides westeri, 451
rongyloidosis, 451
rongylus vulgaris, 438–46
bfertility, definition, 56
ck reflex of foal, 309, 316, 323, 352
cking behaviour of foal, 362–4
rra, 480
abbing, 530–5
'vamp fever', 428–9
eet itch, 456
novial fluid, 398
cytology, 539

achycardia, 195, 292
apeworm, 451
easing, 33, 42–7
emperature, rectal, 293, 352
enosynovitis, 397, 399
eratogenic drugs, influence on fetus, 340
eratomas, ovarian, 66
est, *see specific test*
est mating programme, 79, 80
estes, 120, 124, 139, 154
estosterone, 124, 127, 128
etanus, 432–4
heiler's disease, 471
horax, compression of, 315
hyroid hormones, 305
hyroid-stimulating hormone (TSH), 6
cks, 453, 489
acheotomy, 432
ans-tracheal aspiration, 539
ichophyton equinum, 454
ichophyton verrucosum, 454
Trombicula autumnalis, 453
Trypanosoma brucei, 480
Trypanosoma equinum, 481
Trypanosoma equiperdum, 481
Trypanosoma evansi, 480
Trypanosoma hippicum, 481
Trypanosomiasis, 480
Tuberculosis, 438
Tumour, 62, 456
  abdominal, 459
  granulosa cell, 65, 66
  see also specific tumour
Twins, 177–8, 195, 198, 357
Tympany, 411, 477
Tyzzer's disease, 407–9

Ultrasonic detection of pregnancy, 195, 213
Umbilical cord, 181
  rupture, 247, 280
Ureteral ectopia, 409
Urinary calculi, 486
Urinary clearance ratios, 527–8
Urinary system, 486–8
Urine, 29, 356
  analysis, 529–30
  pregnant mares', 31, 41
Urine tests for pregnancy, 212
Uterine infuser, 71
Uterus, 7–8, 11, 68–99
  abnormal, 68–99
  biopsy, 41, 60, 63, 68, 84, 90, 95, 106, 198, 541–3
  changes during gestation, 181–4
  cytology, 537–8
  endoscopy, 514
  infection, 69, 73, 199
  infusion, 35, 39, 71–3, 93, 95
  involution, delayed, 267–8
  manipulation, 41
  muscle activity, 221
  palpation, 47, 50–1, 97
  partial dilatation, 97
  prolapse, 268–9
  rupture, 269

Uterus (*continued*)
stages in gestation, 207–9
swabs, 69, 70, 79, 531–3
torsion, 269

Vaccines, 204, 424, 432, 455
Vagina, 7, 8, 99–102, 103
artificial, 141, 151
examination, 51–2
Vaginoscopy, 512
Vasopressin, 5, 6
Venereal diseases, 59, 78, 79, 81
Virology, 535
Virus infections, 421–30
see also specific diseases and viruses
Vitamins, 148, 489
Vulva, 7, 8, 11, 29, 52, 99, 1C
228

Warble flies, 457
Weaning, 361, 366–7
White cell count, 356, 379, 4
'Wobbler' disease, 410–11
Worm egg counts, 528–9

Yearling, 361–416

Zinc poisoning, 399
Zygote, 165